Arnold and Boggs's

INTERPERSONAL RELATIONSHIPS

Professional Communication Skills for Canadian Nurses

Arnold and Boggs's

INTERPERSONAL RELATIONSHIPS

Professional Communication Skills for Canadian Nurses

CLAIRE MALLETTE, RN, BScN, MScN, PhD
Associate Professor, School of Nursing, York University, Toronto, ON

OLIVE YONGE, RN, BScN, MEd, PhD, R Psych
Professor, Faculty of Nursing, University of Alberta, Edmonton, AB

US EDITORS:

ELIZABETH C. ARNOLD, PhD, RN, PMHCNS-BC
Associate Professor, Retired, University of Maryland, School of Nursing, Baltimore, Maryland
Family Nurse Psychotherapist, Montgomery Village, Maryland

KATHLEEN UNDERMAN BOGGS, PhD, FNP-CS
Family Nurse Practitioner, Associate Professor Emeritus, College of Health and Human Services,
University of North Carolina Charlotte, Charlotte, North Carolina

ELSEVIER

Elsevier

ARNOLD AND BOGGS'S INTERPERSONAL RELATIONSHIPS:
PROFESSIONAL COMMUNICATION SKILLS FOR CANADIAN NURSES   ISBN: 978-0-323-76366-0

Notice

Practitioners and researchers must always rely on their own experience and knowledge in evaluating and using any information, methods, compounds, or experiments described herein. Because of rapid advances in the health sciences in particular, independent verification of diagnoses and drug dosages should be made. To the fullest extent of the law, no responsibility is assumed by Elsevier or the authours, editors, or contributors for any injury and/or damage to persons or property as a matter of products liability, negligence or otherwise, or from any use or operation of any methods, products, instructions, or ideas contained in the material herein.

Managing Director, Global ERC: Kevonne Holloway
Senior Content Strategist (Acquisitions, Canada): Roberta A. Spinosa-Millman
Director, Content Development Manager: Laurie Gower
Content Development Specialist: Lenore Gray Spence
Publishing Services Manager: Deepthi Unni
Senior Project Manager: Manchu Mohan
Design Direction: Bridget Hoette

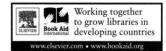

Last digit is the print number: 9   8   7   6   5   4   3   2   1

To students, nurses, and educators: May you use the learnings from this book to provide and advance nursing practice in the delivery of quality, culturally safe, and compassionate care, through communication and interpersonal relationships, in Canada and as global citizens.

Contributor

Dr. Sheila Blackstock, RN, BScN, MScN, COHN, PhD
Assistant Professor, School of Nursing, Thompson
Rivers University, Kamloops, British Columbia

Contributors to US Eighth Edition

Kim Siarkowski Amer, PhD, APRN
Associate Professor, School of Nursing, DePaul
University, Chicago, IL

Shari Kist, PhD, RN, CNE
Assistant Professor, Goldfarb School of Nursing,
Barnes-Jewish College, St. Louis, MO

Pamela E. Marcus, MS, APRN
Associate Professor, Prince George's Community
College, Largo, MD

Eileen O'Brien, PhD, RN
Undergraduate Program Director, Psychology
Department, University of Maryland, Baltimore
County Campus, Baltimore, MD

REVIEWERS

Zoraida Beekhoo, RN, MA
Associate Professor, Teaching Stream
Lawrence S. Bloomberg Faculty of Nursing
University of Toronto
Toronto, Ontario

Sandra Carter, RN, BN, MN
Nurse Educator
Centre for Nursing Studies
St. John's, Newfoundland

Renate Gibbs, BSN, MA
Professor of Nursing
School of Health & Human Services
Camosun College
Victoria, British Columbia

Cheyenne Joseph, RN, BScK, BScN, MPH, CCHN (C)
Rising Sun Treatment Centre
Natoaganeg First Nation
Eel Ground, New Brunswick

Robert Meadus, BN, B.VocEd, MSc(N), PhD, CPMHN(C)
Associate Professor
Faculty of Nursing
Memorial University of Newfoundland
St. John's, Newfoundland

Wilma Schroeder, BN, MMFT
Instructor
Faculty of Nursing
Red River College
Winnipeg, Manitoba

Nicola Thomas, RN, BN, MSc, CAE
Professor
Faculty of Health Science
St. Lawrence College
Kingston, Ontario

Jody Vaughan, RN, BScN, MEd
Nursing Instructor
School of Health Sciences
College of New Caledonia
Prince George, British Columbia

F. Maureen White, RN, MN
Assistant Professor (retired)
School of Nursing
Faculty of Health Professions
Dalhousie University
Halifax, Nova Scotia

Krista Wilkins, RN, PhD
Associate Professor
Faculty of Nursing
University of New Brunswick
Fredericton, New Brunswick

Rachael Wymer, RN, BScN, MScN
School of Community and Health Services
Centennial College
Toronto, Ontario

In 1989, Elsevier published the first US edition of *Interpersonal Relationships: Communication Skills for Nurses*. It was originally developed at the University of Maryland School of Nursing, to accompany a communication seminar course on interpersonal communication skills for nurses. Subsequent editions (now in its 8th edition in the United States), reinforced its salience as a key resource on nurse–person relationships and communication.

This new Canadian edition of *Arnold and Boggs's Interpersonal Relationships: Professional Communication Skills for Canadian Nurses*, First Edition, is designed as a key interactive reference for nursing students and professional nurses in Canada. This first Canadian edition is designed to be relevant to the Canadian health care system and nursing practice. Using Canadian literature and resources, the text emphasizes the important role nurses play through person-centred communication and therapeutic relationships in delivering quality, culturally safe, and compassionate nursing care across the health continuum. This Canadian edition examines how nurses assist people of all ages to engage in various health promotion and disease prevention activities needed to promote maximal personal health and well-being.

In the rapidly changing health care environment, nurses have an unprecedented opportunity to make a difference and shape the future of nursing practice at every level of health care delivery.

Within this text, *Simulation Exercises* with reflective analysis discussions allow students to examine the pros and cons of various approaches and nursing practice issues across clinical settings. Person-centred relationships, health promotion and disease prevention, collaborative interprofessional communication, and team-based approaches are explored within the Canadian context.

Canada is a diverse nation that prides itself on being multicultural. Each person's culture is influenced by socioeconomic factors, values and beliefs, race, gender, ethnicity, sexual orientation, life experiences, spirituality, education, and personal choice. As nurses, we must value each person's individual culture and consider how their culture influences health care experiences. As nurses, we too have our own cultures and need to be aware of the intersections of different perspectives that everyone brings to the health care setting. The complexity of communication in providing culturally safe nursing practice is explored throughout the text, including a chapter on engaging with humility through authentic interpersonal communication in partnership with Indigenous peoples.

Advances in technology that continue to revolutionize health care are explored in relevant chapters. Digital health technologies useful in health education, self-monitoring, and support are rapidly expanding, promoting greater control of a person's own care and potentially improving health outcomes. Nurses play an active role in changing the focus from illness care to health care, through employing the latest in technology to communicate with people requiring care, carry out health promotion, and support people's self-management activities.

ABOUT THE CONTENT

Arnold and Boggs's Interpersonal Relationships: Professional Communication Skills for Canadian Nurses serves as a majour communication and interprofessional resource for Canadian nurses to address the needs of the person, family, community, and health system in a time of significant changes, locally, provincially and territorially, federally, and globally. The text presents a synthesis of relationships in nursing and team-based health communication, with an integrated collaborative approach to person- and family-centred therapeutic interpersonal relationships.

Chapter topics in this book mirror the paradigm shift in health care delivery in Canada, from a focus on disease and illness to primary care delivery, health promotion, and disease prevention. This paradigm shift is based on an integrated, holistic approach to health care that begins with the person's cultural contexts, values, concerns, and preferences. Communication skills and interpersonal relationships, combined with person-centred applications, create the therapeutic partnership that people need to make health decisions and self-manage their care. Health promotion and disease prevention as essential components of health and wellness are discussed in several chapters.

The range of health care applications can follow a person through the life cycle, including end-of-life communication and nursing interventions. The communication content supports health care applications across a broad health continuum that includes primary care, hospitals, long-term care, ambulatory and public health, rehabilitation, palliative care, and home care.

The chapters on person-centred relationships and communication reflect the person- and family-centred focus. As the person and family are the ones who independently care for their health when not engaged with health providers, it is imperative that they be at the centre of care and actively involved in decision making. Therapeutic relationships with people and their families require that nurses integrate people's cultural context, preferences, values, motivations, and hopes with evidenced-informed practices as the basis for shared decision making. This belief is reflected throughout the text and explicitly in several chapters, where appropriate.

A collaborative, practice-ready workforce, offering quality and safe health services, strengthens health care systems and leads to improved health outcomes. Immediately following the opening chapter on conceptual foundations, an entire chapter is devoted to nursing practice with the emphasis on the importance of communication in creating quality and safe health care environments.

Nurses play a key role as collaborative team members and leaders in providing better integrated person-centered care. The central phenomena of professional nursing practice take place within collaborative interprofessional teams that involve health care professionals and the person and family working together, fostering person-centred care. In interprofessional health care environments, where multiple inputs must be considered and coordinated, role clarity and well-defined, clear communication are crucial to ensuring the safety and quality of care delivery. The chapters that discuss characteristics of interprofessional collaboration and teamwork emphasize the Canadian Nurses Association and the Canadian Interprofessional Health Collaborative's (CIHC) National Interprofessional Competency Framework (2010), identifying the integration of each health discipline's focus to achieve coordinated, optimal individual health outcomes and population needs in safe, competent, and cost-effective ways.

With the world becoming better connected through technology, information now gets shared across health care settings in real time. Nurses play a pivotal role in making use of digital health technologies at the point of care and electronic documentation. Relationship-centred communication between people and health care providers is further enhanced through virtual health conferencing and secure patient portals. Two chapters focus on advancing technology and the shifts in care and communication, through examining e-documentation in health information technology systems, digital health, and communication technology.

The text's authors and contributors recognize and acknowledge the diverse histories of the First Peoples of the lands now referred to as Canada. It is recognized that individual communities identify themselves in various ways; within this text, the term *Indigenous* is used to refer to all First Nations, Inuit, and Métis people within Canada.

In the text, gender-neutral language is used to be respectful of and consistent with the values of equality recognized in the *Canadian Charter of Rights and Freedoms*. Using gender-neutral language is professionally responsible and mandated by the Canadian Federal Plan for Gender Equality. Knowledge and language concerning sex, gender, and identity are fluid and continually evolving. The language and terminology presented in this text endeavour to be inclusive of all people and reflect what is, to the best of our knowledge, current at the time of publication.

ABOUT THE CHAPTER ORGANIZATION

The text is divided into six sections containing 27 chapters.

Part I: Theoretical Foundations and Contemporary Dynamics in Person-Centred Relationships and Communication introduces students to basic conceptual information needed for contemporary professional nursing practice in Canada. This section begins with an overview of the origins of nursing, starting with Indigenous healers and the evolution of nursing as a profession in Canada. Theory-based systems, evidence-informed practice, and nursing theories—including those of Canadian theorists—are used to emphasize communication concepts and strategies that nurses need to maintain a safe, quality health care environment. Legal and ethical standards in nursing practice relevant to communication—including social media and the role of critical thinking and clinical judgement processes in providing safe, quality care—are also explored within the Canadian context.

Part II: Essential Communication Competencies identifies the fundamental structure and characteristics of effective, person-centred communication skills and strategies. This section, using a wide application of Canadian literature, explores selected professional approaches and communication strategies required for individuals, diverse populations, and cultural contexts. A chapter on engaging with humility in partnership with Indigenous peoples is included. Group communication skill development is also discussed in this section.

The chapters in *Part III: Relationship Skills in Health Communication* explore the nature of person- and family-centred relationships in health care settings. The chapters discuss communication strategies nurses can use with individuals, groups, and families in health care settings, through developing and implementing person-centred therapeutic relationships. Applying therapeutic communication strategies in conflict situations, and special attention to health promotion community strategies and health teaching within the Canadian context, complete the section.

Part IV: Communication for Health Promotion and Disease Prevention examines resolving conflicts, identification and application of communication strategies for health promotion and disease prevention, how to be effective when providing health teaching, the application of coaching techniques to help families and their loved ones, and how to communicate in stressful situations.

In *Part V: Accommodating People With Special Communication Needs*, the focus is how to communicate with different vulnerable populations such as children, older people, those in palliative care, people who are in crisis, and those with communication disorders.

Part VI: Collaborative Professional Communication examines partnerships in health care agencies with families and people in the community. Nurses do not work alone but are part of interprofessional teams, which means using unique communication strategies based in a philosophy of collaboration with other health care providers or patients and their families. This section also discusses the concept of continuity of care across clinical settings and nursing applications through the use of electronic health records. The influence of rapidly advancing digital technology on health care practices to communicate and manage the person's health information and the Internet of Things, as well as their effects on nurse–person communication and the nursing role, are highlighted.

CHAPTER FEATURES

In this text, chapters can be used as individual teaching modules. The text can also be used as a primary text or as a communication resource, integrated across the curriculum. Chapter text boxes and tables highlight important ideas in each chapter.

Each chapter's format includes learning objectives, concepts, and an application section, connected by a research study or meta-analysis of several studies relevant to the chapter topic. This research, presented in an *Evidence-Informed Practice* box, offers a summary of research findings related to the chapter subject. This feature is intended to strengthen awareness of the link between research and practice.

Simulation Exercises with critical analysis questions provide an interactive component to the student's study of text materials, through experiential understanding of concepts and an opportunity to practise, observe, and critically evaluate professional communication skills from a practice perspective, in a safe learning environment. *Case Examples* help students develop empathy for patients' perspectives and needs. *Questions for Review and Discussion* are at the end of each chapter for student reflective analysis. An exemplar related to *Ethical Dilemmas* is also presented at the end of each chapter.

Through active experiential involvement with relationship-based communication principles, students can develop confidence and skill in their capacity to engage in person-centred communication across clinical settings. The comments and reflections of other students provide a wider, enriching perspective about the person-centred implications of communication in clinical practice. Although the text's content, exercises, and case examples are written in terms of nurse–person relationships, the interactional components are also applicable to clinical practice student relationships entered into by other health care disciplines.

Arnold and Boggs's Interpersonal Relationships: Professional Communication Skills for Canadian Nurses gives voice to the centrality of person-centred relational communication strategies as the basis for ensuring quality, culturally safe, and compassionate care in nursing and health care delivery. Our hope is that this text will serve as a primary Canadian reference resource for nurses seeking to develop and expand their communication and relationship skills in both traditional clinical and nontraditional community-based health care settings.

As the single most consistent health care provider in many people's lives, nurses have the critical responsibility to provide communication that is professional, honest, empathetic, and knowledgeable, in individual and group relationships. As nurses, we are answerable to the people we care for, our profession, and ourselves to communicate with all those involved with a person's care in an authentic, therapeutic manner and to advocate for the person's health, care, and well-being within the larger sociopolitical community.

The opportunity to contribute to the evolving development of communication as a central tenet of professional nursing practice within the Canadian health care landscape has been a privilege as well as a responsibility to our profession. We invite you as students, practicing nurses, and educators to interact with the material in this text, learning from the content and experiential exercises, but also seeking your own truth and understanding in the evolving delivery of nursing practice across Canada and as global citizens.

EVOLVE WEBSITE

Located at http://evolve.elsevier.com/Canada/Mallette/interpersonal/, the Evolve website for this book includes these materials for instructors:

- ExamView® Test Bank, featuring examination format test questions, with rationales and answers for all 27 chapters. The robust ExamView® testing application, provided at no cost to faculty, allows instructors to create new tests; edit, add, and delete test questions; sort questions by category, cognitive level, and nursing process step; and administer and grade tests online, with automated scoring and gradebook functionality.

- PowerPoint® Lecture Slides, consisting of 27 chapters of customizable text slides for instructors to use in lectures.

ELSEVIER EBOOKS

Elsevier eBooks is an exciting program that is available to faculty who adopt a number of Elsevier texts, including *Arnold and Boggs's Interpersonal Relationships: Professional Communication Skills for Canadian Nurses*, First Edition. Elsevier eBooks is an integrated electronic study centre consisting of a collection of textbooks made available online. It is carefully designed to "extend" the textbook for an easier and more efficient teaching and learning experience. It includes study aids such as highlighting, e-note-taking, and cut-and-paste capabilities. Even more importantly, it allows students and instructors to conduct a comprehensive search, within the specific text or across a number of titles. Please check with your Elsevier Educational Solutions Consultant for more information.

SHERPATH

Sherpath book-organized collections offer digital lessons, mapped chapter-by-chapter to the textbook, so the reader can conveniently find applicable digital assignment content. Sherpath features convenient teaching materials that are aligned to the textbook and the lessons are organized by chapter for quick and easy access to invaluable class activities and resources.

ACKNOWLEDGEMENTS

We acknowledge our deep appreciation for the contributions of Sheila Blackstock, who wrote Chapter 8 *Engaging With Humility: Authentic Interpersonal Communication in Partnership With Indigenous Peoples*. Her writings guide our increased awareness and knowledge of the impact of colonization on Indigenous peoples and our understanding and developing applications of critical elements in practice, such as relationally engaging in cultural safety and humility through holistic communication with Indigenous peoples and communities.

We are very grateful to the Elsevier editorial staff, particularly Lenore Gray Spence and Roberta Spinosa-Millman. Their guidance, tangible support, and suggestions were invaluable in the content development of this first edition. Finally, we want to sincerely thank Manchu Mohan from Elsevier and Sherry Hinman for their painstaking, precise copy editing, and editorial support during the production process.

Claire Mallette, RN, BScN, MScN, PhD
Olive Yonge, RN, BScN, MEd, PhD, R Psych

SIMULATION EXERCISES

BOXES

TABLES

EVIDENCE-INFORMED PRACTICE BOXES

CONTENTS

1

Historical Perspectives and Contemporary Dynamics

Claire Mallette

Originating US chapter by *Elizabeth C. Arnold*

OBJECTIVES

At the end of the chapter, the reader will be able to:
1. Discuss the historical evolution of professional nursing.
2. Describe the core components of nursing's metaparadigm.
3. Discuss the role of "ways of knowing," in person-centred nursing care.
4. Compare and contrast linear and transactional models of communication.
5. Explain the use of systems thinking as a foundational construct in professional health care.
6. Discuss the role of health communication in interprofessional communication.

This introductory chapter provides the groundwork for understanding communication and relationship concepts presented in the book chapters. The historical development of professional nursing, communication concepts, and systems thinking offers an evidence-informed foundation for person-centred communication and interprofessional collaborative (IPC) communication as the preferred means for delivering safe, quality health care in contemporary care settings.

BASIC CONCEPTS

Foundations of Professional Nursing Practice

Historically, nursing is as old as humankind. In Canada, the first origins of nursing began with Indigenous healers providing healing and health practices to those in need (Wytenbroek & Vandenberg, 2017). Indigenous healers and midwives treated illnesses using their extensive knowledge of how to harvest and use medicinal plants to care for people in their communities (Wytenbroek & Vandenberg,

2017). Prior to the twentieth century, there are records of Indigenous healers in western Canada also serving as midwives in their communities and settler societies. Following Confederation, as part of the attempt to eradicate Indigenous culture and practices, Indigenous healing knowledge and practices were repressed (Wytenbroek & Vandenberg, 2017). The Canadian Nurses Association [CNA] (2020a) is committed to advancing Indigenous health nursing and providing support where there are inequities in health, social, and educational services.

Starting in the 1600s, nurses trained in religious orders came from Europe to Canada and began establishing hospitals governed by the religious orders. In the 1800s, nonreligious hospitals were also established in Canada (Canadian Association of Schools of Nursing [CASN], 2012).

The "roots of professional nursing as a distinct occupation" began with Florence Nightingale's Notes on Nursing (1859) (Fig. 1.1). Nightingale established the first nursing school (St. Thomas's Hospital of London), in 1860. She

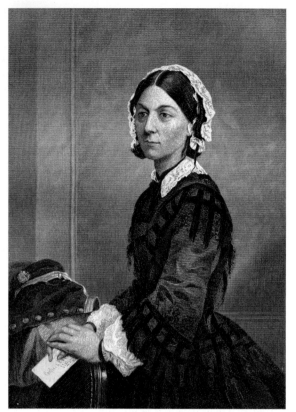

Fig. 1.1 Florence Nightingale is recognized as the first professional nurse. (iStock.com/traveler1116)

introduced the world to roles of professional nursing. Her use of statistical data to document the need for handwashing to prevent infection during the Crimean War marks her as the profession's first nurse researcher. An early advocate for high-quality care, Nightingale viewed nursing as both a science and an art form (Alligood, 2014). Her strong defence of blending scientific evidence with caring about the humanity of those in need lives on to this day.

In 1874, the first nursing training school in Canada was opened in St. Catharines, Ontario, guided by two nurses who were trained by Florence Nightingale (CASN, 2012). Her new hospital apprentice-style training model spread rapidly through Canada, with the introduction of hospital-based schools of nursing, and influenced nursing education for almost a century (CASN, 2012).

While Florence Nightingale is best known as the originator of modern nursing and her work in the Crimean War, Mary Seacole also participated as a nurse in the Crimean War. Mary Seacole was born in 1805, in Kingston, Jamaica. She was of mixed race, with her mother being Jamaican and Black and her father British and White. She became a healer,

using traditional African and Caribbean herbal preparations, and practised nursing skills. When the Crimean War broke out, Seacole applied to join the nursing corps led by Nightingale and was refused. Seacole wrote of her belief that this decision was primarily motivated by the colour of her skin. Not to be discouraged, Seacole made her own way to Crimea and established the British Hotel near the battlefront, which was a boarding house with two rooms where she provided care to the sick and those in need. She also often went to the battlefield to care for wounded soldiers (Sleeth, 2018).

In Canada, Charlotte Edith Anderson Monture (1890–1996) was the first Indigenous registered nurse. Her nursing career path was challenging in that Indigenous women were largely barred from Canadian nursing schools until the 1930s (Wytenbroek & Vandenberg, 2017). Monture applied to nursing schools in Ontario but was not accepted. Undeterred, she then applied to nursing schools in the United States and was finally accepted at the New Rochelle Nursing School in New York, where she graduated in 1914. Upon graduation, she joined the US Army Nurse Corps and served as an army nurse during the First World War. Following the war, she returned to the Six Nations Reserve in Canada and continued as a nurse and midwife for people in her community (Alexander, 2018).

The first Black nurses in Canada also had challenging career paths. Until the late 1940s, those who wanted to be a nurse and were Black were told by Canadian nursing schools to go the United States for their nursing education. When refused entry into Canadian nursing schools, Bernice Redman, born in Toronto, Ontario, went to the United States and earned her nursing diploma in 1945, from the Medical College of Virginia's St. Philip School of Nursing. Upon graduation, she returned to Canada and became the first Black nurse allowed to practise in public health in the Nova Scotia Department of Health and went on to become the first Black woman to be awarded the Victorian Order of Nurses in Canada (Lesmond, 2006). As a result of increasing pressure placed on nursing schools, Black women began to be accepted into Canadian nursing schools, with Ruth Bailey and Gwennyth Barton becoming the first Black women to graduate from a Canadian school of nursing, in 1948 (Ontario Nurses Association, 2021).

Evolution of Nursing as a Profession in Canada

The Canadian nursing profession consists of four regulated nursing groups: licensed/registered practical nurses, **registered nurses**, registered psychiatric nurses, and nurse practitioners (Canadian Nurses Association [CNA], 2015). Nurses work in settings across Canada, in hospitals, nursing homes, rehabilitation centres, clinics, community agencies, homes, academia, research and policy organizations, correctional services, and businesses (CNA, 2020b).

The educational preparation of nurses is imperative in readying them for professional practice (Ross-Kerr, 2011). Professional nursing education has changed in all four regulated nursing groups to better address the more complex health care needs of today that require evidence-informed practice. The programs have expanded to include theory and basic sciences, general and liberal arts and humanities courses, and evidence-informed knowledge and clinical practice concepts.

Educational programs for licensed/registered practical nurses began in the 1940s as a way to address nursing shortages precipitated by World War II (Pringle et al., 2004). Over the next 30 years, programs across the country first were offered through government programs but were then transferred to community colleges (Pringle et al., 2004). Since the 1990s, new knowledge and skill sets were identified for licensed/registered practical nurses to autonomously provide nursing care. They also became a recognized, self-regulated profession in all 13 provinces and territories, whose members work independently, providing health promotion and illness prevention to clients, in collaboration with the health care team (Canadian Institute for Health Information [CIHI], 2018).

For registered nurses' education, nursing leaders in the early 1900s began to look to universities to be involved in nursing education rather than the hospital apprentice-style education model. The University of British Columbia was the first university to offer a five-year baccalaureate nursing program, in 1919 (CASN, 2012). Over the years, the call for university nursing education programs continued, while identifying the need to shift the apprentice style-form of nursing education, to completely separate nursing education from hospitals and service. This resulted, in the late 1960s–'70s, in registered nursing programs being offered in community colleges where students graduated with a diploma in nursing, or in the university programs with an undergraduate degree in nursing (CASN, 2012). As the complexity of registered nursing practice increased, it was recognized that registered nurses needed greater depth in their knowledge and education than a diploma education could provide. Discussions began in the late 1970s, and after much debate, the entry-to-practice Bachelor of Science university requirements were adopted in the late 1990s–early 2000s, in most provinces and territories across Canada (CASN, 2012).

Registered psychiatric nurses are educated and regulated as a separate profession and practice only in Manitoba, Saskatchewan, Alberta, British Columbia, and Yukon (CIHI, 2018; Pringle et al., 2004). Registered psychiatric nurses originated in Manitoba in the 1920s, when the concept arose of preparing nurses to care for people with mental health disorders in asylums (Pringle et al., 2004). Presently, the educational programs to become a registered psychiatric nurse vary in terms of content, length, and prerequisites (Smith & Khanlou, 2013). Registered psychiatric nurses are self-regulated health care providers who coordinate person-centred care, focusing on mental and developmental health, mental health issues, and addictions (CIHI, 2018). They provide holistic care, integrating physical health and biopsychosocial and spiritual models of care through developing therapeutic relationships and using **therapeutic communication** (CIHI, 2018; Registered Psychiatric Nurse Regulators in Canada, 2020).

Nurse practitioners are registered nurses with advanced education that enables them to autonomously diagnose, order and interpret diagnostic tests, prescribe pharmaceuticals, and perform some advanced procedures within their legislated scope of practice (CIHI, 2018). They provide autonomous care in a variety of health care settings, including hospitals and communities across Canada, and work collaboratively with other members of the health care team (Nurse Practitioners' Association of Ontario, 2020).

Nursing Theory Development

Theory development is essential to maintaining the truth of any discipline (Reed & Shearer, 2007). Theory concepts examine the phenomenon of professional nursing in systematic ways. They make visible the nature of the nursing domain, inform clinical practice, and form a framework for research studies. The early definitional theories were described as theoretical frameworks that organized concepts essential to nursing practice that needed to be included in nursing curricula (Thorne, 2011). These theoretical/conceptual frameworks were then used by early nursing scholars to begin to advance nursing knowledge and develop a language that would be recognized by the scientific community (Thorne, 2011). These models were also used to begin to capture the complexity of nursing practice rather than the more simplistic linear, cause and effect models.

In the late 1960s to the mid-1980s, nursing theories were developed to help understand and articulate how knowledge could guide and be applied in nursing practice (Thorne, 2011). These theories had theoretical orientations of being based on practice, basic human needs, interactions, general systems theory, and simultaneity (Thorne, 2011). While many of the nursing theorists were from the United States, Canadian scholars were also developing nursing theories. Margaret Campbell and a team from University of British Columbia (UBC) developed a systems model known as the UBC Model for Nursing. Evelyn Adam of the Université de Montréal developed a model based on the work of Virginia Henderson, examining the nursing process as a helping process. The McGill Model, led by Moyra Allan, theorized nursing as health promotion, primarily at the family level (Thorne, 2011). Sister Simone

Roach described how caring is the human mode of being and is the basis of what nurses do each and every day. Sister Roach developed the model described as the 6 C's of caring: compassion, competence, conscience, confidence, commitment, and comportment, that are at the core of nursing practice (Roach, 1992; Villeneuve et al., 2016).

Theoretical nursing models also provide a foundation for generating hypotheses in research. They offer a common basis for education and act as a guide for nursing praxis. As the profession positions itself to play a key leadership role in a transformational health care system, there is a noticeable shift from theory development to a new era of theory applicability and utilization in nursing praxis (Alligood, 2014).

Nursing's Metaparadigm: The Science of Nursing

Nursing's metaparadigm represents the most abstract form of nursing knowledge (Black, 2017). Fawcett and Desanto-Madeya (2012) describe a **metaparadigm** as the "global concepts that identify the phenomena of central interest to a discipline, the global propositions that describe the concepts, and the global propositions that state the relationships between the concepts" (p. 4.). Four core constructs make up professional nursing's metaparadigm: person/human being, environment, health, and nursing. Each of these four conceptual constructs has an internal consistency related to the knowledge structure of nursing, which is described in different ways across theoretical frameworks (Jarrin, 2012; Karnick, 2013; Marrs & Lowry, 2006).

Concept of Person/Human Being

Knowledge of the person is the start of developing a therapeutic relationship and the delivery of nursing care. The term *human being* is now also being used instead of only using the concept of person. This is to recognize that *person* is not a globally understood term. The term *human beings* has a more transcultural meaning (Fawcett & Desanto-Madeya, 2012). For the purpose of this discussion, the two are used interchangeably.

The metaparadigm concept of person refers to individuals, families, and communities. This interpretation is in recognition that nurses provide holistic care not only at the individual level, but also to families, groups, and communities (Thorne, 2011). The nurse–person relationship is based on the interactions between the nurse and human being. When establishing the therapeutic relationship, the nurse needs to be aware that all individuals are unique, with multiple aspects, such as mental, physical, spiritual, and social health, that are closely interwoven and deeply interdependent (Thorne, 2011; World Health Organization [WHO], 2001). Nurses have a legal and ethical professional responsibility to protect each human being's integrity, well-being,

and rights to self-determination in receiving care. The World Health Organization (WHO) states that "the enjoyment of the highest attainable standard of health is one of the fundamental rights of every human being without distinction of race, religion, political belief, economic, or social condition (WHO, 2014).

Concept of Environment

The term **environment** describes the *context* in which health relationships take place (WHO, 2001). When caring for a human being, the internal and external environmental factors that support or impede health and well-being must be considered. Socioenvironmental factors represent the context that directly and indirectly influence a person's health perceptions and health behaviours. Economic status, education, gender, sexual orientation, culture, religious and spiritual beliefs, type of community (rural or urban), family dynamics, level of social support, health resource availability and ease of access to care, and environmental practices and climate change are all examples of significant environmental determinants of health. Recognition of these contextual factors is important in health promotion, disease prevention, and the capacity of individuals to participate in their care. The importance of environment is highlighted in the CNA (2017a) position statement on climate change and health. The position statement emphasizes that the effects of climate change are evident in shifting ecosystems, food availability, and the frequency and severity of extreme weather events. The CNA (2017b) Code of Ethics for Registered Nurses states that nurses should work individually and collectively to advocate for and support environment preservation and restoration initiatives that reduce environmentally harmful practices to foster the health and well-being of Canadians and the global society.

Concept of Health

The word **health** derives from the word *whole*. *Health* is a relative term, subject to personal interpretation. Cultural contexts and practices, values and beliefs, and previous life experiences influence how a person perceives and interprets health and illness. For example, in some cultures, where poverty is a significant factor, having a robust body size is considered a sign of a healthy lifestyle. In a different culture, a similar body size would be considered a sign of an unhealthy lifestyle (Schiavo, 2014).

The World Health Organization (WHO)'s definition of health, developed in 1948, moved from being "the presence or absence of disease" to describing *health* as "a state of complete physical, mental and social well-being, and not merely the absence of disease or infirmity" (Thompson, 2020). Over the years, there has been wide debate about whether it is realistic to have a state of complete physical, mental, and social well-being. Criticisms were raised that this definition is too broad, ambiguous, and unrealistic. This concern is particularly relevant in the present day, with people who have chronic disease now living longer lives than in the past and still considering themselves healthy (Thompson, 2020).

In the 1980s, with expectations around the world for a new health movement, the WHO held a conference in Ottawa, Canada. The Ottawa Charter for Health Promotion was developed and defined health and health promotion as the "process of enabling people to increase control over, and to improve their health. To reach a state of complete physical, mental and social wellbeing, an individual or group must be able to identify and to realize aspirations, to satisfy needs and to change or cope with environment. Health is therefore a resource for everyday life, not the objective of living. Health is a positive concept emphasizing social and personal resources as well as physical capacities" (WHO, 1986).

Quality of life includes both health and well-being. The term refers to an individual's subjective assessment of well-being (Mount et al., 2007). The term *wellness* is often used in relation to health. Wellness is more than good health as it explores the way a person feels about their health and quality of life (Thompson, 2020). *Wellness* is defined by the WHO as the "optimal state of health of individuals and groups," with two central areas of focus: "the fullest potential of an individual physically, psychologically, socially, spiritually, and economically, and the fulfillment of one's role expectations in the family, community, place of worship, workplace and other settings" (WHO, 2006). Obtaining wellness is the process of making decisions about a person's quality of life, purpose, and good health, keeping in mind that the perception of what good health is, varies from one person to the next. For example, an active 80-year-old can consider themselves quite healthy, despite having osteoporosis and a controlled heart condition. This sense of wellness can be achieved through examining different dimensions of their life that contribute to a perception of wellness. There are many models describing different dimensions of wellness. The 8 dimensions of wellness model is often used and includes physical, social, emotional, environmental, financial, occupational, intellectual, and spiritual (Swarbrick, 2012).

Measuring health on a continuum is one way of assessing a human being's perception of their own health. This continuum is often described as the "health continuum" or "wellness–illness continuum (Fig. 1.2). On one end of the continuum is "optimum health," with the other end labelled "death." The middle of the continuum is considered "fair health" (managing). Individuals can move one way or the other on the continuum, depending on their perception of health, which includes physical, mental, emotional, social, spiritual, and environmental health (Thompson, 2020). This continuum assists health care providers in understanding and assessing how two people with the same chronic illness can view their health on the continuum very differently.

Paradigm shift in health care delivery. Contemporary health initiatives reflect an increasing shift in focus to healthy lifestyle promotion, disease prevention, reducing health disparities, early risk assessments, and chronic disease self-care management strategies. We are seeing dramatic changes in how professional nursing is practiced, and where health care is delivered. Until recent decades, care was delivered primarily in acute-care settings, based on a disease-focused medical model. Many acute disorders that shortened people's lives have been eradicated or are now viewed as manageable chronic conditions. Better diagnostic tools and effective treatments have given rise to improved medical outcomes and longevity. The Public Health Agency of Canada (2017) identifies that, in general, Canada is a healthy nation, with the overall mortality rate and life expectancy improving considerably. More than one in five Canadian adults live longer than in the past, with the chronic diseases of cerebrovascular disease, cancer, chronic respiratory diseases, and diabetes.

Health care now emphasizes health promotion and disease prevention, early intervention for chronic disorders,

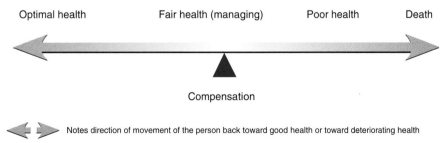

Fig. 1.2 The health or wellness–illness continuum. Source: Thompson, V. D. 2020. *Health and health care delivery in Canada* (3rd ed.). Elsevier. Fig. 7.3, p. 194.

continuity of care, and active participation of the person as part of the health care team. Nurses play an important role in helping people of all ages engage in various health promotion and disease prevention activities needed to promote maximal personal health and well-being.

Simulation Exercise 1.1, The Meaning of Health as a Nursing Concept, provides an opportunity to explore the multidimensional meaning of health.

Concept of Nursing

The International Council of Nurses (ICN) declares that nursing encompasses a continuum of health care services delivered by nurses and that it is found across health care systems and in the community. This document states:

- Nursing encompasses autonomous and collaborative care of individuals of all ages, families, groups, and communities, sick or well, and in all settings.
- Nursing includes the promotion of health; prevention of illness; and the care of ill, disabled, and dying people.
- Advocacy, promotion of a safe environment, research, participation in shaping health policy and in person and health systems management, and education are also key nursing roles (ICN, 2014).

SCIENCE AND ART OF NURSING

Nursing is described as both a science and art. The science of nursing (theory and evidence-informed knowledge, research, clinical guidelines) provides an essential focus and knowledge basis for professional nursing. Evidence-informed nursing actions help people achieve identified health goals through practices ranging from health promotion, preventive care, and health education, to include direct care, rehabilitation, palliative care, research, and health teaching. *The person is at the centre of the model, as its core concept.*

Professional nursing and health care practices are also grounded in human interactions and relationships. The **art of nursing** references a blending of the nurse's ability to adapt to the person's individual needs through processes of understanding the nature of health from the person's perspective through caring, compassion, and therapeutic communication (Henry, 2018; Palos, 2014). Caring practices strengthen person-centred knowledge and therapeutic relationships. The nurse's focus is on developing an individualized understanding of each person as a unique human being. Perceptions are influenced by the nurse's knowledge and professional experiences with other persons. Using this data takes into account the interactive factors that nurses must consider in order to blend their knowledge and skills with scientific understandings to provide safe, quality care. Finkelman and Kenner (2009) differentiate between the science and art of nursing, stating that "knowledge represents the science of nursing, and **caring** represents the art of nursing" (p. 54).

CONTEMPORARY NURSING

Nurses represent the largest group of health care providers in Canada, accounting for almost half of the health workforce (CIHI, 2017). The total number of registered nurses in Canada in 2018 was 431769 (CIHI, 2018). This included 303 146 registered nurses, including 5 697 nurse practitioners; 122 600 licensed/registered practical nurses; and 6 023 registered psychiatric nurses (CNA, 2020c).

SIMULATION EXERCISE 1.1   The Meaning of Health as a Nursing Concept

Purpose

To help students understand the dimensions of health as a nursing concept

Procedure

1. Think of a person whom you think is healthy. In a short report (1–2 paragraphs), identify characteristics that led you to your choice of this person.
2. In groups of three or four, read your stories to each other. As you listen to other students' stories, write down themes that you note.
3. Compare themes, paying attention to similarities and differences, and develop a group definition of health derived from the stories.
4. In a larger group, share your definitions of health and the defining characteristics of a healthy person.

Reflective Analysis Discussion

1. Were you surprised by any of your thoughts about being healthy?
2. Did your peers define health in similar ways?
3. Based on the themes that emerged, how is health determined?
4. Is being ill the opposite of being healthy?
5. In what ways, if any, did you find concepts of health to be related to social determinants or factors such as age, values and beliefs, previous life experiences, culture, or gender?
6. In what specific ways can you as a nurse support the person you are caring for in achieving health and health promotion, based on the Ottawa Charter for Health Promotion?

The CNA has been the national professional voice of registered nurses, including nurse practitioners, since 1908. However, in 2018, voting delegates at the CNA's annual meeting of members voted overwhelmingly to include licensed/registered practical nurses and registered psychiatric nurses to be more inclusive in representing the voices of all nurses in Canada, strongly promote and contribute to intraprofessional collaboration, and gain a stronger advocacy voice (CNA, 2018). Each province and territory has a professional regulatory nursing body, a professional nursing association, or both.

PROFESSIONAL NURSING: A PRACTICE DISCIPLINE

Professional nursing represents a practice discipline. There are many definitions of what makes up a profession; however, the attributes that are regularly used to describe professionalism include knowledge, accountability, autonomy, self-regulation, inquiry, collegiality, collaboration, innovation, ethics, and values (Registered Nurses' Association of Ontario [RNAO], 2007).

As part of being a member of a self-regulated profession, nurses must acquire, maintain, and continually increase their knowledge and skills to guide evidence-informed decision making in their practice. The nursing profession is also held accountable to the public. This accountability is achieved through writing a licensing or registration exam upon graduation from a nursing program. Entry-level standards of practice are based on the conceptual framework that highlights the regulatory purposes of the five competency categories: professional responsibility and accountability; knowledge-based practice; ethical practice; service to the public; and self-regulation (see Fig. 1.3). All provincial and territorial regulatory bodies have continuing competence programs that nurses must meet each year to renew their licensure/registration (CNA, 2015).

Nurses are guided in their practice by the CNA and provincial and territorial regulatory codes of ethics, nursing standards, best practice, research, and laws and regulations that guide practice (CNA, 2017a). Nurses are also expected to integrate evidence-informed care principles, specialized knowledge and skills, and compassion and caring into practice assessments, and to then base their clinical judgements and care decisions on them (Epstein & Street, 2011; Smith & McCarthy, 2010). Professional nursing combines specialized knowledge and critical thinking and judgement to meet person, family, and community health care needs. Both the science and art of nursing are needed to support the safety and quality of professional practice.

Simulation Exercise 1.2, What Is Professional Nursing? can help you look at your philosophy of nursing.

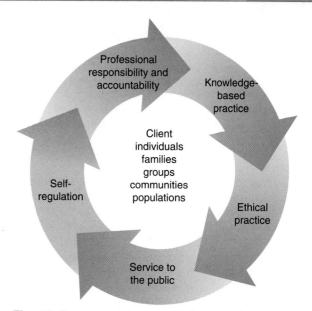

Fig. 1.3 Conceptual framework for organizing competencies. Source: Adapted from Canadian Nurses Association. (2015). *Framework for the practice of registered nurses in Canada.* https://www.cna-aiic.ca/~/media/cna/page-content/pdf-en/framework-for-the-pracice-of-registered-nurses-in-canada.pdf?la=en p.11.

WAYS (PATTERNS) OF KNOWING IN NURSING

Nurses use **patterns of knowing** to bridge the interpersonal space between scientific understandings and person-centred health experiences. It is this dimension of knowledge that helps nurses to individualize nursing and interprofessional care strategies (Zander, 2007). In a seminal work, Carper (1978) described four patterns of knowing embedded in nursing practice: empirical, personal, aesthetic, and ethical. Although these ways of knowing are described as individual patterns of knowing, in practice, nurses use these patterns as an integrated form of knowing about the person. The patterns (ways) of knowing consist of the following:

- *Empirical ways of knowing:* This type of knowledge draws upon verifiable data from science. The process of empirical ways of knowing includes incorporating logical reasoning and problem solving. Nurses use empirical ways of knowing to provide scientific rationales when choosing and supporting appropriate nursing interventions. An evidenced-informed research discussion or study is included in this book, related to

SIMULATION EXERCISE 1.2   What Is Professional Nursing?

Purpose

To help students develop an understanding of professional nursing

Procedure

1. Interview a professional nurse who has been in practice for more than 12 months. Ask for descriptions of what the nurse considers professional nursing to be today; how nurses make a difference; and how the nursing role could evolve and change within the next 10 years.
2. In groups of three to five students, discuss and compare your findings.
3. Develop a group definition of professional nursing.

Reflective Discussion Analysis

1. What does nursing mean to you?
2. In what ways, if any, have your ideas about nursing changed, now that you are actively involved in people care as a nurse?
3. Is your understanding of nursing different from those of the nurse you interviewed?
4. As a new nurse, how would you want to present yourself?

---

the content of each chapter, to better understand how evidence-informed knowledge informs practice.

- **Personal ways of knowing:** Personal ways of knowing refers to knowledge that is characterized as subjective, concrete, and existential (Carper, 1978). Personal knowing is relational. This pattern of knowing occurs when nurses connect with the "humanness" of a person's experience. Personal knowing involves knowing oneself and having the self-awareness to be able to engage and relate with others. Personal knowledge develops when nurses understand and connect with people based on their own experience, expertise, and knowledge as unique human beings. Self-awareness allows nurses to self-check any biases that might prevent the development of an authentic personal connection with a person, as well as to empathetically understand what is happening. Because nurses learn to develop experiential knowledge of their own responses from previous clinical situations, this way of knowing can provide a better interpretation of difficult health situations.

- **Aesthetic ways of knowing:** This type of knowledge links the humanistic components of care with their scientific knowledge. This way of knowing represents a deeper appreciation of the whole person or situation, moving beyond the superficial to see the experience as part of a larger whole to make meaningful connections. The ability to empathize with a person through aesthetic ways of knowing enables nurses to experientially relate to the fear behind a person's angry response, or the courage of a person with stage four cancer facing death. Aesthetic knowing is linked to art, beauty, and sensory and emotional experiences such as suffering (Hartrick Doane & Varcoe, 2015). By including aesthetic ways of knowing, the unseen parts of the story allow everyone, including the person, to learn new information.

- **Ethical ways of knowing:** This type of knowledge refers to principled care, which nurses experience when they confront the moral aspects of nursing care (Porter et al., 2011). Ethical ways of knowing refer to knowledge of what is right and wrong, what ought to be done, attention to **professional standards** and codes in making moral choices, taking responsibility for one's actions, and protecting person autonomy and rights. Carnago and Mast (2015) note, "To make an ethical decision, the nurse must consider the clinical situation, be aware of personal beliefs and values, and determine how to apply ethical and moral principles to the situation" (p. 389). Chinn and Kramer (2015) introduced a fifth pattern, emancipatory ways of knowing.

- **Emancipatory ways of knowing:** Emancipatory ways of knowing include awareness of social problems and social justice issues as contributory determinants of health disparities. This pattern of knowing focuses on social determinants as a context for health care concerns. Health Canada (2019) identifies the main determinants of health as income and social status, employment and working conditions, education and literacy, childhood experiences, physical environments, social supports and coping skills, healthy behaviours, access to health services, biology and genetic endowment, gender, culture, and race and racism. With improved knowledge of social, political, and economic determinants of health and well-being, nurses can serve as better advocates in assisting people, families and communities collectively, to identify and reduce the inequities in health care.

Simulation Exercise 1.3, Patterns of Knowing in Clinical Practice, provides practice with using patterns or ways of knowing in clinical practice.

SIMULATION EXERCISE 1.3   Patterns of Knowing in Clinical Practice

Purpose

To help students understand how patterns of knowing can be used effectively in clinical practice

Procedure

1. Break into groups of three to four students. Identify a record-keeper of the discussion for each student group.
2. Using the following case study, decide how you would use empirical, personal, ethical, aesthetic, and emancipatory ways of knowing to see that Mrs. Jackson's holistic needs are addressed in the next 48 hours.

Case Study

Mrs. Jackson, an 86-year-old widow, was admitted to the hospital with a hip fracture. She has very poor eyesight because of macular degeneration and takes eyedrops for the condition. Her husband died 5 years ago, and she subsequently moved into an assisted seniors residence. She had to give up driving because of her eyesight and sold her car to another resident 5 months ago. Although her daughter lives in the area, Mrs. Jackson has little contact with her. This distresses her greatly, as she describes having been very close with her daughter until 8 years ago. She feels safe in her new environment but complains that she is very lonely and is not interested in joining activities. She has a male friend in the complex, but recently, he has been showing less interest. Her surgery is scheduled for tomorrow, but she has not yet signed her consent form. She does not have advance directives.

Reflective Analysis Discussion

1. In a large group, have each smaller group share their findings.
2. For each pattern of knowing, write the suggestions on the board.
3. Compare and contrast the findings of the different groups.
4. Discuss how the patterns of knowing add to an understanding of the person in this case study.

SIMULATION EXERCISE 1.4   A Caring Moment

Purpose

To help students develop an understanding of the knowledge and actions that occur in caring moments

Procedure

1. Individually read the case study that follows and identify the knowledge, self-awareness of values and biases, and caring actions that occurred. What made them caring actions? What surprised you? Why was this a defining moment for the student nurse?
2. Pair up with another student and share your findings.
3. Summarize the most important points from your discussion, and then share these points with another group of two students. Summarize the most important points to share with the large group.

Case Study

A student nurse describes the following caring moment she had with a person:

"A person who was under palliative care and had a history of substance abuse was on our unit. I was upset about how many of the nurses stigmatized the person and were doing only the most basic of care for him and not going into his room unless they had to. I went into the room and saw that the poor gentleman was having trouble breathing, and I thought, 'You know what? I'm going to offer to give him a bed bath,' because he looked very uncomfortable and he had body odour. I remember giving the gentleman a bath, and all of sudden he opens his eyes, and the way he looked at me was a defining moment for me. I remember thinking, 'Yeah, this is what nursing is all about.'"

Reflective Discussion Analysis

1. In a large group, discuss what were the most important points from your discussions.
2. Why did the nursing student think this is what nursing is all about?
3. What made this a caring moment?

CARING AS A CORE VALUE OF PROFESSIONAL NURSING

Caring is considered an *essential* functional construct in professional nursing practice, which defines the person-centred relationship and the development of interpersonal relationships in practice settings (Wagner & Whaite, 2010). Professional caring is much more than "being kind." Instead, it is a complex relationship that encompasses knowledge, being present with another, and actions focusing on achieving positive outcomes and well-being. Think about the most important relationship you have experienced in health care. What made it meaningful to you? See Simulation Exercise 1.4, A Caring Moment.

The concept of caring has been evolving since the time of Florence Nightingale and is considered at the core of nursing practice. Caring nursing practices are the integration of compassion, empathy, knowledge, and competence and are interdependent in meeting the needs of the people being cared for. Caring moments are often the component of nursing care best remembered by persons, families, and nurses. Caring strengthens person-centred knowledge and adds depth to other nursing competencies that nurses bring to the clinical situation (Rhodes et al., 2011).

Professional caring is about the involvement of the nurse and person in the encounter, and its meaning to the people involved. There are many forms of caring in clinical practice—some visible, others private and personal, known only to the persons who are experiencing feeling cared for. In a qualitative study, when graduate student nurses were asked to describe a professional caring incident in their practice, they identified the attributes of caring as (a) giving of self, (b) involved presence, (c) intuitive knowing and empathy, (d) supporting the person's integrity, and (e) professional competence (Arnold, 1997).

FUNCTIONS OF COMMUNICATION IN HEALTH CARE SYSTEMS

More than any other variable, effective interpersonal communication supports the safety and quality in health care delivery (see Chapter 2).

Definition

The term *communication* derives from the Latin, "communicare," meaning "to share" (Dima et al., 2014). Communication connects people and ideas through words, nonverbal behaviours, and actions. This is known as interpersonal communication. People communicate as a key means to share information, ask questions, and seek assistance. Words are used to persuade others, take a position, and create an understandable story. In fact, "communication represents the very essence of the human condition" (Hargie, 2011, p. 2). Human communication is unique. Only human beings have complex vocabularies and are capable of learning and using multiple language symbols to convey meaning.

Communication between health care providers and the people being cared for impacts the way care is delivered; it is as important as the care itself. Outcomes of effective interpersonal communication in health care relate to higher person satisfaction, quality care, and productive health changes. People are more likely to understand their health conditions through meaningful communication and to alert providers when something feels wrong. Other specific ways interpersonal health communication impacts the quality of care is through the following:

- Development of a collaborative care partnership
- Better understanding of the person's condition
- More effective identification of health issues and earlier recognition of health changes
- Personalized care plans for therapeutic treatments
- More efficient utilization of health services
- Stronger, longer-lasting positive outcomes

Two-way communication provides the opportunity to share information, to be heard, and to be validated. Having the opportunity to provide input empowers persons and families to take a stronger position in contributing to their health care. The two communication models used most frequently are referred to as linear and transactional models (see Chapter 5 for details).

The **linear communication model** (Fig. 1.4) is the simplest communication model, consisting of sender, message, receiver, channels of communication, and context. Linear models focus only on the sending and receiving of messages and do not necessarily consider communication as enabling the development of co-created meanings. They are useful in emergency health situations, when time is of the essence to get immediate information.

Transactional communication models are more complex. These models define interpersonal communication as a reciprocal interaction in which both sender and receiver influence each other's messages and responses as they converse (Fig. 1.5). Each communicator constructs a mental picture of the other during the conversation, including perceptions about the other's attitude and potential reactions to the message. Previous experiences and exposure to concepts and ideas heighten recognition, and influence the interpretation of the message. The outcome of transactional models represents a co-created set of collaborative meanings developed during the conversation.

Transactional models employ systems concepts. A human system (person, family, and provider) receives information from the environment (*input*), internally processes it, and interprets its meaning (*throughput*). The internal process and interpreting meaning are influenced by each person's knowledge, goals, culture values, communication abilities, and internal references. The result is new information or behaviour (*output*). *Feedback loops* (from

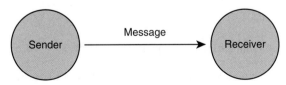

Fig. 1.4 Linear model of communication

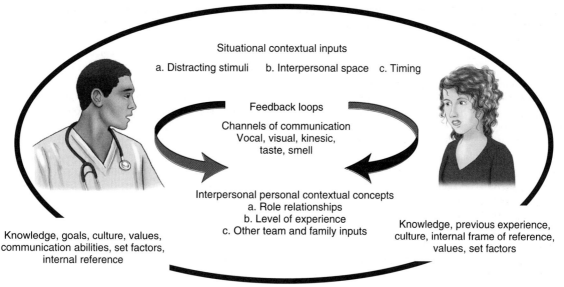

Situational contextual inputs
a. Distracting stimuli   b. Interpersonal space   c. Timing

Feedback loops

Channels of communication
Vocal, visual, kinesic,
taste, smell

Interpersonal personal contextual concepts
a. Role relationships
b. Level of experience
c. Other team and family inputs

Knowledge, goals, culture, values,
communication abilities, set factors,
internal reference

Knowledge, previous experience,
culture, internal frame of reference,
values, set factors

Fig. 1.5 Transactional model of communication

SIMULATION EXERCISE 1.5   Comparing Linear and Transactional Models of Communication

Purpose
To help students see the difference between linear and transactional models of communication.

Procedure
1. Role-play a scenario in which one person provides a scene that might occur in the clinical area using a linear model: sender, message, and receiver.
2. Role-play the same scenario using a transactional model of communication, framing questions that

recognize the context of the message and its potential impact on the receiver, and provide feedback.

Discussion
1. Was there a difference in your level of comfort? If so, in what ways?
2. Was there any difference in the amount of information you gave or received as a result of the communication? If so, in what ways?
3. What implications does this exercise have for your future nursing practice?

---

the receiver or the environment) provide information about the output as it relates to the data received or acted upon (or both). Feedback either validates the received data or reflects a need to correct or modify its original input information. Thus, transactional models draw attention to communication as having purpose and meaning-making attributes. Simulation Exercise 1.5, Comparing Linear and Transactional Models of Communication, provides a simulated exercise to demonstrate the differences between linear and transactional models of communication.

SYSTEMS THEORY FOUNDATIONS

The WHO (2007) defines a health system as consisting of "all organizations, people and actions whose primary intent

is to promote, restore or maintain health" (p. 2). Systems theory provides a foundation for understanding the quality and safety of health care and providing professional nursing practice. It supports competency education for nurses guided by the Canadian Association of Schools of Nursing (CASN) and outlined by provincial or territorial regulatory bodies. Throughout the chapters in this text, knowledge, skills and abilities are explored associated with concepts and applications related to competency-based nursing education and evidence-informed practice within the complex health care system.

Systems theory focuses on the interrelationships within a given system and is based on the whole being greater than the sum of its parts (Weberg, 2012). These systems are made up of patterns and relationships with interactions

EVIDENCE-INFORMED NURSING PRACTICE

Evidence-informed professional nursing serves as a critical foundation for nursing praxis, education, and research. The CNA (2010) defines *evidence-informed nursing practice* as "the ongoing process that incorporates evidence from research, clinical expertise, client preferences, and other available resources to make nursing decisions about clients."

Integrating individual clinical expertise and judgement with objective evidence and collaborative interprofessional consultations is recognized as being critical to safe, quality professional nursing care. "It is a way of practicing owned by all nurses" (Taylor et al., 2016, p. 576). Fueled by professional communication, a strong evidence base represents a blending of the nurse's expertise with research findings and best practices guidelines. Nurses partner with persons and the health care team to merge this data with person preferences, value beliefs, and personal capacity to develop jointly constructed action plans to resolve health issues. Ideally, professional nurses integrate their professional clinical expertise with "patterns of knowing" about people they care for to incorporate research-based findings and clinical guidelines in providing knowledgeable, skilled, person-centred care. Sackett et al. (1996) makes the point, "External clinical evidence can inform, but can never replace, individual clinical expertise, and it is this expertise that decides whether the external evidence applies to the individual person at all and, if so, how it should be integrated into the clinical decision" (p. 72). At the end of each chapter in this book, we have included an evidence-informed research study or suggestions for evidence-informed research to emphasize important praxis or research connections with each chapter's content.

that are nonlinear, interactive, and continually changing, with unpredictable outcomes (Mallette & Rykert, 2018). From a systems perspective, everything within the health care system is interrelated and interdependent (Porter-O'Grady & Malloch, 2014). Health care systems are made up the person, family, and community receiving care; the health care team, including all health care providers; health care organizations where care is provided; and the environment where health relationships exist. These health system patterns and relationships, alongside the interactions with education, service, and research systems are all interrelated and best interpreted within a systems framework.

Systems theory is a fundamental contributor to understanding the functional communication occurring within larger professional health organizations. Care transition guidelines and technology applications are examples of systems approaches to health care across clinical settings (Porter-O'Grady & Malloch, 2014). Systems thinking is also essential to understanding interprofessional team collaboration in health care (Clark, 2016; Dolansky & Moore, 2013).

The person, family, and community are now considered essential team members in an interprofessional collaborative health care relationship. In the past, health care providers would try to "engage" persons and families in their care. Evidence-informed practice now demonstrates that having persons, families, and communities participating as integral members of the health care team in all decision making is central to providing safe and quality care (Canadian Patient Safety Institute [CPSI], 2018). They are considered experts about the meaning of their own health within a personalized life context and are important members in team decision making regarding care (Mead & Bower, 2000).

Systems thinking helps you as a health professional understand *how* the interrelationships among different parts of the health care system contribute to its overall functioning at macro and micro levels. At a macro level, systems thinking reminds nurses to see how changes in one aspect of care provision can produce unexpected consequences for others in the system. Systems thinking also allows nurses to examine individual health care issues and to consider how they link to larger health system care outcomes. Health care systems represent integrated wholes, whose properties cannot be effectively reduced to a single unit (Porter-O'Grady & Malloch, 2014). These interacting parts work together to achieve important goals. Only by looking at the whole system can one fully appreciate the meaning of how its individual parts work together.

Case Application

Systems thinking moves a nurse from individualized care at the micro level, for example of turning a person from side to side to avoid decubiti, to the meso and macro level of monitoring the person's nutrition, hydration, underlying diseases such as diabetes and peripheral vascular disease, mobility, staffing levels, availability of pressure-reducing devices on the unit, and the pressure ulcer rate on the unit compared to that of the health care organization to understand the different influences within the system that impact on the risk of the person developing decubiti (Phillips et al., 2016).

Interprofessional Education and Practice

The CNA (2019) advocates for **interprofessional education** integrated throughout nurses' educational programs and practice, as they are imperative in providing person-centred care and improving health outcomes. A systems perspective can greatly enhance clinically team-based **relational communication**. Each health discipline has different education, focus, and priorities, which must be integrated to achieve coordinated optimal health outcomes. The Canadian Interprofessional Health Collaborative's (CIHC) National Interprofessional Competency Framework (2010) identifies six competency domains that are interdependent of each other in providing interprofessional practice. The domains encompass the knowledge, skills, abilities and **values** that guide communication and judgements necessary for collaborative practice. The six competency domains are as follows:

- Interprofessional communication
- Person/client/family/community-centred care
- Role clarification
- Team functioning
- Collaborative leadership
- Interprofessional conflict resolution

The ways in which health providers implement interprofessional practice in achieving clinical outcomes becomes a measure of systems-based team competence.

APPLICATIONS

Paradigm Shifts in Health Care Delivery

In this introductory chapter, we introduce concepts that influence health care delivery that are explored throughout the text. Health care delivery has "moved from a 'one-professional: one person' care model" (Batalden et al., 2006, p. 549) to interprofessional practice, with the person and family as integral members of the health care team. As the person and family are the ones who independently care for their health when not engaged with health providers, it is imperative that they be at the centre of care and actively involved in decision making (Orchard et al., 2017).

 DEVELOPING AN EVIDENCE-INFORMED PRACTICE TO EXAMINE HEALTH TEAMS AS COMPLEX ADAPTIVE SYSTEMS

Background: This research article explores the functioning of interprofessional teams using the system perspective called complex adaptive systems (CAS). CAS was used as a framework to examine health care providers' interactions to explore factors influencing team functioning. CAS was also used to study complex systems through examining the interrelationships and connections of the system's factors rather than focusing on individual factors. Evidence has indicated that the relationship patterns between individuals in the health care team influence the quality of care delivery, the rate of information flow, and the adaptability of the health care team to respond to changing system demands.

Methods: An interview study was done with 21 palliative home-care nurses, 20 community nurses, and 18 general practitioners, in Flanders, Belgium. Analysis of the data was performed using a two-step deductive analysis, using the CAS principles as a coding framework.

Findings: While all CAS principles were identified in the data, the most predominant findings were related to team functioning. Team members identified that team interactions and behaviours were all influenced by these factors: individual autonomy guided by their internalized basic rules of focusing on the person and quality of care; acting in the best interests of the person; and the acknowledgement of each other's knowledge and expertise. There was also an awareness that, while the general practitioner did have the final responsibility of prescribing medications

and the treatment plan, this decision was made based on the health care team collaboratively exploring options to identify what was optimal for the person. They identified that ensuring the tasks and responsibilities were clear for everybody within the team was important for cohesiveness of team members knowing their own and each other's tasks and responsibilities.

Conclusion: This study examined team interactions and functioning through the lens of CAS. Patterns of team interactions influenced team behaviours and functioning. The interactions between team members also, at times, generated unpredicted new behaviours.

Application to Your Clinical Practice: Studies such as this can inform nursing practice and working within interprofessional teams. This study highlights the interrelationships amongst health care providers in complex adaptive systems. One of the primary findings was the importance of communication amongst team members and how it can influence team behaviours and ultimately quality care. The findings have educational implications for the need for students from different health professions to have interprofessional educational opportunities to better understand each other's roles and enhance working more collaboratively in practice. Future research is also needed to validate these results and further identify the different patterns of team communication that influence team dynamics and effectiveness.

Adapted from Pype, P., Mertens, F., Helewaut, F. et al. (2018). Healthcare teams as complex adaptive systems: Understanding team behaviour through team members' perception of interpersonal interaction. *BMC Health Services Research, 18:*570. https://bmchealthservres.biomedcentral.com/articles/10.1186/s12913-018-3392-3.

Recognizing the health care team as a system composed of skilled interdependent team members, each representing a relevant discipline involved in the person's care, creates a different care paradigm. The various perspectives of each discipline and the person and family provide a deeper understanding of the issues and development of a more comprehensive treatment plan. Instead of caring *for* the person, nurses are charged with working *with* the person to develop and implement action plans that acknowledge the reality of the person's health condition while working to achieve desired clinical outcomes and personal well-being. Everyone—health care providers, persons and their families, researchers, educators and policy makers—will need to continue to make changes to enable interprofessional person-centred care to better meet individual health outcomes and population needs, in safe, competent, and cost effective ways (Canadian Foundation for Healthcare Improvement, n.d). Specific communication and interprofessional collaborative concepts related to community-based continuity of care initiatives are presented throughout subsequent chapters in this text.

Core components of today's health care system include an engaged person and family within the health care team and the dual concepts of person-centredness and person empowerment. This broader shift in orientation has been strengthened through multiple reports and research over the years, evaluating the Canadian health care system and calling for a transformed health care system in which care is person, family, and community driven and delivered within an interprofessional, collaborative care framework. Interprofessional collaboration is described as the most efficient means to deliver accessible, high-quality, person-centred health care that addresses wellness, prevention of illness, adverse events, self-management of chronic illness, and interdependent clinical applications (CNA, 2015). Interprofessional collaboration is essential to the implementation of safe, quality care in a transformed health care system.

Nursing plays an increasing and important role in transforming the health care system with advancing technology and the increased focus on health promotion, primary care, and prevention rather than disease-oriented, episodic acute care practices. New roles for nurses will continue to emerge, focusing on the needs of diverse populations, including people who are Indigenous, in a variety of contexts and practice settings (CNA, 2015). Nurses will contribute to offering care across the lifespan, preventing and treating a wide range of communicable and noncommunicable diseases, and promoting health and well-being through ensuring access to care for vulnerable populations, addressing the social determinants of health through collaborative action, and delivering care in emergencies, pandemics, epidemics, and diseases (WHO, 2020).

SUMMARY

This chapter traces the development of nursing and health communication as a basic foundation for understanding concepts presented in later chapters. It identifies core concepts of nursing's metaparadigm and discusses ways and patterns of knowing through which nurses integrate and apply relational knowledge to benefit persons and families in clinical settings.

The chapter also describes two evidence-informed models of communication—linear and transactional—and begins to explore the contributions of communication theory in developing therapeutic relationships and its use as a primary means of achieving treatment goals while fostering quality and safe practices.

Nursing is recognized as a critical professional body needed to transform the health care system. The rapidly changing health care system creates the need for nurses to clearly "own" the essence of their discipline and redefine their professional nursing role responsibilities, embedded within a collaborative, interprofessional, person-centred health care system. Nurses have an unprecedented opportunity to make a difference and shape the future of nursing practice through communication at every level in health care delivery.

ETHICAL DILEMMA
What Would You Do?

Craig Montague is a difficult person to care for. As his nurse, you find his constant arguing, poor hygiene, and poor treatment of his family very upsetting. It is difficult for you to provide him with anything but the most basic care, and you just want to leave his room as quickly as possible. How could you use a person-centred approach to understanding Craig? How could you apply the ethical pattern of knowing, in caring for Craig?

QUESTIONS FOR REVIEW AND DISCUSSION

1. In what specific ways is your nursing practice influenced by Carper's ways of knowing?
2. In what ways would you envision your leadership role as a nurse being as important as your technical ability to deliver safe, quality care at the bedside?
3. How would you describe your role responsibilities as a nurse representative on an interprofessional care team?
4. What do you see as the major challenges faced by professional nurses today?

REFERENCES

Alexander, K.L. (2018). *Charlotte Edith Anderson Monture*. National Women's History Museum. https://www.womenshistory.org/education-resources/biographies/charlotte-edith-anderson-monture.

Alligood, M. (2014). *Nursing Theory: Utilization and Application* (5th ed.). Mosby Elsevier.

Arnold, E. (1997). Caring from the graduate student perspective. *International Journal for Human Caring, 1*(3), 32–42.

Batalden, P., Orging, G., & Batalden, M. (2006). From one to many. *Journal of Interprofessional Care, 20*(5), 549–551. https://doi.org/10.1080/13561820600953967.

Black, B. (2017). *Professional Nursing: Concepts and Challenges* (8th ed.). Elsevier.

Canadian Association of Schools of Nursing. (2012). Ties that bind: *The evolution of education for professional nursing in Canada from the 17th to the 21st century*. https://www.casn.ca/wp-content/uploads/2016/12/History.pdf.

Canadian Foundation for Healthcare Improvement. (n.d.). *What if: Interprofessional Care was the norm in Canada?* https://www.cna-aiic.ca/~/media/cna/page-content/pdf-en/what_if_interprofessional_care_norm_cfhi_e.pdf?la=en.

Canadian Institute for Health Information. (2017). *Regulated Nurses, 2016: Report*. https://secure.cihi.ca/free_products/regulated-nurses-2016-report-en-web.pdf.

Canadian Institute for Health Information. (2018). *Nursing in Canada, 2018: A lens on supply and workforce*. https://www.cihi.ca/sites/default/files/document/regulated-nurses-2018-report-en-web.pdf.

Canadian Interprofessional Health Collaborative. (2010). *A national interprofessional competency framework*. http://ipcontherun.ca/wp-content/uploads/2014/06/National-Framework.pdf.

Canadian Nurses Association. (2010). *Evidence-informed decision-making and nursing practice*. https://www.cna-aiic.ca/-/media/nurseone/page-content/pdf-en/evidence-informed-decision-making-and-nursing-practice.pdfCanadian.

Canadian Nurses Association. (2015). *Framework for the practice of registered nurses in Canada*. https://www.cna-aiic.ca/~/media/cna/page-content/pdf-en/framework-for-the-pracice-of-registered-nurses-in-canada.pdf?la=en.

Canadian Nurses Association. (2017a). *Position statement: Climate change and health*. https://www.cna-aiic.ca/~/media/cna/page-content/pdf-en/climate-change-and-health-position-statement.pdf.

Canadian Nurses Association. (2017b). *Code of ethics for registered nurses*. https://www.cna-aiic.ca/~/media/cna/page-content/pdf-en/code-of-ethics-2017-edition-secure-interactive.

Canadian Nurses Association. (2018). *Canadian Nurses Association members vote in favour of representing all nurses*. https://www.cna-aiic.ca/en/news-room/news-releases/2018/cna-members-vote-in-favour-of-representing-all-nurses.

Canadian Nurses Association. (2019). *Position statement: Interprofessional collaboration*. https://www.cna-aiic.ca/-/media/cna/page-content/pdf-en/interprofessional-collaboration-ps-2019.pdf.

Canadian Nurses Association. (2020a). *Indigenous health*. https://cna-aiic.ca/en/policy-advocacy/indigenous-health.

Canadian Nurses Association. (2020b). Nursing in Canada. https://www.cna-aiic.ca/en/nursing-practice/nursing-as-a-career/nursing-in-canada.

Canadian Nurses Association. (2020c). Nursing statistics. https://www.cna-aiic.ca/en/nursing-practice/the-practice-of-nursing/health-human-resources/nursing-statistics.

Canadian Patient Safety Institute (2018). Engaging patients in patient safety: A Canadian guide. https://www.patientsafetyinstitute.ca/en/toolsResources/Patient-Engagement-in-Patient-Safety-Guide/Documents/Engaging%20Patients%20in%20Patient%20Safety.pdf.

Carnago, L., & Mast, M. (2015). Using ways of knowing to guide emergency of nursing practice. *Journal of Emergency Nursing, 41*, 387–390.

Carper, B. (1978). Fundamental patterns of knowing in nursing. *Advances in Nursing Science, 1*, 13–23.

Chinn, P., & Kramer, M. (2015). *Knowledge Development in Nursing: Theory and Process* (9th ed.). Mosby.

Clark, K. (2016). Systems thinking IPE/IPP, Team STEPPS and communicating: Are they interconnected? A look with a broad brush. *Nursing and Palliative Care, 1*(4), 85–88.

Dima, I. C., Teodorescu, M., & Gifu, D. (2014). New communication approaches vs. traditional communication. *International Letters of Social and Humanistic Sciences, 20*, 46–55.

Dolansky, M. A., & Moore, S. M. (2013). Quality and safety education for nurses (QSEN): The key is systems thinking. *Online Journal of Issues in Nursing, 18*(3).

Epstein, R., & Street, R. (2011). The values and value of patient-centered care. *Annals of Family Medicine, 9*(2), 100–103.

Fawcett, J., & Desanto-Madeya, S. (2012). *Analysis and evaluation of nursing models and theories: Contemporary nursing knowledge*. F.A. Davis.

Finkelman, A. W., & Kenner, C. (2009). *Teaching the IOM: Implications of the IOM reports for nursing education*. American Nurses Association.

Hargie, O. (2011). *Skilled interpersonal communication: Research, theory and practice*. (5th ed). Routledge.

Hartrick Doane, G., & Varcoe, C. (2015). *How to nurse: Relational inquiry with individuals and families in changing health and healthcare contexts*. Lippincott Williams & Wilkins.

Health Canada. (2019). *Social determinants of health and health inequalities*. https://www.canada.ca/en/public-health/services/health-promotion/population-health/what-determines-health.html.

Henry, D. (2018). Rediscovering the art of nursing to enhance nursing practice. *Nursing Science Quarterly, 31*(1), 47–54.

International Council of Nurses. (2014). Definition of Nursing. http://www.icn.ch/about-icn/icn-definition-of-nursing/.

Jarrin, O. (2012). The integrality of situated caring. *Advances in Nursing Science, 35*(1), 14–24.

Karnick, P. (2013). The importance of defining theory in nursing: Is there a common denominator? *Nursing Science Q, 26*(1), 29–30.

Lesmond, J. (2006). Celebrating Black nurses this February and beyond. *Registered Nurses Journal, 18*(1), 5. https://rnao.ca/sites/rnao-ca/files/Pages_from_Jan-Feb_Pres_View_0.pdf.

Mallette, C., & Rykert, L. (2018). Promoting positive culture change in nursing faculties: Getting to maybe through liberating structures. *Journal of Professional Nursing, 34*(3), 161–166. https://doi.org/10.1016/j.profnurs.2017.08.001.

Marrs, J., & Lowry, L. (2006). Nursing theory and practice: Connecting the dots. *Nursing Science Quarterly, 19*(1), 44–50.

Mead, N., & Bower, P. (2000). Patient-centredness: A conceptual framework and review of the empirical literature. *Social Science & Medicine, 51*, 1087–1110.

Mount, B., Boston, P., & Cohen, R. (2007). Healing connections: On moving from suffering to a sense of wellbeing. *Journal of Pain and Symptom Management, 33*(4), 372–388.

Nurse Practitioners' Association of Ontario. (2020). *What is a nurse practitioner?* https://npao.org/about-npao/what-is-a-np/.

Ontario Nurses Association. February 1, 2021. Black History Month 2021. https://www.ona.org/news-posts/black-history-month/.

Orchard, C. A., Sonibare, O., Morse, A., et al. (2017). Collaborative leadership, Part 2: The role of the nurse leader in interprofessional team-based practice—Shifting from task- to collaborative patient-/family-focused care. *Nursing Leadership, (30)*2, 26–38.

Palos, G. R. (2014). Care, compassion and communication in professional nursing: Art, science or both. *Clinical Journal of Oncology Nursing, 18*(2), 247–248.

Phillips, J., Stalter, A., Dolansky, M. et al. (2016). Fostering future leadership in quality and safety in health care through systems thinking. *Journal of Professional Nursing, 32*, 15–24.

Porter-O'Grady, T., & Malloch, K. (2014). *Quantum leadership: Building better partnerships for sustainable health* (4th ed.). Jones & Bartlett Learning.

Porter, S., O'Halloran, P., & Morrow, E. (2011). Bringing values back into evidenced-based nursing: The role of patients in resisting empiricism. *Advances in Nursing Science, 34*(2), 106–118.

Pringle, D., Green, L., & Johnson, S. (2004). *Nursing education in Canada: Historical review and current capacity*. Ottawa, Ontario: Nursing sector Study Corporation. https://www.mycna.ca/~/media/nurseone/page-content/pdf-en/nursing_education_canada_e.pdf.

Public Health Agency of Canada. (2017). *How healthy are Canadians? A trend analysis of the health of Canadians from a health living and chronic disease perspective.* https://www.canada.ca/content/dam/phac-aspc/documents/services/publications/healthy-living/how-healthy-canadians/pub1-eng.pdf.

Reed, P., & Shearer, N. (2007). *Perspectives on nursing theory*. Lippincott.

Registered Nurses' Association of Ontario. (2007). *Healthy work environments best practice guidelines: Professionalism in nursing.* https://rnao.ca/sites/rnao-ca/files/Professionalism_in_Nursing.pdf.

Registered Psychiatric Nurse Regulators in Canada. (2020). *Registered psychiatric nursing in Canada.* http://www.rpnc.ca/registered-psychiatric-nursing-canada.

Rhodes, M., Morris, A., & Lazenby, R. (2011). Nursing at its best: Competent and caring. *Online Journal of Issues in Nursing, 16*(2), 10.

Roach, S. M. (1992). *The human act of caring*. Canadian Hospital Association Press.

Ross-Kerr, J. C. (2011). Professionalization in Canadian nursing. In J. C. Kerr & M. J. Wood (Eds.), *Canadian nursing: Issues and perspectives* (5th ed., pp. 42–50). Elsevier Mosby.

Sackett, D., Rosenberg, W., Gray, J., et al. (1996). Evidenced based medicine: What it is and what it isn't. *British Medical Journal, 312*(7023), 71–72.

Schiavo, R. (2014). *Health communication: From theory to practice* (2nd ed.). Jossey-Bass.

Sleeth, P. (2018). March 22, 2018. *Mary Seacole: Disease and care of the wounded, from Jamaica to the Crimea.* https://nursingclio.org/2018/03/22/mary-seacole-care-jamaica-to-the-crimea/.

Smith, M., & Khanlou, N. (2013). An analysis of Canadian psychiatric mental health nursing through the junctures of history, gender, nursing education and quality of work life in Ontario, Manitoba, Alberta and Saskatchewan. *ISRN Nursing,* https://doi.org/10.1155/2013/184024.

Smith, M., & McCarthy, M. P. (2010). Disciplinary knowledge in nursing education: Going beyond the blueprints. *Nursing Outlook, 58*, 44–51.

Swarbrick, M. (2012). A wellness approach to mental health recovery. In A. Rudnick (Ed.), *Recovery of people with mental illness: Philosophical and related perspectives*. Oxford University Press.

Taylor, M., Priefer, B., & Alt-White, A. (2016). Evidence-based practice: Embracing integration. Nursing Outlook, (64), 275–282.

Thompson, V. D. (2020). *Health and health care delivery in Canada.* Elsevier.

Thorne. S. (2011). Theoretical issues in nursing. In J. C. Kerr & M. J. Wood (Eds.), *Canadian nursing: Issues and perspectives* (5th ed.) (pp. 85–104). Elsevier Mosby.

Villeneuve, M. J., Tschudin, V., Storch, J. et al. (2016). A very human being: Sister Marie Simone Roach, 1922–2016. *Nursing Inquiry, 23*, 283–289. https://doi.org/10.1111/nin.12168.

Wagner, D., & Whaite, B. (2010). An exploration of the nature of caring relationships in the writings of Florence Nightingale. *Journal of Holistic Nursing, 4*, 225–234.

Weberg, D. (2012). Complexity leadership: A healthcare imperative. *Nursing Forum, 47*(4), 268–277. http://journals1.scholarsportal.info.ezproxy.library.yorku.ca/pdf/00296473/v47i0004/268_clahi.xml.

World Health Organization. (1986). *The Ottawa charter for health promotion.* World Health Organization, Health and Welfare Canada and Canadian Public Health Association. https://www.who.int/healthpromotion/conferences/previous/ottawa/en/.

World Health Organization. (2001). *Mental health, new understanding, new hope*. Geneva, Switzerland.

World Health Organization. (2006). *Health promotion glossary update*. https://www.who.int/healthpromotion/about/HPR%20Glossary_New%20Terms.pdf.

World Health Organization. (2007). Everybody's business: Strengthening health systems to improve health outcomes. WHO's framework for action. https://www.who.int/healthsystems/strategy/everybodys_business.pdf.

World Health Organization. (2014). *The Constitution*. http://apps.who.int/gb/bd/PDF/bd48/basic-documents-48th-edition-en.pdf#page=7.

World Health Organization. (2020). *State of the world's nursing report 2020: Investing in education, jobs and leadership*. https://www.who.int/publications-detail/nursing-report-2020.

Wytenbroek, L., & Vandenberg, H. (2017). *Reconsidering nursing's history during Canada 150. Canadian Nurse, July–August 2017*. https://www.cna-aiic.ca/en/canadian-nurse-home/articles/issues/2017/july-august-2017/reconsidering-nursings-history-during-canada-150.

Zander, P. (2007). Ways of knowing in nursing: The historical evolution of a concept. *Journal of Theory Construction & Testing, 11*(1), 7–11.

Clarity and Safety in Communication

Claire Mallette

Originating US chapter by *Kim Siarkowski Amer*

OBJECTIVES

At the end of the chapter, the reader will be able to:

1. Identify the role of communication in meeting safety goals.
2. Define the role of communication in a "culture of safety."
3. Describe why patient safety is a complex system issue and an individual function.
4. Analyze the relationship between open communication, error reporting, and a culture of safety.
5. Discuss advocacy for safe, high-quality care as a team member.
6. Create simulations to demonstrate use of standardized tools for clear communication affecting patient care, such as using situation, background, assessment, recommendation (SBAR) in a simulated conversation with a physician.

Communication is the key to safe health care. When health care workers communicate effectively, fewer errors occur, and people are more satisfied. The majority of errors in health care are linked to a lack of proper communication. This lack of communication can be between nurses; among interprofessional teams, including physicians; with physiotherapists, occupational therapists, dietitians, social workers, and pharmacists; or with any member of the health care team. Since patient safety is the first priority in nursing care, effective communication should be incorporated in all of the components of planning so that nurses can provide the highest quality of care.

The ability to give safe and effective care is identified in the Canadian Nurses Association [CNA] (2017) Code of Ethics of Nursing, and every province's and territory's regulatory practice standards. Nurses and nursing students must be aware of the need for education regarding error prevention and the potential threats to safe care at multiple levels in the care system. Some examples of errors are wrong site surgery, equipment failure, incorrect labelling of specimens, falls, and medication errors. Research has indicated that miscommunication amongst health care providers has resulted in major patient safety issues and poor quality care (Canadian Patient Safety Institute [CPSI], 2017a).

GOAL

This chapter discusses communication strategies designed to promote a safe environment and focuses on commonly used **standardized communication tools** for clear communication. The tools range from effective communication between nurses and other health care providers—such as using situation, background, assessment, recommendation (SBAR)—to simple templates used when nurses finish a shift and report or "hand off" to the next nurse. Improving communication in health care has become an international priority, as recognized by the World Health Organization (WHO). The aim is to reduce patient mortality, decrease medical errors, and promote effective health care teamwork. A number of agencies and professional organizations are developing and updating guidelines for levels of communication that prevent errors and adverse patient outcomes. The goal is to improve the quality of care and safety of our patients by embedding a "culture of safety" within all levels of health care. Since nurses play a critical role in patient safety, they need to be aware of best practices in communication. Globally, all nurses need to be responsible for making safety a priority (Kowalski & Anthony, 2017).

BASIC CONCEPTS

Safety Definition

Multiple health care organizations have issued definitions of safety. **Safety** is defined by the Canadian Patient Safety Institute [CPSI] (2020a) as "the pursuit of the reduction and mitigation of unsafe acts within the health care system, as well as the use of best practices shown to lead to optimal patient outcomes." The World Health Organization (2020) states that "patient safety is the absence of preventable harm to a patient during the process of health care and reduction of risk of unnecessary harm associated with health care to an acceptable minimum. An acceptable minimum refers to the collective notions of given current knowledge, resources available, and the context in which care was delivered, weighed against the risk of nontreatment or other treatment."

The nursing profession has always had safe practice as a major goal, as identified in each provincial and territorial nursing regulatory body's nursing standards. For example, the College and Association of Registered Nurses of Alberta (CARNA) identifies that the goal of nursing practice in Alberta is to provide safe, competent, and ethical nursing care to Albertans (CARNA, 2013). In British Columbia, the British Columbia College of Nursing Professionals merged with the College of Midwives of BC and, as of September 2020, became the British Columbia College of Nurses and Midwives (BCCNM). Their safety standards for psychiatric nursing includes "a registered psychiatric nurse incorporates evidence-informed knowledge to promote safety and quality in psychiatric nursing practice" (British Columbia College of Nurses and Midwives, 2021); and in New Brunswick, licensed practical nurses are guided by the Canadian Council for Practical Nurse Regulators in that licensed practical nurses are "self-regulating and accountable for providing safe, competent, compassionate, and ethical care within the legal and ethical framework of nursing regulation" (Association of New Brunswick Licensed Practical Nurses, 2013). The CNA (2009) believes that "patient safety is the reduction and mitigation of unsafe acts within the health care system as well as through the use of best practices shown to lead to optimal patient outcomes" (p.1).

Safety Incidence

In 2018–2019, there was at least one harmful event in 18 hospital stays in Canada (Canadian Institute for Health Information [CIHI], 2020). This means there were 132 000 harmful events out of 2.5 million hospital stays. The breakdown of harmful events was as follows: 45% related to health care and medications, 30% infections, 21% procedure related, and 4% patient accidents (CIHI, 2020).

 DEVELOPING AN EVIDENCE-INFORMED PRACTICE

The figures on preventable deaths from errors and miscommunication in health care have continued to increase globally, despite the proven effectiveness of safety-promoting communication tools, such as checklists (TeamSTEPPS Webinar, July 12, 2017).

The use of checklists, for example surgical checklists, creates an expectation that organizations assess effective communication and safe practices during surgery, at three perioperative intervals: prior to administration of anaesthesia, prior to skin incision, and prior to the patient leaving the operating room or procedural area (CPSI, 2020b).

The World Health Organization and the CPSI are committed to encouraging the use of checklists prior to surgical procedures. Such checklists have demonstrated a decrease in the likelihood of complications and improved outcomes, with a reduction of health care costs (CPSI, n.d.).

Application to Your Practice

Analyze patient report procedures, change-of-shift hand-offs, and so on, in your clinical area, and consider whether use of safety tools such as checklists would improve communication and patient safety.

Case Example: Decreased Central Venous Catheter (CVC) Infection in a Cohort Patient Study

In February 2017, a group of researchers explored the impact of a checklist and heightened awareness of nursing staff on central line infection rates. The cohort study showed a dramatic difference.

Data are listed in the following table:

Variables	Test	Control	P-value
Male	57/82 (70%)	47/82 (57%)	0.093
Female	25/82 (30%)	35/82 (43%)	0.093
Age (years)	58.0 ± 20.5	57.0 ± 18.7	0.951

Variables	Test	Control	P-value
Infection present	2/82 (2.50%)	31/82 (37.80%)	0.000
Maintenance (days)	10.0 ± 1.14	10.0 ± 18.2	0.235
Hospitalization time (days)	10.0 ± 1.14	10.0 ± 18.2	0.235
Mortality	32/82 (39%)	39/82 (47.60%)	0.232

Distribution of numbers, percentages, and values of the medians of patients in test and control groups and their *P* values are listed in the following table:

Variables	With Infection	No Infection	P-value	Beta
Test	2.50%	97.50%	.00	−0.442
Control	37.80%	62.20%	0.00	−0.442
Duration of CVC maintenance (days)	22.0 ± 22.3	9.0 ± 9.6	0.00	0.385
Hospitalization time (days)	22.0 ± 22.3	9.0 ± 9.6	0.00	0.385

CVC, Central venous catheter.

The test group had 2.5% infections versus the control group, which had 37.8%, a finding that is dramatically statistically significant. A major part of the study was positive communication and the implementation of the checklist in the experimental group. A working group of multiple health care providers and regular meetings enhanced the collaboration and communication for the study.

Gameiro, A. J. R., Focaccia, R., da Silva, G. M. et al. (2017). A cohort study on nurse-led checklist intervention to reduce catheter-related bloodstream infection in an intensive care unit. *Journal of Intensive and Critical Care, 3,* 1.

Principles Related to the Occurrence of Unsafe Events

Miscommunication

Much has changed in health care practice since the landmark 1999 Institute of Medicine (IOM) study, "To err is human: Building a safer health system," which found that preventable health care errors were responsible for almost 98,000 deaths each year in the United States.

Baker et al.'s (2004) seminal research on adverse events in Canada indicated that 7.5% of all patients experienced an adverse event, where an unintended injury caused by health care led to increased hospital stays, disability, or death. The report also indicated that 37% of these adverse events were identified as being preventable. Since then, awareness of the importance of patient safety and how patients can be harmed by health care have increased. Yet, in 2014–2015, it was determined that one in five hospitalizations in Canada involved more than one occurrence of harm. It is also estimated that on any given day, there are 1600 hospital beds in Canada occupied by patients that had an increased length of stay in hospital due to harm while in hospital (CIHI, 2016).

Multiple studies have pinpointed miscommunication as a major causative agent in sentinel events, that is, errors resulting in unnecessary death and serious injury. The curricula for health professions include interprofessional team communication and present the benefits of rounding and professional hand-offs.

Case Example: Student Nurse Lakesha

After hand-off to the nurse (staff RN), student nurse Lakesha says, "I am assigned to give the meds today. I'll be giving them with my instructor." However, she meant all the oral meds for the team, since her instructor assigned these to her, but not the intravenous (IV) medications. Fortunately, her instructor was there to clarify the message. This is an excellent example of inadequate communication potentially doing harm to the patient. If the IV medications were not given for 8 hours, there could have been serious consequences. How could the student nurse have better communicated what she was assigned to do? What could the staff RN also have done to ensure there wasn't any misunderstanding?

Errors Are Usually System Problems

Most Errors Are Preventable

Many reported errors are preventable. "Preventable" means the error occurs because of confused orders, poor communication of expectations, or a failure to communicate potential risks, such as allergies to medications, infection control, or fall risk (Kear & Ulrich, 2015). Fatigue is repeatedly cited as a factor contributing to errors. One of the most common causes of error is incomplete communication during the very many "hand-offs" transferring responsibility for patient care to another care provider, unit, or agency. It is estimated that in 1 day, a patient may experience up to eight hand-offs. The use of a consistent blueprint, or hand-off sheet or tool, is an excellent way to ensure comprehensive and safer hand-offs (Anderson et al., 2015; Smeulers et al., 2016). Just as the use of checklists for central line insertion decreases infections, the use of a consistent hand-off tool can prevent errors of omission and optimizes nursing care. Errors have a high financial cost, in addition to the human cost. For example, in 2014–2015 in Canada, the hospital costs excluding physician fees associated with harmful events were estimated at an additional $685 million or 1% of Canada's estimated total hospital spending for that year ($63.6 billion for 2014) (CIHI, 2016). Another report estimates that, over the next 30 years, within acute and home care settings, an additional $2.75 billion will be spent treating preventable patient safety incidents (CPSI, 2017b).

GENERAL SAFETY COMMUNICATION GUIDELINES FOR ORGANIZATIONS

Unlike in other countries, such as Great Britain, in Canada there is no one national database for reporting unsafe care, making data less readily accessible. The Canadian Institute for Health Information (CIHI), Statistics Canada Health Reports, and the Canadian Patient Safety Institute (CPSI) are national associations that analyze data to examine patient safety issues. The CPSI was created in 2003 with the support of Health Canada to "work with governments, health organizations, leaders, and healthcare providers to inspire extraordinary improvement in patient safety and quality" (CPSI, n.d.). The CPSI website contains a wealth of information and tools on how to keep people safe (https://www.patientsafety institute.ca/en/About/Pages/default.aspx).

The Health Quality Council of Alberta, Health Quality Ontario, and the Manitoba Institute for Patient Safety are all organizations that have also focused on how to foster patient safety. Professional nursing associations (e.g., Canadian Association of Schools of Nursing [CASN], Registered Nurses' Association of Ontario [RNAO]) have made recommendations for clear communication strategies as a basis for clinical practice to provide safer care that affects communication with other nurses, health team members, and patients and their families.

BARRIERS TO SAFE, EFFECTIVE COMMUNICATION IN THE HEALTH CARE SYSTEM

Fragmentation

The structure of health care organizations is complex. Health care systems can have multiple sites or community organizations with multiple partners and agencies. An example of this is in Ontario, where Ontario Health Teams are forming that connect health care providers (hospitals, doctors, and home and community care providers) to work as one coordinated team to organize and deliver care that is more connected to people in their local communities (Ontario Ministry of Health and Long Term Care, 2020). This organizational complex combination of differing philosophies can impede communication. Fragmentation of systems operations or different basic policies can be a barrier to safer care. To prevent fragmentation and gaps in communication, evidenced-informed practices must be reinforced and implemented at a system wide level. Communication within the health care team is imperative. Fig. 2.1 highlights what is important for excellent team communication to occur. Although most hospitals and agencies have policies on error reports, they may lack a system-wide department for processing safety information.

Hand-offs (also handovers), or transfers of patient care, refer to the transfer of information and responsibility of care from one nurse to the next, which promotes continuity of care and the incoming nurse's plan of care (Thomson et al., 2018). Miscommunication errors can often occur during a hand-off procedure.

Patient care responsibility is transitioned or handed off to the next shift of nurses or when the patient is transferred to another unit. Transition times are at high risk for incomplete communication and consequently result in more errors. This increase in errors has been attributed to frequent interruptions, inconsistent report format, and omission of key information (Cornell & Gervis, 2013). Some agencies have adopted standardized hand-off communication tools, including the use of hand-held devices (Anderson et al., 2015). The most ideal clinical hand-off is between two nurses in the patient's room, with access to the electronic health care record (EHR). Discussing the care of the patient with the patient's input is best. The use of simple summary aids, such as a whiteboard with critical information, such as "patient likes to be called Emma" and ALLERGIC TO SULFA also supports good communication. The most important part of the hand-off is taking the time to adhere to the essential elements, including a thorough review of the assessment and planning of the patient's care.

Underreporting of Errors in a Punitive Climate

Many health care providers express concern about reporting errors or near miss incidents. **Near-miss incidents** are defined as a "patient safety incident that did not reach the patient and therefore no harm resulted" (CPSI, 2020a). If we are to create a culture of safety, the system needs to be redesigned to be a blame-free, nonpunitive culture. A culture of safety is characterized by installing a strong, blame-free, nonpunitive reporting system; supporting care providers

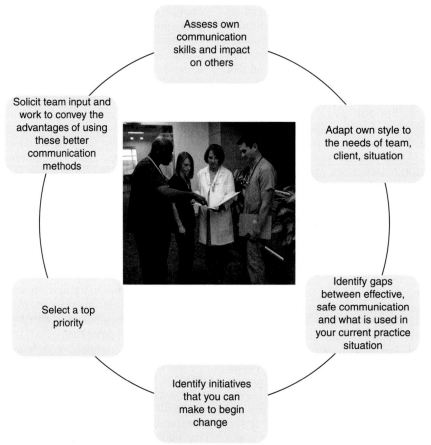

Fig. 2.1 Communication competencies for creating safer care. Adapted from Carey, M., Buchan, H., & Sanson-Fisher, R. (2009). The cycle of change: Implementing best-evidence clinical practice. *Int J Qual Health Care, 21*(1), 37–43; Cronenwett, L., Sherwood, G., Barnsteiner, J. et al. (2007). Quality and safety education for nurses. *Nurs Outlook 55*(3),122–131.

after adverse events; and developing a method to inform and compensate patients who are harmed. Other disciplines have better models for safety. One example is aviation's successful crew resource management (CRM) practice model, which has been used as a template. One necessary step is to require the reporting of near misses so that new, safer policies and procedures can be created. Each time an error or near miss occurs, the team members get together and discuss in a nonjudgemental way to determine improved processes to help decrease future errors. *We need to create this new climate of safety in which agencies, policies, and employees maintain a vigilant, proactive attitude toward adverse events.* Recognizing that human error occurs, everyone's focus needs to be on correcting system flaws to avoid future adverse events, rather than finding out who is to blame.

Fatigue

Errors are more likely to occur during long shifts, with little rest or nutrition. The risk of error nearly doubles when nurses work more than 12 consecutive hours. Specifically, the last two hours of the shift are when nurses are the most fatigued (Amer, 2013). The effect of fatigue in the final hours of a 12-hour shift is important for all nurses to recognize so structures can be created to minimize fatigue. Nurses need to take responsibility to be aware of and recognize signs and symptoms of fatigue and identity strategies to mitigate and manage their fatigue and self-care. Health care organizations also need to take responsibility for promoting a culture of safety by establishing fatigue management policies and programs (CNA & RNAO, 2010).

INNOVATIONS THAT FOSTER SAFETY

Communication problems and communication solution strategies identified as "best practices" for creating a culture of safety are summarized in Table 2.1. Beyond individual changes to create safer climates for our patients, we need to advocate for organizational system changes. Leadership is needed to incorporate the three C's that promote safer clinical practice:

1. Communication clarity
2. Collaboration
3. Cooperation

Create a Culture of Safety

Agencies are working toward promoting a culture of safety in many ways (CIHI, CPSI, and/or Health Quality agencies in each province and territory). A major focus is to improve the clarity of communication. This improvement occurs through the use of standardized communication tools and team training.

Leadership is essential to change to a just culture model, in which the organization creates a balance between accountability of individuals and the institutional system

TABLE 2.1 Safe Communication: Problems and Recommended Best Practices	
Communication Problem	**Best Practice Communication Solution**
Health care system complexity	Agency establishes safety as a priority Agency policies adopt procedures to promote transparency and accountability
Hierarchical status difference with decreased willingness to communicate	Team training such as TeamSTEPPS Canada Clarify duties of each team member
Distraction or preoccupation	Policy that isolates you from interruptions (signal to others not to interrupt, such as wearing vest when administering meds) Team members maintain safety awareness as a priority Control high levels of ambient noise/alarm fatigue Establish policy to limit interruptions during crucial times
Heavy workload	Held accountable for evidence-informed practice Support from administration and colleagues Team members share common safety goals, which each person sees as their responsibility
Stress and practice pressures due to lack of time, leading to use of shortcuts and poor communication	Adherence to safety protocols, especially in med administration Team huddles, meetings, bedside rounds
Staff fail to say what they mean; fail to speak up about safety concerns (lack of assertiveness)	All staff receive continuing education that emphasizes safety promotion, communication, and assertiveness training Use of time-outs, SAFER practice
Attitude of not believing in usefulness of practice guidelines	Ease of access and increased availability of evidence-informed practice guidelines specifically relevant to your patient Value electronic decision-support apps Participate in team meetings, conference calls, and opportunities to share successes
Education in isolation of others, where each health provider has own jargon and assumptions	Use of standardized communication tools Team training Each team member is encouraged to give input
Cultural differences or language issues	Cultural-competence education, especially relevant to adapting communication strategies

(Continued)

TABLE 2.1 **Safe Communication: Problems and Recommended Best Practices**—cont'd.	
Communication Problem	**Best Practice Communication Solution**
Miscommunication	Adapt communication, and verify receipt of message Use standardized communication Participate in simulations and critical event training scenarios to foster clear, efficient communication Read back and record verbal orders immediately With patients, use teach-backs or "show me" techniques Solicit questions
Avoidance of confrontation and communication with the person in conflict	Use conflict-resolution skills Practise open communication Be assertive in confronting the problem
Cognitive difficulty obtaining, processing, or understanding information Lack of training	Continuing education units about effective communication skills Avoidance of factors interfering with decision making such as, fatigue Seek continuing education units, in-service
Patient and/or family are not following recommended guidelines for safe, effective care	Team recognizes that safe outcomes require work and communicates that this must involve patient and family Bedside rounds, briefings, and involving patient in daily care-plan goal setting

Adapted from TeamSTEPPS, Team Strategies and Tools to Enhance Performance and Patient Safety; Adapted from Leonard, M., Graham, S., & Bonacum, D. (2004). The human factor: The critical importance of effective teamwork and communication in providing safe care. *Qual Safe Health Care 13*(Suppl 1),i85–i90.

(Ring & Fairchild, 2013). Establishment of an organizational culture of safety requires us to acknowledge the complexity of any health care system. Strong leaders can change the focus to safety practices as a shared value. Creating a safe environment requires us to communicate openly, be vigilant, and be willing to speak up and be held accountable.

Create a Team Culture of Collaboration and Cooperation

Creating effective health teams means getting all team members to value teamwork more than individual autonomy. Team collaborative communication strategies involve shared responsibility for maintaining open communication and engaging in mutual problem solving, decision making, and coordination of care. Increasing patient safety occurrences have been attributed to communication breakdowns and teamwork failures (CPSI, 2011). Creating a safe environment requires all team members to communicate openly, to be vigilant and accountable, and to express concerns and alert team members to unsafe situations.

Create a Blame-Free, Nonpunitive Culture

Establishing a **just culture** system creates expectations of a work environment in which staff can speak up and express

concerns and alert team members to unsafe situations. A just culture does not mean eliminating individual accountability but rather puts greater emphasis on an analysis of the problems that contribute to adverse events in a system (Rideout, 2013). In a just culture, when something goes wrong or nearly wrong (near miss), health care workers are treated with respect and made to feel supported (Health Quality Council of Alberta, 2019).

Establishing open communication about errors is an important aspect of a just culture. Provincial and territorial regulatory nursing bodies require nurses to report unsafe practice by coworkers; however, nurses may have mixed feelings about reporting an error or colleague. Barriers to reporting include fear, threat to self-esteem, threat to professional livelihood, and lack of timely feedback and support. Ethical reasons to report are for the protection of the patient and for professional protection.

In a blame-free, nonpunitive reporting environment, staff are encouraged to report errors, mistakes, and near misses. They work in a climate in which they feel comfortable making such reports. Compiling a database that includes near-miss situations that could have resulted in injury is important in preventing future errors. A complete error-reporting process should include timely feedback to the person reporting.

Administrators should assume errors will occur and put in place a plan for "recovery" that has well-rehearsed procedures for responding to adverse events.

Best Practice: Communicating Clearly for Quality Care

Health care professions, associations, and health care delivery organizations have undertaken initiatives designed to foster **best practice** safer patient care by designing evidence-informed protocols for care. Evidence-informed care and decision making recognizes that health care providers need to be knowledgeable about evidence not only coming from research but also taking into consideration clinical experience and judgement, clients preferences, and values and beliefs and the context of the situation (Ciliska, 2012; Melnyk, 2014)). Use best practices by increasing the use of evidence-informed best practice versus usual practice. This information is used to develop and distribute protocols for best practice, including formats of standard communication techniques. We need more studies of interventions to promote best communication between nurses and other health care providers, with documented outcomes for patients.

Developing an evidence-informed best practice requires closing the gap between best evidence and the way communication occurs in your current practice. Think of a clinical experience and apply information from evidence-informed best practices for safe practice. The process for development of practice guidelines, protocols, situation checklists, and so on is not transparent or easy. Solutions include gathering more evidence on which to base our practice. When is the "evidence" sufficiently strong to warrant adoption of a standardized form of communication about care? Examples of best practice protocols can be found on the Cochrane Library website https://www.cochranelibrary.com/ and in the Registered Nurses' Association of Ontario Best Practice Guidelines (https://rnao.ca/bpg).

Electronic health records (EHRs) improve the safety of patient care and empower providers to have better-quality care delivery and greater accountability for preventive care and compliance with standard care protocols. EHRs aid in decision support and communication as specialists, health care providers, and health organizations have access to the person's health record. EHRs are discussed in Chapter 26.

Standardized Communication as an Initiative for Safer Care

Health care systems are being restructured to make patient care safer. The consensus is that this change requires improving communication. Good nurse–health provider collaborative communication has empirically been associated with a lower risk for negative patient outcomes and greater satisfaction (Amer, 2013). The renewed focus on improving patient safety is resulting in the standardization of many health care practices. Standardization of communication is an effective tool to avoid incomplete or misleading messages. Safe communication about patient care needs to be clear, explicit, timely, accurate, complete, open, and understood by the recipient to reduce errors.

Patient Safety Outcomes

Standardized communication tools in certain areas of practice can provide a more consistent language that can result in more optimal outcomes and prevent harm to patients.

Nurse-Specific Initiatives

Nurses are often the "last line of defence" against error. Nurses are in a position to prevent, intercept, or correct errors. To prevent errors, nurses need to communicate clearly with other members of the health team. Clarity of communication can prevent safety risks, such as medication errors, patient injuries from falls, and high rehospitalization rates. Poor communication can compromise patient safety. One sample case might be that of Nurse Kay, in the following example.

Case Example: Kay

Ms. Kay, RN, a newly hired staff nurse, has six patients assigned to her on a surgical unit. She calls the resident for additional pain medication for a patient. Dr. Andrews, a first-year resident on a 3-month thoracic surgery rotation, has responsibility for more than 40 patients this weekend, when he is on call. Many of these patients he has never seen. In the phone call, Ms. Kay uses the person's name and then tells Dr. Andrews that she is concerned about the patient's pain. When Dr. Andrews does not seem to recognize the patient, nor understand what she is asking for, Ms. Kay becomes irritated. What could Nurse Kay do to improve the situation?

Interruptions interfere with a nurse's ability to perform a task safely, yet interruptions have become an almost continual occurrence. A study by McGillis Hall et al. (2010) identified that almost a third of the interruptions that nurses experience are from other health care team members. Other nurses account for almost 25% of interruptions. These interruptions are tied to an increased risk of errors. Nonverbal strategies to signal others to avoid distracting communication have been suggested, such as wearing an orange vest when preparing and administering medications.

MEDICATION PROCESS

A particular focus for error reduction is during the entire medication process, ranging from ordering to administration. Medication incidents are defined as "any preventable event that may cause or lead to inappropriate medication use or patient harm while the medication is in the control of the healthcare professional, patient, or consumer. Medication incidents may be related to professional practice, drug products, procedures, and systems, and include prescribing, order communication, product labelling/packaging/nomenclature, compounding, dispensing, distribution, administration, education, monitoring, and use" (Institute for Safe Medication Practices Canada [ISMP], 2016). Near misses should also be considered. For example, a nurse prepares an ordered medication but recognizes that the ordered dose far exceeds safe parameters. Medication errors stem from unclear communication, lack of knowledge about the drug, side effects, incompatibility, administration error, and system issues.

APPLICATIONS

Communication interventions shown to improve safe communication are listed in Table 2.1. These are best practices. For example, when there is conflicting information or a concern about a potential safety breach, nurses can use the "two challenge rule." The nurse states their concern twice. This is theoretically enough cause to stop the action for a reassessment.

A discussion of the standardized tools used to promote safe interprofessional and nursing communication is the main focus of our application section. The mantra for safe communication should be: simplify, clarify, verify.

Attitude

Within health care organizations, an environment that fosters a culture of safety as top priority is needed. A prime goal should be to improve communication about a patient's condition among all the people providing care to that patient. Errors occur when we assume someone else has addressed a situation.

Patient Safety Outcomes

Once nurses understand the use of clinical guidelines and evidence-informed practice procedures and become comfortable accessing this information, they see that they are providing a higher quality of care, improving their decision-making skills, and avoiding errors, resulting in safer care for their patients. They have fewer error incident reports, fewer patient falls, fewer medication events, less delay in treatment for patients, and fewer wound infections, among other outcomes (Saintsing et al.,2011).

TOOLS FOR SAFER CARE

Skills Acquisition Through Simulation

Skills acquisition is described as "a gradual transition from rigid adherence to rules to an intuitive mode of reasoning that relies heavily on deep tacit understanding" (Peña, 2010, p. 3).

Communication and practice skills are developed and refined through clinical situation simulations. Students learn in a safe, low-stakes simulation lab. The simulations can be low fidelity, with model patients, or high fidelity, with computerized human patient simulators. Students can practise their communication, critical thinking, and clinical judgement skills. Since the instructor is present with several students in the lab, there is a more dynamic experience than the one-on-one experience in clinical settings. Students should feel free to attempt assessments and get feedback and can expect to improve over time.

Ideally, the simulations should have an interprofessional group of participants. The simulation allows practice without the risk of potentially devastating outcomes in an actual patient care situation.

Simulation laboratories are integrated into most nursing programs and hospitals. You can view sample scenarios on the Internet (even on sites such as YouTube). Practising clinical assessments and interventions can help build students' confidence and increase their communication and clinical decision-making skills (Hooper et al., 2015). In summary, simulations are designed to increase cognitive decision-making skills, increase technical proficiency, and enhance teamwork, including efficient communication skills.

Patient Safety Outcomes

More research is needed about the impact of practice simulations on nursing communications that affect actual patient safety. Certainly, strong evidence shows increased skill proficiency and increased patient safety.

Introduction to Use of Standardized Communication Tools

Use of Checklists

Checklists are lists of actions that, based on evidence, should be followed by health care providers to improve patient safety and positive outcomes. Checklists have been found to reduce medical errors and adverse events, leading to improved patient safety (Boyd et al., 2017). An example is the surgical safety checklist that is used to "initiate, guide and formalize communication among team members conducting a surgical procedure" (CPSI, 2020b). The user's goal is to follow each step in the process. Following a checklist ensures that key steps will not be omitted and important information will not be missed due to fatigue, pressure, distraction, or other factors.

A checklist is a cognitive guide to accurate task completion or to complete the communication of information. However, one cannot assume that a checklist alone will improve patient safety. Grif Alspach (2017) highlights that just because a checkmark is placed on a checklist, does not mean one can assume the process has been done correctly. In order for checklists to be used appropriately and for the defined purpose, all health care providers need to make a commitment for a culture of safety through using the checklist accurately. When this occurs, it greatly reduces the possibility of miscommunication or slips leading to error.

Operating rooms and urgent care sites are places that can use time-out checklists; these checklists stop everyone in their tasks to verify correctness. Staff verbally run down completion of the list to avoid errors of wrong patient, wrong procedure/surgery, and wrong site.

Unit checklists are used when, for example, the floor nurse uses a preoperative checklist to verify that everything has been completed before sending the patient to the operating room, but this list is again checked when the patient arrives, and before the actual surgery. Such system redundancies are used to prevent errors. However, they have limited and specific uses and do not address underlying communication problems. No standardized protocol exists for checklist development, so use of expert panels with multiple pilot testing is recommended. One example found in most agency preoperative areas is a checklist where standard items are marked as having been done and available in the patient's record or chart. For example, laboratory results are documented regarding blood type, clotting time, and so forth. Adoption of assertion checklists empowers any team members to speak up and state their concerns when they become aware of missing information.

Patient Safety Outcomes

Evidence shows that the use of checklists improves communication and patient safety, especially in areas managing rapid change, such as preoperative areas, emergency departments, and anaesthesiology. According to Amer (2013), use of a simple checklist saved more than 1 500 lives in a recent 18-month test period. However, some nurses in surgical areas have complained that lists are redundant, take too much time, or are not used by all surgeons.

Use of Situation, Background, Assessment, Recommendation (SBAR)

The **SBAR (situation, background, assessment, recommendation)** method uses a standardized verbal communication tool with a structured format to create a common language among nurses, physicians, and other members of the health team. This method is especially useful when brief, clear communication is needed in acute situations, such as emergent declines in patient status or during handoffs. See Table 2.2 for the SBAR format.

TABLE 2.2		**SBAR Structured Communication Format**
S	Situation	Identify yourself; identify the patient and the problem. In 10 seconds, state what is going on. This may include patient's date of birth, hospital ID number, verification that consent forms are present, etc.
B	Background	State relevant context and brief history. Review the chart if possible before speaking to or phoning the physician. Relate the patient's background, including patient's diagnosis, problem list, allergies, relevant vital signs, medications that have been administered, and laboratory results, etc.
A	Assessment	State your conclusion—what you think is wrong. List your opinions about the patient's current status. Examples: patient's level of pain, medical complications, level of consciousness, problem with intake and output, your estimate of blood loss, etc.
R	Recommendation or request	State your informed suggestion for the continued care of this patient. Propose an action. What do you need? In what time frame does it need to be completed? Always include an opportunity for questions. Some sources recommend that any new verbal orders now be repeated for feedback clarity. If no decision is forthcoming, reassert your request.

Adapted from personal interviews: Bonacum, D. (2009). CSP, CPHQ, CPHRM, Vice President, Safety Management, Kaiser Foundation Health Plan, Inc., February 25; Fleischmann, J. A. (2008). *Medical vice president of Franciscan Skemp.* LaCrosse, WS: Mayo HealthCare System.

SBAR is designed to convey only the most critical information by eliminating excessive language. It eliminates the hierarchy gradient by flattening the traditional physician-to-nurse relationship, making it possible for staff to say what they think is going on. This improves communication and creates collaboration. This concise format has gained wide adoption globally (Shahid & Thomas, 2018). SBAR is used as a situational briefing, so the team is "on the same page." It is used across all types of agencies, groups, and even in emails. SBAR simplifies verbal communication between nurses and other health care providers because content is presented in an expected format. Some hospitals use laminated SBAR guidelines at the telephones for nurses to use when calling physicians about changes in patient status and requests for new orders. Refer to Box 2.1 for an example. Then, practice your use of SBAR format in Simulation Exercises 2.1, 2.2, and 2.3.

Patient Safety Outcomes

Evidence-informed reports show that patient adverse events have decreased through the use of SBAR, including decreases in unexpected deaths. Practising the use of standardized communication formats has been found to improve student nurses' ability to effectively communicate with physicians and other health care providers about emergent changes in a patient's condition, and its use has been shown to help develop a mental schema that facilitates

---

BOX 2.1   Situation, Background, Assessment, Recommendation Example

Clinical Example of Use of SBAR Format for Communicating With Patient's Physician

S Situation "Dr. Preston, this is Wendy Obi, evening nurse on 4G at St. Simeon Hospital, calling about Mr. Lakewood, who's having trouble breathing."

B Background "Kyle Lakewood, DOB 7/1/60, a 53-year-old man with chronic lung disease, admitted 12/25, whose condition has been deteriorating × 2 h. Now he's acutely worse: his vital signs are heart rate 92 bpm, respiratory rate 40 breaths/min with gasping, blood pressure 138/94 mm Hg, oxygenation saturation down to 85%."

A Assessment "I don't hear any breath sounds in his right chest. I think he has a pneumothorax."

R Recommendation "I need you to see him right now. I think he needs a chest tube."

Adapted from: Leonard, M., Graham, S., & Bonacum, D. (2004). The human factor: The critical importance of effective teamwork and communication in providing safe care. *Quality and Safety in Health Care, 13*(Suppl 1), i85–i90.

---

rapid decision making by nurses (Vardaman et al., 2012). This format sets expectations about what will be communicated to other members of the health care team.

Using the SBAR tool to communicate patient information amongst health care providers is recognized as a best-practice protocol. In addition to using SBAR when there is a change in a patient's health status, this communication format is used at shift change between nurse colleagues and between nurses and other health care providers during rounds, transfers, and hand-offs from one care setting or unit to another. Some suggest that agencies conduct annual SBAR-competency validations.

A distinct advantage of using SBAR or other standardized communication tools between nurses and other health care providers is that it decreases professional differences in communication styles. In a study to implement and evaluate the effective use of SBAR with interprofessional teams in a rehabilitation setting, the findings indicated that SBAR is an effective way to communicate urgent and non-urgent safety issues within the interprofessional team (Andreoli et al., 2010). In a study by Compton et al. (2012), 78% of physicians surveyed stated they receive enough information to make clinical decisions. Several authors speculate that use of SBAR leads to creation of cognitive schemata in staff. Use of this structured format enables less-experienced nurses to give as complete a report as experienced nurses.

Use of the electronic SBAR format when transferring patients to another unit or during change-of-shift report has been shown to enhance the amount, consistency, and comprehensiveness of information conveyed, yet not take any longer than a traditional shift report (Cornell & Gervis, 2013).

Crew Resource Management (CRM)-Based Tools

Crew Resource Management (CRM) is another communication tool similar to SBAR, which was adapted from the field of aviation. This tool provides rules of conduct for communication, especially during hand-off care transitions. Just prior to an event, such as surgery, all members of the team stop and summarize what is happening. Each team member has an obligation to voice safety concerns.

Briefing. In team situations, such as in the operating room, the team may use another sort of standardized format: a briefing. The leader (the surgeon, in this case) presents a brief overview of the procedure about to happen and identifies roles and responsibilities, plans for the unexpected, and increases each team member's awareness of the situation. The leader asks anyone who sees a potential problem to speak up. In this manner, the leader encourages every team member to voice their concerns. This can include the patient, as many patients will not speak unless specifically invited to do so.

SIMULATION EXERCISE 2.1   Using Standardized Communication Formats

Purpose
To practise the situation, background, assessment, recommendation (SBAR) technique.

Case Study
Mrs. Robin, date of birth January 5, 1950, is a preoperative patient of Dr. Hu's. She is scheduled for an abdominal hysterectomy at 9 a.m. She has been NPO (fasting) since midnight. She is allergic to penicillin. The night nurse reported that she got little sleep and expressed a great deal of anxiety about this surgery immediately after her surgeon and anesthesiologist examined her at the time of admission. Preoperative medication consisting of atropine, which was administered at 8:40 a.m. instead of 8:30 a.m. as per order. Abdominal skin was scrubbed with Betadine per order, and an intravenous (IV) drip of 1 L 0.45 saline was started at 7 a.m. in her left forearm. She has a history of chronic obstructive pulmonary disease, controlled with an albuterol inhaler, but has not used this since admission yesterday.

Directions
In triads, organize this information into the SBAR format. Student #1 gives the report. Student #2 role-plays the nurse receiving the report. Student #3 acts as the observer and evaluates the accuracy of the report.

SIMULATION EXERCISE 2.2   Telephone Simulation: Conversation Between Nurse and Physician About a Critically Ill Patient

Purpose
To improve your telephone communication technique using structured formats.

Procedure
Read the case, and then simulate making a phone call to the physician on call. It is midnight.

Case
Ms. Babs Pointer, date of birth January 14, 1942, is 6 h post-op for knee reconstruction, complaining of pain and thirst. Her leg swelling has increased 4 cm in circumference, lower leg has notable ecchymosis spreading rapidly. Temperature 37.2°C; respiratory rate 20 breaths/min; pedal pulse absent.

Discussion/Written Paper
Record your conversation for later analysis. In your analysis, write up an evaluation of this communication for accurate use of situation, background, assessment, recommendation (SBAR) format, effectiveness, and clarity.

SIMULATION EXERCISE 2.3   Situation, Background, Assessment, Recommendation for Change-of-Shift Simulation

Purpose
To practise use of situation, background, assessment, recommendation (SBAR) procedure.

Procedure
In post-conference, have Student A be the day-shift nurse reporting to Student B, who is acting as the evening nurse. Practise reporting on their assigned patients' conditions, or simulate four or five postoperative patients' status. Use the SBAR format.

Discussion
Have the entire post-conference group of students critique the advantages and disadvantages of using this type of communication.

Debriefing. A debriefing is usually led by someone other than the leader. It occurs toward the end of a procedure—a surgery or critical incident—and is a recap or summary as to what went well or what might be changed. It is a callback or review, during which each team member has an opportunity to voice problems that arose, identify what went well, and suggest changes that can be made in future. This is similar to the feedback nurses ask patients to do after they have presented some educational health teaching, which verifies that the patient understood the material.

Patient Safety Outcomes

Mortality rates have decreased using this tool in the surgical area. Staff identify adverse events that were avoided due to the information communicated during the briefing (Bagian, 2010). Use of structured hand-off tools increases perceptions of adequate communication (Jukkala et al., 2012).

TEAM TRAINING MODELS

Teamwork is described in Chapters 24 and 25 on continuity of the nurse–health provider communication.

The majority of reported errors have been found to stem from poor teamwork and poor communication. An effective team has clear, accurate communication understood by all. All team members work together to promote a climate of patient safety. To improve **interprofessional health team collaboration** and communication, it is recommended that nurses and other health care providers jointly share communication training and team-building sessions to develop an "us" rather than "them" work philosophy. When conflict occurs, differences need to be addressed. Specific conflict-resolution techniques are discussed in Chapter 24.

Ideally, the health care team would provide the patient with more resources, allow for greater flexibility, promote a "learning from each other" climate, and promote collective creativity in problem solving. Use of standardized communication tools fosters collaborative practice by creating shared communication expectations. Obstacles to effective teamwork include a lack of time, a culture of autonomy, heavy workloads, and the different terminologies and communication styles used by each discipline. Building in standardized communication methods cuts errors, but it takes extra time to develop these types of communication practices in interprofessional teams.

The Interprofessional Collaborator Assessment Rubric (ICAR) is an assessment tool available in both English and French, developed for use in the assessment of interprofessional collaborator competencies (Curran et al., 2011). Development of the rubric was informed by an interprofessional advisory committee of Canadian educators from the fields of medicine, nursing, and the rehabilitation sciences (Memorial University, n.d.). The rubric can be used for both formative and summative assessments of the interprofessional collaborator competencies of communication, collaboration, roles and responsibilities, a collaborative patient/client/family-centred approach, team functioning, and conflict management and resolution (Curran et al., n.d.).

TeamSTEPPS Model

One prominent safety model is Team Strategies and Tools to Enhance Performance and Patient Safety (Team-STEPPS). TeamSTEPPS was developed by the United States Department of Defense and the Agency for Healthcare Research and Quality (CPSI, 2016). In CPSI's efforts to improve patient safety through effective teamwork, communication, and patient safety culture, **TeamSTEPPS™** has been adopted, adapted, and made available in Canada (CPSI). This program emphasizes improving patient outcomes by improving communication using evidence-informed techniques. Communication skills include briefing and debriefing, conveying respect, clarifying team leadership, cross-monitoring, situational monitoring feedback, assertion in a climate valuing everyone's input, and use of standard communication formats, such as SBAR (TeamSTEPPS National Conference, 2017). Creating a team culture means each member is committed to the following:

- Open communication, with frequent, timely feedback
- Protecting others from work overload
- Asking for and offering assistance

TeamSTEPPS With "I PASS the BATON"

The TeamSTEPPS program recommends that all team members use the "I PASS the BATON" mnemonic during any transition by staff in patient care. Table 2.3 explains this

TABLE 2.3	I PASS the BATON	
I	Introduction	Introduce yourself and your role
P	Patient	State patient's name, identifiers, age, sex, location
A	Assessment	Present chief complaint, vital signs, symptoms, diagnosis
S	Situation	Current status, level of certainty, recent changes, response to treatment
S	Safety concerns	Critical laboratory reports, allergies, alerts (e.g., falls)
B	Background	Comorbidities, previous episodes, current medications, family history
A	Actions	State what actions were taken and why
T	Timing	Level of urgency, explicit timing and priorities
O	Ownership	State who is responsible
N	Next	State the plan: what will happen next, any anticipated changes

Developed by the US Department of Defense: Department of Defense Patient Safety Program. (2005). *Healthcare communications toolkit to improve transitions in care.* Falls Church, VA: TRICARE Management Activity.

communication strategy. I PASS hand-off provides a structured communication method for health care providers that can significantly improve patient safety. After the Hospital for Sick Children in Toronto, Ontario, implemented the I PASS hand-off communication method, harmful medical errors decreased by 30% (Sick Kids, 2017). The I PASS method is being used by health care organizations globally (Starmer et al., 2017).

Saskatchewan Health Quality Council Safety Alert/Stop the Line

The Safety Alert/Stop the Line initiative's goal is to eliminate harm to patients and staff. This is achieved through encouraging patients, visitors, and staff to identify harmful incidents in the moment and "stop the line" by calling for additional support to restore safety. This initiative includes processes, policies, and behavioural expectations to create a safety culture where everyone takes responsibility for making health care settings S.A.F.E.R. The acronym S.A.F.E.R. stands for the following:

Stop if you see something unsafe.

Assess the situation. Ask for support from others (i.e., peers, supervisors, leaders).

Fix the unsafe situation if you can. If you can't, then …

Escalate your concern. Call in help from a team member or leader.

Report unsafe situations, environments, and practices, including both instances of no harm and incidents that have resulted in harm to patients or staff. Safety factors can't be improved if they are not known (CPSI, 2017b; Saskatchewan Health Quality Council, 2017).

PATIENT SAFETY OUTCOMES OF TEAM TRAINING PROGRAMS

Multiple studies tend to demonstrate increased satisfaction, primarily from nurses, when team communication strategies are implemented.

Nursing Teamwork

The traditional patient report from one nurse handing over care to another needs to be accurate, specific, and clear and allow time for questions to foster a culture of patient safety. Team training is one tool used to increase collaboration between nurses and other health providers. The use of teams is a concept that has been around for years within nursing and other health providers. For example, medicine has used medical rounds to share information among physicians. Nursing has end-of-shift reports, when responsibility is handed over to the next group of nurses. Using SBAR or any other standardized communication format

for reports, especially if these reports are at the bedside, has been shown to increase patient safety, with evidence indicating decreased patient falls, shorter lengths of stay, and decreased overtime costs while improving team communication and collaboration (Tobiano et al., 2018). In a systematic mixed-methods review of patient participation in nursing bedside handover, Tobiano et al. recommend that to foster patient involvement in handovers, tools like SBAR provide a standard way of reporting information, but nurses need to be flexible in their approach to support each patient's situation and preferences.

Interprofessional Rounds and Team Meetings

Contemporary health care teams use "interprofessional rounds" to increase communication among the whole team, which can include nurses, physicians, pharmacists, therapists, social workers, and dietitians. This strategy may increase communication and positively affect patient outcomes. For example, daily discharge interprofessional rounds have been correlated with decreased length of hospital stay. Interprofessional team meetings can be held daily or weekly to also explore common goals, concerns, and options; address issues before they escalate into conflicts; or provide support.

A **huddle** is a brief, informal gathering of the team to decide on a course of action. Huddles reinforce the existing plan of care or inform team members of changes to the plan. A team huddle can be called by any team member.

Callouts and **time-outs** allow staff to stop and review. As mentioned earlier, the surgical checklist has a time out in which all team members review the details of the surgery about to take place, to prevent wrong patient and wrong site surgeries. In callouts, assertive language may need to be used. The CUS guideline can guide any member calling out concerns and succinct escalation. The **CUS** guideline consists of three statements: "I'm **C**oncerned," "I'm **U**ncomfortable," and "This is a **S**afety issue" (CPSI, 2011).

Patient Safety Outcomes

Strategies to improve interprofessional communication are found to break down barriers, increase staff satisfaction (Rosenthal, 2013), decrease night pager calls to residents, and hopefully help to improve the quality of care.

Technology-Oriented Solutions Create a Climate of Patient Safety

Health information technologies (HITs) are a key tool for increasing safety and a means to decrease health care costs and increase quality of care. HITs, text messaging, and dedicated smart phones are some of the technological innovations discussed in Chapters 26 and 27, as are clinical decision support systems, electronic clinical pathways and care plans, and computerized registries or national data-banks that monitor treatment and outcomes.

Electronic transmission of prescriptions involves sending medication orders directly to the patient's pharmacy in the community. This can help decrease errors caused by misinterpretation of handwritten prescriptions.

Radiofrequency identification (RFID), which puts a computer chip in identity cards or even into some people, is an emerging technology that allows you to locate a certain nurse, identify a patient or medical equipment, or even locate an individual medication. RFID may be able to be incorporated into a nurse's hand-held computer and has been shown to improve patient safety (Paaske et al., 2017).

Prevention of misidentification of the patient is an obvious error-prevention strategy. Before administering medication, the nurse needs to verify patient allergies, use another nurse to verify accuracy for certain stock medications, and reverify the patient's identity. Best practice recommendations include completing the medication safety checks, checking the patient's name band, and then asking the patient to verbally confirm their name and give a second identifier, such as date of birth.

Use of technology such as barcoded name bands (Fig. 2.2) offers protection against misidentification (Institute for Safe Medication Practices Canada [ISMP], 2013). Some barcoded name bands include the patient's picture, along with the patient's name, date of birth, and barcode, for verification of patient identity.

Whiteboards have long been used at the central nursing station to list the census and the staff assigned to care, in labour and delivery units to list labour status, and in

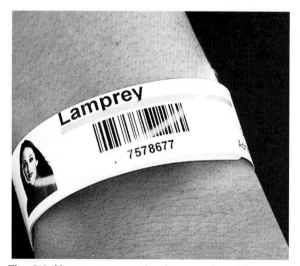

Fig. 2.2 Nurse scans patient's name band for accurate identification.

operating rooms to track procedures and staff. In some areas, there are electronic whiteboards, and patients are invited to add to the information displayed on them.

Patient Safety Outcomes

Many agencies have used barcodes for years. When a new medication is ordered by a physician, it is transmitted to the pharmacy, where it is labelled with the same barcode as is on the patient's name band. The nurse administering the medication must first verify both codes by scanning with the battery-operated barcode reader, similar to when you buy something at a store. In a review of the literature on barcode medication administration technology from 2007–2017, it was found that this technology reduces medication administration errors by 50–70 percent (Baiden, 2018). In a similar fashion, barcoded labels on laboratory specimens also prevent mix-ups.

OTHER SPECIFIC NURSING EFFORTS

Following Safety Policies

Implementing unit-based safety programs, such as S.A.F.E.R., and following policy helps decrease errors and improve the efficiency of care. Measures to improve efficiency may also increase the time you have for communication with patients. Examples of safety redundant processes that can improve patient safety are the two identifiers required before administering a procedure or medicine or the use of the two-challenge rule.

Workarounds are shortcuts. Nurses under pressure of time constraints have sometimes developed these shortcuts. Workarounds are nonapproved methods to expedite one's work and are not recommended. An example is printing an extra set of barcodes for all your patients who are scheduled to receive medication at 10 a.m. and scanning them all at once rather than scanning each patient's barcode name band when in their room administering the medication.

Patient Safety Outcomes

Deviating from safety protocols inherently introduces risks. While in the short term, time may be saved, in the long run, mistakes cost millions of dollars each year, harm patients, and put you at risk for liability or malpractice.

Transforming Care at the Bedside

An example of how patient safety can be improved at the bedside is the Transforming Care at the Bedside (**TCAB**; pronounced *tee-cab*) initiative that was an Institute for Healthcare Improvement initiative from 2003–2008. This initiative was funded by the Robert Wood Johnson Foundation to improve patient safety and the quality of hospital bedside care by empowering nurses at the bedside to make system changes and could be considered to use in your practice (Amer, 2013; Robert Wood Johnson Foundation, 2008).

This program has four core concepts to improve care:

1. Create a climate of safe, reliable patient care. Uses practices such as brainstorming and retreats for staff nurses, to develop better practice and better communication ideas. One example would be for nurses to initiate presentation of the patients' status to physicians at morning rounds using a standard format. Another strategy is to empower staff nurses to make decisions.
2. Establish unit-based vital teams. Interprofessional, supportive care teams foster a sense of increased professionalism for point-of-care nurses. This, together with better nurse–physician communication, should positively affect patient outcomes.
3. Develop patient-centred care. This ensures continuity of care and respects family and patient choices.
4. Provide value-added care. This eliminates inefficiencies, for example, by placing high-use supplies in drawers in each patient's room.

Patient Safety Outcomes

Evaluation in more than 60 project hospitals showed that units using this method cut their mortality rate by 25% and reduced nosocomial infections significantly (Amer, 2013). The TCAB program was implemented in eight units in a multihospital centre in Montreal, Quebec, which resulted in an increase in team effectiveness and a decrease in nosocomial infections (Lavoie-Tremblay et al., 2017).

Patient–Provider Collaborations

Patients and families have been described as being the eyes and ears in health care practices as they are invested in their own care and well-being, know their symptoms and treatment responses, and have insights on how care can be provided (CPSI, 2017b). Evidence increasingly indicates that patient and family collaborations are important in fostering patient safety. Patients and their families should be specifically invited to be an integral part of the care process.

Emphasize to Patients and Families That They Are Valued Members of the Health Team

Let your patients know they are encouraged to actively participate in their care. Safe care is a top goal shared by patient and care provider. Empowering your patients and families to be collaborators in their own care enhances error prevention. Emphasize this health provider–patient partnership, and increase open communication through bedside rounds,

bedside change-of-shift hand-offs, and patient access to their own records. In building the relationship, to establish rapport, nurses can follow the mnemonic PEARLS (*p*artnership; *e*mpathy; *a*pology, such as "sorry you had to wait"; *r*espect; *l*egitimize or validate your patient's feelings and concerns with comments; and offering *s*upport.

Use Written Materials

In one hospital system, pamphlets are given to patients upon admission, instructing them to become partners in their care. A nurse comes into the patient's room at a certain time each day, sits, and makes eye contact. Together, nurse and patient make a list of the day's goals, which are written on a whiteboard in the patient's room. As a part of safety and communication, awareness of language barriers can be signalled to everyone entering the room by posting a logo on the chart, in the room, or on the bed. Use of interpreters and information materials written in the patient's primary language may also reduce safety risks.

Assess Patients' Level of Health Literacy

As mentioned, it is important to make verbal and written information as simple as possible. As a nurse, you need to assess the health literacy level of each patient. Provide privacy to avoid embarrassment. Obtain feedback or teach-backs (ask the patient to describe in their own words what has been discussed) to determine the patient's understanding of the information you have provided: simplify, clarify, verify!

Patient Safety Outcomes

We need more data regarding patient involvement effects on safety. When McGill University Health Centre in Montreal, Quebec, introduced patient representative participation on quality improvement teams with staff, alongside redesigned processes such as use of whiteboards and better nursing hand-offs, there was 60% reduction in medication incidents, decreased infection rates, and an 8% increase in registered nurses' direct time in care (CPSI, 2018). Placing information such as fall prevention posters in the room of a patient at risk has also been reported by agencies to reduce the number of falls.

▌ SUMMARY

Major efforts to transform the health care system are ongoing. We maximize patient safety by minimizing the risk for errors made by all health care workers. Because miscommunication has been documented to be one of the most significant factors in error occurrence, this chapter focused on communication solutions. It described some individual and system solutions that should help all nurses practise more safely and effectively.

👤 ETHICAL DILEMMA

What Would You Do?

You are a new nurse working for a hospice, providing in-home care for Ms. Wendy, a 34-year-old woman with recurrent spinal cancer. At an interprofessional care-planning conference 2 months ago, Dr. Chi, the oncologist; Dr. Spenski, the family physician; hospice staff; and Ms. Wendy agreed to admit her when her condition deteriorated to the point where she would require ventilator assistance. Today, however, when you arrive at her home, she states a desire to forego further hospitalization. Her family physician agrees to increase her morphine to handle her increased pain, even though you feel that such a large dose will further compromise her respiratory status.

1. What are the possibilities for miscommunication?
2. What would you do to ensure Ms. Wendy and the health care team are understanding what the next steps should be?

QUESTIONS FOR REVIEW AND DISCUSSION

1. Examine Table 2.1, and give one example you have seen for each of the best-practice communication solutions provided.
2. Complete the SBAR exercises (Simulation Exercises 2.1, 2.2, 2.3). What was the easiest and hardest part? Role play the exercises with each other.

REFERENCES

Amer, K. S. (2013). *Quality and safety for transformational nursing: Care competencies*. Pearson Publishing.

Anderson, J., Malone, L., Shanahan, K. et al. (2015). Nursing bedside clinical handover—an integrated review of issues and tools. *Journal of Clinical Nursing, 24*, 662–671.

Andreoli, A., Fancott, C., Karima, V. et al. (2010). Using SBAR to communicate falls risks and management in interprofessional rehabilitation teams. *Healthcare Quarterly, 13*(Sp.). 94–101.

Association of New Brunswick Licensed Practical Nurses. (2013). *Standards of Practice for Licensed Practical Nurses in Canada*. https://www.anblpn.ca/resources/STANDARDS_OF_PRACTICE.pdf.

Bagian, J. P. (2010). Medical team communication training before, during and after surgery improves patient outcomes. *JAMA, 304*(5), 1693–1700.

Baiden, D. (2018). Factors affecting the impact of barcode medication administration technology in reducing medication administration errors by nurses. *Canadian Journal of Nursing Informatics, 13*(1). https://cjni.net/journal/?p=5368.

Baker, G. R., Norton, P. G., Flintoft, V. et al. (2004). The Canadian adverse events study: The incidence of adverse events among hospital patients in Canada. *Canadian Medical Association Journal, 170*(11), 1678–1686.

Boyd, J. M., Wu, G., & Stelfox, H. T. (2017). The impact of checklists on inpatient safety outcomes: A systematic review of randomized controlled trials. *Journal of Hospital Medicine, 12*(8), 675–682. https://www.journalofhospitalmedicine.com/jhospmed/article/143603/hospital-medicine/impact-checklists-inpatient-safety-outcomes-systematic.

British Columbia College of Nurses & Midwives (2021). *Professional Standards for Psychiatric Nursing*. https://www.bccnm.ca/RPN/ProfessionalStandards/Pages/Default.aspx.

Canadian Institute for Health Information. (2016). *Measuring patient harm in Canadian hospitals*. https://secure.cihi.ca/free_products/cihi_cpsi_hospital_harm_en.pdf.

Canadian Institute for Health Information. (2020). *Patient harm in Canadian hospitals? It does happen*. https://www.cihi.ca/en/patient-harm-in-canadian-hospitals-it-does-happen.

Canadian Nurses Association. (2009). *Position statement: Patient safety*. https://nurses.ab.ca/docs/default-source/document-library/endorsed-publications/ps102_patient_safety_e.pdf?sfvrsn=2b595357_12.

Canadian Nurses Association. (2017). *Code of ethics for registered nurses*. https://www.cna-aiic.ca/~/media/cna/page-content/pdf-en/code-of-ethics-2017-edition-secure-interactive.

Canadian Nurses Association & Registered Nurses' Association of Ontario. (2010). *Nurse fatigue and patient safety: Research report-Executive summary*. https://cna-aiic.ca/-/media/cna/page-content/pdf-en/fatigue_safety_2010_summary_e.pdf?la=en&hash=71247D396E270A4F69AB85CCF2B1AC50ABB6B4DF.

Canadian Patient Safety Institute. (n.d). *Joint position statement: Advocacy and support for use of a surgical safety checklist*. https://www.patientsafetyinstitute.ca/en/toolsResources/Surgical-Safety-Checklist-Position-Statement/Documents/SurgicalSafetyChecklist_PositionStatement_FINAL_E.pdf.

Canadian Patient Safety Institute. (2011). *Canadian framework for teamwork and communication: Literature review, needs assessment, evaluation of training tools and expert consultations*. https://www.patientsafetyinstitute.ca/en/toolsResources/teamworkCommunication/Pages/default.aspx.

Canadian Patient Safety Institute. (2016). *TeamSTEPPS Canada™*. https://www.patientsafetyinstitute.ca/en/education/TeamSTEPPS/Pages/default.aspx.

Canadian Patient Safety Institute. (2017a). *The patient safety education program™ Canada.* https://www.patientsafety institute.ca/en/education/PatientSafetyEducationProgram/ PatientSafetyEducationCurriculum/Documents/Module%20 03%20-%20Communications.pdf.

Canadian Patient Safety Institute. (2017b). *The case for investing in patient safety in Canada.* https://www. patientsafetyinstitute.ca/en/About/Documents/The%20 Case%20for%20Investing%20in%20Patient%20Safety.pdf.

Canadian Patient Safety Institute. (2018). *Engaging patients in patient safety: A Canadian guide.* https://www. patientsafetyinstitute.ca/en/toolsResources/Patient- Engagement-in-Patient-Safety-Guide/Documents/ Engaging%20Patients%20in%20Patient%20Safety.pdf.

Canadian Patient Safety Institute. (2020a). *Glossary.* https:// www.patientsafetyinstitute.ca/en/toolsResources/ PatientSafetyIncidentManagementToolkit/Pages/Glossary.aspx.

Canadian Patient Safety Institute. (2020b). *Surgical safety checklist.* https://www.patientsafetyinstitute.ca/en/Topic/ Pages/Surgical-Safety-Checklist.aspx.

Ciliska, D. (2012). *Introduction to evidence-informed decision making.* https://cihr-irsc.gc.ca/e/45245.html#b1.

College & Association of Registered Nurses of Alberta. (2013). *Practice standards for regulated members.* https:// nurses.ab.ca/docs/default-source/document-library/ standards/practice-standards-for-regulated-members. pdf?sfvrsn=d4893bb4_12.

Compton, J., Copeland, K., Flanders, S. et al. (2012). Implementing SBAR across a large multihospital health system. *Joint Commission Journal on Quality and Patient Safety, 38*(6), 261–268.

Cornell, P., & Gervis, M. T. (2013). Improving shift report focus and consistency with the situation, background, assessment, recommendation protocol. *The Journal of Nursing Administration, 43*(7/8), 422–428.

Curran, V., Hollett, A., Casimiro, L.M. et al. (n.d.). *Interprofessional Collaborator Assessment Rubric.* https:// www.med.mun.ca/getdoc/b78eb859-6c13-4f2f-9712- f50f1c67c863/ICAR.aspx.

Curran, V., Hollett, A., Casimiro, L. M. et al. (2011). Development and validation of the interprofessional collaborator assessment rubric (ICAR). *Journal of Interprofessional Care, 25,* 339–344. https://doi.org/10.3109/1 3561820.2011.589542.

Grif Alspach, J. (2017). The checklist: Recognize limits, but harness its power. *Critical Care Nurse, 37*(5). https://doi. org/10.4037/ccn2017603.

Health Quality Council of Alberta. (2019). *Just culture beliefs and attitudes.* https://justculture.hqca.ca/what-is-a-just-culture/.

Hooper, B., Shaw, L., & Zamzam, R. (2015). Implementing high- fidelity simulations with large groups of nursing students. *Nurse Educator, 40*(2), 87–90. https://doi.org/10.1097/ NNE.0000000000000101.

Institute for Safe Medication Practices Canada. (2013). *Canadian pharmaceutical bar coding project: Medication bar code system implementation planning-a resource guide.*

https://www.ismp-canada.org/barcoding/download/ ResourceGuide/BarCodingResourceGuideFINAL.pdf.

Institute for Safe Medication Practices Canada. (2016). *Definitions of terms.* https://www.ismp-canada.org/ definitions.htm.

Institute of Medicine. (1999). *To err is human: Building a safer health system.* Washington, DC: The National Academies Press.

Jukkala, A. M., James, D., Autrey, P. et al. (2012). Developing a standardized tool to improve nurse communication during shift report. *Journal of Nursing Care Quality, 27*(3), 240–246.

Kear, T., & Ulrich, B. (2015). Patient safety and patient safety culture in nephrology nurse practice settings: Issues, solutions and best practices. *Nephrology Nursing Journal, 42*(2), 113–122.

Kowalski, S. L., & Anthony, M. (2017). Nursing's evolving role in patient safety. *American Journal of Nursing, 117,* 34–38.

Lavoie-Tremblay, M., O'Connor, P., Biron, A. et al. (2017). The effects of the Transforming Care at the Bedside Program on perceived team effectiveness and patient outcomes. *The Health Care Manager, 36*(1), 10–20. https://doi.org/10.1097/ HCM.0000000000000142.

McGillis Hall, L., Pedersen, C., & Fairley, L. (2010). Losing the moment: Understanding interruptions to nurses' work. *Journal of Nursing Administration, 40*(4), 169–176.

Melnyk, B. M. (2014). Evidence-based practice versus evidence- informed practice: A debate that could stall forward momentum in improving healthcare quality, safety, patient outcomes and costs. *Worldviews on Evidence-Based Nursing, 11*(6), 347–349. https://doi.org/10.1111/wvn.12070.

Memorial University. (n.d.). *Centre for Collaborative Health Professional Education: Interprofessional Collaborator Assessment Rubric (ICAR).* https://www.med.mun.ca/getdoc/ a2dd2960-4ab5-49d8-a0b1-2602def08081/ICAR-Synopsis- Handout.aspx.

Ontario Ministry of Health and Long-Term Care. (2020). *Ontario Health Teams.* http://health.gov.on.ca/en/pro/programs/ connectedcare/oht/#OHT.

Paaske, S., Bauer, A., Moser, T., et al. (2017). The benefits and barriers to RFID technology in healthcare. *Online Journals of Nursing Informatics, 21*(2)http://www.himss.org/ojni.

Peña, A. (2010). The Dreyfus model of clinical problem-solving skills acquisition: A critical perspective. *Medical Education Online, 15*(1), 4846. https://doi.org/10.3402/meo.v15i0.4846.

Rideout. D. (2013). "Just Culture" encourages error reporting, improves patient safety. *OR Manager, 29*(7), 1.

Ring, L., & Fairchild, R. M. (2013). Leadership and patient safety: A review of the literature. *Journal of Nursing Regulation, 4*(1), 52–56.

Robert Wood Johnson Foundation. (2008). *The Transforming Care at the Bedside (TCAB) Toolkit.* http://www.rwjf.org/ en/research-publications/find-rwjf-research/2008/06/the- transforming-care-at-the-bedside-tcab-toolkit.html.

Rosenthal, L. (2013). Enhancing communication between nightshift RNs and hospitalists. *Journal of Nursing Administration, 43*(2), 59–61.

Saintsing, D., Gibson, L. M., & Pennington, A. W. (2011). The novice nurse and clinical decision-making: How to avoid errors. *Journal of Nursing Management, 19*, 354–359.

Saskatchewan Health Quality Council. (February 2, 2017). *HQC news: Provincial initiative aims to improve health care safety*. https://www.hqc.sk.ca/en-us/news-events/hqc-news/provincial-initiative-aims-to-improve-health-care-safety.

Shahid, S., & Thomas, S. (2018). Situation, background, assessment, recommendation (SBAR) communication tool for handoff in healthcare: A narrative review. *Safety in Health, 4*(7). https://doi.org/10.1186/s40886-018-0073-1.

Sick Kids. (2017). Shift-change handoff program recognized for improving patient safety through standardization of provider-to-provider communication. http://www.sickkids.ca/AboutSickKids/Newsroom/Past-News/2017/shift-change-handoff-program-recognized-improving-patient-safety.html.

Smeulers, M., Dolman, C. D., Atema, D. et al. (2016). Safe and effective nursing shift handover with NURSEPASS: An interrupted time series. *Applied Nursing Research, 32*, 199–205.

Starmer, A. J., Spector, N. D., West, D. C. et al. (2017). Integrating research, quality improvement, and medical education for better handoffs and safer care: Disseminating, adapting and implementing the I-PASS Program. *The Joint Commission Journal on Quality and Patient Safety, 43*, 319–329. https://www.jointcommissionjournal.com/article/S1553-7250(17)30176-9/pdf.

TeamSTEPPS National Conference. (June 2017). Cleveland: Ohio.

TeamSTEPPS, Webinar. (July 2017). www.ahrq.gov/teamstepps/webinars/index.html.

Thomson, H., Tourangeau, A., Jeffs, L. et al. (2018). Factors affecting quality of nurse shift handover in the emergency department. *Journal of Advanced Nursing, 74*(4), 876–886. https://doi.org/10.1111/jan.13499.

Tobiano, G., Bucknall, T., Sladdin, I. et al. (2018). Patient participation in nursing bedside handover: A systematic mixed-methods review. *International Journal of Nursing Studies, 77*, 243–258.

Vardaman, J. M., Cornell, P., Gondo, M. B. et al. (2012). Beyond communication: The role of standardized protocols in a changing health care environment. *Health Care Management Review, 37*(1), 88–97.

World Health Organization. (2020). *Patient safety*. https://www.who.int/patientsafety/en/.

3

Professional Guides for Nursing Communication

Claire Mallette

Originating US chapter by *Kathleen Underman Boggs*

OBJECTIVES

At the end of the chapter, the reader will be able to:

1. Describe the impact on nursing communication of standards and guidelines for care and communication issued by multiple organizations.
2. Discuss competencies expected of the newly graduated nurse, as listed by the Canadian Association of Schools of Nursing (CASN), provincial and territorial regulatory bodies and other organizations, specifically as they affect communication.
3. Discuss legal and ethical standards in nursing practice relevant to communication, including social media.
4. Construct examples of communications that meet privacy legal requirements related to access to personal health information in provinces and territories.
5. Translate empirical knowledge into clinical practice by applying evidence-informed practice (EIP) information to construct a case study.

This chapter introduces the student to standards and guidelines that influence nursing care, with the focus on communication in both academia and clinical practice. It provides a brief overview of communication as a component of the nursing process. Globally, standards mandate that nurses provide care with compassion and respect for the inherent dignity, worth, and uniqueness of every individual. (Fig. 3.1).

BASIC CONCEPTS

Standards as Guides to Communication in Clinical Nursing

As nurses, we are guided by standards, policies, ethical codes, regulations, and laws. Factors external to the nursing profession, such as technology innovations, research reports, and government mandates, are driving major changes in the way nurses communicate. As described in Chapter 1, our focus is not only on laws but also on standards and guidelines from professional organizations affecting communications in our practice.

In an ideal work environment, nurses demonstrate professional conduct by using established evidence-informed "best practices" to provide safe, high-quality compassionate care for the people we care for. We also have excellent communication with the person, their families, and all members of the interprofessional health care team. Effective communication is essential to workplace efficiency and effective delivery of care.

Effective Communication Concepts

Effective communication is defined as a two-way exchange of information, verbally and nonverbally, among the person and health providers, ensuring that the expectations and responsibilities of all are clearly understood. It is an active process for all involved. Two-way communication provides feedback, which enables both senders and receivers to understand. It is timely, accurate, and usable. Messages are processed by all parties until the information is clearly understood by all and integrated into care. A number of international, national, and professional associations have issued standards, guidelines, and recommendations impacting the way nurses communicate. Let's consider a general summary of these recommendations for effective, safe communication, with many of these recommendations starting with "C."

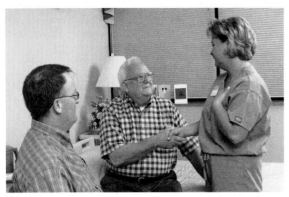

Fig. 3.1 The nurse in all professional relationships practices with compassion and respect for the inherent dignity, worth, and uniqueness of every individual.

- Correct/accurate (Canadian Nurses Association [CNA], 2017; International Council of Nurses [ICN], 2012)
- Concise, concrete, complete (CNA, 2017; ICN, 2012))
- Confidential (ICN, 2012; Nurses Association of New Brunswick [NANB], 2019)
- Culturally competent (CNA, 2017; College of Registered Psychiatric Nurses of Manitoba [CRPNM], 2019)
- Compassionate (CNA, 2017; College of Licensed Practical Nurses of Prince Edward Island, [CLPNPEI], 2013)
- Client-centred (British Columbia College of Nursing Professionals [BCCNP], 2019; ICN, 2012)
- Competent (CNA, 2017; College of Registered Nurses of Newfoundland and Labrador [CRNNL], 2019)
- Collaborate (CNA, 2017; College & Association of Registered Nurses of Alberta [CARNA], 2013).

Alongside these are timely communication and advocacy, which are also important for effective, safe communication.

Communication problems occur when there are failures in one or more categories: the system, the transmission, or the reception. Communication errors have been found to be the most common adverse event during care of the person (Shahid & Thomas, 2018).

- System failures occur when the necessary channels of communication are absent or not functioning.
- Transmission failures occur when the channels exist but the message is never sent or is not clearly sent.
- Reception failures occur when channels exist and necessary information is sent, but the recipient misinterprets the message.

Outcomes

Why are nurses interested in using communication standards to modify and clarify their own communication? Ideally, because we are motivated to provide the best, safest possible care. Outcomes for failure to adhere to established nursing practice and professional practice standards range from harm to persons all the way to professional and legal ramifications, potentially including malpractice lawsuits. Consider the case of Kay Smite.

Case Example: Nurse Kay Smite

Immediately following graduation from her nursing program and becoming a registered nurse, Kay Smite takes an entry position on a busy surgical unit in a small community hospital. With no orientation, she is assigned to work evening shift, with one registered nurse and two personal support workers. During her second week, when the other experienced registered nurse calls in sick, Kay is told by the nursing supervisor that she is "charge nurse" this evening, and a float nurse will be sent as soon as possible to help with the workload. A surgeon arrives and rapidly gives verbal instructions, telling her that Mr. Omar's preoperative preparation for a craniotomy tomorrow will be limited to shaving his head at the incision site only, in the operating suite. As a student, Kay has never spoken to a physician. The physician writes an order, stating, "Mr. Omar will be shaved according to charge nurse's instructions." He asks Kay to call the operating room to relay these instructions, which she does. Nothing is in the record describing the area to be shaved. When the day shift arrives in the surgical suite, the telephone message from Kay is not passed on. Mr. Omar's head is completely shaved, and he threatens a lawsuit.

---

1. What standards of communication were violated?
2. What system, transmission, and reception failures occurred within this work environment?
3. What would you change in this unfortunate, but true situation?

PROFESSIONAL NURSING ORGANIZATIONS ISSUING HEALTH CARE COMMUNICATION GUIDELINES

Professional standards of practice serve the dual purpose of providing a standardized benchmark for evaluating the quality of nursing care and offering the person a common means of understanding nursing as a professional relationship. In this way, standards are used to communicate with the public as to what can be expected from professional nurses. Globally, professional practice organizations are issuing practice standards for nursing care that specify clear, comprehensive communication as a requirement. Examples include The Australian Practice Standards for Specialist Critical Care Nurses (Gill et al., 2016); Registered Nurses Association of Ontario (RNAO); Nursing & Midwifery Council (2015); and the American Nurses Association (ANA) (2010).

Curriculum for Quality and Safety in Communication

Clear communication is a priority competency, deemed essential for nurses (Clark et al., 2016). Application of professional communication standards necessitates the use of critical thinking and problem-solving skills in all aspects of care (described in Chapter 4). Practice related to communication standards is outlined by each province or territory's professional nursing regulatory bodies. Nursing curriculums also have communication knowledge, skills, attitudes and abilities as core competencies woven throughout the different nursing programs.

Canadian Association of Schools of Nursing (CASN)

CASN (n.d.) is the "national voice of nursing education, research, and scholarship and represents baccalaureate and graduate nursing programs in Canada." In 2015, CASN developed a National Nursing Education Framework, conveying core competencies for baccalaureate, master's, and doctoral programs. The purpose of the framework is to provide schools of nursing with national guidelines for each of the nursing programs, outlined through six domains of knowledge and learning (CASN, 2015). Each domain consists of guiding principles and related outcomes expected in nursing practice and increases in expectations and scope from one degree level to the next. The domains are not independent of one another. Instead, they are interrelated and integral in implementing nursing practice. The six domains are as follows:

1. Knowledge—the theoretical, conceptual, and factual content that is taught and learned in the programs
2. Research, methodologies, critical inquiry, and evidence—thinking and inquiry skills, and the processes used to appraise, generate, synthesize, translate, and implement knowledge
3. Nursing practice—activities related to a broad range of roles in nursing practice, including research and scholarship
4. Communication and collaboration—the interactions and relationships between the nurse and persons, the health care team, and key stakeholders

5. Professionalism—accountability, ethics, and values of the nurse as a member of the nursing profession
6. Leadership—processes of social influence with others to create, coordinate, and enable the achievement of goals and tasks (CASN, 2015)

While the communication domain outlines specific expected communication outcomes, the other five domains are also influenced by nurses' communication practices. The essential components for Domain 4: Communication and Collaboration can be found in Table 3.1.

TABLE 3.1 **CASN's Baccalaureate Competencies**
Domain 4: Communication and Collaboration
Guiding Principle: Programs prepare students to communicate and collaborate effectively with clients and members of the health care team
Essential Components: The program prepares the student to demonstrate the following:
4.1 The ability to communicate and collaborate effectively with diverse clients and members of the health care team to provide high quality nursing care
4.2 The ability to self-monitor one's beliefs, values, and assumptions and recognize their impact on interpersonal relationships with clients and team members
4.3 The ability to communicate using information technologies to support engagement with persons/clients and the interprofessional team
4.4 The ability to coarticulate a nursing perspective and the scope of practice of the registered nurse in the context of the health care team
4.5 The ability to collaborate with diverse clients, adapt relational approaches appropriately and accommodate varying contextual factors in diverse practice situations.
4.6 The ability to contribute to positive health care team functioning through consultation, application of group communication theory, principles, and group process skills

Adapted from Canadian Association of Schools of Nursing. (2015). *National nursing education framework: Final report.* https://www.casn.ca/wp-content/uploads/2014/12/Framwork-FINAL-SB-Nov-30-20151.pdf.

Patient Safety Communication in Nursing Education

As discussed, CASN's National Nursing Framework (2015) identified core competencies for nursing practice for baccalaureate, master's, and doctoral nursing programs. There was also the recognition that health care provider education has a responsibility to educate future professionals specifically on how to ensure and improve patient safety. To address this need, CASN (2018) developed learning outcomes for patient safety competencies in undergraduate nursing curricula.

Learning Outcomes for Patient Safety in Undergraduate Curricula (2018) were developed so that nursing graduates would enter practice with the knowledge, skills, attitudes, and abilities to work with persons, families, and interprofessional teams, specifically to increase patient safety. There is also an expectation that nurses in practice should be contributing to a just and no-blame patient safety culture.

The learning outcomes and core competencies were based on the Canadian Patient Safety Institute [CPSI] (2008) domains for safety competencies, which are as follows:

- Contribute to a culture of patient safety
- Work in teams for patient safety
- Communicate effectively for patient safety
- Manage safety risks
- Optimize human and environmental factors
- Recognize and respond to and disclose adverse events and near misses

Domain 3 of the CASN learning outcomes recognizes the importance of communicating effectively for patient safety. The specific learning outcomes can be found in Box 3.1. While Domain 3 outlines explicit communication practices for patient safety, communication learning outcomes for patient safety are also included in the other domains listed previously (CASN, 2018).

Central to nursing education, being a professional nurse and communication is person-centred practice, also called *patient and family-centred care* or *client and family-centred care* (discussed in every chapter); teamwork and collaboration (discussed in Chapters 2, 3, 6, 22, 23, and 24); cultural contexts, and cultural competence, humility, and safety (Chapters 7 & 8); evidence-informed practice (discussed in Chapters 1, 2, 3, and 23, with examples and application to practice in every chapter); safety and quality improvement (discussed in Chapters 2 and 25); and advancing technology and informatics (discussed in Chapters 2, 25, and 26). Communication is a key component of each of these areas of practice. Provincial and territorial regulatory bodies all have core competencies expected of nurses in these areas. All stress excellent communication, coordination, and collaborative skills.

> **BOX 3.1   CASN Learning Outcomes for Patient Safety in Undergraduate Nursing Curricula: Domain 3: Communicate Effectively for Patient Safety**
>
> - Use a patient-centred approach to communication
> - Describe attributes of effective team communication
> - Identify how health literacy affects patient safety
> - Tailor their communication to respect cultural diversity and health literacy
> - Articulate how protecting patient privacy and confidentiality relate to patient safety
> - Engage person and families in decision making
> - Facilitate safe transfers of care
> - Use team communication tools
> - Ask questions and seek help from others
> - Advocate for individual persons and for appropriate resources to ensure safety

Adapted from Canadian Association of Schools of Nursing. (2018). *Learning outcomes for patient safety in undergraduate nursing curricula.* p. 8. https://www.casn.ca/wp-content/uploads/2018/08/CPSI-EN-FINAL-r-Apr-2019.pdf.

CODES CONTAINING ETHICAL STANDARDS

Ethics is a critical part of everyday nursing practice in providing nursing care (CNA, 2017). Nurses have an ethical accountability to the people they serve that extends beyond their legal responsibility in everyday nursing situations. Nurses have consistently been rated very highly in public opinion polls for honest, trustworthy and ethical behaviour (CNA, n.d.-a). The process for applying ethical decision making is described in Chapter 4.

Ethical Codes

All legitimate professions have standards of conduct. A code of ethics for nurses provides a broad conceptual framework outlining the principled behaviours and value beliefs expected of professional nurses in delivering health care to individuals, families, and communities. Embodied in ethical codes are nursing's core values. Written codes of ethics are found in most nations. An international code of ethics, *The ICN Code of Ethics for Nurses*, was adopted by the International Council of Nurses (ICN) in 1953 and revised in 2012. This code identifies four fundamental nursing responsibilities of promoting health, preventing illness, restoring health, and alleviating suffering. Moreover, the code says that each nurse has the responsibility to maintain a clinical practice that promotes ethical behaviour while sustaining collaborative, respectful relationships with coworkers. Among many elements of the code, those addressing communication state that we need to ensure that each person receives accurate, sufficient communication in a timely manner and to maintain confidentiality (ICN, 2012).

Professional nurses, regardless of the setting, are expected to follow ethical guidelines in their practice. The Canadian Nurses Association *Code of Ethics for Registered Nurses* (2017) establishes principled guidelines designed to protect the integrity of the person related to their care, health, safety, and rights. It provides guidelines for your ethical practice and decision making to protect persons' rights and provides a mechanism for professional accountability. Listed in Box 3.2 are the primary values in the Code of Ethics, with a few examples of communication responsibilities within each value. For a complete description of the values and responsibilities within the CNA Code of Ethics (2017), go to https://www.cna-aiic.ca/~/media/cna/page-content/pdf-en/code-of-ethics-2017-edition-secure-interactive.

Ethical standards of behaviour require a clear understanding of the multidimensional aspects of an ethical dilemma, including intangible human factors that make each situation unique (e.g., personal and cultural values or resources). Chapter 4 discusses nurses and ethics in more depth, while Simulation Exercise 3.1 provides an opportunity to consider the many elements in an ethical nursing dilemma. Ethical committees can assist nurses when ethical challenges arise, through providing education, advice, and guidelines. Committee membership can include nurses, physicians, spiritual advisors, lawyers, administrators, and members of the interprofessional team (Keatings & Adams, 2020). Of particular importance to the nurse–person relationship are ethical directives related to the nurse's primary commitment to the following:

- Persons welfare
- Persons autonomy
- Recognition that an individual is unique and worthy of respect
- Truth-telling and advocacy

BOX 3.2   CNA Code of Ethics With Communication Responsibility Examples

Part 1. Nursing Values and Ethical Responsibilities and Selected Communication Related Examples:

Nurses in all contexts and domains of practice and at all levels of decision making bear the ethical responsibilities identified under each of the seven primary nursing values that are related to communication practices.

A. Providing Safe, Compassionate, Competent, and Ethical Care

- Nurses engage in compassionate care through their speech and body language and through their efforts to understand and care about others' health care needs
- Nurses build trustworthy relationships with persons receiving care as the foundation of meaningful communication, recognizing that building these relationships involves a conscious effort. Such relationships are critical to understanding people's needs and concerns.

B. Promoting Health and Well-Being

- Nurses work with persons receiving care to explore the range of health care choices available to them, recognizing that some have limited choices because of social, economic, geographic, or other factors that lead to inequities.
- When a community health intervention interferes with the individual rights of persons, nurses use and advocate for the use of the least restrictive measures possible for those in their care.

C. Promoting and Respecting Informed Decision Making

- Nurses provide persons receiving care with the information they need to make informed and autonomous decisions related to their health and well-being. They also work to ensure that health information is given to those persons in an open, accurate, understandable, and transparent manner.
- Nurses respect the wishes of capable persons receiving care to decline to receive information about their health condition.

D. Honouring Dignity

- Nurses, in their professional capacity, relate to all persons receiving care, with respect.
- Nurses utilize practice standards, best practice guidelines, policies, and research to minimize risk and maximize safety, well-being and dignity for persons receiving care.
- Nurses maintain appropriate professional boundaries and ensure their relationships are always for the benefit of the person.
- Nurses treat each other, colleagues, students, and other health care providers in a respectful manner. They work with others to honour dignity and resolve differences in a constructive way.

E. Maintaining Privacy and Confidentiality

- Nurses respect policies that protect and preserve the privacy of persons receiving care, including security safeguards in information technology.

(Continued)

BOX 3.2   CNA Code of Ethics With Communication Responsibility Examples—cont'd.

- In the use of social media, nurses safeguard the privacy and confidentiality of persons and other colleagues.

F. Promoting Justice

- Nurses do not discriminate on the basis of a person's race, ethnicity, culture, political and spiritual beliefs, social or marital status, gender, gender identity, gender expression, sexual orientation, age, health status, place of origin, lifestyle, mental or physical ability, socioeconomic status, or any other attribute.
- Nurses respect the special history and interests of Indigenous peoples as articulated in the Truth and Reconciliation Commission of Canada's (TRC) Calls to Action (2012).

G. Being Accountable

- Nurses are honest and practise with integrity in all of their professional interactions. Nurses represent themselves clearly with respect to name, title, and role.
- Nurses practise within the limits of their competence.

- Nurses advocate for more comprehensive and equitable mental health care services across age groups, sociocultural backgrounds and geographic regions.

Part II: Ethical Endeavors Related to Broad Societal Issues

Ethical nursing practice addresses broad aspects of social justice that are associated with health and well-being.

- Advocating for publicly administered health systems that ensure accessibility, universality, portability, and comprehensiveness in necessary health care services
- Advocating for a full continuum of accessible health care services at the right time, in the right place, and by the right provider
- Becoming well-informed about laws (e.g., privacy, safe contraception, medical assistance in dying) and advocating for and working with others to create policies and processes that provide ethical guidance to all nurses

Adapted from Canadian Nurses Association. (2017). *Code of ethics for registered nurses.* https://www.cna-aiic.ca/~/media/cna/page-content/pdf-en/code-of-ethics-2017-edition-secure-interactive.

SIMULATION EXERCISE 3.1   Applying the Code of Ethics for Nurses to Professional and Clinical Situations

Purpose

To help students identify applications of the CNA *Code of Ethics for Registered Nurses*

Procedure

Break into groups of four or five students and role-play the following clinical scenarios.

Refer to the Canadian Nurses Association Code of Ethics. (2017). https://www.cna-aiic.ca/~/media/cna/page-content/pdf-en/code-of-ethics-2017-edition-secure-interactive

1. Barbara Kohn is a 75-year-old woman who lives with her son and daughter-in-law. She reveals to you that her daughter-in-law keeps her locked in her room when the daughter-in-law has to go out, to prevent Mrs. Kohn from getting into trouble. She asks you not to say anything as her family will get angry at her.
2. The nursing supervisor asks you to "float" to another unit that will require some types of tasks that you believe you do not have the knowledge or skills to perform. When you explain your problem, the nursing supervisor tells you that she understands, but the unit is short staffed and she really needs you to do this.

3. Bill Jackson is an elderly patient who suffered a stroke and is unable to communicate or swallow. He is under palliative care. The health care team is considering placement of a feeding tube based on his wife's wishes. Mrs. Jackson agrees that he probably will not survive but wants the feeding tube just in case the doctors are wrong.
4. Dr. Holle criticizes a nurse in front of the patient, Mrs. DiTupper, and her family.

Reflective Analysis and Discussion

Share each ethical dilemma with the group and collaboratively come up with a resolution that the group agrees on, using the nurse's code of ethics to work through the situations.

1. Describe some of the challenges your group encountered in resolving different scenarios.
2. Select a situation that offers the most challenge ethically, and explain your choice.
3. Justify any problems in which the code of ethics was not helpful.
4. Create a scenario depicting how you have used the knowledge gained from this exercise in your nursing practice.

LEGAL STANDARDS

As stressed in every provincial and territorial set of nursing standards, nurses must be accountable for their own contributions to the delivery of high-quality care. As professional nurses, we are held legally accountable for all aspects of the nursing care we provide to persons and families, including documentation and referral. Of special relevance to communication within the nurse–person relationship are issues of confidentially, informed consent, and professional liability.

Classifications of Laws in Canadian Health Care

Canadian Common Law

While Canada is an independent country from Britain, all of Canada except for Quebec is still guided by English common law. Common law is guided by rules, principles, and doctrine that form precedents. The rules and principles are established from decisions made at trials and appeal courts over hundreds of years. These decisions are reviewed for the principles and precedents that then guide decisions in presentday cases (Keatings & Adams, 2020).

Civil laws

Civil laws in Quebec are based on French civil law. In civil law, judges follow comprehensive sets of rules and the laws as written in relation to the circumstances of the present case. Historical decisions and precedents are not considered.

Civil law in provinces and territories other than Quebec is separate and distinct from criminal law. Civil law is described as a body of rules and legal principles that oversee relations and rights and obligations among individuals, corporations, or other institutions. Most significant for nurses are tort laws. A tort is a civil wrong (not a criminal one) committed by one person against another, such as when negligence occurs, but when deliberate intent is not present (Keatings & Adams, 2020).

Four elements are necessary to qualify for a claim of malpractice or negligence:
- The professional duty was owed to the person (professional relationship).
- A breach of duty occurred in which the nurse failed to conform to an accepted standard of care.
- Causality in which a failure to act by professional standards was a proximate cause of the resulting injury.
- Actual damage or injuries resulted from breach of duty (Canadian Nurses Protective Society [CNPS], 2004).

As nurses, we are legally bound by the principles of civil tort law to provide the care that any reasonably prudent nurse would provide in a similar situation. If taken to court, this standard would be the benchmark against which our actions would be judged.

Statutory Laws. **Statutory laws** (also called legislation), in both English common law and French civil law, are formal written sets of rules passed by a legislative body to regulate a particular area. For example, the acts that regulate the nursing profession in each province and territory is a statute law. Statute law is a method of changing common law to achieve a favourable consequence (Keatings & Adams, 2020).

Criminal Law. Criminal law is when fundamental values and practices are purposely violated, resulting in the endangerment of peace, stability, well-being, and order. Examples of violation of criminal law include murder, theft, and criminal negligence (Keatings & Adams, 2020).

Malpractice and Legal Liability in Nurse–Person Relationships

In the nurse–person relationship, the nurse is responsible for maintaining the professional conduct of the relationship. Examples of unprofessional conduct include the following:
- Breaching the person's confidentiality
- Verbally or physically abusing a person
- Assuming nursing responsibility for actions without having competence
- Inappropriately delegating care to unlicensed personnel, which could result in injury
- Following a doctor's order that would result in harm to the person
- Failing to assess, report, or document changes in the person's health status
- Falsifying records
- Failing to obtain informed consent
- Failure to question a physician's orders if they are not clear
- Not following hospital policies
- Failure to provide for patient safety (e.g., not putting the side rails up for a person with a stroke)

Effective and frequent communication with persons and other providers is one of the best ways to avoid or minimize the possibility of harm leading to legal liability.

Documentation as a Legal Record

As described in Chapter 25, nurses are responsible for the accurate and timely documentation of nursing assessments, the care given, and the outcome responses. This documentation represents a permanent record of health care experiences. In the eyes of the law, failure to document in written form any of these elements means the actions were not taken.

APPLICATIONS

As illustrated in Fig. 3.2, Communication in the nursing process, communication standards and skills are an integral component of the knowledge, experience, skills, and

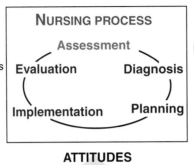

KNOWLEDGE
Underlying disease process
Normal growth and development
Normal physiology and psychology
Normal assessment findings
Health promotion
Assessment skills
Communication skills

EXPERIENCE
Previous patient care experience
Validation of assessment findings
Observation of assessment techniques

NURSING PROCESS
Assessment
Evaluation   Diagnosis
Implementation   Planning

STANDARDS
Provincial and territorial standards of practice

ATTITUDES
Perseverance
Fairness
Integrity
Confidence
Creativity

Fig. 3.2 Communication in the nursing process. From Harris, K. (2015). Nursing practice implications of the year of ethics. AWHONN, 19(2), 1. Modified from Potter, P., Perry, A., Stockert, P. et al. (2019). *Canadian Fundamentals of nursing* (6th ed.). Mosby.

attitudes encompassed in using the nursing process to deliver care. As emphasized, standards for clear, complete communication are specified in professional codes and guidelines. Nursing students need opportunities to practise communicating effectively, before entering the workforce. Throughout this book, emphasis is placed on the importance of guiding your practice through the application of both professional standards and evidence-informed practices in your nursing care. Discussing case studies and exercises offers opportunities to improve communication skills.

EVIDENCE-INFORMED PRACTICE (EIP)

Evidence-informed practice (EIP) is a conscious choice to use the most current research to provide "best care." The terms *evidence-based* and *evidence-informed practice* are defined in many ways and are often used interchangeably. **Evidence-based practice** was originally defined as "the conscientious, explicit, and judicious use of current best evidence in making decisions about the care of individual patients" (Sackett et al., 1996, p. 71). Evidence-based practice in nursing has been defined by Melnyk et al. (2010) as a "problem-solving approach to the delivery of health care that integrates the best evidence from well-designed studies and patient care data and combines it

with clinical expertise and patient preferences and values" (p. 51). Evidence-informed practice is viewed as moving beyond evidence-based practice to be a holistic approach that incorporates both research and practice knowledge and evidence from local ways of knowing, Indigenous knowledge, cultural and religious norms, and clinical judgement (LoBiondo-Wood et al., 2018; Mackey & Bassendowski, 2017). In Canada, the term *evidence-informed practice* is used more often than *evidence-based*, in recognizing that health care providers need to not only be knowledgeable about evidence coming from research but also take into consideration clinical experience and judgement as well as persons' preferences, values, and beliefs, and the context of the situation (Ciliska, 2012; Melynk, 2014).

Translating knowledge into practice using findings from multiple empirical studies to help solve clinical problems is universally advocated (Al-Mowani et al., 2016). EIP guidelines are clinical behaviours compiled from the best current research evidence available and the expertise of clinicians. Nursing education provides opportunities for students to develop competency in the use of EIP and collaborative teamwork to ensure the delivery of safe, person-centred care across settings (Leung et al., 2016). Saunders et al.'s (2016) findings show student use of EIP results in increased use as they become more experienced.

Use of EIP is an expectation of nursing practice standards across Canada. Each nurse is expected to be able to integrate "best current evidence" with clinical expertise and person/family preferences and values to deliver optimal care (Barnsteiner et al., 2013). In developing this skill, you learn to determine which data are scientifically valid and useful in guiding your practice. By consulting EIP guidelines, your ability to make specific clinical decisions about care for the person is enhanced, so you can provide the highest quality care. Do you have a clinical question? Many sources are available to you through databases such as the Cochrane Library and CINAHL, professional associations such as the Registered Nurses' Association of Ontario (RNAO) (e.g., for RNAO's Best Practice Guidelines), and government websites.

Assets That Support Use of Evidence-Informed Practice Information

Accessibility of Information

Taking ownership of improving your practice means continuing to increase your awareness of what credible evidence is available. When a policy or guideline is not yet available, you can access specific journal research articles using any of several databases such as CINAHL. Careful critical thinking is needed when relying on just one study's findings. The "Best evidence for best practice" motto encourages us to use the EIP samples provided in this book to stimulate discussion and encourage seeking out findings you can apply in your clinical practice.

Repeated study findings show staff nurses are unaware of evidence that could improve their care. One reason for this is that, traditionally, nurses use information passed down through instruction, rituals, tradition, and personal choice (Mick, 2017). This can also occur when nurses lack the knowledge to do Internet literature searches and interpret the evidence; access to journal articles is limited or non-existent; and educational preparation and negative beliefs and attitudes exist about the use of EIP by nurses (CNA, n.d.-b). Other organizational system issues such as workload time constraints, leadership, and organizational culture (discussed below) can influence nurses' ability to provide evidence-informed practice (CNA, n.d.-b).

Workload Time Constraints

With higher patient acuity and decreased resources to complete assigned tasks, staff nurses are challenged to find time to seek out evidence (Jun et al., 2016). Yet, maintaining competency depends on valuing this clinical inquiry (Leung et al., 2016).

Leadership

It helps when nurses are exposed to leaders who value EIP and when they are members of a health team that values

getting current evidence to set clear goals and using recommended interventions (White & Spruce, 2015).

Organizational Culture

A culture respecting "best practice" must be created. Administrators who build consensus toward use of EIP are likely to work with nurses who value and use clinical practice guidelines. Clear interprofessional communication is also an important component (Jun et al., 2016).

 DEVELOPING AN EVIDENCE-INFORMED PRACTICE (EIP)

EIP is built on finding, analyzing, and applying empirical findings alongside clinical expertise and person/family preferences and values that will help solve person-care problems. Acceptance of new care techniques is based on analysis of multiple findings. For teaching purposes, the authors often present findings from just one study. So let's consider a study from Atlantic Canada. See if you can find other sources to validate these study findings. This study was designed to assess nursing students' Facebook activity and their perceptions about accountability, confidentiality, and e-professionalism in relation to Facebook. Barnable et al., (2018) conducted a descriptive study design using a revised survey based on the Cain Survey, Pharmacy Students Use of and Attitudes toward Facebook. The survey questions explored students' perceptions of accountability, e-professionalism, and confidentiality related to Facebook. Students in years 1 through 4 were recruited, with 97 completing the survey. For comparative analysis and as a result of low sample size, student responses were examined in two groups (students completing years 1 and 2 in one group with those in years 3 and 4 in the second group), and T-tests were performed.

Findings: The findings indicated that most students (96.9%) had a Facebook account and recognized they needed to be accountable for unprofessional behaviour posted on their personal site. Half of the students (49%) believed that employers should not access and use information posted on their personal Facebook sites to inform hiring decisions. Findings also demonstrated that students might not fully understand what type of behaviours are unprofessional on Facebook and the consequences of breaching the person's confidentiality.

These findings suggest that content and strategies on how to appropriately use and be aware of professional violations, potential risks, and safeguards on social media sites such as Facebook need to be incorporated into nursing education programs throughout the years of the program.

(Continued)

DEVELOPING AN EVIDENCE-INFORMED PRACTICE (EIP)—cont'd

Application to Your Clinical Practice

Examine the quality of this research. Are these findings valid? Do you have a Facebook site? Try Googling your name and find out what information about you and how many pictures of you appear. Do any of the pictures reflect an unprofessional image? Are privacy issues and professionalism covered in your nursing courses in a way that made an impact on behaviour? Authors such as Sinclair et al. (2015) write that social media platforms are very useful to students, both for learning and for support. In fact, empirical data show student use of social media helps coping with stress (Warshawski et al., 2017). With constant advances in social media, the blurring of boundaries between personal and professional roles is happening in many professions. Reflect on whether a person's posts could lead to harm. Apply the guidelines in Table 3.2 to your practice.

Social media sites are increasingly being used for health education, knowledge translation, and support groups. What do you need to know about these social media sites before using them and recommending them to others?

Nursing Process

The **nursing process** consists of five progressive phases: assessment, issue identification and diagnosis, outcome identification and planning, implementation, and evaluation. Fig. 3.2 illustrates how this process is central to the care of persons. As a dynamic, systematic clinical management tool, it functions as a primary means of assessing, identifying the presenting issues, planning, implementation, and evaluation of nursing care to achieve specific health goals. Continual and timely communication is a component of each step in the nursing process. Specifically, communication plays a role in the following:

- Establishing and maintaining a therapeutic relationship
- Helping the person to promote, maintain, or restore health or to achieve a peaceful death
- Facilitating the person's management of difficult health care issues
- Providing quality nursing care in a safe and efficient manner

The nursing process is closely aligned with meeting professional nursing standards in providing total care. Table 3.3 illustrates the relationship. The nursing process begins with your first encounter with a person and family and ends with discharge or referral. Although there is an ordered sequence of nursing activities, each phase is flexible, flowing into and overlapping with other phases of the nursing process. For example, in providing a designated nursing intervention, you might discover a more complex need than what was originally assessed. This could require a modification in the identification of the issues and nursing diagnosis, the identified outcome, the intervention, or the need for a referral.

You employ communication skills in each step. From introducing yourself and explaining the purpose during initial assessment all the way through the nurse–person interaction. Refer to any nursing fundamentals textbook for a full discussion on the nursing process.

TABLE 3.2 Guidelines for Nurses Using Social Media	
Principles	**Actions**
Posts are bound by confidentiality and privacy laws within each province and territory.	Refrain from posting identifiable personal information. This absolutely applies to photos and videos. It applies even if you do not show the person's face.
Professional ethical standards need to be followed.	Separate personal from professional information; use two separate accounts. Observe professional boundaries. Do not cross from professional into social friendships.
Social media sites are public forums. Legal liability laws apply. Clicking on "restricted access" does not qualify as a private site.	Any disparaging comments are considered cyber bullying." Use the highest privacy settings. Understand that colleagues, employers, and even people you care for may read your posts.
Laws and nursing ethical codes and standards apply to online information. Provincial and territorial regulatory associations act on complaints.	Social media is permanent and universal. For example, Tweets may be retweeted. Civil, criminal, and professional penalties may apply.

TABLE 3.3 Relationship of the Nursing Process to Professional Nursing Standards in the Nurse–Person Relationship

Nursing Process	Related Nursing Standard
Nursing Process: Assessment Collects data/information from: • Person's history/interview • Observations, physical examination • Family members • Past records and tests • Other members of health team	The nurse collects data throughout the nursing process related to the person's strengths, limitations, available resources, and changes in the person's condition.
Analyzes data	The nurse organizes cluster behaviours and makes inferences based on subjective and objective data, combined with personal and scientific nursing knowledge.
Verifies data	The nurse verifies data and inferences with the person to ensure validity.
Nursing Process: Diagnosis Identifies health care needs and issues and formulates a statement describing the identified health care needs and issues	The nurse develops comprehensive statements that capture the essence of the person's health care needs and problems. The nurse validates the accuracy of the statement with the person and family; these statement becomes the basis for nursing interventions.
Nursing Process: Outcome Identification and Planning Prioritizes health care needs and issues	The nurse prioritizes health care needs and issues based on the most immediate needs in the current health care situation.
Identifies health goals and outcomes Selects nursing interventions Communicates nursing care plan	The nurse and person mutually and realistically develop expected outcomes based on the person's needs, strengths, and resources. Considers the consequences of each nursing intervention and chooses dependent, independent, and collaborative interventions to achieve the stated goal. Communicates with the intra- and interprofessional health care team on the nursing care plan.
Nursing Process: Implementation Takes appropriate nursing action interventions Nursing interventions alter person's status and symptoms	The nurse encourages, supports, and validates the person in taking agreed-on action to achieve goals and expected outcomes through integrated, therapeutic nursing interventions and communication strategies.
Nursing Process: Evaluation Evaluates goal achievement Nurse states expected outcome and is quickly able to identify the person's current status	The nurse and person mutually evaluate attainment of expected outcomes and survey each step of the nursing process for appropriateness, effectiveness, adequacy, and time efficiency. Modifies the plan if evaluation shows expected outcome not achieved.

Adapted from NANDA, North American Nursing Diagnosis Association; *NOC,* Nursing Outcomes Classification. (2015). Gregory, D., Raymond-Seniuk, C., Patrick, L. et al. *Fundamentals: Perspectives on the Art and Science of Canadian Nursing.* Wolters Kluwer.

Prioritize

One method to assist nurses to assess and identify goals and objectives is through using Maslow's hierarchy of needs as a framework to identify client needs and prioritize nursing interventions. Examples of nursing issues associated with each level of Maslow's hierarchy are included in Table 3.4. Priority attention should be given to the most immediate, life-threatening problems. Use communication skills to validate these priorities with the person and health team. Try Simulation Exercise 3.2 to practise considering cultural contexts, age, and gender-related themes when using the nursing process with different people.

Use communication skills to collaborate with health team members and with the person and family members as you implement the nursing process. Your communication skills help you collaborate with the person to provide safe, quality care.

After using your communication skills to obtain feedback from the person, contrasting actual progress with expected outcomes, analyze factors that might have effected goal achievement. Communicate with team members to modify interventions, as needed.

ISSUES IN APPLICATION OF ETHICAL AND LEGAL GUIDELINES

Moral Distress

The Canadian Nurses Association (2017) describes **moral distress** occurring when nurses, guided by their own moral judgement, are not able to do what they believe is the right thing to do. This can happen as a result of system structures, issues related to the person, personal limitations, or a combination of these reasons. Nurses can then experience physical and emotional suffering, resulting in feelings of anger, frustration, and guilt. While negative consequences can occur, moral distress can also lead to self-reflection, growth, and advocacy.

TABLE 3.4   Identifying Nursing Problems and Issues Associated with Maslow's Hierarchy of Needs

Physiological survival needs	Circulation, food, intake and output, physical comfort, rest
Safety and security needs	Domestic abuse, fear, anxiety, environmental hazards, housing
Love and belonging	Lack of social support, loss of significant person or pet, grief
Self-esteem needs	Loss of job, inability to perform normal activities, change in position or expectations
Self-actualization	Inability to achieve personal goals

SIMULATION EXERCISE 3.2   Using the Nursing Process as a Framework in Clinical Situations

Purpose

To help develop skills in considering cultural, age, and gender role issues in assessing each person's situation and identifying health care needs and issues

Procedure

1. In groups of three to four students, role-play how you might assess and incorporate differences in person and family values, knowledge, beliefs, and cultural background in delivery of care for each of the people described below. Indicate what other types of information you would need to make a complete assessment.
2. Identify and prioritize health care needs and issues for each to ensure person-centred care.
   - Michael Sterns was in a skiing accident. He is suffering from multiple internal injuries, including a head injury. His parents have been notified and are flying in to be with him.
   - Lo Sun Chen is a young Chinese woman admitted for abdominal surgery. She has been in this country for only 8 weeks and speaks very little English.
   - Maris LaFonte is a 17-year-old woman admitted for the delivery of her first baby. She has had no prenatal care.
   - Stella Watkins is an 85-year-old woman admitted to a nursing home after she broke a hip.

Analytical Reflection and Discussion

1. The needs of each person can be different, based on age, gender role, and cultural background. Explain how you account for these differences.
2. Describe any common themes in the types of information each group decided it needed to make a complete assessment.
3. Construct a scenario demonstrating your use of the knowledge gained from this exercise to show how you would apply information in your clinical practice.

Protecting the Person's Privacy

Legal and ethical standards to protect personal health information and keep it confidential can be found in federal, provincial, and territorial legislation, governing personal health information, regulated health professions acts, health facilities, health insurance, occupational health and privacy (CNPS, 2008). Provincial and territorial nursing practice standards and the CNA Code of Ethics (2017) also specifically address the nurse's responsibility to safeguard the person's right to privacy.

Personal Health Information Acts

The CNA Code of Ethics (2017) highlights that **privacy** is a fundamental right of all individuals, and it is nurses' responsibility to recognize the importance of privacy and confidentiality in safeguarding personal, family, and community information obtained in the context of the therapeutic relationship. Nursing practice in each province and territory is guided by standards related to privacy and confidentiality associated with personal health information.

All provinces and territories have legislation regulating access to personal health information—for example, Alberta's *Health Information Act*, British Columbia's *Personal Information Protection Act*, Newfoundland and Labrador's *Personal Health Information Act*, and Ontario's *Personal Health Information Protection Act* (Keatings & Adams, 2020). Alberta Government's *Health Information Act* (2018) governs and regulates access to and the collection, use, and disclosure of health information. The Act also protects the privacy and confidentiality of health information, while enabling health information to be accessed and shared, to facilitate health services to be provided and to manage the health system. In Ontario, under the *Personal Health Information Protection Act* (PHIPA), personal health is described as any information about the client in verbal, written, or electronic form. Examples include physical and or mental health information of the person and their family history; any care provided, including the names of the care providers; or a person's health card number (College of Nurses of Ontario [CNO], 2019).

These acts guide the disclosure of health information that can only be released with express or implied consent. *Express consent* is when an individual provides an informed consent, and it cannot be obtained under fraud, deception, or coercion. An example of an *implied consent* is when the nurse provides health information to another health care provider who is involved in the person's care. This is called being in the "circle of care" (Keatings & Adams, 2020).

Ethical Responsibility to Protect the Person's Privacy in Clinical Situations

In addition to legally mandated informational privacy, informal protection of the person's right to control the access to one's person in clinical situations is an ethical responsibility. Simple strategies that nurses can use to protect the person's right to privacy in clinical situations include the following:

- Providing privacy for the person and family when disturbing matters are to be discussed
- Explaining procedures to the person before implementing them
- Providing a warning before entering another person's personal space (e.g., knocking or calling the person's name) and, preferably, waiting for permission to enter
- Providing an identified space for personal belongings
- Encouraging the inclusion of personal and familiar objects on the nightstand
- Decreasing direct eye contact during hands-on care
- Minimizing body exposure to what is absolutely necessary for care
- Using only the necessary number of people during any procedure
- Using touch appropriately

Confidentiality

Protecting the privacy of the person's information and confidentiality are related but separate concepts. **Confidentiality** is defined as providing *only* the information needed to provide care for the person to other health professionals who are directly involved in their care. The assurance of confidentiality reflects ethical principles such as autonomy and beneficence (Alderman, 2017). These are discussed in Chapter 4. This information on a "need to know" basis should be made clear to each person as they enter the clinical setting. Other than these individuals, the nurse must have the person's written permission to share their private communication, unless the withholding of information would result in harm to them or to someone else, or in cases where abuse is suspected. Confidential information about the person cannot be shared with the family or other interested parties without the person or designated legal substitute decision maker's written permission. Shared confidential information, unrelated to identified health care needs, should not be communicated or charted in the person's health record.

Confidentiality within the nurse–person relationship involves the nurse's legal responsibility to guard against invasion of the person's privacy related to the following:

- Releasing information to unauthorized parties

- Discussing the person's problems in public places or with people not directly involved within the circle of care or on any social media platform
- Taking pictures without consent or using the photographs without the person's permission
- Publishing data about a person in any way that makes them identifiable, without their permission

Professional Sharing of Confidential Information

Nursing reports and interdisciplinary team case conferences are acceptable forums for the discussion of health-related communications shared by persons or families. Other venues include change-of-shift reports, one-on-one conversations with other health professionals about specific care issues, and the person's approved consultations with their families. Discussion of the person's care should take place in a private room with the door closed. Only relevant information specifically related to assessment or treatment should be shared. Discussing private information casually with other health professionals, such as in the lunchroom or on social media, is an abuse of confidentiality. The ethical responsibility to maintain the person's confidentiality continues even after discharge.

Mandatory Reporting

Under certain circumstances, you are required to report the person's personal health information. Examples are child protection legislation requiring the reporting of child abuse or neglect; public health and communicable disease legislation, and disclosure of information to protect public health and safety (CNPS, 2008). A court order is needed to release information in a police investigation, such as a blood alcohol level. However, under the *Gunshot and Wounds Mandatory Reporting Act*, 2007, police must be notified about people with gunshot wounds (Keatings & Adams, 2020). Legally required mandatory disclosures may differ slightly across provinces and territories. This duty to report supersedes the person's right to confidentiality or privileged communication with a health provider. Relevant data should be released only to the appropriate agency and handled as confidential information. The information provided must be the minimum amount needed to accomplish the purposes of disclosure, and the person should be informed about what information will be disclosed, to whom, and for what reason(s).

Informed Consent

Informed consent is a focused communication process defined as when a capable person consents to a specific medical treatment after being informed by a health care practitioner of the nature and purpose of the treatment, possible alternatives, the risks and benefits of having or not having the treatment, and the opportunity to ask questions about the treatment prior to signing the consent (CNPS, 2018; Keatings & Adams, 2020).

Ethical principles such as autonomy (self-determination) and beneficence (nurse's actions promote good) are the basis for **informed consent**. Informed consent is a safety issue and a person-centred care issue, but primarily, it is a legal right. In some cases, a substitute decision maker—someone appointed or authorized by law to give consent for a specified treatment or procedure on behalf of another when the person is unable to give a consent because of physical or mental incapacity—will provide the consent (Keatings & Adams, 2020).

Responsibility for Obtaining the Consent

Whoever is performing the treatment should be the one to provide the necessary information related to the treatment, answer any questions, and obtain the consent from the person prior to performing the treatment. For example, the physician should provide the information and obtain the consent for medical or surgical interventions. Nurses implementing invasive procedures are required to provide information about the procedure to the person, answer questions, and obtain their consent. They should then document the information provided and that consent was obtained.

EIP indicates that you use more than one method for educating each person about the procedure (Mahjoub & Rutledge, 2011). Unless there is a life-threatening emergency, all persons have the right to decide about whether to consent. Internationally, part of the ICN Code of Ethics says that nurses ensure that the individual receives accurate, sufficient, and timely information, in a culturally appropriate manner, on which to base consent for care and related treatment, supporting their right to choose or refuse treatments (ICN, 2012). Box 3.3 lists elements that must be part of an informed consent for it to be legal.

Allowing the person to sign a consent form without fully understanding the meaning invalidates the legality of consent. Ending the conversation leading to the actual signing of the consent form should always include the question, "Is there anything else that you think might be helpful in making your decision?" This type of dialogue gives the person permission to ask a question or address concerns.

Nurses are accountable for verifying whether the person is able to understand and appreciate the nature and consequences of providing consent. A person who has reached the legal statutory age based on provincial or territorial legislation can consent to treatment. Some provinces and territories have created legislation lowering the age for consent in some circumstances. Some minor children who are

BOX 3.3   Elements of a Legally Valid Informed Consent

- The consent must be genuine and voluntary.
- The procedure must not be an illegal procedure.
- The consent must authorize the particular treatment or care as well as the particular caregiver.
- The consenter must have the legal capacity to consent.
- The consenter must have the necessary mental competency to consent.
- The consenter must be informed.
- The consent should be obtained without coercion, threat, or undue influence and without influence of drugs or alcohol.

Adapted from Canadian Nurses Protective Society. (2018). *Consent to treatment: The role of the nurse.* https://cnps.ca/index.php?page=101.

able to demonstrate an appreciation of the nature and consequences of treatment may be able to sign a consent for themselves (CNPS, 2018).

Substitute Decision Maker. Legislation globally stipulates that a legal guardian or substitute decision maker can provide consent for the medical treatment of adults who lack the capacity to consent on their own behalf. In most cases, legal guardians or parents must give legal consent for minor children. When assessing for mental competence, factors such as age, disease, level of consciousness, and the presence of drugs or other substances should be considered (CNPS, 2018).

Duration. There is no recommended duration of consent unless it is stipulated in the document, so a form could address repeated procedures. But a new consent form should be signed if the person's condition changes. Many agencies require that the signature on a consent form be witnessed.

Negligence. Negligence is described as the failure to take the care that a reasonable nurse in similar situations would have taken. For a nurse to be deemed negligent, not meeting the elements of duty of care, breaching standard care, and causing foreseeable harm need to have occurred (CNPS, 2004). All nurses are advised to carry their own malpractice insurance, even if their employer has coverage. Remember to document everything about changes in the person's condition, including who was notified and what outcome followed this notification.

Use of Social Media

Many people post frequently on social media platforms. Powerful sites such as Facebook, Twitter, Instagram, LinkedIn, Myspace, Snapchat, TikTok use the Internet to connect people, transforming the way they interact.

Advances

Social media is transforming traditional nurse–person interactions. Allowing us to communicate with hundreds of people simultaneously, gives us the power to provide health care information and support. We do need to differentiate between general open-to-all social sites, even with privacy settings, and secure restricted sites such as those created by care agencies for internal professional staff use. "A post is forever" is a useful mantra.

Privacy Cautions

Privacy regulations apply to you in your off-duty time as well as during clinical time. Students cannot, at any time, reveal private health information. This includes posting any pictures on social media taken in a clinical facility or during a home health care visit. Read about Cassie in the case example.

Case Example

Cassie takes great pleasure in the semester-long home visit assignment caring for Syed, age 4, who has severe cerebral palsy. She feels this is a great learning experience and that she is contributing to Syed's progress. Today, she uses her smartphone to snap a really cute picture of him enjoying his first ice cream cone and shares it with her friends, later posting it on her Facebook page.

Provincial and territorial regulatory bodies and the CNA Code of Ethics (2017) all identify the importance of a person's privacy and state that posts on social media are bound by practice standards, confidentiality, and privacy laws. Consequences for violations can be severe. Student nurses have been involuntarily withdrawn from their schools. The misuse of electronic communication also has consequences for educational programs, placing in jeopardy the school's relationship with a community agency they rely on for clinical experiences. Ensure that you review and enact your school's social media policies and your provinces or territory's professional association or regulatory body's social media standards and guidelines.

Blurring Between Professional Role and Personal Life

People have become accustomed to posting so much on social media sites that they sometimes don't stop to think about whether a posting violates a person's privacy laws or ethical nurse conduct. We need to differentiate between our personal posts and our professional duty to protect a person's privacy and confidentially, and to avoid potential harm to the person, coworkers, or employers. As Westrick (2016) comments, we need to use extreme caution when discussing any person-related experience related to our professional role. Refer to Table 3.2, which lists social media use guidelines compiled from multiple organizations to help you reflect on this issue. Beginning nursing students can have difficulty in translating a cautionary lecture about social media use into behaviour. One recommendation is to include using senior students as peer teachers as their experiences with social media problems will have greater credibility and relevance (Marnocha et al., 2017).

SUMMARY

This chapter addresses major factors affecting current nursing communication. Standards issued by various professional associations and organizations guide nurses in their communications with and about persons. Standards provide a measurement benchmark, which is used to assess nursing competency as they apply evidence-informed practice and clinical guidelines. Ethical and legal aspects of nursing communication, especially privacy regulations in each province or territory, have been described. The CASN standards related to communication and CNA's *Code of Ethics for Registered Nurses* provide important guides to the choice of communication. The nursing process serves as a clinical management framework as communication is woven into each of the steps. All phases are person-centred, where the person and family are active participants and decision makers. The importance of maintaining the person's privacy and confidentiality have been stressed, especially with regard to posts on social media platforms.

🔍 ETHICAL DILEMMA

What Would You Do?

As a student nurse, you observe a staff nurse making a medication error, but you are not able to intervene. She is visibly upset by her error. The person was not actually harmed by the medication error, but the nurse hesitates to report the error. What would you do?

QUESTIONS FOR REVIEW AND DISCUSSION

1. Identify three ways to communicate effectively with each member of the person's health care team.

2. Assemble some examples of nurses choosing not to follow written standards for communication, and then critique these examples.

REFERENCES

Alberta Government. (2018). *Health Information Act.* https://open.alberta.ca/publications/h05.

Alderman, E. M. (2017). Confidentiality in pediatric and adolescent gynecology: When we can, when we can't, and when we're challenged. *Journal of Pediatric & Adolescent Gynecology, 30*(2), 176–183.

Al-Mowani, M., Al-Barmawi, M. A., Al-Hadid, L. et al. (2016). Developing a tool that explores factors influencing the adoption of evidence-based principles in nursing practice in Jordan. *Applied Nursing Research, 32,* 122–127.

American Nurses Association. (2010). *Nursing: Scope and standards of practice* (2nd ed.). Author. www.nursingworld.org/practice-policy/nursing_excellence/ethicsfornurses/code-of-ethics.

Barnable, A., Cunning, G., & Parcon, M. (2018). Nursing students' perceptions of confidentiality, accountability and e-professionalism in relation to Facebook. *Nurse Educator, 43*(1), 28–31.

Barnsteiner, J., Disch, J., Johnson, J. et al. (2013). Diffusing QSEN competencies across Schools of Nursing: The AACN/RWJF faculty development institutes. *Journal of Professional Nursing, 29*(2), 1–8.

British Columbia College of Nursing Professionals. (2019). Standards: Harmonized standards. https://www.bccnp.ca/Standards/all_nurses/harmonized/Pages/Default.aspx.

Canadian Association of Schools of Nursing. (n.d.). *CASN Mission.* https://www.casn.ca/about-casn/casnacesi-mission/.

Canadian Association of Schools of Nursing. (2015). *National nursing education framework: Final report.* https://www.casn.ca/wp-content/uploads/2014/12/Framwork-FINAL-SB-Nov-30-20151.pdf.

Canadian Association of Schools of Nursing. 2018. *Learning outcomes for patient safety in undergraduate nursing curricula.* https://www.casn.ca/wp-content/uploads/2018/08/CPSI-EN-FINAL-r-Apr-2019.pdf.

Canadian Nurses Association. (n.d.-a). *Our members.* https://www.cna-aiic.ca/en/about-us/our-members.

Canadian Nurses Association. (n.d.-b). *Barriers to nursing: Evidence-based practice/evidence-informed decision making.* https://www.cna-aiic.ca/en/nursing-practice/evidence-based-practice/barriers-to-nursing.

Canadian Nurses Association. (2017). *Code of ethics for registered nurses.* https://www.cna-aiic.ca/~/media/cna/page-content/pdf-en/code-of-ethics-2017-edition-secure-interactive.

Canadian Nurses Protective Society. (2004). Negligence. https://cnps.ca/index.php?page=78.

Canadian Nurses Protective Society. (2008). Confidentiality of Health Information. https://www.cnps.ca/index.php?page=104..

Canadian Nurses Protective Society. (2018). Consent to treatment: The role of the nurse. https://cnps.ca/index.php?page=101.

Canadian Patient Safety Institute. (2008). The safety competencies: Enhancing patient safety across the health professions. https://www.patientsafetyinstitute.ca/en/toolsResources/safetyCompetencies/Documents/CPSI-SafetyCompetencies_EN_Digital.pdf.

Ciliska, D. (2012). *Introduction to evidence-informed decision making.* Canadian Institute of Health Research. https://cihr-irsc.gc.ca/e/documents/Introduction_to_EIDM.pdf.

Clark, M., Raffray, M., Hendricks, K. et al. (2016). Global and public health core competencies for nursing education: A systematic review of essential competencies. *Nurse Education Today, 40,* 173–180.

College & Association of Registered Nurses of Alberta. (2013). *Practice standards for regulated members.* https://nurses.ab.ca/docs/default-source/document-library/standards/practice-standards-for-regulated-members.pdf?sfvrsn=d4893bb4_12.

College of Licensed Practical Nurses of Prince Edward Island. (2013). *Standards of practice for licensed practical nurses in Canada.* http://clpnpei.ca/wp-content/uploads/2018/04/LPN-Standards-of-Practice-CLPNPEI.pdf.

College of Nurses of Ontario. (2019). Practice standard: Confidentiality and privacy—Personal health information. https://www.cno.org/globalassets/docs/prac/41069_privacy.pdf.

College of Registered Nurses of Newfoundland and Labrador. (2019). *Standards of practice for registered nurses and nurse practitioners.* https://www.crnnl.ca/sites/default/files/documents/Standards_of_Practice_for%20RNs_and_NPs.pdf.

College of Registered Psychiatric Nurses of Manitoba. (2019). *Standards of psychiatric nursing practice.* https://www.crpnm.mb.ca/wp-content/uploads/2019/10/Standards-of-Psychiatric-Nursing-Practice-FINAL-October-2019.pdf.

Gill, F. J., Kendrick, T., Davies, H., et al. (2016). A two phase study to revise the Australian Practice Standards for specialist critical care nurses. *Australian Critical Care,* e1–e9. www.elsevier.com/locate/aucc.

International Council of Nurses. (2012). *The ICN code of ethics for nurses: Revised 2012.* http://www.old.icn.ch/images/stories/documents/about/icncode_english.pdf.

Jun, J., Kovner, C. T., & Stimpfel, A. W. (2016). Barriers and facilitators of nurses' use of clinical practice guidelines: An integrative review. *International Journal of Nursing Studies, 60,* 54–68.

Keatings, M., & Adams, P. (2020). *Ethical and legal issues in Canadian nursing* (4th ed.). Elsevier.

Leung, K., Trevena, L., & Waters, D. (2016). Development of a competency framework for evidence-based practice in nursing. *Nurse Education Today, 39,* 189–196.

LoBiondo-Wood, G., Haber, J., Cameron, C., et al. (2018). *Nursing research in Canada: Methods, critical appraisal and utilization* (4th ed.). Elsevier.

Mackey, A., & Bassendowski, S. (2017). The history of evidence-based practice in nursing education and practice. *Journal of Professional Nursing, 33*(1), 51–54. https://doi.org/10.1016/j.profnurs.2016.05.009.

Mahjoub, R., & Rutledge, D. N. (2011). Perceptions of informed consent for care practices: Hospitalized patients and nurses. *Applied Nursing Research, 24*(4), 1–6.

Marnocha, S., Marnocha, M., Cleveland, R. et al. (2017). A peer-delivered educational intervention to improve nursing student cyberprofessionalism. *Nurse Educator, 42*(5), 245–249.

Melynk, B. M. (2014). Evidence-based practice versus evidence-informed practice: A debate that could stall forward momentum in improving healthcare quality, safety, patient outcomes and cost. *Worldviews on Evidence-Based Nursing, 11*(6), 347–349.

Melnyk, B. M., Fineout-Overholt, E., Stillwell, S. B. et al. (2010). Evidence-based practice: Step by step: The seven steps of evidence-based practice. *American Journal of Nursing, 110*(1), 51–53.

Mick, J. (2017). Call to action: How to implement evidence-based nursing practice. *Nursing 2017, 47*(4). www.Nursing2017.com.

Nurses Association of New Brunswick. (2019). *Nursing Standards.* http://www.nanb.nb.ca/media/resource/NANB2019-RNPracticeStandards-E-web.pdf

Nursing & Midwifery Council. (2015). *The code: Professional standards of practice and behaviour for nurses, midwives and nursing associates.* https://www.nmc.org.uk/globalassets/sitedocuments/nmc-publications/nmc-code.pdf.

Sackett, D., Rosenberg, W. M., Muir, G. J. A. et al. (1996). Evidence-based medicine: What it is and what it isn't. *British Medical Journal, 312,* 71–72. http://www.bmj.com/content/312/7023/71.

Saunders, H., Vehvilainen-Julkunen, K., & Stevens, K. R. (2016). Effectiveness of an educational intervention to strengthen nurses' readiness for evidence-based practice: A single-blind randomized controlled study. *Applied Nursing Research, 31,* 175–185.

Shahid, S., & Thomas, S. (2018). Situation, background, assessment, recommendation (SBAR) communication tool for handoff in health care: A narrative review. *Safety in Health, 4*(7)https://doi.org/10.1186/s40886-018-0073-1.

Sinclair, W., McLoughlin, M., & Warne, T. (2015). To Twitter to woo: Harnessing the power of social media (So Me) in nurse education to enhance the student's experience. *Nurse Education in Practice, 15,* 507–511.

Warshawski, S., Barnoy, S., & Itzhaki, M. (2017). Factors associated with nursing students' resilience: Communication skills course, use of social media, and satisfaction with clinical placement. *Journal of Professional Nursing, 33*(2), 153–161.

Westrick, S. J. (2016). Nursing students' use of electronic and social media: Law, ethics, and e-professionalism. *Nursing Education Perspectives, 37*(1), 16–22.

White, S., & Spruce, L. (2015). Perioperative nursing leaders implement clinical practice guidelines using Iowa Model of Evidence-Based Practice. *AORN Journal, 102*(1), 50–59.

4

Clinical Judgement
Critical Thinking and Ethical Decision Making

Claire Mallette

Originating US chapter by *Kathleen Underman Boggs*

OBJECTIVES

At the end of the chapter, the reader will be able to:

1. Define person-centred care communication terms related to thinking, ethical reasoning, and critical thinking.
2. Discuss three principles of ethics underlying bioethical reasoning, and apply within the nurse–person relationship.
3. Describe the 10 steps of critical thinking.
4. Analyze and apply the critical thinking process used in making clinical decisions.
5. Demonstrate ability to analyse, synthesise, and evaluate a complex simulated case situation to make a clinical judgement.
6. Utilize evidenced-informed practice competency by discussing the application of findings from research to clinical practice.

This chapter examines the principles of ethical decision making and the process for critical thinking. You will need both types of essential foundational knowledge to make effective nursing clinical judgements and deliver safe, competent care (Kaya et al., 2017). In addition to developing technical nursing skills, you will need to be able to use critical thinking and ethical reasoning skills and to communicate; these will be determining factors in your competency as a nurse (Trobec & Starcic, 2015). Successfully developing these abilities also contributes to success on the registration examinations (Romeo, 2010). Ethical responsibility is a large aspect of nursing care. It is a much wider concept than legal responsibility, engaging not only the person but also your entire community (Tschudin, 2013). Making ethical decisions requires that you understand the process. In this book, the focus is on the current literature in bioethics as held in Western society. In addition to basic content presented in this chapter, an ethical dilemma is included in each subsequent chapter to help you to begin applying your reasoning process.

Critical thinking is a learned skill that teaches you how to use a systematic process to make your clinical decisions. In the past, expert nurses accumulated this skill with on-the-job experience, through trial and error. But this essential nursing skill can be learned with continual practice and conscientious applications while in school. The Applications section of this chapter specifically walks you through the reasoning process in applying the 10 steps of critical thinking. Simulation exercises in each chapter help you practise applying these skills.

BASIC CONCEPTS

Types of Thinking

There are many methods of thinking (Fig. 4.1). Students often attempt to use total recall by simply memorizing a bunch of facts (e.g., memorizing the cranial nerves by using a mnemonic such as "On Old Olympus Towering Top . . ."). At other times, we rely on developing habits through repetition, such as practising cardiopulmonary resuscitation (CPR) techniques. More structured methods of thinking, such as inquiry, have been developed in disciplines related to nursing. For example, you are probably familiar with the scientific method. As used in research, this is a logical, linear method of systematically gaining new information, often by setting up an experiment to test an idea. The nursing process uses a method of systematic steps: assessment before planning, planning before intervention, and finally, evaluation.

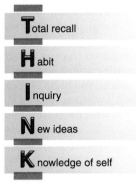

Total recall

Habit

Inquiry

New ideas

Knowledge of self

Fig. 4.1 Mnemonics can be useful tools.

TABLE 4.1 Characteristics of a Critical Thinker	
KNOWLEDGE [thought processes]	• Be reflective and anticipate consequences • Combine existing knowledge and standards with new information (transformation) • Incorporate creative thinking • Recognize when information is missing and seek new input • Discard irrelevant information (discrimination) • Effectively interpret existing data • Consider alternative solutions
SKILLS	• Think in an orderly way, using logical reasoning in complex problem situations • Thoroughly persevere in seeking relevant information • Recognize deviations from expected patterns • Revise actions based on new input • Evaluate solutions and outcomes
ATTITUDE	• Be inquisitive, desire to seek the truth • Seek to develop analytical thinking • Maintain open-mindedness and flexibility

This chapter focuses on the most important concepts that help you develop your clinical judgement abilities.

Critical Thinking

Critical thinking is the basis of all our clinical reasoning, problem solving, and decision making. Critical thinking is a complex, analytical method of thinking, in which you purposefully use specific thinking skills to make clinical decisions. You are able to reflect on your own thinking process to make effective interventions that improve the person's outcome. Although no consensus has been reached on a definition for critical thinking in nursing, we generally define it as the purposeful use of a specific cognitive framework to identify and analyze problems. Critical thinking enables us to recognize emergent situations; make clear, objective, clinical decisions; and intervene appropriately to give safe, effective care. It encompasses the steps of the nursing process, but possibly in a more circular loop than we usually envision the nursing process to involve. By thinking critically, we can modify our care based on responses to these nursing interventions.

Characteristics of a Critical Thinker in Making Clinical Decisions

PROCESS. Critical thinkers are skilled at using inquiry methods. They approach problem solutions in a systematic, organized, and goal-directed way when making clinical decisions. They continually use past knowledge, communication skills, new information, and observations to make these clinical judgements. Table 4.1 summarizes the characteristics of a critical thinker.

ACT. Expert nurses recognize that priorities change continually, requiring constant assessment and alternative interventions. Expert nurses use knowledge, evidence-informed practice, skill level, personal characteristics, and

relationships with the people they care for to inform the critical thinking steps described in this chapter when they make their clinical judgements, even though they were not always able to verbally state the components of their thinking processes (Melin-Johansson et al., 2017). Expert nurses organized each input of the person's information and quickly distinguished relevant from irrelevant information. They seemed to categorize each new fact into a problem format, obtaining supplementary data and arriving at a decision about the issues and intervention. Often, they commented about comparing this new information with prior knowledge, sometimes from academic sources and "best practice protocols" but most often from information gained from other nurses. They constantly scan for new information and constantly reassess the person's situation. This kind of thinking is not linear; new input is always being added. This contrasts with the thinking of novice nurses who tend to think in a linear way, collect lots of facts but not logically organize them, and fail to make as many connections with past knowledge as more experienced nurses. Novice nurses' assessments are more generalized and less focused, and they tend to jump too quickly to identification of an issue without recognizing the need to obtain more information.

REFLECT. Critical thinking is more than just a cognitive process of following steps. It also has an affective component—the willingness to engage in self-reflective inquiry. Most nurse educators say this sense of inquiry is crucial (Carter et al., 2016). As you learn to be a critical thinker, you improve and clarify your thinking process skills, reflect on this process, and learn from the situation so that you are more accurately able to solve problems based on available evidence (Johnsen et al., 2016). An attitude of openness to new learning is essential. Although cognitive thinking skills can be taught, you also need to be willing to consciously choose to apply this process.

Barriers to Thinking Critically and Reasoning Ethically

Attitudes and Habits

Barriers that decrease a nurse's ability to think critically, including attitudes such as "my way is better," interfere with our ability to empower persons to make their own decisions. Our values and beliefs and our conscious and unconscious biases can also impede communication with persons or families making complex bioethical choices. Examples include becoming accustomed to acknowledging "only one right answer" or selecting only one option. Behaviours that act as barriers include automatically responding defensively when challenged, resisting changes, and desiring to conform to expectations. Cognitive barriers, such as thinking in stereotypes, also interfere with our ability to treat a person as an individual.

Cognitive Dissonance

Cognitive dissonance refers to the mental discomfort you feel when there is a discrepancy between what you already believe and some new information that does not go along with your thinking. In this book, we use the term to refer to the holding of two or more conflicting values at the same time.

Personal Values Versus Professional Values

We all have a personal value system developed over a lifetime that has been extensively shaped by forces such as race, culture, gender, age, sexual orientation, economic and political forces, and years of life experiences (this will be discussed in greater detail in Chapter 7). Our values

change as we mature in our ability to think critically, logically, and morally. Strongly held values become a part of our self-concept.

Our education as nurses helps us acquire a professional value system. In nursing school, as you advance through your clinical experiences, you begin to take on some of the values of the nursing profession (Box 4.1). You are acquiring these values as you learn the nursing role. The process of this role socialization is discussed in Chapter 23. For example, maintaining confidentiality is a professional value, with both a legal and a moral requirement. We must take care that we do not allow our personal values to obstruct care for a person who holds differing values.

Values Clarification and the Nursing Process

The nursing process offers many opportunities to incorporate values clarification into your care. During the assessment phase, you can obtain an assessment of the person's values in regard to the health system. For example, you interview Mr. Fletcher for the first time and learn that he has chronic obstructive pulmonary disease and is having difficulty breathing, but he insists on smoking. Is it appropriate to intervene? In this example, you know that smoking is detrimental to a person's health and you, as a nurse, find the value of health in conflict with his value of smoking. It is important to understand the person's values. When your values differ, you attempt to care for this person within their reality. In this example, Mr. Fletcher has the right to make decisions that are not always congruent with those of health care providers.

When identifying specific health issues, it is important that your assessments and identification of issues or

---

BOX 4.1   Seven Core Values and Ethical Responsibilities of Professional Nursing

Seven core values and ethical responsibilities of professional nursing have been identified by the Canadian Nurses Association (2017):

1. Providing safe, compassionate, competent, and ethical care
2. Promoting health and well-being
3. Promoting and respecting informed decision-making
4. Honouring dignity
5. Maintaining privacy and confidentiality
6. Promoting justice
7. Being accountable

Canadian Nurses Association. (2017). *Code of Ethics for registered nurses.* (p.3). https://www.cna-aiic.ca/~/media/cna/page-content/pdf-en/code-of-ethics-2017-edition-secure-interactive.

problems are not biased by your own personal values. An example of a value conflict might be spiritual distress related to a conflict between spiritual beliefs and prescribed health treatments. In the planning phase, it is important to identify and understand the person's value system as the foundation for developing the most appropriate interventions. Plans of care that support rather than ignore the person's health care beliefs are more likely to be received favourably. Your interventions include values clarification as a guideline for care. You help people examine alternatives. During the evaluation phase, examine how well the nursing and person goals were met while keeping within the guidelines of the person's value system.

To summarize, in case of conflict (with their own personal ethical values and beliefs), nurses must put these aside to provide necessary assistance in a case of emergency, when there is imminent risk to a person's life. Critical thinking and ethical reasoning skills are essential competencies for making clinical judgements, in an increasingly complex health care system. To apply critical thinking to a clinical decision, we need to base our intervention on the best evidence available. Developing higher levels of critical thinking is a learned ability (Van Graan et al., 2016).

ETHICAL REASONING

Quality nursing care, in part, depends on nursing values and ethics (Trobec & Starcic, 2015). Nurses identify persons' well-being and dignity as an important value related to giving care. They report feeling distress when forced to act in a way that is contrary to what they believe is the person's best interests (Gronlund et al., 2015). Yet, we nurses often face moral dilemmas while giving care. Most nurses report facing ethical dilemmas at least on a weekly basis. As care becomes even more complex, we will be confronted even more often (Sinclair et al., 2016). The three most commonly reported issues involve a person's choice, quality of life, and end-of-life decisions. As a nurse, you will frequently have to act in value-laden situations. For example, you may have a person who requests a "do not resuscitate" (DNR; "no code") order or refuses a lifesaving treatment. Willingness to comply with ethical and professional standards is a hallmark of a professional.

Many professions have difficulty applying ethical principles to clinical care situations. When tested, health care providers, including nurses, often do not respond correctly to questions about how to address ethical dilemmas. Is not being ethically correct acceptable? Practice in applying ethical principles is important. Although most health care organizations now have ethics committees that often have the primary responsibility of resolving difficult ethical

dilemmas, you, the nurse, will be called on to make ethical decisions.

As nurses, we need to have a clear understanding of the ethics of the nursing profession. Most if not all nursing organizations have formally published ethical codes to promote ethical care and protect person rights. Examples include the Canadian Nurses Association [CNA] (2017); the Nursing & Midwifery Council (2015); and the American Nurses Association (ANA) (2015).

Refer to your provincial or territorial regulatory association's ethics practice standards and CNA's Code of Ethics, described in Chapter 3.

Case Example

During the coronavirus (COVID-19) disease pandemic in 2020, Ivan Holder, RN, is reassigned to work on an unfamiliar pulmonary intensive care unit. Persons on the unit have the COVID-19 virus and some are receiving mechanical ventilation. He worries that if he refuses to care for these persons, he could lose his job or even his nursing registration. But he also fears carrying this infection home to his two preschool children.

This case highlights conflicting duties: employer–person versus self–family. According to the CNA and provincial and territorial nursing standards, nurses are obligated to care for all persons, but there are limits to the personal risk of harm nurses can be expected to accept. It is their moral duty to care for people if they are at significant risk for harm that nursing care can prevent. Choosing not to provide care becomes a moral option only if there are alternative sources of care (i.e., other nurses available).

Ethical Theories and Decision-Making Models

Ethics is study of questions that are morally good or bad or are morally right or wrong. Ethical theories provide the bedrock from which we derive the principles that guide our decision making. There is no one "right" answer to an ethical dilemma—the decision may vary depending on which theory the involved people subscribe to. The following section briefly describes the most common decision-making models currently used in bioethics. They are, for the most part, representative of a Western European and Judeo-Christian viewpoint. As we are more culturally diverse, other equally worthwhile viewpoints will need to be considered. This discussion focuses on three decision-making models: utilitarian or goal-based, duty-based, and rights-based models.

The **utilitarian or goal-based model** says that the "rightness" or "wrongness" of an action is always a function of its consequences. Rightness is the extent to which performing or omitting an action will contribute to the overall good of the person. *Good* is defined as maximum welfare or happiness. The rights of persons and the responsibilities of a nurse are determined by what will achieve maximum welfare. When a conflict in possible outcomes occurs, the correct action is the one that will result in the greatest good for the majority. An example of a decision made according to the goal-based model is vaccinating people against communicable diseases to protect the individual and other members of the community. Vaccinating people produces the greatest balance of good over harm for the majority. Thus, the "goodness" of an action is determined solely by its outcome.

The **deontological model (duty-based model)** is person centred. It incorporates Immanuel Kant's deontological philosophy, which holds that the "rightness" of an action is determined by other factors in addition to its outcome. Respect for every person's inherent dignity is a consideration. For example, a straightforward implication would be that a nurse or other health care provider will always be honest with a person. Do you agree? Decisions based on this duty-based model have a spiritual–social foundation. Rightness is determined by moral worth, regardless of the circumstances or the individual involved. In making decisions or implementing actions, the nurse cannot violate the basic responsibilities and rights of individuals. Decisions about what is in the best interests of the person require consensus among all parties involved. Examples are the code "do no harm" and the nursing responsibility to "help save lives."

The **human rights–based model** is based on the belief that each person has basic rights. Our responsibilities as health care providers arise from these basic rights. For example, a person has the right to refuse care. Conflict arises when the provider's duty is not in the best interests of the person. The person has the right to life and the nurse has the responsibility to care for the person, but what if the quality of life is intolerable and there is no hope for a positive outcome?

Feminist ethics recognizes that moral dilemmas involve human relationships, with a greater emphasis on values, feelings, and desires and on creating a path to end social and political oppression of women. Moral perspectives are also important when caring for Indigenous peoples. Regardless of the ethical theory being followed, when caring for any individual, what is most important is that nurses cannot assume that there are common moral values and beliefs assumed by all people within a community (Keatings & Adams, 2020).

Ethical dilemma (also moral dilemma) arise when an actual or potential conflict occurs regarding principles, duties, or rights. Of course, many ethical or moral concepts have been codified into law. Laws may vary by country and region, but a moral principle should be universally applied. Moral principles are shared by most members of a group, such as nurses and other health care providers, and represent the professional values of the group. Conflict arises when a nurse's professional values differ from the law. Conflict may also arise when you have not come to terms with situations in which your personal values differ from the profession's values or the person's values. One example is medical assistance in dying (MAID).

Case Example

Si Wu has a diagnosis of pancreatic cancer that will gradually leave her unable to do any activities of daily living. She believes she has the right to choose when she will end her life. *Legally*, Ms. Wu may qualify for medical assistance in dying (MAID). *Professionally*, the CNA Code of Ethics (2017) guides you to work with a person to attain their highest possible level of health and well-being. *Personally*, you believe medically assisted dying is morally wrong. Can you assist Ms. Wu by providing information on MAID?

Bioethical Principles

Ethics questions how human beings should treat one another, shape societies, explore how to respond in certain situations, and examine moral actions and judgements. Bioethics focuses on ethical issues in health care, with advances in scientific knowledge, technology, and practice (Collier & Haliburton, 2015). To practise nursing in an ethical manner, you must be able to recognize the existence of a moral issue. Once you recognize a situation that puts the person in jeopardy, you must be able to take action. Three essential guiding, ethical principles have been developed from the theories cited earlier. The three principles that can assist us in decision making are autonomy, beneficence (maleficence), nonmaleficence, and justice (Fig. 4.2).

Autonomy and the Illness Experience. **Autonomy** is the person's right to self-determination. In the health care context, respect for autonomy is a fundamental ethical principle. It is the basis for the concept of informed consent, which means the person makes a rational, informed decision without coercion. In the past, nurses and other health care providers often made decisions for persons based on what they thought was best for them. This authoritarianism discounted the wishes of persons and their families. The ethical concept of autonomy has emerged strongly as a right. Aspects involving the individual's right to participate in health care decisions about their own care are now recognized as part of ethical standards of practice.

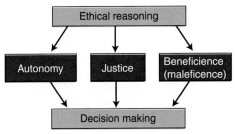

Fig. 4.2 Guiding ethical principles that assist in decision making

This moral principle of autonomy means that persons have the right to decide about their health care. Persons who are empowered to make such decisions are more likely to participate in the treatment plan. Internal factors, such as pain, may interfere with a person's ability to choose. External factors, such as coercion by a care provider or family member, may also interfere. As a nurse, you and your employer must legally obtain the person's permission for all treatment procedures. In Canada, each province and territory has legislation related to consent of health care treatments, such as the *Health Care Consent Act* (1996), in Ontario. Nurses, as well as other health care providers, must provide persons with all the relevant and accurate information, such as benefits, risks, and expected outcomes; they need to make an "informed" decision about whether they agree to treatments (College of Nurses of Ontario [CNO], 2017). Nursing codes, such as the CNA Code of Ethics (2017), state that the "nurse recognizes, respects, and promotes a person's right to be informed to make the right decisions" (p. 11), as discussed in Chapter 3 (see section "Informed Consent").

Many of the nursing theories incorporate concepts about autonomy and empowering the person to be responsible for self-care, so you may find this easy to accept as part of your nursing role. However, what happens if the person's right to autonomy puts others at risk? Whose rights take precedence?

The concept of autonomy also has been applied to the way we practise nursing, but our professional autonomy has limitations. According to the CNA Code of Ethics (2017) and provincial and territorial standards of practice, nurses are ethically obligated to care for persons in need of health care. A nurse has autonomy in caring for a person, but this is somewhat limited because, legally, nurses must also follow physician orders and be subject to policies and regulations. Before the nurse or other health care providers can override a person's right to autonomy, they must be able to present a strong case for their point of view, based on either or both of the following principles: beneficence and justice.

Autonomy Case Example

Mrs. Dorothy Newt, 72 years of age, refuses to be placed in a long-term care facility after being diagnosed with early onset Alzheimer's disease. Instead, she wants to rely on her aged, disabled spouse to provide her total care as she deteriorates physically and mentally. As her home health nurse, you find her husband is unable to provide the needed care and both are deteriorating in health. What do you do?

Beneficence and Nonmaleficence

Beneficence implies that a decision results in the greatest good or benefit to the person and for the greatest number of people. Avoiding actions that bring harm—"do no harm"—to another person is known as **nonmaleficence**. Nonmaleficence involves providing competent care and minimizing harm.

In health care, beneficence is the underlying principle in nursing codes of ethics, saying that the good of the person is your primary responsibility. Nursing theorists have incorporated this concept into the nursing role, so you may find this easy to accept. Helping others may be why you chose to become a nurse. In nursing, you have the obligation to provide the best nursing care, avoid harming the people you care for, and advocate for their best interests.

Beneficence can be challenged in many clinical situations (e.g., a person requesting all lifesaving treatments be stopped). Currently, some of the most difficult ethical dilemmas involve situations where decisions may be made to withhold treatment. These types of decisions then need to be justified in that such violations of beneficence are done guided by ethics and person autonomy.

Beneficence can be challenged when the involved parties hold different viewpoints about what is best for the person. Consider a case in which the family of a person who is older, post-stroke, comatose, and ventilator-dependent wants all forms of treatment continued, but the health care team does not believe it will benefit the person. The initial step toward resolution may be to hold a family conference and really listen to the viewpoints of family members, asking them whether their relative ever expressed wishes verbally or in writing in the form of an advance directive or living will. Maintaining a trusting, open, mutually respectful communication may help avoid an adversarial situation.

Beneficence Case Example

Mr. Rossi, 62 years of age, is admitted with end-stage organ failure (damage to major organs such as the heart, kidney or brain). You are expected to assess for any pain he may have and treat it. Do you seek a palliative order even though his liver cannot process drugs?

It is estimated that more than 50% of conscious persons spend their last week of life in moderate to severe pain. Who is advocating for them?

Justice

Justice refers to fairness for individuals and groups. A related concept is equality (e.g., the just distribution of goods or resources, sometimes called *social justice* or *distributive justice*). Within the health care arena, this distributive justice concept might be applied to scarce treatment resources. As new and more expensive technologies that can prolong life become available, who has a right to them? Who should pay for them? If resources are scarce, how do we decide who gets them? Should a limited resource be spread out equally to everyone? Or should it be allocated based on who has the greatest need (equity)?

Unnecessary Treatment. Decisions made based on the principle of justice may also involve the concept of unnecessary treatment. Are all operations that are performed truly necessary? Why do some persons receive antibiotics for viral infections, when we know they do not kill viruses? Are unnecessary diagnostic tests ever ordered solely to document that a person does not have a specific condition, in case questions arise in the future related to errors of omission or malpractice?

Social Worth. Another justice concept to consider in making decisions is that of social worth. Are all people equal? Are some more deserving than others? If Nasrin is 7 years old instead of 77 years old, and the expensive medication would cure his condition, should these factors affect the decision to give him the medication? If there is only one liver available for a transplant, and there are two equally viable potential recipients—Daryus, age 54 years, whose alcoholism destroyed his own liver; or Esohe, age 32 years, whose liver was destroyed by hepatitis she got while on a life-saving mission abroad—who should get the liver?

Veracity. Truthfulness is the bedrock of trust. And trust is an essential component of the professional nurse–person relationship. Not only is there a moral imperative against not telling the truth, but it is also destructive to any professional relationship. Generally, nurses would agree that a nurse should always be truthful with a person. However, there can be ethical dilemmas in relation to withholding information. For example, other than nurse practitioners, nurses are guided by their provincial or territorial Regulated Health Professions Act, which does not allow them to communicate a diagnosis to a person. Situations occur where the nurse knows important information about the person, such as someone returning from surgery with a terminal cancer diagnosis, yet the nurse cannot say anything about the diagnosis until the physician has spoken to the person. Nurses then may face an ethical dilemma, when the person, or family members, or both ask if the nurse has heard any results from the surgery. Nurses have evaded questions like this by responding, "You will have to ask your physician about this." Nurses may feel that they are not being truthful, yet they are bound by their professional standards of practice. Can you suggest another response when asked questions such as this?

Justice Case Example

Lee, age 18 years, is admitted to the emergency department (ED) bleeding from a chest wound. His blood pressure is falling, and shock is imminent. Taranpreet, Sue, and Zohra were registered ahead of Lee but do not have life-threatening concerns. ED's **triage** protocol says that care for the least stable person is a priority. Is this a "just distribution" of ED resources?

Steps in Ethical Decision Making

The process of moral reasoning and making ethical decisions has been broken down into steps. These steps are only a part of the larger model for critical thinking. If you are the moral agent making this decision, you must be skillful enough to implement the actions in a morally correct way.

In deciding how to spend your limited time with the people you are caring for, do you base your decision entirely on how much good you can do for each one? Under distributive justice, what should happen when the needs of the people you are caring for conflict? You could base your decision on the principle of beneficence and do the greatest good for the most persons, but this is a very subjective judgement. In using an ethical decision-making processes, nurses must be able to tolerate ambiguity and uncertainty. One of the most difficult aspects for the novice nurse to accept is that there often is no one "right" answer; rather, usually several options may be selected, depending on the person or situation. Apply these questions to the following ethical decision-making case.

Ethical Decision-Making Case Example

You are assigned to four persons in critical condition, on your unit. Mrs. Wang, 83 years of age, is unconscious and dying, and needs suctioning every 10 minutes. Mr. Kowalczyk, 47 years of age, has been admitted for observation for severe bloody stools. Mr. Hernandez, 52 years of age, has newly diagnosed diabetes and is receiving intravenous (IV) drip insulin; he requires monitoring of vital signs every 15 minutes. Mr. Singh, 35 years of age, is experiencing suicidal thoughts and has been told today he has inoperable cancer. Would one of them benefit more from nursing care than the others?

DEVELOPING AN EVIDENCE-INFORMED PRACTICE

A study was conducted with the purpose of comparing the impact of two teaching methods on ethical reasoning. Active online learning outcomes were compared with classroom teaching outcomes for 436 Slovenian nursing students. Pre- and post-tests measured comprehension and application to real-life ethical problems.

Results: After initial lectures, students developed their abilities through active engagement in group work, role-play, and discussion, either online or in the classroom. No differences were found between groups. Both methods resulted in the development of ethical competencies, communication competencies, interpersonal skills, critical thinking, and collaboration. Online students reported that they missed face-to-face contact, which reveals much via nonverbal communication.

Application to practice: This type of active learning has also been shown to help students develop their critical thinking skills needed for clinical reasoning (Costello, 2017). In this study's active learning environment, students cited the importance of collaboration and communication in developing their own learning. If we apply this factor to a person's learning, it suggests a need to actively engage persons in their learning process.

Clinical decision: We need to base our intervention on *the best evidence available* to provide quality care. As health care becomes increasingly complex, and care shifts from hospital to home, nurses need to use high levels of thinking (Johnsen et al., 2016). Your ability to use the critical thinking process in making difficult clinical decisions is a learned ability (Van Graan et al., 2016).

Skills can be learned by participating in simulated case situations. According to Nelson (2017) and others, accepted teaching–learning methods for assessing critical thinking include use of case studies, questioning, reflective journalism, portfolios, concept maps, and problem-based learning.

From Trobec, I., & Starcic, A. I. (2015). Developing nursing ethical competencies online versus in the traditional classroom. *Nursing Ethics, 22*(3), 352–366.

APPLICATIONS

Schools of nursing curriculum require the inclusion of content on critical thinking. Accepted methods for accessing your critical thinking abilities include case study analysis, questioning, reflective journalling, person simulations, portfolios, concept mapping, and problem-based learning.

SOLVING ETHICAL DILEMMAS AS PART OF CLINICAL DECISION MAKING

Nurses indicate a need for more information about dealing with the ethical dilemmas they encounter, yet most say they receive little education in doing so. Simulation Exercises 4.1 (autonomy), 4.2 (beneficence), and 4.3 (justice) give you this opportunity.

The ethical issues that nurses commonly face today can be placed in three general categories: moral uncertainty, moral or ethical dilemmas, and moral distress. **Moral uncertainty** occurs when a nurse is uncertain as to which moral rules (i.e., values, beliefs, or ethical principles) apply to a given situation. For example, should a terminally ill person who is in and out of a coma and chooses not to eat or drink anything be required to have IV therapy for hydration purposes? Does giving IV therapy constitute giving the person extraordinary measures to prolong life? Is it more comfortable or less comfortable for the dying person to maintain a high hydration level? When there is no clear definition of the problem, moral uncertainty develops because the nurse is unable to identify the situation as a moral problem or to define specific moral rules that apply. Strategies that might be useful in dealing with moral uncertainty include using the values clarification process, developing a specific philosophy of nursing, and acquiring knowledge about ethical principles.

Ethical or moral dilemmas arise when two or more moral issues are in conflict. An ethical dilemma is a problem in which there are two or more conflicting but equally right answers. Organ harvesting of an infant with severe brain damage is an example of an ethical dilemma. Removal of organs from one infant may save the lives of several other infants. However, even though the infant with brain damage is definitely going to die, is it right to remove organs before the child's death? It is important for the nurse to understand that, in many ethical dilemmas, there is often no single "right" solution. Some decisions may be "more right" than others, but often what one nurse decides is best differs significantly from what another nurse would decide.

The third common kind of ethical problem seen in nursing today is moral distress. Moral distress results when the nurse knows what is "right" but is bound to do otherwise because of legal, regulatory, or institutional constraints. When such situations arise (e.g., a terminally ill person who does not have a "do not resuscitate" medical order, and therefore resuscitation attempts must be made), nurses may experience inner turmoil, leading to feelings of anger, frustration, and guilt (CNA, 2017).

Nurses have reported that three of their most commonly encountered ethics problems have to do with the following situations: resuscitation decisions for dying persons lacking clear code orders; persons and families who want more

SIMULATION EXERCISE 4.1   **Autonomy**

Purpose

To stimulate class discussion about the moral principle of autonomy

Procedure

In small groups, read the three case examples in this chapter (Autonomy Case Example (p. 59); Beneficence Case

Example (p. 59); and Justice Case Example (p. 60) and discuss whether the person has the autonomous right to refuse treatment if it affects the life of another person.

Reflective Analysis

Prepare your argument for an in-class discussion

SIMULATION EXERCISE 4.2   **Beneficence**

Purpose

To stimulate discussion about the moral principle of beneficence

Procedure

Read the following case example and prepare for discussion:

Tegan, a staff nurse, answers the telephone and receives a verbal order from Dr. Kakar. Ms. Patton was admitted this morning with ventricular arrhythmia. Dr. Kakar orders Tegan to administer a potent diuretic, furosemide (Lasix) 80 mg, IV, STAT. This is such a large dose that she has to order it up from pharmacy.

As described in the text, you are legally obliged to carry out a doctor's orders unless they threaten the welfare of the person. How often do nurses question orders? What would happen to a nurse who questioned orders too often? In a research study using this case simulation, nearly 95% of the time, the nurses participating in the study attempted to implement this potentially lethal medication order before being stopped by the researcher!

Reflective Analysis

1. What principles are involved?
2. What would you do if you were this staff nurse?

SIMULATION EXERCISE 4.3   **Justice**

Purpose

To encourage discussion about the concept of justice

Procedure

Read the following case example and, in a small group, answer the discussion questions:

Mr. Diaz, aged 74 years, has has been diagnosed with cancer. He has led an active life and continues to be the sole support for his wife and his daughter with a disability.

The doctors think his cancer may respond to a very expensive new drug, which is not paid for under his province's health insurance coverage.

Discussion

1. Does everyone have a right to all recommended treatments, with the costs covered under the Canadian health care system?

aggressive treatment; and colleagues who discuss persons inappropriately.

Because values underlie all ethical decision making, nurses must understand their own values thoroughly before making an ethical decision. Instead of responding in an emotional manner on the spur of the moment (as people often do when faced with an ethical dilemma), the nurse who uses the values clarification process can respond rationally. It is not an easy task to have sufficient knowledge of oneself, the situation, and legal and moral constraints to be able to implement ethical decision making quickly. Expert nurses still struggle and still have uncertainties (Gronlund et al., 2015). Taking time to examine situations can help

you develop skills in dealing with ethical dilemmas in nursing, and the exercises in this book will give you a chance to practise these skills. Each chapter in this book includes at least one ethical dilemma, so you can discuss what you would do.

As nurses, we advocate for the person's best interests. To do so, we avoid imposing what we think is in their best interests, instead listening and finding out their preferences so we can work collaboratively with the health care team in developing an ethical, person-centred plan of care. Issues most frequently necessitating ethical decisions occur at the beginning of life and at the close of life.

Finally, reflect on your own ethical practice. How important is it for the person to be able to always count on you? Consider the following personal reflection of a person receiving care (Milton, 2002):

I ask for information, share my needs, to no avail. You come and go . . .
"Could you find out for me?" "Sure, I'll check on it."
[But] check on it never comes . . .
Who can I trust? I thought you'd be here for me . . .
You weren't. What can I do?
Betrayal permeates . . .

PROFESSIONAL VALUES ACQUISITION

Professional values or ethics consist of the values held in common by the members of a profession. Professional values are formally stated in professional codes. One example already mentioned is the CNA Code of Ethics for Nurses (2017). Often, professional values are transmitted by tradition, in nursing classes and clinical experiences. They are modelled by expert nurses and assimilated as part of the role socialization process during your years as a student and new graduate. Professional **values acquisition** should be the result of conscious choice by a nursing student.

APPLYING CRITICAL THINKING TO THE CLINICAL DECISION-MAKING PROCESS

This section discusses a procedure for developing critical thinking skills as applied to solving clinical problems. Different examples illustrate the reasoning process developed by several disciplines. Unfortunately, each discipline has its own vocabulary. Table 4.2 shows that we are talking about concepts with which you are already familiar. It also contrasts terms used in education, nursing, and philosophy to specify 10 steps to help you develop your critical thinking skills. For example, the nurse performs a "health assessment," which in education is referred to as "collecting information" or in philosophy may be called "identifying claims."

The process of critical thinking is systematic, organized, and goal directed. As critical thinkers, nurses are able to explore all aspects of a complex clinical situation. This is a learned process. Among many teaching–learning techniques helping you develop critical thinking skills, most are included in this book: reflective journalling, concept maps, role-playing, guided small group discussion, and case study discussion. An extensive case application follows. During your learning phase, the critical thinking skills are divided

TABLE 4.2 Reasoning Process

Generic Reasoning Process	Identifies Health Care Needs/ Issues in the Nursing Process	Ethical Reasoning	Critical Thinking Skill
Collect and interpret information	Collects information from a variety of sources (person history, physical assessment, family, other health team members)	Identify ethical problem (parties, claim, basis)	1. Clarify concepts 2. Identify own, person's, and professional values and differentiate
Identify problem	Statement of identified health care issues or problems	Consider ethical dilemma State the problem Collect additional information Develop alternatives for analysis	3. Integrate data and identify missing data 4. Collect new data 5. Identify problem 6. Examine skeptically 7. Apply criteria 8. Generate options and look at alternatives 9. Check for change in context
Plan for problem solving	Prioritization of problems and interventions	Prioritized claims	10. Make decision, select best action plan, and make the intervention
Implement plan	Nursing action	Take moral action	
Evaluate	Outcome evaluation	Moral evaluation of outcome and reflect on the process used	Evaluate the outcome and reflect on the process

into 10 specific steps. Each step includes a discussion of application to the clinical case example provided.

To help you understand how to apply critical thinking steps, read the following case and then see how each of the steps can be used in making clinical decisions. Components of this case are applied to illustrate the steps and to stimulate discussion in the critical thinking process; many more points may be raised. From the outset, understand that, although these are listed as steps, they do not occur in a rigid, linear way in real life. The model is best thought of as circular. New data are constantly being sought and added to the process.

Case Example

Day 1—Mrs. Vlios, a 72-year-old widowed teacher, has been admitted to your unit. Her daughter, Sara, lives 2 hours away from her mother, but she arrives soon after admission. According to Sara, her mother lived an active life before admission, taking care of herself in an apartment in a retirement residence. Sara noticed that for about 3 weeks now, telephone conversations with her mother did not make sense or she seemed to have a hard time concentrating, although her pronunciation was clear. The admitting diagnosis is dehydration and dementia; rule out Alzheimer's disease, neurocognitive disorder, and depression. An IV drip of 1000 mL dextrose/0.45 normal saline is ordered at 50 drops/hour. Mrs. Vlios's history is unremarkable except for a recent 10-pound weight loss. She has no allergies and is known to take acetaminophen regularly for minor pain.

Day 2—When Sara visits her mother's apartment to bring personal items to the hospital, she finds the refrigerator and food pantry empty. A neighbour tells her that Mrs. Vlios was seen roaming the halls aimlessly 2 days ago and, when asked, could not remember whether she had eaten. As Mrs. Vlios's nurse, you notice that she is oriented today (to time and person). A soft diet is ordered, and her urinary output is now normal.

Day 5—In the morning report, the night nurse states that Mrs. Vlios was hallucinating. A nasogastric tube was ordered to suction out stomach contents because of repeated vomiting. Dr. Patel tells Sara and her brother, Todos, that their mother's prognosis is guarded; she has acquired a serious systemic infection, is semi-comatose, is not taking nourishment, and needs antibiotics and hyperalimentation. Sara reminds the doctor that her mother signed a living will in which she stated that she refuses all treatment except IVs to keep her alive. Todos is upset, yelling at Sara that he wants the doctor to do everything possible to keep their mother alive.

Step 1: Clarify Concepts

The first step in making a clinical judgement is to identify whether a problem actually exists. Poor decision makers often skip this step. To figure out whether there is a problem, you need to think about what to observe and what basic information to gather. If it is an ethical dilemma, you need to identify not only the existence of the moral problem, but also all the stakeholders who are involved in the decision. Figuring out exactly what the problem or issue is may not be as easy as it sounds.

Look for Clues

Are there hidden meanings to the words being spoken? Are there nonverbal clues?

Identify Assumptions

What assumptions are being made?

Case Discussion

This case is designed to present both physiological and ethical dilemmas. In clarifying the problem, address both domains.

- Physiological concerns: Based on the diagnosis, the initial treatment goal was to restore homeostasis. By day 5, is it clear whether Mrs. Vlios's condition is reversible?
- Ethical concerns: When is a decision made to initiate treatment or to abide by the advance directive and respect Mrs. Vlios's wishes regarding no treatment?
- What are the wishes of the family? What happens when there is no consensus?
- Assumptions: Is the diagnosis correct? Does she have dementia? Or was her confusion a result of dehydration or delirium from being hospitalized?

Step 2: Identify Your Own Person and Professional Values

Values clarification helps you identify and prioritize your values. It also serves as a base for helping persons being cared for identify the values they hold as important. Unless you are able to identify the person's values and can appreciate the validity of those values, you run the risk for imposing your own values. It is not necessary for your values and the person's values to coincide; this is an unrealistic expectation. However, whenever possible, the person's values should be taken into consideration during every aspect of nursing care. Discussion of the case of Mrs. Vlios presented in this section may help you with the clarification process.

Having just completed the exercises given earlier should help your understanding of your own personal values and the professional values of nursing. Now apply this information to this case.

Case Discussion

Identify the values of each person involved:

- Family: Mrs. Vlios signed an advance directive. Sara wants it adhered to; Todos wants it ignored. Why? (Missing information: Are there religious beliefs that contribute? Is there unclear communication? Is there guilt about previous troubles in the relationship?)
- Personal values: What are yours?
- Professional values: Nurses are advocates for the person; beneficence implies nonmaleficence ("do no harm"), but does autonomy mean the right to refuse treatment? What is the organization's policy? What are the legal considerations? Practise refining your professional values acquisition by completing the values exercises in this chapter.

In summary, you need to identify which values are involved in a situation or which moral principles can be cited to support each of the positions advocated by the involved individuals.

Step 3: Integrate Data and Identify Missing Data

Think about knowledge gained in prior courses and during clinical experiences. Try to make connections between different subject areas and clinical nursing practice.

- Identify what data are needed. Obtain all possible information and gather facts or evidence (evaluate whether data are true, relevant, and sufficient). Situations are often complicated. It is important to figure out what information is significant to this situation. Synthesize prior information you already have with similarities in the current situation. Conflicting data may indicate a need to search for more information.
- Compare existing information with past knowledge. Has this person complained of difficulty thinking before? Does she have a history of dementia?
- Look for gaps in the information. Actively work to recognize whether there is missing information. For example, was Mrs. Vlios previously taking medications for depression? For a nurse, this is an important part of critical thinking.
- Collect information systematically. Use an organized framework to obtain information. Nurses often obtain a health history by asking questions about each body system. They could just as systematically ask about basic needs.
- Organize your information. Clustering information into relevant categories is helpful. For example, gathering all the facts about a person's breathing may

help focus your attention on whether they are having respiratory difficulty. In your assessment, you note the rate and character of respirations, the colour of nails and lips, the use of accessory muscles, and grunting noises. At the same time, you exclude information about bowel sounds or deep tendon reflexes as not being immediately relevant to this person's respiratory status. Categorizing information also helps you notice whether there are missing data. A second strategy that will help you organize information is to look for patterns. It has been indicated that experienced nurses intuitively note recurrent meaningful aspects of a clinical situation.

Case Discussion

Rely on prior knowledge or clinical experience. Cluster the data. What was Mrs. Vlios's status immediately before hospitalization? What was her status at the time of hospitalization? What information is missing? What additional data do you need?

- Physiology: Consider pathophysiological knowledge about the effects of hypovolemia and electrolyte imbalances on systems such as the brain, kidneys, and vascular system. What is her temperature? What are her laboratory values? What is her 24-hour intake and output? Is she still dehydrated?
- Psychological/cognitive: How does hospitalization affect older persons?
- Social/economic: Was weight loss a result of dehydration? Why was she without food? Could it be due to economic factors or cognitive issues?
- Legal: What constitutes a binding advance directive to not resuscitate, drawn up by Mrs. Vlios, in your province or territory? Where would you find this information?

Step 4: Collect New Data

Critical thinking is not a linear process. Expert nurses often modify interventions based on the response to the event, or a change in the person's physical condition. Constantly consider whether you need more information. Establish an attitude of inquiry and obtain more information as needed. Ask questions; search for evidence; and check reference books, journals, the ethics sources on the Internet, or written professional or organization protocols.

Evaluate conflicting information. There may be time constraints. If a person has suspected "respiratory difficulties," you may need to set priorities. Obtain data that are most useful or are easily available. It would be useful to know oxygenation levels; you may not have time to have laboratory tests ordered, but you could obtain an oxygen saturation measurement.

Sometimes you may need to change your approach to improve your chances of obtaining information. For example, when the charge nurse caring for Mrs. Vlios used an authoritarian tone to try to get the sister and brother to provide more information about possible drug overdose, they did not respond. However, when the charge nurse changed his approach, exhibiting empathy, the daughter volunteered that on several occasions her mother had forgotten what pills she had taken.

Case Discussion

List sources from which you can obtain missing information. Physiological data such as temperature, vital signs, or laboratory test results can be obtained quickly; however, some of the ethical information may take longer to consider.

Step 5: Identify the Significant Problems

- Analyze existing information: Examine all the information you have. Identify all the possible scenarios.
- Question what is occurring: What might be going on? What are the possible issues? Make a list of the issues.
- Prioritize: Which issues are most urgently in need of your intervention? What are the appropriate interventions?

Case Discussion

A significant physiological concern is sepsis (body's extreme response to infection), regardless of whether it is an iatrogenic (health care–associated) infection or one resulting from immobility and weakness. A significant ethical concern is the conflict among family members and Mrs. Vlios (as expressed through her living will). At what point do spiritual concerns take priority over a worsening physical concern?

Step 6: Examine Skeptically

Thinking about a situation may involve weighing positive and negative factors, and differentiating facts that are credible from opinions that are biased or not grounded in facts.
- Keep an open mind.
- Challenge your own assumptions.
- Consider whether any of your assumptions are unwarranted. Does the available evidence really support your assumption?
- Discriminate between facts and assumptions. Your assumptions need to be logical and possible, based on the available facts.
- Are there any problems that you have not considered?
  In trying to evaluate a situation, consciously raising questions becomes an important part of thinking critically.

At times, there will be alternative explanations or different lines of reasoning that are equally valid. The challenge is to examine your own and others' perspectives for important ideas, complicating factors, other possible interpretations, and new insights. Some nurses view examining information skeptically as part of each step in the critical thinking process rather than as a step by itself.

Case Discussion

Challenge assumptions about the cause of Mrs. Vlios's condition. For example, did you eliminate the possibility that she had a head injury caused by a fall? Could she have liver failure as a result of acetaminophen overdosing? Have all the possibilities been explored? Challenge your assumptions about outcome: Are they influenced by expected probable versus possible outcomes for this client? If she, indeed, has irreversible dementia, what will the quality of her life be if she recovers from her physical problems?

Step 7: Apply Criteria

In evaluating a situation, think about appropriate responses.
- Assess standards for "best practices" related to the person's situation.
- Laws: There may be laws, nursing practice standards, and policies that can be applied to guide your actions and decisions. For example, if you suspect elder abuse, you will need to report your concerns following professional standards, regulations, organization policies, and laws in your province or territory.
- Legal precedents: Legal decisions do guide health care practices. In end-of-life decisions, when there is no legally binding health care power of attorney, you will need to find out the most frequent hierarchy of family members who are consulted for decision making in your province or territory. In Ontario, the most frequent hierarchy is the spouse, and then the adult children, parents, brother or sister, any other relative (Community Legal Education in Ontario, 2016).
- Policies and procedures: There may be standard protocols for managing certain situations. Your organization may have standing orders for caring for Mrs. Vlios if she develops respiratory distress, such as administering oxygen per face mask at 5 L/min.

Case Discussion

Many criteria could be used to examine this case, including the professional code of ethics or general ethical principles of beneficence and autonomy; the organization's written protocols and policies; provincial or territorial laws regarding living wills; and prior court decisions about living wills. Remember that advance directives are designed to take effect only when individuals become unable to make their own wishes known.

Step 8: Generate Options and Look at Alternatives

- Evaluate the major alternative points of view.
- Involve experienced peers as soon as you can to assist you in making your decision.
- Use information from others to help you "put the picture together."
- Can you identify all the arguments—pros and cons—to explain this situation? Almost all situations have strong counterarguments or competing hypotheses.

Case Discussion

The important concept is that the nurse or other health care providers should not handle this situation alone; rather, others should be involved (e.g., the hospital bioethics committee, the ombudsman client representative, the family's spiritual counsellor, and other health care experts such as a gerontologist, psychologist, and clinical nurse specialist).

Step 9: Consider Whether Factors Change if the Context Changes

Consider whether your decision would be different if there were a change in circumstances. For example, a change in the person's age, the site of the situation, or their culture may affect your decision. A competent nurse prioritizes the aspects of a situation that are most relevant and can modify their actions based on the person's responses. A competent nurse anticipates consequences.

Case Discussion

If you knew the outcome from the beginning, would your decisions be the same? What if you knew Mrs. Vlios had terminal cancer? What if Mrs. Vlios had remained in her retirement residence and you were the home health nurse? What if Mrs. Vlios had remained alert during her hospitalization and refused IVs, hyperalimentation, a nasogastric tube, and so on? What if the family and Mrs. Vlios were in agreement about no treatment? Would you make more assertive interventions to save her life if she were 7 years old, or a 35-year-old mother of five young children?

Step 10: Make the Decision, Implement, and Evaluate the Outcome

After analyzing available information in this systematic way, you need to make a judgement or decision. An important part of your decision is your ability to communicate it clearly to others and to reflect on health status outcomes.

- Justify your conclusion.
- Evaluate outcomes.
- Test out your decision or conclusion by implementing appropriate actions.

As a critical thinker, you need to be able to accept that there may be multiple solutions that can be equally acceptable. In other situations, you may need to make a decision even when there is incomplete knowledge. Be able to cite your rationale or present your arguments to others for your decision choice and interventions. Revise interventions as necessary.

Clinical Decision Making

While we have yet to arrive at a universal consensus for understanding clinical decision making, many articles cite components of models developed by Levett-Jones et al. (2010), Tanner (2006), Hunter and Arthur (2016), and others. Making clinical decisions is complex. As illustrated in Fig. 4.3, we could perhaps think of decision making and intervention as striving to achieve (PAR)—we need to Process, Act, and Reflect in order to provide safe, competent, nursing care.

PROCESS. Nurses are faced with processing large amounts of information quickly in using their critical thinking skills; we assess person status and notice factors that characterize the person's current situation. We incorporate our existing clinical knowledge to help us understand what is happening. This includes processing information from our assessment, from biophysical and psychosocial data, from our knowledge of the person's preferences, and from our understanding of current circumstances.

ACT. Applying our clinical knowledge to identify problems, incorporate ethical values, and set goals, we make appropriate interventions. We recognize the need to continually gather and analyze new information.

REFLECT. After you implement interventions, you examine outcomes. Was your assessment correct? Did you obtain enough information? Did the benefits to the person and family outweigh the harm that may have occurred? In retrospect, do you know you made the correct decision? Did you anticipate possibilities and complications correctly? Did you communicate with the health team in a timely manner? This kind of self-examination can foster self-correction and learning. Reflecting on one's own thinking is the hallmark of a critical thinker. This self-reflection facilitates our learning.

This is a cyclical nursing care process in which constant re-evaluation and reflection on one's actions and subsequent outcomes becomes new input (Lee et al., 2016).

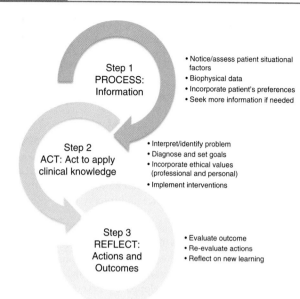

Step 1
PROCESS:
Information

- Notice/assess patient situational factors
- Biophysical data
- Incorporate patient's preferences
- Seek more information if needed

Step 2
ACT: Act to apply clinical knowledge

- Interpret/identify problem
- Diagnose and set goals
- Incorporate ethical values (professional and personal)
- Implement interventions

Step 3
REFLECT:
Actions and Outcomes

- Evaluate outcome
- Re-evaluate actions
- Reflect on new learning

Fig. 4.3 The clinical decision-making process

While the example of Mrs. Vlios described a hospital situation, it is even more essential that nurses in the community be able to apply critical thinking to clinical decision making so they may implement safer, evidence-informed high-quality care in independent situations. Recognizing and treating deteriorations might prevent hospitalization (Johnsen et al., 2016).

Summarizing the Learning Process

Learning these steps in critical thinking results from repeated application. In addition to using peer discussions of the case studies, recording role-playing of simulated case situations using standardized person models or computer-generated problems give opportunity for practice. A new graduate nurse must, at a minimum, be able to identify essential clinical data, know when to initiate interventions, know why a particular intervention is relevant, and differentiate between problems that need immediate intervention versus problems that can wait for action. Repeated practice in applying critical thinking can help a new graduate fit into the expectations of employers. In addition to simulation situations, learning can occur through the analysis of interviews with experienced nurses about their decision making, as described in Simulation Exercise 4.4.

Try responding to the Gonzales case example.

Case Example

Mr. Gonzales has terminal cancer. His family defers to the attending physician, who prescribes aggressive cancer treatment, including surgery and chemotherapy. The hospice nurse is an expert in the expressed and unexpressed needs of persons with a terminal cancer diagnosis. She advocates for a conservative and supportive palliative plan of care. A logical case could be built for each position.

SIMULATION EXERCISE 4.4   Your Analysis of an Expert's Critical Thinking: Interview of Expert Nurse's Case

Purpose
To develop awareness of critical thinking in the clinical judgement process

Procedure
Find an experienced nurse in your community and record them, after asking permission to do so, describing a person they cared for (ensuring to maintain person confidentiality). You can use your phone to record an interview that takes only a few minutes. During the interview, have the nurse describe an actual case in which there was a significant change in the person's health status. Have the nurse describe the interventions and thinking process that took place during this situation. Ask what nursing knowledge,

laboratory data, or experience helped the nurse make their decision. You can work with a partner. Remember to protect confidentiality by omitting all names and other identifiers.

Reflective Analysis
Analyze the recording using an outline of the 10 steps in critical thinking. Discussion should first include citation examples of each step noted during their review of the recorded interview, followed by application of the broad principles. Discussion of steps missed by the interviewed nurse can inform your own learning, as long as care is taken to avoid any criticism of the nurse.

SUMMARY

Ethical reasoning and critical thinking are systematic, comprehensive processes to aid you in making clinical decisions. An important concept is to forget the idea that there is only one right answer in discussing ethical dilemmas. Accept that there may be several equally correct solutions, depending on each individual's point of view.

Critical thinking is not a linear process. Analysis of the thinking processes of expert nurses reveals that they continually scan new data and simultaneously apply these steps in clinical decision making. They monitor the effectiveness of their interventions in achieving desired outcomes for their person. A nurse's moral reasoning and critical thinking abilities often have a profound effect on the quality of care given, which affects health outcomes. Functioning as a competent nurse requires you to have knowledge of biomedical, psychosocial, and nursing content; knowledge of best practice guidelines; an accumulation of clinical experiences; and an ability to think critically.

Almost daily, we confront ethical dilemmas and complicated clinical situations that require expertise as a decision maker. We can follow the 10 steps of the critical thinking process described in this chapter to help us respond to such situations. Developing clinical judgement is a learned process, one that requires repeated application.

⚖ ETHICAL DILEMMA

What Would You Do?

The Moyers family has power of attorney over hospitalized, terminally ill Gail Midge, aged 42 years. They are consistently at her bedside and refuse to allow you and other nurses to administer pain medication ordered by Mrs. Midge's physician, since they fear it will overdose her, causing her death. Gail often moans, cries with pain, and begs you for pain medications. The family threatens a lawsuit if she is given anything and then dies. What would you do?

This example is based on a case reported by Pavlish et al., (2011, p. 390). The nurse in that case considered conflicting variables from each point of view and assumed responsibility for initiating action, calling the palliative care team and the ethics consultation team.

QUESTIONS FOR REVIEW AND DISCUSSION

1. In the CNA Code of Ethics (2017), find within each of the nursing values and ethical responsibilities the statements related to person-centred care and autonomy. Apply these statements in discussing the question, When does a person have the right to refuse treatment?
2. Analyze the characteristics of a critical thinker listed in Table 4.1. How do or did you develop these characteristics? Are they innate or how and when did you acquire them?
3. Construct an example showing when a nurse has an ethical obligation. By choosing to become a nurse, do you assume an ethical obligation to treat any person assigned to you? When are there exceptions?

REFERENCES

American Nurses Association. (2015). *Code of ethics for nurses with interpretive statements (View only for members and nonmembers)*. https://www.nursingworld.org/coe-view-only.

Canadian Nurses Association. (2017). *Code of ethics for registered nurses*. https://www.cna-aiic.ca/~/media/cna/page-content/pdf-en/code-of-ethics-2017-edition-secure-interactive.

Carter, A. G., Creedy, D. K., & Sidebotham, M. (2016). Efficacy of teaching methods used to develop critical thinking in nursing and midwifery undergraduate students: A systematic review of the literature. *Nurse Education Today, 40,* 209–218.

College of Nurses of Ontario. (2017). *Practice guideline: Consent.* http://www.cno.org/globalassets/docs/policy/41020_consent.pdf.

Collier, C. & Haliburton, R. (2015). *Bioethics in Canada: A philosophical introduction.* (2nd ed.). Canadian Scholars' Press Inc.

Community Legal Education in Ontario. (2016). *What if I do not have a power of attorney for personal care?* https://www.cleo.on.ca/en/publications/power/what-if-i-do-not-have-power-attorney-personal-care.

Costello, M. (2017). The benefits of active learning: Applying Brunner's discovery theory to the classroom: Teaching clinical decision-making to senior nursing students. *Teaching and Learning in Nursing, 12,* 212–213. https://doi.org/10.1016/j.teln.2017.02.005.

Gronlund, C. E. C. F., Soderberg, A. I. S., Zingmarken, K. M. et al. (2015). Ethically difficult situations in hemodialysis care-nurses' narratives. *Nursing Ethics, 26*(6), 711–722.

Hunter, S., & Arthur, C. (2016). Clinical reasoning of nursing students on clinical placement: Clinical educators' perceptions. *Nurse Education in Practice, 18,* 73–79.

Johnsen, H. M., Fossum, M., Vivekananda-Schmidt, P., et al. (2016). Teaching clinical reasoning and decision-making skills to nursing students: Design, development, and usability evaluation of a serious game. *International Journal of Medical Informatics, 94,* 39–48.

Kaya, H., Senyuva, E., & Brodur, G. (2017). Developing critical thinking disposition and emotional intelligence of nursing students: A longitudinal research. *Nurse Education Today, 48,* 72–77.

Keatings, M., & Adams, P. (2020). *Ethical and legal issues in Canadian nursing.* (4th ed.). Elsevier; Canadian Scholars' Press Inc.

Lee, J., Lee, Y. J., Bae, J., et al. (2016). Registered nurses' clinical reasoning skills and reasoning process: A think-aloud study. *Nurse Education Today, 46*, 75–80.

Levett-Jones, T., Hoffman, K., Dempsey, J., et al. (2010). The 'five rights' of clinical reasoning: An educational model to enhance nursing students' ability to identify and manage clinically 'at risk' patients. *Nurse Education Today, 30*, 515–520.

Melin-Johansson, C., Palmqvist, R., & Rönnberg, L. (2017). Clinical intuition in the nursing process and decision-making—A mixed-studies review. *Journal of Clinical Nursing, 26*, 3936–3949. https://doi.org/10.1111/jocn.13814.

Milton, C. (2002). Ethical implications for acting faithfully in nurse-person relationships. *Nursing Science Quarterly, 15*, 21–24.

Nelson, A. E. (2017). Methods faculty use to facilitate nursing students' critical thinking. *Teaching and Learning in Nursing, 12*, 62–66.

Nursing & Midwifery Council. (2015). *The Code: Professional standards of practice and behaviour for nurses, midwives and nursing associates*. https://www.nmc.org.uk/globalassets/sitedocuments/nmc-publications/nmc-code.pdf.

Pavlish, C., Brown-Sullivan, K., Herish, M., et al. (2011). Nursing priorities, actions, and regrets for ethical situations in clinical practice. *Journal of Nursing Scholarship, 43*(4), 385–395.

Romeo, E. M. (2010). Quantitative research on CT and predicting nursing students' NCLEX-RN performance. *The Journal of Nursing Education, 49*(7), 378–386.

Sinclair, J., Pappas, E., & Marshall, B. (2016). Nursing students' experiences of ethical issues in clinical practice: A New Zealand study. *Nurse Education in Practice, 17*, 1–7.

Tanner, C. A. (2006). Thinking like a nurse: A research-based model of clinical judgment in nursing. *The Journal of Nursing Education, 45*, 204–211.

Trobec, I., & Starcic, A. I. (2015). Developing ethical competencies online versus in the traditional classroom. *Nursing Ethics, 22*(3), 352–366.

Tschudin, V. (2013). Two decades of nursing ethics: Some thoughts on changes. *Nursing Ethics, 20*(2), 123–125.

Van Graan, A. C., Williams, M. J. S., & Koen, M. P. (2016). Professional nurses' understanding of clinical judgment: A contextual inquiry. *Health SA Gesondheid, 21*, 280–293.

5

Developing Person-Centred Communication Skills

Claire Mallette

Originating US chapter by *Elizabeth C. Arnold*

OBJECTIVES

At the end of the chapter, the reader will be able to:

1. Discuss the concept of health communication.
2. Describe the elements of person-centred communication.
3. Apply communication strategies and skills in person-centred relationships.
4. Discuss active listening responses used in therapeutic communication.
5. Discuss the use of verbal responses as a communication strategy.
6. Describe other forms of communication used in nurse–person relationships.

Nurses communicate on many different levels—with people, their families, other professional disciplines, and a variety of external care providers involved with a person's care. Although professional communication uses many of the same strategies as social communication, professional communication represents a specialized form of communication. It always has goals and a health-related purpose. This chapter focuses on knowledge and skills related to person-centred communication and describes communication strategies that nurses can use to inform, support, care, educate, and empower people to effectively self-manage their health-related issues.

Communicating as a professional nurse can be a challenge. Relational and informational aspects do not exist in the words themselves but rather in their potential interpretations by the communicators engaged in the dialogue. Consequently, professional communication is carefully thought out and always considerate of how the recipient might respond to it. Keep in mind that effective communication represents a combination of relationship building, information sharing, and decision making in communication, all of which are needed to achieve critically important clinical outcomes.

Professional conversations differ from social conversations. Nurses must learn to be equally skilled at communicating with professional audiences and at knowing how to translate technical and medical information into a way that the person and family members can understand. They also need to competently communicate with physicians and other health provider colleagues, using professional, technical, and medical language. Talking with people who need care requires a different skill set that bridges the medical and technical dialogue needed for health and social care with a socially understandable exchange of ideas. Professional conversations have health-related expectations and legal and ethical boundaries about what can and cannot be shared with others. This chapter focuses on the development of communication knowledge and skills in health care circumstances.

Schiavo (2013) notes, "Being sick is among one of the most vulnerable times in people's lives, especially in the case of severe, chronic, or life threatening diseases" (p. 116).

People respond best when they believe their care providers are placing full attention on their concerns as a high priority. Incorporating the person's preferences and values while providing care demonstrates that this characteristic lies at the heart of person-centred care. Other indicators involve accurate clinical assessments, fully informed consent, shared decision making, and effective health teaching geared to the person and family needs and preferences. Ongoing collaborative conversations between the person and family and their health care providers have a direct impact on the quality and safety of clinical care, the achievement of meaningful clinical outcomes, and satisfaction with the care received. The person and family are expected to be active partners in their health care journey, to whatever extent possible, with health care providers (Errasti-Ibarrondo et al., 2015). Frequent consultation with other team professionals involved in a person's care also helps ensure continuity of care. This, in turn, acts to promote personal health efficacy and to strengthen trust in the person–health care provider partnership required for self-management of chronic disorders. The importance of the person and family's involvement and satisfaction are further emphasized by their inclusion as a measurable quality and safety indicator in health organizations, and they are considered critical outcomes, intimately tied to communication (Health Quality Ontario, 2017).

BASIC CONCEPTS

Definitions

Communication refers to each transmission of information, whether intentional or not. Nonverbal behaviours, written communication, tone of voice, and words are all forms of communication. The concept takes into consideration the values and beliefs, words and ideas, emotions, and body language of the sender, receiver, and context. Increasingly, people also use media and other technology to communicate messages formally and informally.

Each **message** is meant to convey an intended meaning, to exchange or strengthen ideas and feelings, and to share significant life experiences. Accompanying the message are nonverbal qualifiers in the form of gestures, body movements, eye contact, and personal or cultural symbols.

Person-centred communication refers to more than just having communications about health issues with health providers. Instead, it is a way of being, where the person, family, and support network are valued and placed at the centre of care and decision making. Person-centred care and communication moves beyond focusing on the person as a patient. Instead, person-centred care not only focuses on health issues, but also considers the person's social care influenced by cultural contexts, values, family, diversity, social circumstances, and lifestyles (Hafskjold et al., 2015; Kuluski et al., 2016).

Functions of Professional Communication in Health Care Systems

More than any other variable, effective interpersonal communication skills support safety and quality in health care delivery (see Chapter 2). Professional communication skills connect virtually all concepts and activities related to human health and well-being. Today's nurses should be equipped with a strong understanding of human biopsychosocial issues, medical and nursing care required for diverse health concerns, health-related ethical and legal issues, end-of-life care, and intra- and interprofessional team collaboration, among other topics.

Professional communication is defined as a complex interactive process, used in clinical settings to help people achieve health-related goals (Street & Mazor, 2017). The outcomes of effective interpersonal communication in health care relate to person satisfaction, addressing health issues, safety, and better quality care. People are more likely to understand their health conditions through meaningful communication and be able to alert health providers when they have concerns. Other specific ways that professional health communication impacts quality compassionate care is through these outcomes:

- Development of person-centred health partnerships
- Increased person and family satisfaction
- More effective diagnosis and earlier recognition of health changes
- Better understanding of the person's condition
- Personalized, meaningful, person-centred therapeutic regimes
- More efficient utilization of health services
- Stronger, longer-lasting positive outcomes

As discussed in Chapter 3, the Canadian Association of Schools of Nursing [CASN] (2015) Code of Ethics, the Canadian Nurses Association [CNA] (2017) Code of Ethics, and each provincial and territorial regulatory body's nursing standards all address person-centred communication.

Communication Models

This chapter builds on basic concepts of linear and transactional communication that were introduced in Chapter 1. The application section describes the use of active listening responses, verbal communication strategies, and other communication techniques that nurses and other health providers consciously use to facilitate person- and family-centred health care. Communication concepts and strategies presented in this chapter provide a practical methodology for connecting with the person and family to improve health outcomes.

Overview of Linear Model and Transactional Model

The *linear model* is the simplest communication model, which consists of sender, message, receiver, channels of communication, and context. Linear models focus only on the sending and receiving of messages. *Transactional communication models* are more complex in defining communication as a reciprocal interaction process in which sender and receiver influence each other's messages and responses simultaneously as they converse. Each communicator constructs a mental picture of the other during the conversation, including **perceptions** about the other's attitude and potential reactions to the message. Individual perceptions influence the transmission of the message and its meaning to one or both of the communicators, leading to a new, co-created set of collaborative meanings.

PROFESSIONAL COMMUNICATION SKILLS

Therapeutic communication, a term introduced by Jurgen Ruesch in 1961, refers to a dynamic interactive process entered into by health care providers, with the person and significant others, for the purpose of achieving identified, health-related goals (Ruesch, 1961). Therapeutic communication occurs in a variety of ways: through words, facial expressions, body language, digitally, through documentation, and through behaviours. With the person, nurses implement treatment activities, collaborate with those involved in the person's care, exchange information, and make shared decisions about all aspects of care with the person and family. Therapeutic communication has purpose, active engagement of the person as a full partner in a health-related interactive process, and inclusion of relevant values and goals of the person and family emphasized throughout the dialogue. Additionally, the message takes into account the person's and family's values, beliefs, cultural contexts, developmental level, interest, and general health condition (Rosenberg & Gallo-Silver, 2011).

Each therapeutic conversation is unique because the people holding them have different insights, personal strengths, values, and beliefs. The interaction also continually changes based on internal and external factors of the people engaged in the therapeutic conversation (Registered Nurses' Association of Ontario [RNAO], 2015).

At first glance, it may appear that therapeutic communication doesn't require extra or specialized study—this is not true. In therapeutic conversations, health care providers must maintain a skilled mindfulness, which allows them to consider each person's unique situation while simultaneously monitoring their own personal responses and reactions and other corroborative evidence. This is what Peplau (1960) meant by the nurse being a "participant observer" in therapeutic relationships.

Person-centred Communication Skills

Person-centred communication skills in health care are imperative in delivering nursing practice, such as obtaining a health assessment, explaining a diagnosis, and providing competent, compassionate nursing care with related health teaching. Communication competency offers a primary means for establishing a trusting, collaborative relationship with people being cared for and their families. Communication is embedded within all professional relationships.

The quality of health care relationships strongly affects the outcome of the health encounter (Van Dalen, 2013; Watzlawick et al., 1967). "Positive" clinical experiences involve human communication encounters in which a person's human needs and values are respected, and the humanity of the health provider is transparent. Interestingly, the human connection sometimes influences a person's health care impression of a care experience as much, if not more, than the level of the provider's competence. With "negative" clinical encounters, the person's experience disconnects with the knowledge and interpersonal care the person and family expect from the provider, in part because of the way the information is presented. It becomes an uncomfortable, rather than a productive, encounter. Poor communication is implicated as a key factor in clinical safety errors and quality (Gluyas, 2015).

CHARACTERISTICS OF PERSON-CENTRED COMMUNICATION

Honesty, clarity, and empathy are fundamental elements of effective therapeutic conversations. In clinical practice, **empathy** refers to being emotionally attuned to a person's perspective of a situation, as well as to its reality (see Chapter 13). Referred to as the person's frame of reference or **world view**, a person's "perception" of their health may differ significantly from the nurse's frame of reference. Therapeutic communication helps to link the different perspectives into a workable common ground for discussion, therapeutic relationship, and the development of constructive goals and actions. Reflective responses based on the nurse's knowledge and integration with ways of knowing are designed to encourage further dialogue.

Defined Interpersonal Boundaries

Professional conversations have defined interpersonal boundaries, related to their purpose, discussion topics, focus, sharing of thoughts and feelings, time, and prescribed settings (see also Chapter 12). Unlike social conversations, in which each participant spontaneously expresses thoughts and feelings, professional therapeutic conversations focus only on the person and family health care needs. Interactions are person and family centred, and the

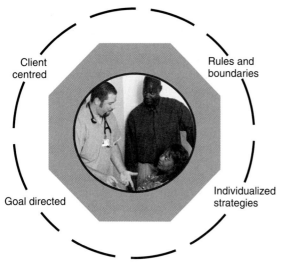

Fig. 5.1 Characteristics of therapeutic communication

associated dialogue is health related. Only the person and family are expected to consistently reveal personal information related to the health situation. See Fig. 5.1, which shows the characteristics of therapeutic conversation.

With interprofessional boundaries, the health provider should avoid disclosing personal information about themselves. However, there may be times when the nurse may choose to self-disclose personal information to strengthen the therapeutic relationship. Reasons for doing this could be to develop a relationship with the person and family, **role modelling** appropriate behaviours, fostering trust, or a way to make the relationship more reciprocal and equal (Steuber & Pollard, 2018; Unhjem et al., 2018). Types of information disclosed can include demographic and biographical information, personal insights, and coping strategies (Unhjem et al.). While self-disclosure can be beneficial, it should be used only to benefit the therapeutic relationship, infrequent, and carefully worded. The self-disclosure should be in response to the person's needs and the context of the situation. Following the self-disclosure, the focus should return immediately to the person (Unhjem et al.).

Health-Related Purpose

Professional therapeutic conversations take place within a defined health care format and terminate when the health-related purpose is achieved or the person is no longer in need of care. Characteristics of professional therapeutic conversations include the following:
- Specific rules and boundaries, related to function and privacy of the conversation

- Defined therapeutic goals
- Person-centred
- Individualized strategies related to health-related goals

All professional conversations are subject to federal, provincial, or territorial privacy guidelines and professional standards regarding confidentiality and protected health information, which are discussed in Chapter 3.

Nonverbal Communication Supports

Nonverbal communication refers to behaviours not expressed in words but that can indicate how the person is emotionally feeling. When having therapeutic conversations, it is important for nurses to be aware of and assess whether what the person is saying is congruent with what their behaviours are indicating (RNAO, 2015). Behavioural signals, found in the tone of voice, inflections and intonations, facial expression, and body language, accompany verbal messages. This is true for both the nurse and person. As nurses, we sometimes forget that the people we care for are assessing us at the same time as we are assessing them.

In face-to-face interactions, nurses have a rich range of visual and vocal cues, which provide additional data about the person, if read correctly. Knowledge of a person's habits, beliefs, preferences, cultural contexts, and attitudes can support or contradict the spoken words. Facial expressions, body postures and movements, or agitation can often suggest what the person may be feeling about the verbal message. However, these cues may be easily misinterpreted, so asking for clarifying feedback to ensure that all parties are looking at a situation from a similar perspective is essential.

ACTIVE LISTENING

Active listening is a dynamically focused, interpersonal process in which a nurse hears a person's message, decodes its meaning, asks questions for clarification, and provides feedback to the person. It is a transactional process that integrates the verbal and nonverbal components of a message. Nurses demonstrate active listening through their body language, asking open-ended questions, and expressing nonjudgemental and careful observational listening prompts. Leaning slightly forward with the upper part of your body, maintaining eye contact, restating the person's concerns, nodding, and summarizing conceptually are important communication connectors.

The goal of active listening is to understand what the person is trying to communicate through their story. Active listening requires full attention to understanding the person's perspective without making any judgements. Using the listening responses presented later in the chapter increases understanding. As you ask clarifying questions, and share your own thinking responses about what you are seeing or hearing, you can develop a more in-depth understanding of the health care situation from the person's perspective.

Included with each verbal message are important non-verbal instructions (metacommunication) about how to interpret the message (see Chapter 6). If a nurse sits down in a relaxed position with full attention and good eye contact and actively listens, these verbal and nonverbal activities indicate interest and commitment. The same verbal message, delivered while looking at the clock or your watch, provides a nonverbal message that the person does not have your full attention.

Sometimes, the emotional nonverbal component of a message differs from that of the verbal message. Nurses need to be sensitive to what is left out of the message, as well as to what is included—this too is important information to explore and consider. If you notice nonverbal behaviours that seem to contradict words, it is appropriate to call the person's attention to the discrepancy with a simple statement, such as, "I notice that you seemed very quiet when we talked about . . . . Is something going on that we should discuss?"

Verbal Responses

Verbal responses refer to the spoken words in a professional conversation. Words are a meaning-making basic tool that enable the health care provider and person to organize data about their health issues, explore different options, resolve issues, make common meaning of their experiences, and dialogue with each other. Unlike the written word, verbal dialogue cannot be erased, although words can be explained or modified.

The meaning of words resides in the person who uses them, not in the words themselves. When languages or word meanings differ, their significance changes. Nurses should pay close attention to the words and language the person is using and clarify what the person is saying to ensure the nurse understands the message. Nurses also need to adjust their communication style (for example, tone and loudness of voice) based on the person's needs (age, cognitive status, health issue, and language) (RNAO, 2015).

Choice of words matters. Terminology should be clear, complete, concrete, and easily understandable to the listener. Words should neither overstate nor understate the situation. Since both words and nonverbal behaviours are subject to misinterpretation, nurses need to check in with the person to ensure the accuracy of their perceptions. For example, "I'd just like to check in with you to make sure that I understand. Are you saying that . . .?"

Factors That Influence Communication

Personal Factors

Developing a common understanding of the dialogue that occurs between nurses and the person is a critical outcome of professional communication. Personal and environmental factors influence communication availability and readiness. For example, eye contact and full attention on the person, coupled with genuine respect and clear, concise messages, encourage the person being cared for to participate. Words that respect a person's cultural contexts (Chapter 7), spiritual beliefs, and educational level are more likely to capture their attention. Factors that affect the accurate transmission of communicated messages are found in Fig. 5.2.

People communicate nonverbally through body language, eye contact, and level of attention. The nurse should consciously use body language, gestures, and

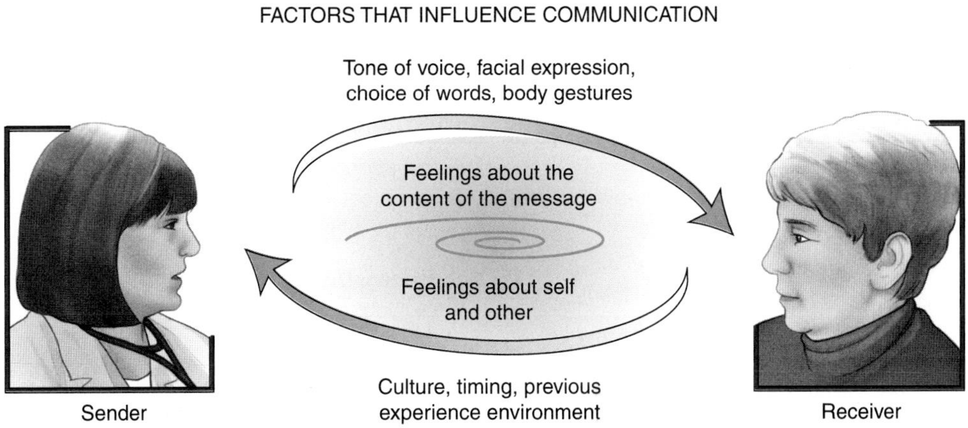

FACTORS THAT INFLUENCE COMMUNICATION

Tone of voice, facial expression, choice of words, body gestures

Feelings about the content of the message

Feelings about self and other

Culture, timing, previous experience environment

Sender

Receiver

Fig. 5.2 Factors that influence communication

minimal verbal cues to encourage further communication. Physical cues are used to support or contradict the meaning of words.

Barriers to Effective Communication Within the Person

Barriers to effective communication can occur within people when they are in these circumstances:
- Preoccupied with pain, physical discomfort, worry, or contradictory personal beliefs
- Unable to understand the nurse's use of language, terminology, or frame of reference
- Struggling with a personal, emotionally laden, topic
- Feeling defensive, insecure, or judged
- Confused by the complexity of the message—too many issues, unrelated comments
- Deprived of privacy, especially if the topic is a sensitive one
- Have sensory or cognitive deficits that limit or compromise their ability to receive accurate messages

Barriers Within the Nurse

Barriers to effective communication within the nurse occur when the nurse is not fully engaged with the person for one or more of the following reasons:
- Preoccupation with personal concerns
- Being in a hurry to complete physical care
- Making assumptions about the person's motivations
- Cultural stereotypes
- Defensiveness or personal insecurity about being able to help the person
- Thinking ahead to the next question
- Intense emotion or aggressiveness by the person
- Comments that do not add value to the conversation

Simulation Exercise 5.1 is designed to help students identify difficult communication issues in nursing practice.

Self-Awareness

Self-awareness is a person's ability to understand their own personal strengths, weaknesses, and influence on others (Shirey, 2015). Research has demonstrated that when we have self-awareness, we make better decisions, build stronger relationships, communicate more effectively, understand others better, and are happier in what we are doing (Eurich, 2018; Macleod, 2019). To become more self-aware, it is important to reflect on your own attitudes, behaviours, preferences, biases, values, strengths, and limitations (Rasheed, 2015). Being self-aware of personal vulnerabilities, values and beliefs, and biases allows nurses to maintain the authenticity, patience, neutrality, and understanding needed for therapeutic exploration of health issues with the people being cared for. Nurses also have an ethical and professional responsibility to resolve personal issues so that countertransference feelings do not affect communication. *Countertransference* is defined as the nurse's "unconscious personal response to a person" (Jordan Halter & Benner Carson, 2014, p. 28). For example, if the person reminds the nurse of someone that is not liked, the nurse may unconsciously respond in a negative way to the person being cared for.

Person-centred communication requires greater self-awareness. Before you begin communicating with someone, think about the goals you want to achieve with the person, and remember to include the person's areas of importance and concern. As you do this, make sure that your nonverbal behaviours support rather than contradict your words. Also, staying flexible in your communication based on what the person tells you promotes a more in-depth interaction than if you use only focused questioning as conversational prompts.

Environmental Factors

Privacy, space, and timing affect therapeutic conversations. People need privacy, free from interruption and environmental noise, for meaningful dialogue to take place. **Noise** refers to any distraction that interferes with being able to

---

SIMULATION EXERCISE 5.1   Complicated Communication Issues With a Person

Purpose
To help students identify common, complicated communication issues with a person

Procedure
In groups of three to four students:
1. Each student shares a brief description of a nursing or personal experience that illustrates a challenging communication encounter you have had or witnessed in a nurse–person exchange.

2. Identify what components made the conversation difficult.
3. If you could have the conversation again, what might you do differently?

Reflective Discussion Analysis
1. Did your group find any common themes in the identified communication challenges?
2. Explore the insights you gained from doing this exercise.
3. How could you use what you learned from doing this exercise in your future nursing practice?

pay full attention to the discussion. Noise can be physical—for example, call bells, background conversations; even TV or music can be distracting. Noise is also considered physiological in the form of environmental distractions, such as pain, fatigue, or being tired. Semantic noise can also occur in the form of language barriers or using medical terminology, and psychological noise is associated when stereotypes, biases, emotions, fear, grief, or stress influence communication (Chute, 2015).

People require different amounts of personal space to communicate. **Personal space** is important as it allows a person to maintain their own space while providing them with the ability to keep a sense of identity, security, and control (Jakubec & Astle, 2019). When considering a person's personal space, it is important to remember that every individual is unique. Cultural contexts, personal preference, nature of the relationship, and the topic will influence personal space needs. Four areas of personal space have been identified: the intimate zone (0–45 cm), personal zone (45 cm–1 m), social zone (1 m–4 m), and public zone (4 m and greater) (Jakubec & Astle). Examples of nursing activities in each of these zones are the following: the intimate zone is when changing a person's dressing or bathing; sitting at the person's bedside or having professional communication with the person is within the personal zone; the social zone would be conducting a group session or sitting a conference table; and a public zone example is teaching a class of students (Jakubec & Astle).

People experiencing anxiety usually need more physical space, whereas those experiencing a sudden physical injury or undergoing a painful procedure may appreciate having the nurse in closer proximity, as in the intimate or personal zone.

Timing is important. Planning communication for periods when the person is able to participate physically and emotionally is time-efficient and respectful of the person's needs. Give the people you care for enough time to absorb material, to share their impressions, and to ask questions. The person's behaviour can cue the nurse about emotional readiness and available energy. The presence of pain or variations in energy levels, anger, or anxiety will require extra time for the nurse to inquire about how the person is feeling and its meaning before proceeding with the health care dialogue.

Communication as a Shared Partnership

Person-centred care and collaborative partnerships require a broader span of collaborative communication skills to accomplish the active partnership needed for managing complex health issues. Through verbal and nonverbal communication and active listening, while demonstrating empathy and caring, the nurse focuses on the person's health issues, recognizing the person's unique experience.

People expect to be listened to and to play a key role in managing their own care (Kuluski et al., 2016). But they also need support to do so. Person-centred communication includes the following:

- Partnerships with sharing power, responsibility, information, and decisions
- Being sensitive and responding to the person's needs, uncertainties, and emotions
- Attention to the whole person
- Empowering the person in self-management activities
- Respecting the person as an expert on themselves and their life (Hafskjold et al., 2015; RNAO, 2015).

Person-centred communication is an interactive, reciprocal exchange of ideas in which nurses try to understand what it is like to be this person, in this situation, with this health issue. Each person and family has a unique set of values, patterns of behaviour, and preferences that must be taken into account. How people communicate with the nurse varies, based on culture, diversity, values, beliefs, and social background factors. Their readiness to learn, personal ways of relating to others, physical and emotional conditions, life and social experiences, and their place in the life cycle are related factors in planning and implementing nursing care through therapeutic conversations.

Person-centred conversations include discussions needed for collaborative decision making. Talking about complex personal health problems with a health provider allows people and families to hear themselves, as they put health concerns into words. Feedback provided by the health provider ideally helps people to realistically sort out their priorities and determine the actions they want to take to effectively cope with their health circumstances.

APPLICATIONS

Effective communication is an art as well as a professional competency. It is not only what you say but also how you say it. Certain personality traits and attitudes—for example, a nonjudgemental respectful attitude; having a good sense of humour; and maintaining a calm, thoughtful manner throughout the communication process—are intangible characteristics of communication ease.

Engaging the Person

A person-centred communication process starts with the first encounter. Your initial presentation of yourself will influence the communication that follows. Each person you communicate with should have your full attention. This means clearing your own mind of any preconceived notions, biases, and even your own thoughts. Entering the person's space with an open, welcoming facial expression, respectful tone, and direct eye

DEVELOPING AN EVIDENCE-INFORMED PRACTICE

Purpose: To investigate which communication factors correlate with the constructs of positive therapeutic communication.

Method: Systematic review assessment of communication factors included interaction styles and verbal and nonverbal factors, while factors associated with the therapeutic relationship included collaboration, affective bond, agreement, trust, and empathy. Participants included health clinicians and people in primary, secondary, and tertiary care settings. Over 3000 published research papers were identified from the initial search of seven online databases. Twelve studies met the inclusion criteria, which yielded 67 communication factors related to interaction styles and verbal and nonverbal factors.

Findings: The interaction factors that showed the greatest strength related to the provision of emotional support, asking questions, and listening to what people have to say.

Application to Your Practice: Using person-centred interaction styles, with careful listening, and encouraging involvement of the person with a focus on emotional issues can enhance therapeutic communication.

Pinto, R. Z., Ferreira, M., Oliveira, V. et al. (2012). Patient-centred communication is associated with positive therapeutic alliance: A systematic review. *Journal of Physiotherapy, 58,* 77–87.

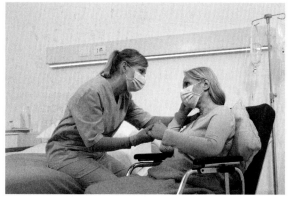

Fig. 5.3 Whether you are sitting or standing, your posture should be relaxed, with the upper part of your body inclined slightly toward the client. iStock.com/Visivasnc

contact indicates your interest and intent to know this person. Your posture immediately gives the person a message, either inviting trust or conveying disinterest. Whether you are sitting or standing, your posture should be relaxed, facing the person and leaning slightly forward (Fig. 5.3). Shaking the person's hand (if appropriate) with an open facial expression and a smile, signals to the person that they are the most important person for the moment.

Introductions are important, especially if many health providers are involved in the person's care. Failure to give your full name (first and last name) and role can create uncertainty within the person about who you are and what you want to discuss with them (Jakubec & Astle, 2019). Make eye contact when you introduce yourself as it is an important inclusive gesture. Ask for the person's name and how they would like to be addressed and what pronoun they would like to use (he, she, or they). It is better to be more formal than informal until you get to know the person better. Using the person's name conveys caring and respect for the person. When others (family or other health team members) are involved in a discussion, expand the introductions. Centre your attention on the person, but do not ignore other participants. You can include family members with eye contact and physical cues and can do so throughout the conversation.

Building Rapport

Begin with asking routine questions about the reason for seeking out health care, along with asking for other common information. Routine questions help to put the person and family members at ease. However, when you ask the person to tell you about their health concerns and what prompted them to seek help at this time, keep this part of the conversation open. Allow the person to tell you about their personal situation from a personal perspective, with few interruptions. Sequence questions going from general to more specific, complex questions.

Keep in mind that persons will vary in their ability to effectively communicate their feelings, preferences, and concerns. Personal characteristics, culture, previous life and health experiences, language, and education level create differences. Considering these factors allows you to phrase questions and interpret answers in more meaningful ways.

Being attentively present, providing relevant information, and actively listening to the person's concerns help to build rapport. People who feel safe, accepted, and validated by their health care providers find it easier to collaborate and communicate with them. Although rapport building begins with the initial encounter, it continues as a thread throughout the nurse–person relationship. Remember that people are looking to you not only for competence but also for sincerity and genuine interest in them as individuals. Simulation Exercise 5.2 provides an opportunity to practise an initial person-centred interview.

SIMULATION EXERCISE 5.2 Using Person-Centred Communication Role-Play

Purpose

To use person-centred communication strategies in an assessment interview

Procedure

1. Develop a one-paragraph scenario of a person-centred situation that you are familiar with from before class.
2. Pair off as person and nurse.
3. Conduct an initial person-centred 5-minute assessment interview using one of the scenarios, with the author of the paragraph taking the role of the nurse and the other student taking the role of the person being interviewed.
4. Reverse roles and repeat with the second student's scenario.

Reflective Discussion Analysis

1. In what ways were person-centred communication strategies used in this role-play?
2. How awkward was it for you in the nursing role to incorporate queries about the person's preferences, values, and so on?
3. What parts of the interview experience were of greatest value to you when you assumed the person role?
4. If you were conducting an assessment interview with a person in the future, what modifications might you make?
5. How could you use what you learned from doing this exercise in future nurse–person interviews?

SIMULATION EXERCISE 5.3 Establishing Rapport: "What Makes Me Comfortable"

Purpose

To help students identify personal communication features, which make it easier for people to establish rapport in new situations

Procedure

In groups of three to five students, each student should individually describe a firsthand interpersonal situation in which they felt comfortable with people they were meeting for the first time.

1. Individually, write down the factors that you feel accounted for your comfort in communicating with people in this

situation. What made the situation different from other first encounters?
2. Share your findings with the other members in your student group.

Reflective Discussion Analysis

1. What words, actions, and attitudes contributed to your feelings of comfort? Which of the three was most important to your comfort?
2. Were there any common communication features that facilitated initial rapport?
3. How could you use findings from this exercise to facilitate connection with new people?

Developing a Shared Partnership

The idea of health care as a shared partnership, in which the person is an equal stakeholder and partner in ensuring quality health care, is relatively new. Building a shared, workable partnership requires these elements:

- Empathetic objectivity, which allows you to experience persons as they are, not the way you would like them to be
- A "here and now" focus on the current issues and concerns important to the person
- Demonstration of respect, and asking questions about cultural and social differences that can influence care
- Authentic interest in the person and a confident manner that communicates competence
- The ability to consider competing goals and alternative ways to meet them

Finding Common Ground

Person-centred communication strategies allow the person and nurse to find common ground related to the person's explanations of the issues, their priorities, and their treatment goals. Before you can participate in the development of a shared approach to a problem, you have to give your full attention to what you are hearing from the person.

The aspects of care that are most important to a person and family, and what helps or hinders their capability to self-manage their health issues, is critical information. Look for themes revealing fears, feelings, and level of engagement. The person and family also need to understand the full range of therapeutic choices available to them in treating and self-managing their health. This is critical information, particularly for situations requiring informed consent. Simulation Exercise 5.3 is designed to increase the student's understanding of communication strategies in building rapport.

Observing Nonverbal Cues

Nonverbal communication involves all five senses and refers to communication other than through speaking. Research has identified that nonverbal communication is made up by approximately 38% vocal cues and 55% nonverbal body cues (Jakubec & Astle, 2019). People cannot always put their concerns into words. Some are not even aware of what is worrying them or what to do about their concerns. Others experience powerful emotions that make verbalizing personal concerns difficult.

Watch for nonverbal cues from the person. There are different "channels" of nonverbal communication (e.g., facial expressions, vocal tones, gestures and body positions, body movements, touch, and personal space). Take note of whether cues such as the person's facial expression, body movements, posture, and breathing rate support or contradict the meaning of their spoken message (See Box 5.1).

Changes in body language and nonverbal cues can indicate discomfort with the discussion. The person who declares that he is ready for surgery and seems calm may

---

BOX 5.1   Physical Behavioural Cues

Emblems: Gestures or body motions having a common verbal interpretation (e.g., handshaking, baby waving bye-bye, sign language).

Illustrators: Actions that accompany and emphasize the meaning of the verbal message (e.g., smiling, a stern facial expression, pounding a fist on the table).

Affect Displays: Facial presentation of emotional affect. Affect displays have a large range of meaning and act to support or contradict the meaning of the verbal message. (Nurses need to validate accuracy of perception with the person.)

Regulators: Nonverbal means of communication, such as nodding, facial expression, and hand gestures to stop conversation or reinforce or modify what is being said in the course of the conversation.

Adaptors: Person-specific, repetitive, nonverbal actions that are part of a person's usual response to emotional issues. Examples include nervous foot tapping, blushing, and hair twirling.

Physical Characteristics: Nonverbal information about the person observed in the outward appearance of the person (e.g., body odour, physical appearance [dirty hair, unshaven]).

Adapted from Blondis, M., & Jackson, B. (1982). *Nonverbal communication with patients: Back to the human touch* (pp. 9–10), (2nd ed.). New York: Wiley.

---

be sending a different message through the tense muscles the nurse touches when providing care. The differences between the person's words and body language cues can suggest that he may be worried about the surgery. Environmental cues, such as a half-eaten lunch or tapping of a foot, can provide other nonverbal evidence that perhaps the person is in distress but not verbalizing it. When this happens, you can comment on your perception—for example, "I'm wondering what you are feeling right now about what I am saying as I notice you didn't finish your lunch," or, "I noticed when I mentioned _____, your expression changed." Like verbal communication, nonverbal behaviours and signals are culture bound so they may mean different things in different cultures (see also Chapter 7; Samovar, Porter, & McDaniel, 2008). Simulation Exercise 5.4 provides practice with observing for nonverbal cues.

Active Listening

Active listening is defined as an intentional form of listening. It involves more than simply hearing words. Instead, it involves being aware of what the person is communicating, both verbally and nonverbally. Nonverbal skills that enhance your active listening ability can be applied by using the acronym SOLER (Townsend, 2013).

S: *Sit* facing the person, as this posture indicates that you want to listen and are interested in what the person has to say.

O: Keep an *open* posture, meaning that your arms and legs are uncrossed, which that you are open to what the person is saying. Crossed arms and legs can convey that you are uncomfortable and are closed to hearing what the person is telling you.

L: *Lean* toward the person, which conveys that you are interested and engaged in the conversation.

E: Initiate and maintain *eye contact* as this shows you are listening to what the person is telling you. Not maintaining eye contact or shifting your eyes away can indicate you are being distracted or not listening to what the person is saying.

R: *Relax.* As you communicate with the person, try to relax. Being restless can portray that you are uncomfortable or show a lack of interest.

The importance of listening in health care communication cannot be overestimated. When a person is ill, listening requires extra effort. It also involves the nurse noting feelings and looking for underlying themes. The goal is mutual understanding of facts and emotions.

Listening responses in a person-centred health environment ask about *all* the person's relevant health concerns. They take into account the person's values, culture, preferences, and expectations related to treatment goals, priorities, and

---

SIMULATION EXERCISE 5.4   Observing for Nonverbal Cues

Purpose

To develop skill in interpreting nonverbal cues

Procedure

1. Watch a dramatic movie (that you haven't seen before) with the sound off, for 5–15 minutes.
2. As you watch the movie, write down the emotions you see expressed, the associated nonverbal behaviour, and your interpretations of the meaning and the other person's response.

Reflective Discussion Analysis

In a large group, share your observations and interpretations of the scenes watched. Discussion should focus on the variations in the interpretations of the nonverbal communication. Discuss ways in which the nurse can use observations of nonverbal communication with a person in a therapeutic manner to gain a better understanding of the person. Time permitting, the movie segment could be shown again, this time with the sound. Discuss any variations in the interpretations without sound versus with verbal dialogue. Discuss the importance of validation of nonverbal cues.

---

attitudes about treatment suggestions. Open-ended questions, such as the ones identified below, are core clinical questions:

- "What is important to you now?"
- "What do you see as the next step?"
- "What are you hoping will happen with this treatment?"
- "What is most important for you to know?"

Listening responses can be integrated with asking for validation of person preferences—for example, asking the person, "How does the idea of _____ sound to you?" or "What concerns you about learning to use your crutches?" Each of these questions, and others along the same line, can encourage a person to explore potential concerns, expand on an idea, or voice confusion. This information is essential to achieve a shared understanding and realistic clinical expectations.

A person-centred interview begins with the nurse encouraging the person to tell their story in an authentic way, while demonstrating caring and being open in understanding the person's lived experience (RNAO, 2015). Open-ended questions are a major means of helping people tell their story, of obtaining relevant information, and of reducing misunderstandings. There are different ways of asking questions. Questions fall into three categories: open-ended, closed-ended, and circular.

Open-Ended Questions

Open-ended questions are defined as questions that are open to interpretation and cannot be answered by "yes" or "no," or a one-word response. They allow the person to express their problems or health concerns in their own words. Open-ended questions usually begin with words such as "what," "how," or "can you describe for me . . .," etc. They provide a broader context for each person's unique health concerns and are likely to yield more complete information. Open-ended questions invite the person to think and reflect on their situation. They help connect relevant elements of the person's experience (e.g., relationships, impact of the illness on self or others, environmental and social barriers, and potential resources or concerns).

Open-ended questions are used to elicit the person's thoughts and perspectives without influencing the direction of an acceptable response, for example:

"Can you tell me what brought you to the clinic today?"

"Describe for me what it has been like for you since the accident."

"Where would you like to begin today?"

"How can I help you?"

"What would you like to see happen today?"

"Can you tell me how you get relief from your pain at home?"

Ending the dialogue with a general open-ended question, such as "Is there anything else concerning you right now or that you would like to tell me?" or "Is there anything that we've left out today?" can provide relevant information that might otherwise be overlooked. Simulation Exercise 5.5 provides an opportunity to practise the use of open-ended questions.

Focused Questions

Focused questions require more than a yes or no answer, but they place limitations on the topic to be addressed. They are useful in emergencies and in other situations when immediate, concise information is required. Focused questions can clarify the timing and sequence of symptoms and concentrate on details about a person's health concerns. For example, they can include when symptoms began, what other symptoms the person is having, and what a person has done to date to resolve the problem.

People with limited verbal skills sometimes respond better to focused questions because they require less interpretation. Examples of focused questions include the following:

"Can you tell me more about the pain in your arm?"

"Can you give me a specific example of what you mean by . . . ?"

"When did your stomach pain begin?"

SIMULATION EXERCISE 5.5 **Asking Open-Ended Questions**

Purpose

To develop skill in the use of open-ended questions to facilitate information sharing

Procedure

1. Break up into pairs. Role-play a situation in which one student takes the role of the facilitator and the other the sharer. (If you work in the clinical area, you may want to choose a clinical situation.)
2. As a pair, select a topic. The facilitator begins asking open-ended questions.
3. Dialogue for 5–10 min on the topic.
4. In pairs, discuss perceptions of the dialogue and determine what questions were comfortable and open-ended.

The student facilitator should reflect on the comfort level experienced with asking each question. The sharing student should reflect on the efficacy of the listening responses in helping to move the conversation toward their perspective.

Reflective Discussion Analysis

As a class, each pair should contribute examples of open-ended questions that facilitated the sharing of information. Compile these examples on the board. Formulate a collaborative summation of what an open-ended question is and how it is used. Discuss how open-ended questions can be used sensitively with uncomfortable topics.

Focused questions help the person organize data and prioritize immediate concerns—for example, you might ask a question at the end of the conversation such as, "Of the concerns we talked about today, which has been the most difficult for you or is the most important for you?"

Circular questions are a form of focused questions that look at how other people within the person's support circle respond to the person's health issues. These questions are designed to identify differences in the impact of an illness on individual family members and explore changes in relationships brought about by the health circumstances. For example, "When your dad says he doesn't want hospice care because he is a fighter, what is that like for you?"

Closed-Ended Questions

Closed-ended questions are defined as narrowly focused questions for which a single answer—for example, "yes," "no," or a simple phrase—serves as a valid response. They are useful in emergency situations, when the goal is to obtain information quickly and the context or person's emotional reactions are of secondary importance because of the seriousness of the immediate situation. Examples of closed-ended questions include the following: "Does the pain radiate down your left shoulder and arm?" "When was your last meal?"

What the Nurse Listens for: Themes

Behind the actual words exist themes. *Themes* refer to the underlying message, present but not identified in the person's words. Listening for themes requires observing and understanding what the person is not saying as well as what the person actually reveals through words. Identifying the underlying themes in a therapeutic conversation can relieve anxiety and provide direction for

individualized nursing interventions. For example, the person might say to the nurse, "I'm worried about my surgery tomorrow." This is one way of framing the problem. If the same person presents his concern as, "I'm not sure I will make it through the surgery tomorrow," the underlying theme of the communication changes from a generalized worry to a more personal theme of survival. Alternatively, a person might say, "I don't know whether my husband should stay tomorrow when I have my surgery. It is going to be a long procedure, and he gets so worried." The theme (focus) here expresses a concern about how her husband is dealing with her surgery. In each communication, the person expresses a theme of concern related to a statement, but the emphasis in each requires a different response.

When listening for themes, it is important to remain objective and not make judgements or assumptions. Instead, the nurse should try to understand what the person is conveying in their words and actions to better understand the person's concerns, attitudes, beliefs, and values at that moment. Simulation Exercise 5.6 provides practice in listening for themes.

ACTIVE LISTENING RESPONSES

Active listening responses are essential components of person-centred communication. Through active listening, a new level of understanding can develop; potential or actual problems can be reframed and resolved with the development of collaborative, shared goals. The minimal verbal cues, clarification, restatement, paraphrasing, reflection, summarization, silence, and touch are examples of skilled listening responses that nurses can use to guide therapeutic interventions (Table 5.1).

SIMULATION EXERCISE 5.6 **Listening for Themes**

Purpose
To help students identify underlying themes in messages

Procedure
1. Divide into groups of three to five students.
2. Take turns telling a short story about yourself—about growing up, important people or events in your life, or significant accomplishments (e.g., getting your first job).
3. As each student presents a story, listen carefully to be prepared to ask questions for clarification, if needed. Write them down so you will not be tempted to change them as you hear the other stories. Notice nonverbal behaviours accompanying the verbal message. Are they consistent with the verbal message of the sharer?
4. When the story is completed, each person in the group shares their observations with the sharer.

5. After all students have shared their observations, validate their accuracy with the sharer.

Reflective Discussion Analysis
1. Were the underlying themes recorded by the group consistent with the sharer's understanding of their own communication?
2. As others related their interpretations of significant words or phrases, did you change your mind about the nature of the underlying theme?
3. Were student interpretations of pertinent information relatively similar or significantly different from each other?
4. If they were different, what implications do you think such differences have for nurse–person relationships in nursing practice?
5. What did you learn from doing this exercise?

TABLE 5.1 **Active Listening Responses**

Listening Response	Example
Minimal cues and leads	Body actions: smiling, nodding, leaning forward
	Words: "mm," "uh-huh," "oh, really," "go on"
Clarification	"Could you describe what happened in sequence?" "I'm not sure I understand what you mean. Can you give me an example?"
Restatement	"Are you saying that . . . (repeat person's words)?" "You mean . . . (repeat person's words)?"
Paraphrasing	Person: "I can't take this anymore. The chemo is worse than the cancer. I just want to die."
	Nurse: "It sounds as though you're saying you've had enough."
Reflection	"It sounds as though you feel guilty because you weren't home at the time of the accident." "You sound really frustrated because the treatment is taking longer than you thought it would."
Summarizing	"Before moving on, I would like to go over with you what I think we've accomplished thus far."
Silence	Briefly disconnecting with a brief pause but continuing to use attending behaviours after an important idea, thought, or feeling has been expressed.
Touch	Gently rubbing a person's arm during a painful procedure or holding their hand.

Listening Responses

Minimal Cues and Leads

Nonverbal communication is transmitted through body action (smiling, nodding, and leaning forward, encouraging the person to continue their story). Short phrases such as "Go on" or "And then?" or "Can you say more about . . .?" are useful verbal prompts. Simulation Exercise 5.7 provides an opportunity to practise **minimal cues** and verbal prompts in person-centred communication.

Clarification

Clarification is defined as a brief question or a request for validation. It is used to better understand a person's message—for example, "You stated earlier that you were concerned about your blood pressure. Tell me more about what concerns you." The tone of voice used with a clarification response should be neutral, not accusatory or demanding. Failure to ask for clarification when part of the communication is poorly understood means that

---

SIMULATION EXERCISE 5.7   Minimal Cues and Leads

Purpose
To practise and evaluate the efficacy of minimal cues and leads

Procedure
1. Initiate a conversation with someone outside of class and attempt to tell the person about something with which you are familiar, for 5–10 minutes.
2. Make note of all the cues that the person puts forth that either promote or inhibit conversation.
3. Now try this with another person and write down the different cues and leads you observe as you are speaking, as well as your emotional response to them (e.g., what most encouraged you to continue speaking?).

Reflective Discussion Analysis
As a class, share your experience and observations. Compile the different cues and responses on the board.

Discuss the impact of different cues and leads on your comfort and willingness to share about yourself. What cues and leads promoted communication? What cues and leads inhibited sharing?

Variation
This exercise can be practised with a clinical problem simulation in which one student takes the role of the professional helper and the other takes the role of the person. Perform the same scenario with and without the use of minimum encouragers. What were the differences when encouragers were not used? Was the communication as lively? How did it feel to you when telling your story when this strategy was used by the helping person?

SIMULATION EXERCISE 5.8   Using Clarification

Purpose
To develop skill in the use of clarification

Procedure
1. Write a paragraph related to a clinical experience you have had.
2. Place all the student paragraphs together and then pick one (not your own).

3. Develop clarification questions you might ask about the selected clinical experience.

Reflective Discussion Analysis
Share with the class your chosen paragraph and the clarification questions you developed. Discuss how effective the questions are in clarifying information. Other students can suggest additional clarification.

---

you might act on incomplete or inaccurate information. You can practise the clarification response in Simulation Exercise 5.8.

Restatement

Restatement is an active listening strategy used to broaden a person's perspective or when the nurse needs to validate or clarify the person's statement. For example, a person may say, "I am so sad" and the nurse would respond, "You're sad?" When sparingly implemented in a questioning manner, a restatement strategy can help the person clarify and expand upon what they are trying to convey.

Paraphrasing

Paraphrasing is a listening response used to check whether the nurse's translation of the person's words represents an accurate interpretation of the message. The strategy involves the nurse taking the person's original message and transforming it into their own words, without losing the meaning. A paraphrase should be shorter and more specific than the person's initial statement so that the focus is on the core elements of the original statement. Your objective in using paraphrasing as an active listening response is to find a common understanding of issues important to the person. Paraphrasing allows you to summarize or streamline a message, and highlight key points of the longer message. For example, the person tells you that they are "so tired of being told something different by different health providers on what they need to do to get better." The nurse using paraphrasing could respond, "It sounds to me like you're feeling overwhelmed right now with all the information you're receiving."

Reflection

Reflection is an active listening response that focuses on the emotional part of a message. It offers nurses a way to

SIMULATION EXERCISE 5.9   Role-Play Practice With Paraphrasing and Reflection

Purpose

To practise the use of paraphrasing and reflection as listening responses

Procedure

1. The class forms into groups of three students each. One student takes the role of person, one the role of nurse, and one the role of observer.
2. The person shares with the nurse a recent health problem they encountered and describes the details of the situation and the emotions experienced. The nurse responds, using paraphrasing and reflection in a dialogue that lasts at least 5 minutes. The observer records the statements made by the helper. At the end of the dialogue, the person writes their perception of how the helper's statements affected the conversation, including what comments were most helpful.

The helper writes a short summary of the listening responses they used, with comments on how successful the responses were.

Discussion

1. Share your summary and discuss the differences in using the techniques from the helper, person, and observer perspectives.
2. Discuss how these differences related to influencing the flow of dialogue, helping the person feel heard, and the impact on the helper's understanding of the person, from both the person and the helper positions.
3. Identify places in the dialogue where one form of questioning might be preferable to another.
4. How could you use this exercise to understand the concerns of the person in your scenario?
5. Were you surprised by any of the summaries?

empathetically mirror their sense of how a person may be emotionally experiencing their health situation. There are several ways to use reflection, for example:

- Reflection on vocal tone: "You seem to have some anger and frustration in your voice as you describe your accident" or "You sound happy when you talk about your grandson."
- Reflection example, linking feelings with content: "It sounds like you feel _____ because _____."
- Linking current feelings with past experiences: "This experience seems to remind you of feelings you had with other health care providers, when you didn't feel understood."

A reflective listening response should be a simple observational comment, expressed tentatively, not an exhaustive comment about the person's emotional reaction. It offers an opportunity for the person to validate or to change the narrative. When reflecting on an emotional observation, students sometimes feel they are putting words into the person's mouth when they "choose" an emotion from their perception of a person's message. This would be true if you were choosing an emotion out of thin air but not when you empathetically mirror what you are hearing from the person. You can simply present potential or observable underlying feelings present in the person's narrative, without interpreting its meaning. Simulation Exercise 5.9 provides practice in using paraphrasing and reflection as listening responses.

Summarization

Summarization is an active listening skill used to review content and process. Summarization pulls several ideas and feelings together, either from one interaction or from a series of interactions, into a few brief sentences. This would be followed by a comment seeking validation, such as, "Tell me if my understanding of this agrees with yours." A summary statement can also be useful as a bridge to changing the topic or focus of the conversation. The summarization should be completed before the end of the conversation, but with enough time before you leave the room, for validation or questions. Simulation Exercise 5.10 is designed to provide insight into the use of summarization as a listening response.

Silence

Silence, delivered as a brief pause, is a powerful listening response. Intentional pauses can allow the person to think. A short pause lets the nurse step back momentarily and process what has been heard, before responding. Silence can be used to emphasize important points that you want the person to reflect on. By pausing briefly after presenting a key idea and before proceeding to the next topic, it encourages a person to reflect on what has just been discussed.

When a person falls silent, it can mean many things: something has touched the person, the person is angry or does not know how to respond, or the person is thinking about *how* to respond. A verbal comment to check on the meaning of the message is helpful.

SIMULATION EXERCISE 5.10   **Practising Summarization**

Purpose

To provide practice in summarizing interactions

Procedure

1. Choose a partner for a pair's discussion. Choose one person to be Participant A and one to be Participant B.
2. For 5 minutes, discuss why you decided to become a nurse.
3. After 5 minutes, both partners must stop talking until Participant A summarizes what Participant B said, to Participant B's satisfaction, and vice versa.

Discussion

After both partners have completed their summarization, discuss the process of summarization and answering the following questions:

1. Did knowing you had to summarize the other person's point of view encourage you to listen more closely?
2. Did the act of summarizing help clarify any discussion points? Did you find any points of agreement? What points of disagreement did you find?
3. Did the exercise help you to understand the other person's point of view?
4. How did you determine which points to focus on in your summarization?

TABLE 5.2   **Negative Listening Responses**

Category of Response	Explanation of Category	Examples
False reassurance	Using pseudo-comforting phrases in an attempt to offer reassurance	"It will be okay." "Everything will work out." "Don't worry."
Giving advice	Making a decision for a person; offering personal opinions; telling a person what to do (using phrases such as "ought to," "should")	"If I were you, I would . . ." "I feel you should . . ."
False inferences	Making an unsubstantiated assumption about what a person means; interpreting the person's behaviour without asking for validation; jumping to conclusions	"What you really mean is you don't like your physician." "Subconsciously, you are blaming your husband for the accident."
Moralizing	Expressing your own values about what is right and wrong, especially on a topic that concerns the person	"Medical assistance in dying (MAID) is wrong." "It is wrong to refuse to have the operation."
Value judgements	Conveying your approval or disapproval about the person's behaviour or about what the person has said using words such as "good," "bad," or "nice"	"I'm glad you decided to . . ." "That really wasn't a nice way to behave." "She's a good person."

Not all listening responses are helpful. Nurses need to recognize when their responses are interfering with objectivity or are inviting premature closure. Table 5.2 provides definitions of negative listening responses that block communication.

MIRRORING COMMUNICATION PATTERNS

Communication patterns provide a different type of information. Being respectful of the person's communication pattern involves accepting the person's communication style as a part of who the person is, without expecting that person to be different (see also Chapter 6). Some people can exaggerate information; others characteristically leave out highly relevant details. Some talk a lot, using dramatic language and multiple examples; others say very little and have to be encouraged to provide details. When adapting to people's communication patterns, it is recommended to start where the person is, and to mirror the person's communication style.

Evaluation of the person's present overall pattern of interaction with others includes strengths and limitations, family communication dynamics, and developmental and educational levels. Culture, role, ways of handling conflict, and ways of dealing with emotions also reflect and influence communication patterns. For example, AJ frequently interrupts and presents with a loud, strong opinion on most things. This is AJ's communication pattern. To engage successfully with her, you would need to listen while accepting her way of communicating as a part of who she is, without being judgemental, joining in with arguing the validity of her position, or getting lost in detail. Remember that when some people are anxious or worried, they can use a controlling form of communication. They may have difficulty listening to or understanding information. Taking a little extra time to establish rapport and understand what is concerning AJ can foster the interactions and help determine what to focus on in your therapeutic communication. Box 5.2 describes what the nurse listens for when communicating with the person.

BOX 5.2 What the Nurse Listens For

- Content themes
- Communication patterns
- Discrepancies in message content, body language, and verbalization
- Feelings revealed in a person's voice, body movements, and facial expressions
- What is not being said as well as what is being said
- The person's preferred representational system (auditory, visual, tactile)
- The nurse's own inner responses and personal ways of knowing
- The effect communication produces in others involved with the person

---

VERBAL COMMUNICATION AND RESPONSES

Active listening and verbal responses are inseparable from each other; each informs and reinforces the other. Simulation Exercise 5.11 presents a summary of the therapeutic interviewing skills presented in this chapter as they apply to the phases of the nurse–person relationship, using verbal and active listening skills. With shorter time frames for contact with the person, nurses need to verbally connect with the person, beginning with the first encounter. As the relationship develops, it is important to make room for questions that the person may have to ensure that care remains person-centred. You can use a simple lead, such as, "I'm wondering what questions you might have about what we've been discussing." If the person replies with, "I don't have any questions," you could follow up with a short statement—for example, "One question I am frequently asked is . . ."

Most people are seeking feedback and want caring support that suggests a compassionate understanding of their particular situation. No matter what level of communication exists in the relationship, the same needs—"hear me," "touch me," "respond to me," "feel my pain and experience my joys with me"—are fundamental themes. These are the themes addressed by person-centred communication.

Words help people assess their strengths and enable them to use these elements in coping with their current health issues. Nurses use verbal responses to teach, encourage, support, provide, and gather and validate provided information in guiding a person toward goal achievement. Nurses should offer guidance and support but no judgement.

SIMULATION EXERCISE 5.11 Active Listening and Verbal Responses

Purpose
To develop skill in active listening and verbal responses and an awareness of the elements involved

Procedure
1. Students break up into pairs. Each takes a turn reflecting on and describing an important experience they have had in their lives. The person who shares should describe the details, emotions, and outcomes of their experience. During the interaction, the listening partner should use listening responses such as clarification, paraphrasing, reflection, and focusing, as well as attending cues, eye contact, and alert body posture to carry the conversation forward. Verbal responses such as open-ended, focused, and closed-ended questions should also be incorporated into the interaction.

2. After the sharing partner finishes their story, the listening partner indicates understanding by (a) stating in their own words what the sharing partner said and (b) summarizing perceptions of the sharing partner's feelings associated with the story and asking for validation. If the sharing partner agrees, then the listening partner can be sure they correctly utilized active listening skills.

Reflective Discussion Analysis
In the large group, have pairs of students share their discoveries about active listening. As a class, discuss aspects of nursing behaviour that will foster active listening in person interactions.

Verbal response strategies include mirroring, focusing, metaphors, humour, reframing, feedback, and validation, all of which are designed to strengthen the coping abilities of the person, alone or in relationship with others. Nurses use active listening, observation, validation, and patterns of knowing to gauge the effectiveness of verbal interventions. On the basis of the person's reaction, the nurse may decide to use simpler language or to try a different strategy in collaboratively working with the person. Another strategy is to make a simple statement, such as "Let me think about that a bit and get back to you." Obviously, it is important to return to the topic later if you use this strategy.

When making verbal responses or providing information, do not overload the person with too many ideas or too much information. If you find you are doing most of the talking, start using more listening responses to elicit the person's perspective. It is important to provide the necessary information, ensure they understand what is being said, and then support them in their decision making on how to proceed with addressing their health concerns.

People can absorb only so much information at one time, particularly if they are tired, fearful, in pain, overwhelmed, or discouraged. Introducing new ideas *one at a time* allows the person to more easily process what is being conveyed. Repeating key ideas and reinforcing information with concrete examples facilitate understanding and provide an additional opportunity for the person to ask questions. Paying attention to nonverbal response cues from the person that support understanding or that reflect a need for further attention is an important dimension of successful communication.

Matching Responses

Responses that encourage a person to explore feelings about strengths and areas of concern at a slightly deeper but related level of conversation are likely to meet with more success.

Verbal responses should neither expand nor diminish the meaning of the person's remarks. Notice the differences in the nature of the following responses to a person.

Case Example

Person: "I feel so discouraged. No matter how hard I try, I still can't walk without pain on the two parallel bars."

Nurse: "You want to give up because you don't think you will be able to walk again."

At this point, it is unclear that the person wants to give up, so the nurse's comment expands on the person's meaning without having sufficient data to support it. Although it is possible that this is what the person means, it is not the only possibility. The more

---

important dilemma for the person may be whether their efforts have any purpose.

The next response focuses only on the negative aspects of the person's communication, lacks compassion, and ignores the person's comment about their efforts.

Nurse: "So you think you won't be able to walk independently again."

In the final response example below, the nurse addresses both parts of the person's message and makes the appropriate connection. The nurse's statement invites the person to validate the nurse's perception.

Nurse: "It sounds to me as if you don't feel your efforts are helping you regain control over your walking without pain."

Using Plain Language

Plain language refers to the use of clear-cut, simple, easy to understand words to convey ideas, particularly those that use medical terminology or are more theoretical. To develop trust with the person, it is important to speak with a general spirit of inquiry and concern for the person. Verbal messages should address core issues in an understandable, concise manner, taking into account the guidelines for effective verbal expressions, listed in Box 5.3.

Before responding or giving information, consider who the person is, including their health issues, concerns, values, family, diversity, social circumstances, and lifestyles. Also consider the level of anxiety and potential culture or language issues—both your own and those of the person. Remember that your frame of reference may be quite different from theirs.

Avoid using medical jargon or clinical language that people may have trouble understanding. Unless the person or family members can associate new ideas with familiar words and ideas, you might as well be speaking in a different language. People and their families may not tell you that they do not understand what is being said for fear of offending you or of revealing they don't understand what is being said.

Start with finding out what the person already knows or believes about their health situation. Giving information that fails to take into account a person's previous experiences, or assumes that they have knowledge they do not possess, will be ineffective. Frequent check-ins related to content and validation with the person during the conversation help reduce this problem.

Focusing

In today's health care delivery system, nurses must make every second count. It is important for nurses to ask the

BOX 5.3   Guidelines to Effective Verbal Communication in the Nurse–Person Relationship

- Use plain language and vocabulary familiar to the person.
- Simplify and define unfamiliar terms and concepts to improve comprehension.
- Validate the understanding of word meanings.
- Match content and delivery with the person's developmental and literacy level.
- Keep in mind the person's experiential frame of reference, learning readiness, and general medical condition.
- Keep messages clear, concrete, honest, and simple to understand.
- Put ideas in a logical sequence of related material.
- Relate new ideas to familiar ones when presenting new information.
- Repeat key ideas.
- Reinforce key points with vocal emphasis and pauses.
- Focus only on essential elements; present one idea at a time.
- Use as many sensory communication channels as possible for key ideas.
- Make sure that nonverbal behaviours support verbal messages.
- Seek frequent feedback to validate accurate reception of information.

person what are the most pressing or relevant health care concerns for discussion.

Sensitivity to the person's needs and preferences should be taken into consideration. You should not force a person to focus on an issue that they are not yet willing to discuss unless it is an emergency situation. You can always go back to a topic when the person is more receptive. For example, you might say, "I can understand that this is a difficult topic for you, but I'm here for you if you'd like to discuss [identified topic] later."

Presenting Reality

Presenting reality to a person who is misinterpreting it can be helpful, as long as the person does not perceive that the nurse is criticizing the person's perception of reality. A simple statement such as "I know that you feel strongly about _____, but I see it in this way___," is an effective way for the nurse to express a different interpretation of the situation. Another strategy is to put into words the underlying feeling that is being implied but is not stated.

Giving Feedback

Feedback is a message a nurse gives to the person in response to a question, verbal message, or observed behaviour. Feedback can focus on the content, the relationship between people and events, the feelings generated by the message, or parts of the communication that are not clear. Feedback should be specific and directed to the behaviour. It should not be an analysis of the person's motivations. Verbal feedback provides the receiver's understanding of the sender's message and personal reaction to it. Effective feedback offers a neutral mirror, which allows a person to view an issue or behaviour from a different perspective. Feedback is most relevant when it addresses only the topics under discussion and does not go beyond the data the person presents. Effective feedback is clear, honest, and reflective. Feedback supported with realistic examples is believable, whereas feedback without specific instances to support it can lack credibility.

Case Example

After giving birth to her first child in the hospital, a new mother was feeding her newborn 90 ml of formula or more, every 4 hours. She was concerned that her child vomited a considerable amount of the undigested formula after each feeding, so she wanted to make sure her infant was getting enough food. Initially, the nursing student gave the mother instructions about feeding the infant no more than 60 ml at each feeding in the first few days of life, but the mother's behaviour persisted, and so did that of her infant. The nursing student began to question the new mother and discovered that the mother's friend had fed her baby 90 ml right from birth, with no problem and considered this to be the norm. This additional information helped the nursing student work with the new mother in seeing the uniqueness of her child and understanding what the infant was telling her through the behaviour of not tolerating the feedings. The mother began to feel more comfortable and confident in feeding her infant a smaller amount of formula, consistent with his needs.

Effective feedback is specific rather than general. Telling a person they didn't do as expected is less helpful than providing a behavioural description—for example, "I noticed, when the anaesthesiologist was in the room, you didn't ask any of the questions you had about receiving anaesthesia tomorrow. Can we talk about what you might want to know, so you can get the information you need?" With this response, the nurse provides precise information about an observed behaviour and offers a potential solution.

The person is more likely to respond with validation or correction, and the nurse can provide specific guidance.

Feedback can be about the nurse's observations of nonverbal behaviours—for example, "You seem (angry, upset, confused, happy, sad, etc.) when . . ." Request for feedback can be framed as a question, requiring the person to describe their understanding of what has been communicated in their own words; for example, "I want to be sure that we have the same understanding of what we've talked about. Can you tell me in your own words what we discussed?"

Not all feedback is equally relevant, nor is it always accepted. A benchmark for deciding whether feedback is appropriate is to ask yourself, "Does this feedback advance the goals of the relationship?" and "Does it consider the individualized needs of the person?" If the answer to either question is "no," then while the feedback may be accurate, it may be inappropriate in the current context. Most people find "why" questions difficult to answer. In general, avoid asking "why" questions as an initial questioning strategy. Typically, motivation and actions are multidimensional, so "why" questions can be more difficult to answer. "How" or "what" questions are usually focused and more easily answered.

Timing is a critical element. Giving feedback as soon as possible after you observe a behaviour is most effective. Other factors (e.g., a person's readiness to hear feedback, privacy, and the availability of support from others) contribute to effectiveness. Providing feedback about behaviours over which the person has little control only increases the personalized feelings of perhaps low self-esteem and can lead to frustration. Feedback should be to the point and empathetic.

People also give nonverbal feedback. Reactions such as surprise, boredom, anxiety, or anger send a message about how the listener is responding internally to the message. When you receive nonverbal messages suggesting uncertainty, concern, or inattention, it is important to ask for validation.

Validation

Validation is a special form of feedback, which is used to ensure that both participants have the same basic understanding of messages. Word meanings can be different for people. Some words have cultural and contextual implications that can lead to different meanings for each communicator. For example, in Indonesia, the word "air" means water. So someone may ask you for "a glass of air."

Simply asking the person whether they understand what was said is not an adequate method of validating message content. Instead, you might ask, "How do you feel about what I just said?" or "I'm curious what your thoughts are about what I just told you." You can also ask them to repeat what you said, to make sure they understood and heard what you said. If the person does not have any response,

you can suggest that the person can respond later, by saying, "Many people find they have reactions or questions about [the issue] after they've had a chance to think about it. I would be glad to discuss this further." Validation can provide new information that helps the nurse frame comments that are more responsive to the person's need.

OTHER FORMS OF COMMUNICATION

Touch

Touch, the first of our senses to develop and the last to lose, is a nurturing form of communication and validation. Intentional touch can provide a strong connection with the person in providing comfort and improving their experience (Dean & Ferguson, 2016). Touch is a powerful listening response used when words fail to convey the depth of empathy needed. Touch can also enhance person-centred communication and build upon the person–nurse relationship. A hand placed on a frightened mother's shoulder or a squeeze of the hand can speak far more eloquently than words, in times of deep emotion. Touch stimulates comfort, security, well-being, and a sense of feeling valued (Herrington & Chioda, 2014; Sundin & Jansson, 2003). People in pain; those who feel diminished or not valued, lonely, or who are dying; and those experiencing sensory deprivation or feeling confused respond positively to the nurse who is unafraid to enter their world and touch them. (Fig. 5.4).

How you touch a person in providing everyday nursing care is a form of communication. For example, gentle massage of a painful area helps a person relax. Holding the hand of a person with dementia can reduce agitation. Touch also conveys the sense that the nurse is with the person and supporting them in their experience when there is nothing left to do or say.

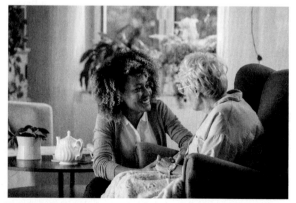

Fig. 5.4 Touch is an important form of communication, particularly when people are stressed. iStock.com/izusek

While touch is a very powerful method of communication, it is important to remember that people can vary in their comfort with touch. In some cultures, touch is used as a common form of communication, whereas in others, it is viewed differently or is seldom used. Touch can also be contraindicated in some health issues or because of a person's experiences, such as someone who has been assaulted. You will need to learn to be sensitive and assess for the person's response and receptiveness to being touched.

Case Example

Brendan's grandfather has dementia. He is in the hospital, which terrifies him. When Brendan visits him, he sits quietly beside the bed at eye level and gently massages his hand. The confused, wild look in his grandfather's eyes disappears as he listens to his grandson recall special moments they have shared, and he peacefully closes his eyes.

SPECIALIZED COMMUNICATION STRATEGIES

Figurative Language

Familiar images promote understanding. Figurative language is a way of representing information in a way that can help people and their family members process difficult, new, or abstract information by comparing it with more familiar images from ordinary life experiences. Laundau, Arndt & Cameron (2018) suggest that a simile example can be easier to understand than a medical explanation. For example, chronic lung disease described as "Emphysema is like having lungs similar to 'Swiss cheese.'" Analogies are also helpful—for example, to compare a coronary artery being occluded with plaque to a pipe that is partially blocked and needs to be cleared. A familiar concrete image can help a person connect with an abstract medical diagnosis that is harder to understand. Data supported by a explanation using figurative language can be more persuasive than a literal explanation. The choice of wording is important. As discussed throughout this chapter, the nurse has to ensure that when figurative language is used, it is age appropriate and the person will understand what the nurse is describing. Examples related to battles have often been used, such as a person diagnosed with cancer is described as "fighting the battle." The Canadian Cancer Society (2019) recently decided to reframe the cancer conversation, to focus on, "Life is Bigger than Cancer." They made this decision recognizing that people with cancer are much more than the disease. It was also a deliberate move away from the potential message that should a person die, saying they lost the battle with cancer could imply that the person did not work hard enough or didn't do something else differently to win the battle and live.

Humour

Humour is a powerful, person-centred communication technique when used for a specific therapeutic purpose. Humour is an important part of life and can assist as a coping strategy when dealing with difficult situations. Nurses can use humour appropriately in lightening the mood and providing comfort and compassionate care (Balzar Riley, 2017). Humour has also demonstrated positive effects on both a person's emotional and physiological well-being (Jakubec & Astle, 2019). A good laugh can bond communicators together in a shared conversation in ways that might not happen otherwise. Using humour needs to be suitable for the situation; the people being cared for indicate that they are open to humour; and it is culturally appropriate (Balzar Riley). A humourous comment should fit the situation, not dominate it. When using humour, it is best to focus on an idea, event, or situation. It should never be used in relation to a person's personal characteristics.

The surprise element in humour can cut through an overly intense situation and put it into perspective.

The following factors contribute to the successful use of humour:

- Knowledge of the person's response pattern
- An overly intense situation
- Timing
- A situation that lends itself to an imaginative or paradoxical solution
- Gearing the humour dynamics to the person's developmental level and interests
- A focus on the humour in a situation or change in circumstance

---

Case Example

A person was walking down the hospital hallway wearing a walking aircast boot. As the nurse went by, she stopped and said, "I love your footwear. I hope you got it while doing something adventurous, like skiing in the Rockies." The person laughed and told the nurse that they wish they had, but it was actually as a result of falling down the stairs.

USING TECHNOLOGY IN PERSON-CENTRED RELATIONSHIPS

The many uses of technology in communication are detailed in Chapters 26 and 27. Increasingly, nurses are incorporating technology to communicate in digital encounters with people and families (Collins, 2014). Although technology can never replace face-to-face time with a person, voice mail, email, social media platforms, and telehealth or virtual conferencing home visits help connect people with care providers and provide critical information. During the COVID-19 pandemic that began in 2020, with the need for social distancing (2 meters apart or the length of a hockey stick), virtual video conferencing became a common method of communicating with health providers in non-emergency situations.

Technology is transforming person–nurse relationships and the way we communicate. For example, routine laboratory results, appointment scheduling, and links to information on the Web can be transmitted through technology. Present-day technology allows people to use the Internet as a communication means to share common experiences with others who have a disease condition, to consult with experts about symptoms and treatment, and to learn up-to-date information about their condition. It is important to assist people in assessing the value of Web health information and what is accurate information on Internet sites.

The electronic nurse–person relationship begins when the nurse comes online or begins speaking to the person. From that point forward, the nurse needs to follow defined standards related to social media platforms and communication principles identified in this chapter and guided by your provincial or territorial regulatory standards and privacy legislation. At the end of each encounter, nurses need to provide the person with clear directions and contact information should additional assistance be required. Confidentiality and protection of identifiable personal information is an essential component of conversations used on social media platforms.

Communication via phone, email, video, or social media platforms can also be an essential communication link. Nurses can connect with people and their families to find out how they are doing and whether they have any questions or concerns related to their health issues.

SUMMARY

This chapter discusses basic therapeutic communication strategies that nurses can use with people across clinical settings. Nurses use active listening responses, such as paraphrasing, reflection, clarification, silence, summarization, and touch, to elicit information and convey caring and compassion. Observation is a primary source of information, but all nonverbal behaviours need to be validated with the person for accuracy.

Open-ended questions give the nurse the most information because they allow the person to express ideas and feelings as they are experiencing them. Focused or closed-ended questions are more appropriate in emergency clinical situations, when precise information is needed quickly or to confirm information obtained through asking open-ended questions.

Nurses use verbal communication strategies that fit the person's communication patterns in terms of level, meaning, and language to help the person meet treatment goals. Other strategies include the use of figurative language, reframing, humour, confirming responses, feedback, and validation. Feedback provides a person with needed information. Simulation Exercise 5.12 provides you with the

---

SIMULATION EXERCISE 5.12 Putting it All Together Using Verbal, Nonverbal, and Active Listening

Purpose

To use all the person-centred communication strategies discussed in this chapter in an assessment interview

Procedure

1. Use the same one-paragraph scenario of a person-centred situation that you created in Simulation Exercise 5.2.
2. Pair off with a different person than the first time to enact the scenarios.
3. Conduct an initial person-centred 5- to 10- minute assessment interview using one of the scenarios, with the author of the paragraph taking the role of the nurse and the other student taking the role of the person being interviewed.
4. Ensure that you are using as many as possible of the person-centred communication strategies you have learned.
5. Reverse roles and repeat with the second student's scenario.

Reflective Discussion Analysis

1. In what ways were person-centred communication strategies used in this role-play?
2. How awkward was it for you in the nursing role to incorporate queries about the person's preferences, values, and so on?
3. What parts of the interview experience were of greatest value to you when you assumed the person role?
4. Explore what different person-centred communication strategies you used this time that you didn't use the previous time? Identify what components made the conversation different and why?
5. Which of these strategies were easier to apply and why? Which ones were more difficult to use? Reflect on why this occurred.
6. How could you use what you learned from doing this exercise in future nurse–person interviews?

opportunity to put all that you have learned about therapeutic communication strategies discussed in this chapter into practice.

DEVELOPING AN EVIDENCE-INFORMED PRACTICE

Purpose: The purpose of this research was to answer the question, "What exactly is patient- or person-centred communication?" (p. 2131)

Method: This research project was designed to examine and critique different approaches to patient-centred communication related to the conceptualization of patient-centred communication and measurement approach. The research focused on seven different measures of patient-centred communication.

Results: Measures differed, relating to whether the measures yielded information about behaviour or how well the behaviour was performed and whether it focused on the patient, clinician, or the interaction as a whole. The article presented a multidimensional framework for developing patient-centred communication measures but recommended development of a better understanding of the specific domains of patient-centred communication.

Application to Your Clinical Practice: As representatives of the profession, nurses need to contribute to the evidence-informed development of person-centred communication, based on continued dialogue with a person and other professional colleagues. The measure is not simply that the person talks more than the clinician or shows interest in the person's concerns.

Street, R. L. (2017). The many disguises of patient-centred communication: Problems of conceptualization and measurement. *Person Education and Counseling*, 100, 2131–2134.

Case Example: Paraphrasing to Understand What Are the Person's Concerns

Person: "I don't know about taking this medication the doctor is putting me on. I've never had to take medication before, and now I have to take it twice a day."

Nurse: "It sounds like you have concerns about taking the medication. Can you tell me more?"

Case Example: Asking for Validation Can Present a Fuller Explanation

Mr. Gupta: "I can't stand that medication. It doesn't sit well." (He grimaces and holds his stomach.)

Nurse: "Are you saying this medication upsets your stomach?"

Mr. Gupta: "No, I just don't like the taste of it."

Sometimes validation is observational rather than expressed through words.

Case Example: Inviting Active Participation by the Person in Mutually Developed Self-Management Strategies

Rose Cheung has been coming to the clinic to lose weight. At first, she was quite successful, losing 2 pounds per week. This week, she has gained 3 pounds. The nurse validates the weight change with Rose and asks for input.

Nurse: "Rose, over the past 6 weeks you have lost 2 pounds per week, but this week you gained 3 pounds. Let's discuss what was different about this week and how you can get back on track with your goal of losing weight."

Case Example

Touch is particularly useful with people who are not in a position to have a verbal discussion, for example in the intensive care unit (ICU).

Nurse: "When caring for persons in the ICU, I observed in some that when I used interpersonal touch such as holding their hand or gently massaging their skin, their blood pressure, respiratory rate, and reported stress and pain level would decrease."

ETHICAL DILEMMA

What Would You Do?

You have had an excellent relationship with a person and the person's family. They have revealed issues they had never talked about before and raised questions that extended beyond the health care situation that they did not have the time to finish. You are about to end your clinical rotation. What do you see as your professional and ethical responsibility to this person and family?

QUESTIONS FOR REVIEW AND DISCUSSION

1. In what ways do person-centred interactions and effective team collaboration intersect to meet the person's needs?

2. What are some ways you can demonstrate that you value the person's experience in the health care setting?

REFERENCES

Balzar Riley, R. (2017). *Communication in Nursing* (8th ed.). Elsevier.

Canadian Association of Schools of Nursing. (2015). *National nursing education framework: Final report.* https://www.casn.ca/wp-content/uploads/2014/12/Framwork-FINAL-SB-Nov-30-20151.pdf.

Canadian Cancer Society. (2019). *Reframing the cancer conversation.* https://www.cancer.ca/en/about-us/for-media/media-releases/national/2019/reframing-the-cancer-conversation/?region=on.

Canadian Nurses Association. (2017). *Code of ethics for registered nurses.* https://www.cna-aiic.ca/~/media/cna/page-content/pdf-en/code-of-ethics-2017-edition-secure-interactive.

Chute, A. (2015). Communication at the heart of nursing practice. In D. Gregory, C. Raymond-Seniuk, & L. Patrick (Eds.), *Fundamentals perspectives on the art and science of Canadian nursing* (pp. 599–636). Wolters Kluwer.

Collins, R. (2014). Best practices for integrating technology into nurse communication processes: Technology can close communication gaps that separate nurses from patients and families. *American Nurse Today, 9*(11)

Dean, S., & Ferguson, C. (2016). Editorial: Is technology responsible for losing touch? *Journal of Clinical Nursing, 20,* 583–585. https://doi.org/10.1111/jocn.13470.

Errasti-Ibarrondo, B., Perez, M., Carrasco, J., et al. (2015). Essential elements of the relationship between the nurse and the person with advanced and terminal cancer: A meta-ethnography. *Nursing Outlook, 63*(3), 255–268.

Eurich, T. (2018). What self-awareness really is (and how to cultivate it). *Harvard Business Review, January, 4,* 2018. https://hbr.org/2018/01/what-self-awareness-really-is-and-how-to-cultivate-it.

Gluyas, H. (2015). Effective communication and teamwork promotes patient safety. *Nursing Standard, 29*(49), 50–57.

Hafskjold, L., Sundler, A. J., Homstrom, I. K., et al. (2015). A cross-sectional study on person-centred communication in the care of older people: The COMHOME study protocol. *BMJ Open, 5*(4) https://bmjopen.bmj.com/content/5/4/e007864.long.

Health Quality Ontario. (2017). *Quality matters: Realizing excellent care for all. A report by Health Quality Ontario's System Quality Advisory Committee.* http://www.hqontario.ca/Portals/0/documents/health-quality/realizing-excellent-care-for-all-1704-en.pdf.

Herrington, C., & Chioda, L. (2014). Human touch effectively and safely reduces pain in the newborn intensive care unit. *Pain Management Nursing, 15*(1), 107–115.

Jakubec, S. L., & Astle, B. J. (2019). Communication and relational practice. In P. A. Potter, A. G. Perry, & J. C. Ross-Jerr (Eds.), *Canadian Fundamentals of Nursing* (6th ed.). Elsevier. [E-reader edition].

Jordan Halter, M., & Benner Carson, V. (2014). Relevant theories and therapies for nursing practice. In C. L. Pollard, S. L. Ray,

& M. Haase (Eds.), *Varcarolis's Canadian psychiatric mental health nursing: A clinical approach* (pp. 28). Elsevier.

Kuluski, K., Peckham, A., Williams, A. P., et al. (2016). What gets in the way of person-centred care for people with multimorbidity? Lessons from Ontario, Canada. *Healthcare Quarterly, 19*(2), 17–23. https://www.longwoods.com/content/24694.

Laundau, M. J., Arndt, J., & Cameron, L. D. (2018). Do metaphors in health messages work? Exploring emotional and cognitive factors. *Journal of Experimental Social Psychology, 74,* 135–149. https://doi.org/10.1016/j.jesp.2017.09.006.

Macleod, H. (2019). *Humanizing leadership: Reflection fuels, people matter, relationships make the difference.* Friesen Press.

Peplau, H. (1960). Peplau's theory of interpersonal relations. *Nursing Science Quarterly, 10,* 162–167.

Rasheed, S. P. (2015). Self-awareness as a therapeutic tool for nurse/client relationship. *International Journal of Caring Sciences, 8*(1), 211–216. http://www.internationaljournalofcaringsciences.org/docs/24-%20Review-Parveen.pdf.

Registered Nurses' Association of Ontario. (2015). Clinical best practice guidelines: Person-and family-centered care. https://rnao.ca/sites/rnao-ca/files/FINAL_Web_Version_0.pdf.

Rosenberg, S., & Gallo-Silver, L. (2011). Therapeutic communication skills and student nurses in the clinical setting. *Teaching and Learning in Nursing, 6,* 2–8.

Ruesch, J. (1961). *Therapeutic communication.* Norton.

Samovar, L., Porter, R., & Roy, C. (2008). *Intercultural communication: A reader* (12th ed.). Wadsworth.

Schiavo, R. (2013). *Health communication: From theory to practice* (2nd ed.). Jossey Bass.

Shirey, M. R. (2015). Enhance your self-awareness to be an authentic leader. *American Nurse Today, 10*(8).https://www.americannursetoday.com/enhance-self-awareness-authentic-leader/.

Steuber, P., & Pollard, C. (2018). Building a therapeutic relationship: How much is too much self-disclosure? *International Journal of Caring Science, 11*(2), 651–657.

Street, R., & Mazor, K. (2017). Clinician-patient communication measures: Drilling down into assumption, approaches, and analyses. *Patient Education and Counseling, 100,* 1612–1618.

Sundin, K., & Jansson, L. (2003). "Understanding and being understood" as a creative caring phenomenon: In care of patients with stroke and aphasia. *Journal of Clinical Nursing, 12,* 107–116.

Townsend, M. (2013). *Essentials of psychiatric mental health nursing: Concepts of care in evidence-based practice* (7th ed.). F. A. Davis.

Unhjem, J. V., Vatne, S., & Hem, M. H. (2018). Transforming nurse-patient relationships: A qualitative study of nurse self-disclosure in mental health care. *Journal of Clinical Nursing, 27*(5–6), e798–807. https://doi.org/10.1111/jocn.14191.

Van Dalen, J. (2013). Communication skills in context: Trends and perspectives. *Patient Education and Counseling, 92,* 292–295.

Watzlawick, P., Beavin, J. H., & Jackson, D. D. (1967). *Pragmatics of human communication.* WW Norton & Company.

6

Variation in Communication Styles

Claire Mallette

Originating US chapter by *Kathleen Underman Boggs*

OBJECTIVES

At the end of this chapter, the reader will be able to:

1. Describe the component systems of communication, describing congruence between verbal and nonverbal messages.
2. Reflect on how communication style influences the nurse–person relationship.
3. Discuss how metacommunication messages may affect the person's responses.
4. Cite examples of body cues that convey nonverbal messages.
5. Apply findings of research studies for evidence-informed clinical practice.

Every individual has different preferred methods for giving and receiving communication. These vary depending on the particular individual and specific situation. This chapter explores styles of communication that serve as a basis for building a relationship to provide safe, effective, person-centred care. Person-centred communication is an essential competency outlined in the Canadian Association of Schools of Nursing [CASN] (2015), Canadian Nurses Association [CNA] (2017) Codes of Ethics, and in each provincial and territorial regulatory body nursing standards, which are discussed in Chapter 3.

Communication style is defined as a set of specific, speech-related characteristics, cueing others as to how to interpret a message. You can and should learn to modify your communication style in your clinical practice (White et al., 2016). Effective communication has been shown to produce better health outcomes, greater satisfaction, increased understanding, shorter hospital stays, and decreased costs (Kee et al., 2018). *Style* is defined as the manner in which one communicates. It is important to learn as much as possible about your own communication style. Some of us tend to be more assertive, more forceful, and even dominant in our relationships, imposing our desires on others, whereas others seek more of an equal partnership, bargaining or negotiating in a give-and-take, win-win fashion. At the other end of the personal style spectrum, some individuals tend to withdraw or

even put all of the other person's desires ahead of their own needs. In developing a style suitable to professional nurse–person or nurse–team–person relationships, we modify our personal style to fit our professional role. As learners, students are guided in the clinical setting as they learn to demonstrate expected communication styles that convey caring, trustworthiness, and respectful assertiveness, and their newly acquired therapeutic communication skills.

Verbal style includes the actual words spoken. Nonverbal style includes pitch (high or low), tone, facial expression, gestures, body posture and movement, eye contact, distance from the other person, and so on. These nonverbal behaviours are clues people give us to help understand their words. Sharpening our observational skills helps us gather data needed for nursing assessments and interventions. Both people, the person and nurse, enter this new relationship with their own specific styles of communication.

Some individuals depend on a mostly verbal style to convey their meaning, whereas others rely more on nonverbal strategies to send their message. Warren (2015) estimates that approximately 90% of messages are conveyed not with words but via verbal pitch and nonverbal cues. Some communicators emphasize giving information; others have as a priority the conveying of interpersonal sensitivity. Longer nurse–person relationships permit each person to better understand the other's communication style.

BASIC CONCEPTS

Metacommunication

Communication is a combination of verbal and nonverbal behaviours integrated for the purpose of sharing information. Within the nurse–person relationship, any exchange of information between two individuals also carries messages about how to interpret the communication.

Metacommunication is a broad term used to describe all of the factors that influence how messages are perceived (Fig. 6.1). It provides information about how to interpret what is going on. Metacommunicated messages may be hidden within verbalizations or be conveyed as nonverbal communication, gestures and expressions. Some studies report greater agreement to requests when they are accompanied by a metacommunication message asking for a response to the appropriateness of the request. Sydney's case example can assist in clarifying this concept.

Case Example: Student Nurse Sydney

Student (smiling, making eye contact, and using a caring tone): Hi, I am Sydney. We nursing students are trying to encourage community awareness in promoting environmental health and are looking for people to hand out fliers. Would you be willing?

(Metacommunication): I realize that this is a strange request, seeing that you do not know who I am, but I would really appreciate your help. I am a concerned individual about environmental health.

In this metacommunicated message about how to interpret meaning, the student nurse used both verbal and nonverbal cues. She conveyed a verbal message of caring; making appropriate, encouraging

---

responses; and sending a nonverbal message by maintaining direct eye contact, smiling, and using a relaxed and fluid body posture without fidgeting.

In a professional relationship, verbal and nonverbal components of communication are intimately related. A student studying sign language for the Deaf was surprised that it was not sufficient merely to make the sign for "smile" but that the student had to actually show a smile at the same time. This congruence helped to convey the message. You can communicate your acceptance, interest, and respect, nonverbally.

VERBAL COMMUNICATION

Words are symbols used by people to think about ideas and to communicate with others. Choice of words is influenced by many factors (e.g., your age, sociocultural factors, educational background, and gender) and by the situation in which the communication is taking place.

The interpretation of the meaning of words may vary according to the individual's background, cultural context, and experiences. It is unsafe to assume that words have the same meaning for everyone who hears them. Language is useful only to the extent that it accurately reflects the experience it is designed to portray. Consider, for example, the difficulty in an English-speaking person communicating with a person who speaks only Vietnamese, or the dilemma of a young child with a limited vocabulary who is trying to tell you where it hurts. One's voice can also be a therapeutic part of treatment, as with Mrs. Garcia, in the case example.

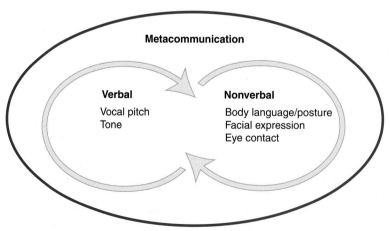

Fig. 6.1 Factors in communication styles

Case Example: Mrs. Garcia

For weeks, while giving care to Mrs. Garcia, a 42-year-old unconscious woman, her nurse used soothing touch and conversation. She also encouraged Mr. Garcia to do the same. When the woman later regained consciousness, she told the nurse that she recognized her voice.

Meaning

There are two levels of meaning in language: denotation and connotation. Both are affected by one's cultural context. **Denotation** refers to the generalized meaning assigned to a word; **connotation** points to a more personalized meaning of the word or phrase. For example, most people would agree that a dog is a four-legged creature, domesticated, with a characteristic vocalization referred to as a bark. This would be the denotative, or explicit, meaning of the word. When the word is used in a more personalized way, it reveals the connotative level of meaning. "His bark is worse than his bite" or "Working like a dog" are phrases some people use to describe personal characteristics of human beings rather than animals. We need to be aware that many messages convey only a part of the intended meaning. Do not assume that the meaning of a message is the same for the sender and the receiver until mutual understanding is verified. To be sure you are getting your message across, ask for feedback.

VERBAL STYLE FACTORS THAT INFLUENCE NURSE–PERSON PROFESSIONAL COMMUNICATION

The following six verbal styles of communication are summarized in Table 6.1 and Fig. 6.2:

1. *Moderate pitch and tone in vocalization.* The oral delivery of a verbal message, expressed through tone of voice, inflection, sighing, and so on, is referred to as **paralanguage**. It is important to understand this component of communication because it affects how the verbal message is likely to be interpreted. For example, you might say, "I would like to hear more about what you are feeling" in a tone that sounds rushed, high-pitched, or harsh. Or you might make this same statement in a soft, unhurried voice that expresses genuine interest. In the first instance, the message is likely to be misinterpreted by the person, despite your good intentions. Your caring intent is more apparent to the person in the second instance. Voice inflection (pitch and tone), loudness, and rate of speaking either support or contradict the content

TABLE 6.1	Styles That Influen... Professional Communications in ... Person Relationships	
Verbal	**Nonverbal**
	Moderate pitch and tone
Allows therapeutic silences	Listens
Varies vocalizations	Uses congruent nonverbal behaviours
Encourages involvement	Uses facilitative body language
Validates worth	Uses touch appropriately
Advocates for the person as necessary	Proxemics—respects the person's space
Appropriately provides needed information—briefly and clearly, avoiding slang	Attends to nonverbal cues

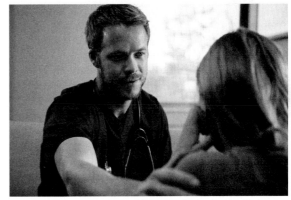

Fig. 6.2 Nurse talks with depressed teen. (iStock. com/monkeybusinessimages)

of the verbal message. Varying your pitch helps others perceive you more positively (Ahmadian et al., 2017). Ideas may be conveyed merely by emphasizing different portions of your statement. When the tone of voice does not fit the words, the message is less easily understood and is less likely to be believed. Some people, especially when upset, communicate in an emotional rather than intellectual manner. A message conveyed in a firm, steady tone is more reassuring than one conveyed in a loud, emotional, abrasive, or uncertain manner. In contrast, if you speak in a flat, monotone voice when you are upset, as though the matter were of no consequence, you can confuse the person, making it difficult to respond appropriately.

2. *Vary vocalizations.* In some cultures and languages, sounds are punctuated, whereas in others, sounds have a lyrical or singsong quality. We need to be aware of the characteristic vocal tones associated with other cultures and languages.

3. *Encourage involvement.* Professional styles of communication have changed over time. We now partner with people in promoting their optimal health. We expect and encourage them to be actively involved in their care and assume responsibility for their own health. Consequently, provider–person communication has changed. Paternalistic styles, exemplified by examples like, "I'll tell you what to do," are no longer acceptable. Reflect on Ms. Grenier's case to see how the person becomes a partner in their own care.

Case Example

Primary health care nurse practitioner Navadeep Ahmed, sitting in the exam room with Ms. Grenier, is typing into the electronic health record (EHR) on her tablet. She says "Your blood pressure is still considered high, but it is much better than where it was." She shares the screen to show a graph of Ms. Grenier's blood pressure recordings. Is this paternalistic? Or is this potentially a way of engaging Ms. Grenier in her blood pressure discussion? Initial studies show that when providers gazed at computer screens instead of maintaining eye contact with the person, the person became detached. Recent literature has suggested that sharing pertinent screen images with the person being cared for is a strategy for getting them to be feel more involved in their care and engaged (Asan et al., 2015).

---

4. *Validate the person's worth.* Styles that convey caring send a message of individual worth that sustains the relationship. For example, some people prefer providers who use a sincere communication style to show caring, give information, and talk about their own feelings. Confirming responses validate the intrinsic worth of the person. These are responses that affirm the right of the individual to be treated with respect. They also affirm autonomy (i.e., the person's right, ultimately, to make their own decisions). Uncaring responses, in contrast, disregard the validity of the person's feelings by either ignoring them or by imposing a value judgement. Such responses take the form of changing the topic, offering reassurance without supporting evidence, or presuming

to know what the person means without verifying the message with them. Learning to validate a person's worth and convey caring in your nursing practice is a communication skill that is learned with experience.

5. *Advocate for the person when necessary.* Our personalities affect our style of social communication; some of us are naturally shy or have an introvert personality style. But in our professional relationships, we must often assume an assertive style of communicating with other health providers or agencies to obtain the best care or services for the people we care for.

6. *Provide needed information appropriately.* Providing accurate information in a timely manner in understandable amounts is discussed throughout this book. In our social conversations, there is often a rhythm: "You talk, I listen," then, "I get to talk, you listen." However, in professional communications, the content is more goal-focused. Self-disclosure from the nurse must be limited. It is not appropriate to tell a person about yourself and your personal life.

NONVERBAL COMMUNICATION

Most of our person-to-person communication is nonverbal. All our words are accompanied by nonverbal cues that offer meaning about how to interpret the message. Think of the most interesting lecturer you ever had. Did this person lecture by making eye contact? By using hand gestures? By moving among the students? By conveying enthusiasm?

The function of nonverbal communication is to give us cues about what is being communicated. We give meaning about the purpose or context of our message nonverbally; this can increase the accuracy and efficiency of its impact on the listener. Some of these nonverbal cues are conveyed by tone of voice, facial expression, and body gestures or movement. Skilled use of nonverbal communication through therapeutic silences, use of congruent nonverbal behaviours, body language, touch, proxemics (amount of space between people), and attention to nonverbal cues such as facial expression can build rapport. Emotional meanings are communicated through body language (Fig. 6.3).

Aspects of Nonverbal Style That Influence Nurse–Person Professional Communication

We must be aware of the ways in which our nonverbal messages are conveyed. The position of your hands, the look on your face, and the movement of your body may give cues regarding your meaning. Attending behaviours can be used, such as leaning forward slightly, to convey to the person that their conversation is worth listening to. Think

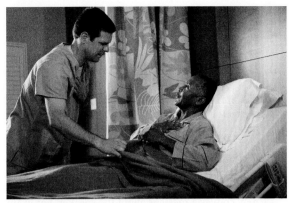

Fig. 6.3 Emotional meanings are communicated through body language, particularly facial expression. (iStock.com/kali9)

of the last time an interviewer kept fidgeting in his seat, glanced frequently at his clock, or shuffled his papers while you were speaking. How did this make you feel? What nonverbal message was being conveyed?

Following is a description of six nonverbal behaviours nurses generally use. However, when communicating with others, it is important to be aware that nonverbal communication is different from person to person, based on each person's cultural contexts. The topic of cultural contexts is discussed in Chapter 7.

1. Allow silences. In our social communications, the norm is a question–response sequence. The goal is to have no overlap and no gap between turns (Sicoli et al., 2015). We often become uncomfortable if silence occurs; there is a tendency to rush in to fill the void. But in our professional nurse–person communication, we use silence therapeutically, allowing needed time to think about things before responding.

2. Use congruent nonverbal behaviours. Nonverbal behaviour should be congruent with the message and should reinforce it. If you knock on your instructor's office door to seek help, do you believe them when they say they would love to talk if you see them grimace and look at their watch? In another example, if you smile while telling your clinical instructor that your assignment is too much to handle, the seriousness of your message may be negated. Try to give nonverbal cues that are congruent with the message you are verbally communicating. When nonverbal cues are incongruent with the verbal information, messages are likely to be misinterpreted. When your verbal message is inconsistent with the nonverbal expression of the message, the nonverbal expression assumes prominence and is generally perceived as

more trustworthy than the verbal content. You need to comment on any incongruence to better understand what is trying to be conveyed. For example, when you enter a room to ask Mr. Sala if he is having any postoperative pain, he may say "No," but he grimaces and clutches his incision. After you comment on the incongruent message, he may then tell you that he is having some discomfort. Can you think of a clinical situation in which you changed the meaning of a verbal message by giving nonverbal cues that conveyed a message of "Don't believe what I say."?

3. Use facilitative body language. Kinesics is an important component of nonverbal communication. Commonly referred to as "body language," *kinesics* is defined as the communicator's conscious or unconscious body positioning or actions. Words direct the content of a message, whereas emotions accentuate and clarify the meaning of the words. Some nonverbal behaviours, such as tilting your head or facing the person at an angle, promote communication. Lange (2016) urges us to pay attention to our body position. He suggests viewing Amy Cuddy's (n.d.) TED talk: (https://www.ted.com/talks/amy_cuddy_your_body_language_may_shape_who_you_are?language=en.)

- **Posture**. Leaning forward slightly can communicate interest and encourages the person to keep the conversation going. Keep your arms uncrossed, with palms open, knees uncrossed, and body loose, not tight and tense. Turning away may indicate lack of interest, whereas directly and closely facing the person, crossing your arms and staring unblinkingly, or jabbing your finger in the air could suggest aggression.

- **Facial expression**. Six common facial expressions (to show surprise, sadness, anger, happiness/joy, disgust/contempt, and fear) represent global, generalised interpretations of emotions common to all cultures, though the expressions themselves may vary. Facial expression either reinforces or modifies the message the listener hears. The power of facial expressions far outweighs the power of the actual words. So try to maintain an open, friendly expression. Avoid furrowing your forehead or assuming a distracted or bored expression.

- **Eye contact**. Making direct eye contact, though not staring, generally conveys a positive message. Most people interpret direct eye contact as an indication of your interest in what they have to say, although there are cultural differences.

- **Gestures**. Some gestures, such as affirmative head nodding, help to facilitate conversation by showing interest and attention. The use of open-handed gestures can also facilitate communication. Avoid folding your arms across your chest or fidgeting. Hargestam et al. (2016) showed that team leaders use gestures to reinforce verbal directions to team members, thus speeding up intervention in a crisis situation.

4. *Touch.* Touching is one of the most powerful ways you have of communicating nonverbally. Within a professional relationship, affective touch can convey caring, empathy, comfort, and reassurance. When a nurse touches a person, this contact can be perceived by the person as either an expression of caring or negatively, as a threat. Care must be taken to abide by the person's cultural values and beliefs and their life experiences, when using touch. The literature cites variations across cultures—for example, some Muslim and Orthodox Jewish men are not allowed to touch or be touched by women other than family members. They might be uncomfortable shaking the hand of a female health care provider. Someone who has been physically assaulted also may not want to be touched. However, many people report feeling comforted when a professional health provider touches them (Atenstaedt, 2012). The "best" type of touch cited by people being cared for is holding one of their hands (Kozlowska & Doboszynska, 2012). All nurses giving direct care use touch to assess and to assist. We touch to help the person walk or roll over in bed, and in doing a physical assessment. However, just as you would be careful about invading someone's personal space, you must be careful about when and where on the body you touch the person. Your use of touch can elicit misunderstanding if it is perceived as invasive or inappropriate. Gender identity and culture can also determine perceptions about being touched. The use of touch in the nurse–person relationship is discussed in Chapter 5.

5. *Proxemics.* We can use physical space to improve our interactions. **Proxemics** refers to the perception of what is a proper distance to be maintained between oneself and others. The way in which we use space communicates messages. You probably have heard the phrase, "You are invading my personal space," used when someone stands too close; such closeness can make people feel uncomfortable.
   - There are generalised guidelines for appropriate distance, depending on the context of the communication. The interaction's purpose determines the appropriate space, so that appropriate distance for intimate interaction would be zero distance, with increased space needed for personal distance, social distance, and public distance; details around the different types of distance are outlined in Chapter 5. In almost all contexts, zero distance is avoided except for loving or caring interactions. In giving physical care, nurses enter this "intimate" space. Violating personal space can be threatening. Nurses need to be aware of this, and caution is needed when you are at this closer distance so your actions don't make the person feel uncomfortable and are not misinterpreted.

6. Attend to Nonverbal Body Cues in Others
   - *Posture.* Often, the emotional component of a message can be indirectly interpreted by observing **body language**. Rhythm of movement and body stance may convey a message about the speaker. For example, when a person speaks while directly facing you, this can convey more confidence than if they turn their bodies away from you at an angle. A slumped, head-down posture and slow movements might give you an impression of fatigue or low self-esteem, whereas an erect posture and decisive movement can suggest confidence. Rapid, diffuse, agitated body movements may indicate anxiety. Forceful body movements may symbolize anger. When someone bows their head or slumps their body after receiving bad news, it may be conveying sadness. Can you think of other cues that body posture might give you?
   - *Facial expression.* Facial characteristics such as frowning or smiling add to the verbal message conveyed. Almost instinctively, we use facial expression as a barometer of another person's feelings, motivations, approachability, and mood. From infancy, we respond to the expressive qualities of another's face, often without even being aware of it. Therefore, assessing facial expression together with other nonverbal cues may reveal vital information that will affect the nurse–person relationship. For example, a worried facial expression and lip biting may suggest anxiety. Absence of a smile in greeting or grimacing may convey a message about how ill the person feels.
   - *Eye contact.* Research suggests that individuals who make direct eye contact while talking or listening create a sense of confidence and credibility, whereas downward glances or averted eyes can signal submission, powerlessness, or shame. Failure to maintain eye contact, known as *gaze aversion*, can be perceived as a nonverbal cue meaning that the person may be feeling uncomfortable, distracted, low self-esteem, fear, insecure, anxious, or possible psychological issues. If a person's eyes wander around

during a conversation, you may wonder whether there is something the person doesn't want to tell you or discuss. The amount of eye contact a person gives can also be influenced by cultural norms, values, and beliefs.

- *Gestures.* Movements of the extremities may give cues. Making a fist can convey how angry someone is, just as the use of stabbing, abrupt hand gestures may suggest distress, whereas hugging one's arms closely (self-embracing gestures) may suggest fear or anxiety.

Assessing the extent to which nonverbal cues communicate emotions can help you to communicate better. Studies repeatedly show that a failure to acknowledge nonverbal cues is often associated with miscommunication by the health provider. Table 6.1 summarizes both the verbal and nonverbal styles that influence professional communication in nurse–person relationships.

Wearing a face mask while providing care can be a barrier to nonverbal communication. When the COVID-19 pandemic began in 2020, wearing face masks was compulsory where social distancing was not possible for health care providers. Wearing a face mask can make it difficult for people who are hard of hearing or deaf and those with dementia. Those who are hard of hearing or deaf often rely on lip reading to assist in understanding what is being said. People with dementia may lose their ability to understand verbal language but are still able to interpret facial signs such as a smile (Carter, 2020; Schlogl & Jones, 2020).

To communicate effectively wearing a face mask, it is important to first be self-aware of how you can reflect a positive calm manner in your voice, body language, hand gestures, and eyes. Approach the person from the front, maintaining eye contact. When you smile, even though the person cannot see your mouth, your smile will be reflected in your eyes and eyebrows. Ensure that you speak clearly, slowly, and loudly enough for the person to hear what you are saying but not perceiving you as shouting. You can also underline your words with the tone of your voice and using hand gestures. As you are speaking, observe the person carefully and listen to what they are conveying both verbally and nonverbally in their responses to your communication. This will enable you to assess whether they appear to be understanding what you are saying. You can also subtly mimic the person's gestures to help them feel understood (Carter, 2020; Schlogl & Jones, 2020).

It is best if we verify our assessment of the meaning of observed nonverbal behaviours since our own and the person's cultural contexts, values, and beliefs influence nonverbal communication. Body cues, although suggestive, are imprecise. When communication is limited by the state of a person's health, it is important to pay even closer attention to nonverbal cues. The person's pain, for example, can be assessed through facial expression even when they are only partially conscious. What would you say to Mr. Geeze?

Case Example: Mr. Geeze

Mr. Geeze smiles but narrows his eyes and stares at the nurse. An appropriate comment for the nurse to make might be, "I notice you're smiling, but the way you're looking at me, it seems like you might be angry or there's something wrong."

Use of an incompatible communication style, making assumptions of what the person is communicating and failing to validate what people are communicating nonverbally, can negatively impact the care provided. This can then result in the person feeling uncared for, anxious, fearful or misunderstood, leading to a sense of hopelessness (Hawthorn, 2015).

COMMUNICATION ACCOMMODATION THEORY

Howard Giles (n.d.) theorized that people adapt or adjust their speech, vocal patterns (diction, tone, rate of speaking), language, word choice, and gestures to accommodate others. This theory, the Communication Accommodation Theory, suggests that it is desirable to adjust one's speech to our conversational partners to help facilitate our interaction, increase our acceptance, and improve trust and rapport. This accommodation is known as *convergence.* Convergence is thought to increase the effectiveness of your communication.

Accommodation can occur unconsciously or can be a conscious choice. For example, when you are speaking to a child, you might deliberately assume a less assertive style, speaking quietly and getting down to the child's eye level to appear less threatening. Conversely, you might choose convergence when you want to teach something about a health issue. You might attempt to match the person's speed and speech style. You definitely adapt or accommodate by choosing to match your vocabulary, in an effort to be better understood. In general, if the person choosing to use convergence has more power in the relationship, they may be perceived as patronizing or having power. Choice of a distinctly different style from the person you are speaking to is known as *divergence.* In divergence, the verbal and nonverbal differences between the people's communication are highlighted. This theory assumes that people are communicating in a collaborative manner.

EFFECTS OF SOCIOCULTURAL FACTORS ON COMMUNICATION

Communication is also affected by such style factors as cultural contexts, age cohort, gender, ethnicity, socioeconomic level, and location. Of course, not everyone communicates in the manner described; these are broad generalizations as described in the literature.

Culture

We must communicate in a culturally safe manner. There is clear evidence that effective communication is associated with the person having better health outcomes and greater satisfaction. In promoting cultural safety, the nurse acknowledges and respects a person's unique cultural context. You must develop an awareness of the person's unique cultural contexts to adapt your communication through cultural competence and humility. Chapter 7 deals in depth with concepts of cultural context communication.

Age Cohort and Generational Diversity

The members of today's nursing workforce now span four generations. As might be expected, members of different generations may hold differing views regarding work motivation, personal values, and attitudes toward their work; they may also have differing communication styles and preferences. Differences can also exist in people's communication styles when they are interacting with each other. If ignored, generational differences can become a source of conflict in the workplace.

Age cohorts are made up of people born within approximately a 20-year period. Each age cohort has some communication style characteristics in common, which differentiate each group from other generations. Communication Accommodation Theory, as described earlier, has been used to explore intergenerational communication problems. In considering the generation gap, beliefs about communication and goals for interactions differ among cohorts. For example, accommodation theory has been used to explore ageism, the negative evaluation of those who are older by those who are younger. In society, youth may use divergence by using different styles, such as by talking more rapidly, using social media platforms, or focusing on other values. Some nurses might prefer digital communication via secure texting on cell phones, Instagram, and Twitter, whereas others might prefer face-to-face communication.

Younger nurses and physicians, raised in the digital age, may rely on the Internet and social medial for information,

social interaction, and communication. The nursing literature suggests that nurses need to determine a person's preferred method of communication as research indicates that miscommunication outcomes can occur in intergenerational interactions between providers and people being cared for. People learn and communicate best if they are engaged in their preferred communication style.

Gender

Communication patterns have traditionally been integrated into gender roles of male or female, which are defined by an individual's culture context. In communication studies, gender differences have been shown to be greatest in terms of the use and interpretation of nonverbal cues. This may reflect gender differences in intellectual style as well as culturally reinforced standards of acceptable role-related behaviours. There are wide variations within gender roles. We are now questioning whether traditional ideas about male and female differences in communication are as prevalent as previously thought.

We also need to consider that persons may identify as one of a range of genders (e.g., female, male, transgender). *Transgender*, or *trans*, is an overarching term describing individuals whose gender identity differs from the sex they were assigned at birth. Trans people can include those who identify as transgender, transsexual, nonbinary, or gender nonconforming (The 519, n.d.). Is there really a major difference in communication according to gender? What is factual and what is a stereotype? Because traditional thinking about gender-related differences in communication content and process in both nonverbal and verbal communication are being revised, consider critically what you read. When caring for people, you can also acknowledge and respect who they are by asking them, "What name would you like to be called and what pronouns would you prefer being used?"

Gender Differences in Communication in Health Care Settings

The effects of gender on communication have long been discussed in the literature. But do these differences actually affect how a nurse delivers care? It has been suggested that more effective communication occurs when the health care provider and person are of the same gender, although this was not found to be true in some studies. What other reasons may be guiding persons wanting to be cared for by someone of the same gender? Try Simulation Exercise 6.1, Gender Bias, to explore and create discussion about gender bias.

SIMULATION EXERCISE 6.1   Gender Bias

Purpose

To create discussion about gender bias

Procedure

In small groups, read and discuss the following comments made about care delivery on a geriatric psychiatric unit by staff and students: "Nurses who are male tend to be slightly more confident and to make quicker decisions, while nurses who are female are better at the feeling things, like conveying warmth."

Analytical Reflection

1. Reflect on the effect of gender on perceptions of these comments. Determine whether these comments are appropriate, considering tht nurses can be identified as female, transgender, or male.

2. Analyze the accuracy of these statements. Be sure to support your answer with evidence, by looking for a recent (in the last 5 years) peer-reviewed scholarly paper on gender bias in nursing.

3. Can you truly generalize attributes to individuals by gender?

 DEVELOPING AN EVIDENCE-INFORMED PRACTICE

Canada has one of the world's most diverse populations, with one in five people having been born in another country. This study explored the use of English and communication challenges in new Canadian immigrants working in entry-level positions.

Participants

Fourteen newcomers to Canada were interviewed who were working within entry-level positions, earning minimum wages, and where English was spoken. The participants immigrated to Canada from countries such as China, Korea, Egypt, Syria, Dominican Republic and Bangladesh. Examples of positions they held were as a waitress, hairstylist, cleaner, salesperson, and others.

Method and Analysis

Two semi-structured interviews were conducted to gain information about the participants' use of English and communication challenges within the workplace. The data were analysed using thematic analysis, using Braun and Clark's (2006) six steps.

Results

Four key themes emerged from the data, with three related to communication challenges and the fourth theme related to communication strategies for coping. The three themes related to communication challenges were topical knowledge (conversational topics, Canadian culture, and workplace communication); language knowledge (grammar, vocabulary, Canadian and diverse English accents, speaking rate too fast to understand, and the application of vocabulary in the workplace); and personal attributes (age, cultural contexts, shyness, or nervousness). Communication strategies used when they had communication issues were asking the person to repeat what they said, avoiding topics they didn't have the knowledge or vocabulary needed to participate in the discussion, having the person slow down their speech rate and use simple language, and preferring face-to-face interactions.

Application to Your Clinical Practice

By using this knowledge you can prepare for interactions by increasing your awareness of the person's ability to speak English and how you can best communicate with them. You can also be aware of the speed of your speech, and slow it down where appropriate. It is important to use therapeutic skills such as active listening, nonverbal communication, demonstrating respect, and focusing on the person's concerns. These findings may also have implications for meeting and communicating virtually. While every person has unique needs, if they have access and the ability to meet virtually, they may be better able to meet those needs virtually than by phone conversations.

Cheng, L., Gwan-Hyeok, I., Doe, C, et al. (2020). Identifying English language use and communication challenges facing "entry-level" workplace immigrants in Canada. *Journal of International Migration and Integration.* https://doi.org/10.1007/s12134-020-00779-w.

APPLICATIONS

Knowing Your Own Communication Style

The style of communication you use can influence people's behaviours and their ability to reach their health goals. An aggressive communication style from a health care provider can create hostility, anxiety, or dislike, whereas the use of an assertive, empathic style while seeking to make a point may lead to best outcomes. Users of a passive communication style are basically not active in helping people to achieve their goals, whereas users of a more collaborative supportive style wait to listen before trying to make their points.

People report being dissatisfied with poor communication more than with other aspects of their care. Simulation exercises in prior chapters should give you the basic skills you need in your nurse–person relationships, but remember that you bring your own communication style with you, as does the person being cared for. Because we differ widely in our personal communication styles, it is important for you to be self-aware and identify your style and know how to modify it, depending on the persons you are caring for. Try Simulation Exercise 6.2 for a quick profile of your personal communication style. How does your affective style come across? Do people view you as empathic, caring, and reassuring? Experienced nurses adapt their innate personal style so that their professional communications fit the person and the situation. You too must modify your style to be sure that it is compatible with the person's needs. Think about the potential for incompatibility in the following case example.

Case Example: Mr. Holtz

Nurse (in a firm tone, speaking quickly): Mr. Holtz, it's time to take your medication now!

Mr. Holtz (in a complaining tone): Why are you rushing me?

Empathic communication is crucial to your nursing care and may improve a person's health outcome. Recognize how others perceive you. Consider all the nonverbal factors that affect their perceptions of you. These could include your age, role (student nurse versus nurse), your tone of voice, and the manner in which you present yourself as confident, uncertain, or nervous.

The initial step in identifying your own communication style may be to compare your style with those of others. Ask yourself, "What makes someone perceive a nurse either as authoritarian or as accepting and caring?" The Simulation Exercise 6.3 video may help you to compare your style with those of others.

Develop an awareness of alternative styles that you can comfortably assume if the occasion warrants. For example, Watts et al. (2017) suggests assessing whether changing your style to speak more slowly, use more nonverbal communication, and involve family members will help get the message across to the people being cared for. It is important to identify whether some other factors may be influencing your style toward a particular person and if that is appropriate. How might your own cultural contexts; conscious

---

SIMULATION EXERCISE 6.2   My Communication Style: Quick Profile

Purpose
To develop self-reflection

Procedure
Answer the following:
1. I prefer to
   - Get my way.
   - Work with others.
   - Follow the rules.
   - Avoid confrontation.
2. My verbal tone is most often
   - Open and approachable.
   - Enthusiastic.
   - Determined.
3. If we have a difference of opinion, I usually want to
   - Dominate.
   - Collaborate.
   - Compromise.
   - Give in.
4. In a social group situation, I sometimes
   - Fail to give my opinion.
   - Am very polite.
   - Digress from the topic.
   - Become irritated with those who disagree with me.
5. My friends have told me that
   - I provide good eye contact.
   - I talk using my hands.
   - I smile a lot.
   - I can't sit still.

Analytical Reflection
Compare your answers with the content in this chapter and the book content on communication style. Analyze how these factors might affect your nurse–person relationships.

SIMULATION EXERCISE 6.3   Self-Analysis of Video Recording

Purpose

To increase awareness of students' own communication style

Procedure

With a partner, role-play an interaction between nurse and person. Use a cell phone to record a 1- to 2-minute video interview, with the camera focused on you. The topic

of the interview could be "identifying health promotion behaviours" or something similar.

Reflective Analysis

Analyze playback of your videos in a group. What postures were used? What nonverbal messages were communicated? How? Were verbal and nonverbal messages congruent?

---

and unconscious biases; values and beliefs; and the other person's age, race, culture, socioeconomic status, or gender affect communication?

We must continually work to update our communication competencies, including being aware that organizational communication is also rapidly becoming electronic, with advancing technology. Some hospital agencies are increasingly relying on digital communication, eliminating many of the nuances communicated nonverbally.

INTERPERSONAL COMPETENCE

Nurse–person communication processes are based on the nurse's interpersonal competence and the situations that nurses find themselves in. Higher levels of anxiety affect your communication (Fletcher et al., 2016). **Interpersonal competence** develops as you come to understand the complex cognitive, behavioural, and sociocultural factors that influence communication. This understanding, together with the use of a broad range of communication skills, can help you to interact positively with the person as they attempt to cope with multiple demands. Developing good communication skills increases your competent communication. Such skills are identified as being among the attributes of expert nurses with the most clinical credibility. In caring for a person in the sociocultural context of the health care system, two kinds of abilities are required: social cognitive competency and message competency.

Social cognitive competency is the ability to interpret message content within interactions from the point of view of each of the participants. By embracing the person's perspectives, you begin to understand how best to assist them in meeting their health needs. This is especially important when the person's ability to communicate is impaired, for example by a mechanical barrier such as a ventilator. Those who have recovered from critical illnesses requiring

ventilator support report that they felt fear, anxiety, and distress during this experience, being unable to communicate.

Message competency refers to the ability to use language and nonverbal behaviours strategically in the intervention phase of the nursing process to achieve the goals of the interaction. Communication skills are used as a tool to support the person in meeting their health care goals. Think how it feels when the person sees you smile and hears you say, "That's impressive; you have successfully self-injected your insulin!"

STYLE FACTORS THAT INFLUENCE RELATIONSHIPS

The establishment of trust and respect in an interpersonal relationship with a person and family is dependent on an effective, ongoing communication style. Having knowledge is not sufficient to guarantee its successful application. For example, providers who sit at eye level, at an optimal distance (proxemics), and without furniture in between (special configuration) will likely have more eye contact and use more nonverbal techniques such as therapeutic touching (when appropriate). Adapting your style to fit the person's needs encourages them to better understand what you are saying (Hawthorn, 2015). Box 6.1 contains suggestions to improve your own professional style of communicating.

Medical Terminology Communication

Beginning nursing students often report confusion while learning all the medical terminology required for their new role. Remembering our own experiences, we can empathize with people who are attempting to understand the medical terminology involved in health care. Careful explanations help overcome this communication barrier. For successful communication, the words we use should have a similar meaning to both individuals in an interaction. An important part of the communication process is the search for a common vocabulary so that the message sent is the same

BOX 6.1   Suggestions to Improve Your Communication Style

- Adapt yourself to the person's cultural values.
- Use nonverbal communication strategies, such as the following:
  - Maintaining eye contact
  - Displaying open, approachable, animated facial expressions
  - Smiling often
  - Nodding your head to encourage talking
  - Maintaining an attentive, upright posture and sitting at the person's level, leaning forward slightly
  - Attending to proper proximity and increasing space if the person shows signs of discomfort, such as averting their gaze, or swinging their legs
- Use touch if appropriate to the situation.
- Use active listening and respond to the person's cues.
- Use verbal strategies to engage the person:
  - Using humour appropriately
  - Attending to proper tone and pitch, avoiding an overly loud voice
  - Avoiding jargon and medical terminology
  - Using nonjudgemental language and open-ended questions
  - Listening and avoiding jumping in too soon with problem solving
  - Verbalizing respect
  - Asking permission before addressing a client by their first name
  - Conveying caring comments
  - Using confirming, positive comments

as the one received. An example of this is when the oncology nurse develops a computer databank of cancer treatment terms. While the nurse is admitting Ms. Hassan for treatment, the nurse uses an existing template model on the computer to create an individualized terminology sheet, with just the words Ms. Hassan will encounter during the course of chemotherapy.

Openness of Participants

How open participants are affects the depth and breadth of communication. Reciprocity affects not only the relationship process but also the person's health outcomes. Some people are naturally more verbal than others. It is easier to have a therapeutic conversation with people who do not have difficulty communicating and want to communicate. It is a good idea to encourage the openness of those

who are less verbal to understand their concerns and provide the best nursing practice. Verbal and nonverbal support encourages people to express themselves. Elsewhere, we discuss knowledge and skills that promote openness, such as active listening, demonstrations of empathy, and acknowledgment of the content and feelings of messages. Sometimes, acknowledging the difficulty the person is having in expressing their feelings, praising their efforts, and encouraging them to use more than one route of communication can help. Such strategies demonstrate interpersonal sensitivity. Listening to the person's care experience, responding to verbal or nonverbal cues, and avoiding "talking down" encourage communication and strengthen the nurse–person partnership in successfully and positively addressing health issues. Simulation Exercise 6.4 will help you practise the use of confirming responses.

Roles of Participants

Paying attention to the roles relationship among the communicators may be just as important as deciphering the content and meaning of the message. The relationships between the roles of the sender and receiver influence how the communication is likely to be received and interpreted. The same constructive criticism made by a good friend and by one's immediate supervisor is likely to be interpreted differently, even though the content and style are similar. Communication between a nurse and nurse manager is far more likely to be influenced by power and style. When roles are unequal in terms of power, the more powerful individual may communicate in a more dominant style. This concept is discussed in Chapters 24 and 25.

Context of the Message

Communication is always influenced by the environment in which the interaction takes place; it does not occur in isolation. Taking time to evaluate the physical setting and the time and space in which the contact takes place—as well as the psychological, social, and cultural characteristics of each individual involved—gives you flexibility in choosing the most appropriate context.

Involvement in the Relationship

Relationships generally need to develop over time because communication changes during different phases of the relationship. Studies show that nurses and other health care providers respond less than half the time to the person's concerns. Responses tend to focus on physical care and often do not address social emotional care. In today's health care environment, nurses often have less time to develop relationships. To begin to explore ethical problems in your nursing relationships, consider the ethical dilemma provided.

SIMULATION EXERCISE 6.4 Confirming Responses

Purpose
To increase students' skills in using confirming communication

Procedure
Formulate a better way to rephrase messages positively. Evaluate whether it is easier for you to send a positive, confirming message or a disconfirming, negative message:
1. "Three of your 14 blood sugars this week were too high. Were you eating a lot of sugary foods?"

2. "Your blood pressure is dangerously high. Are you eating salty foods again?"
3. "You gained 5 pounds this week. Can't you stick to a simple diet?"

Reflective Analysis
Suggest better rephrasing to communicate these messages. Was it relatively easy to send a positive, confirming message?

Use of Humour

As discussed elsewhere (Chapter 5), research has associated the use of humour with stress relief, diffusion of conflict, enhancement of learning, and improved communication in nurse–person relationships (Canha, 2016). How can you incorporate humour into your relationships appropriately?

ADVOCATE FOR CONTINUITY OF CARE

We have learned that people's evaluation of positive health care communication is higher when they consistently relate to the same individuals providing their care. These providers are more likely to listen to them, explain things clearly, spend enough time with them, and show them respect. Because nurses and other health team members communicate differently with people being cared for, it is crucial for the health care team to communicate amongst each other and share information about the person's care.

SUMMARY

Communication involves more than an exchange of verbal and nonverbal information. As our population becomes more diverse, we are challenged to provide person-centred care that is sensitive to sociocultural factors, race, ethnicity, gender, and sexual orientation. The recurring theme in this chapter is that you adapt your communication style to better suit each individual person. Modifying your style to provide more effective communication promotes safer care and better health outcomes. This chapter offers suggestions for styles of verbal and nonverbal communication as well as a discussion of learning to vary your communication style to meet persons' unique communication and health needs. Style factors that affect the communication process include the responsiveness and role relationships of the participants, the types of responses and context of

the relationships, and the level of involvement in the relationship. Skills are suggested, such as using confirming responses to acknowledge the value of a person's communication. More nonverbal strategies to facilitate nurse–person communication are discussed in later chapters.

ETHICAL DILEMMA
What Would You Do?

Gavin Kaur, RN, is a new grad who learns that a serious error that harmed a person has occurred on his unit. He realizes that if staff continue to follow the existing protocol, this error could occur again. In a team meeting led by an administrator, Gavin raises this issue in a cautious, hesitant, and unsure manner. The leader speaks in a loud, decisive voice and states that he wants input from all staff nurses. However, he glances at the clock, gazes over Gavin's head, and maintains a bored expression. Gavin gets the message that the administrator wants to smooth over the error, bury it, and go on as usual rather than using resources and time to correct the underlying problem.
1. What ethical principle(s) is/are being violated in this situation?
2. What message may the administrator's behaviour convey?
3. Explain the congruence of Gavin and the administrator's communication. Draw conclusions about how you would change the nonverbal message to make it congruent.

QUESTIONS FOR REVIEW AND DISCUSSION

1. How may different factors such as age, values and beliefs, role, race, and sociocultural factors influence communication?

2. In a loud, commanding voice, a nurse tells an immediate postoperative person to take deep breaths every 20 minutes despite the pain it causes. Describe three possible reactions that might occur. Formulate ways to make this intervention more effective.

REFERENCES

Ahmadian, S., Azarshahi, S., & Paulhus, D. L. (2017). Explaining Donald Trump via communication style. *Personality & Individual Differences, 107*, 49–53.

Asan, O., Young, H. N., Chewing, B. et al. (2015). How physician HER screen sharing affects patient and doctor nonverbal communication in primary care. *Patient Education Counseling, 98*(3), 1–11.

Atenstaedt, R. (2012). Touch in the consultation. *British Journal of General Practice, 62*(596), 147–148.

Braun, V., & Clarke, V. (2006). Using thematic analysis in psychology. *Qualitative Research in Psychology, 3*(2), 77–101. https://doi.org/10.1191/1478088706qp063oa.

Canadian Association of Schools of Nursing. (2015). *National Nursing Education Framework: Final Report.* https://www.casn.ca/wp-content/uploads/2014/12/Framwork-FINAL-SB-Nov-30-20151.pdf.

Canadian Nurses Association. (2017). *Code of ethics for registered nurses.* https://www.cna-aiic.ca/~/media/cna/page-content/pdf-en/code-of-ethics-2017-edition-secure-interactive.

Canha, B. (2016). Using humor in treatment of substance use disorders: Worthy of further investigation. *Open Nursing Journal, 10*, 37–44.

Carter, L. (July 8, 2020). Face masks: How nurses can overcome the communication barrier and reassure patients. *Primary Health Care: RCNi.* https://rcni.com/primary-health-care/opinion/comment/face-masks-how-nurses-can-overcome-communication-barrier-and-reassure-patients-163116.

Cuddy, A. (n.d.) *Your body language may shape what you are* [Video]. TED Talks. www.ted.com/search?q=amy+cuddy.

Fletcher, I., McCallum, R., & Peters, S. (2016). Attachment styles and clinical communication performance in trainee doctors. *Patient Education & Counseling, 99*, 1852–1857.

Giles, H. (n.d.). *Communication accommodation theory.* www.public.iastate.edu/~mredmond/SpAccT.htm.

Hargestam, M., Hultin, M., Brulin, C. et al. (2016). Trauma team leaders' nonverbal communication: Video registration during trauma team training. *Scandinavian Journal of Trauma, Resuscitation and Emergency Medicine, 24*, 1–2.

Hawthorn, M. (2015). The importance of communication in sustaining hope at the end of life. *British Journal of Nursing, 24*(13), 702–705.

Kee, J. W. Y., Khoo, H. S., Lim, I. et al. (2018). Communication skills in patient-doctor interactions. *Health Professions Education, 4*(2), 97–106.

Kozlowska, L., & Doboszynska, A. (2012). Nurses' nonverbal methods of communicating with patients in the terminal phase. *International Journal of Palliative Nursing, 18*(1), 40–46.

Lange, C. (2016). Nursing and the importance of body language. *Nursing, 46*(4), 48–49.

Schlogl, M., & Jones, C. A. (2020). Maintaining our humanity through the mask: Mindful communication during COVID-19. *Journal of the American Geriatrics Society, 68*(5), E12–13. https://onlinelibrary.wiley.com/doi/full/10.1111/jgs.16488.

Sicoli, M. A., Stivers, T., Enfield, N. J., et al. (2015). Marked initial pitch in questions signals marked communication function. *Language & Speech, 58*(2), 204–223.

The 519. (n.d.). *The 519 glossary of terms.* https://www.the519.org/education-training/glossary.

Warren, E. (2015). Communication with patients. *Practice Nurse, 45*(9), 1–6.

Watts, K. J., Meiser, B., Zilliacus, E. et al. (2017). Communication with patients from minority backgrounds: Individual challenges experienced by oncology health professionals. *European Journal of Oncology Nursing, 26*, 83–90.

White, R. O., Chakkalakal, R. J., Presley, C. A., et al. (2016). Perceptions of provider communication among vulnerable patients with diabetes: Influences of medical mistrust and health literacy. *Journal of Health Communication, 21*(suppl), 127–134.

7

Cultural Contexts and Communication

Claire Mallette

OBJECTIVES

At the end of the chapter, the reader will be able to:
1. Describe the influence of multiple contexts in defining culture.
2. Define *culture* and related terms.
3. Discuss key dimensions of cultural communication and relational practice.
4. Discuss the importance of reflexivity in culturally safe nursing practice.
5. Describe the concepts related to cultural safety.

Canada is described as being multicultural, with multiple **cultures** coexisting in society while maintaining their cultural differences (Srivastava, 2007; Vandenberg, 2010). Each person's culture is influenced by socioeconomic factors, values and beliefs, race, gender, ethnicity, sexual orientation, life experiences, spirituality, education, and personal choices (Douglas et al., 2014; Registered Nurses' Association of Ontario (2007). The Canadian Nurses Association [CNA], (2018) states that nurses must be respectful and have the professional and ethical accountability to be aware of the culture of the person being cared for. Nurses must also value each person's individual culture and consider how the person's culture influence's their health care experience.

Providing culturally competent nursing practice using communication is a critical nursing competency in the CNA Code of Ethics (2017) and in all provincial and territorial nursing standards. The purpose of this chapter is to explore the complexity of communication in providing culturally safe nursing practice.

BASIC CONCEPTS

Overview: Canadian Demographics

In 2019, Canada's population was approximately 37 million (Statistics Canada, 2019). The 2016 Statistics Canada census data indicates over 250 ethnic and cultural origins, with British Isles, French, European, Chinese, East Indian, and Filipino origins being among the 20 most common ancestries in Canada. Four in 10 people reported more than one origin. The census data also indicated that 6.2% of the total Canadian population (2.1 million people) are of Indigenous ancestry, including First Nations, Métis and Inuit peoples (Statistics Canada, 2017a).

Also, 21.9% (approximately 7.5 million) of people identified as either being or having been a landed immigrant or permanent resident (Statistics Canada, 2017b). Of this group, 60.3% were new immigrants who entered Canada under the economic category (having specific occupational skills that will contribute to Canada's economy), 26.8% entered to join family already in Canada, and 11.6% were admitted as refugees (Statistics Canada, 2017b). Those who identified as having refugee status had been forced to leave their home countries due to persecution, oppression, war, or conflict. Canada welcomed more refugees than any other nation during 2018, with 28100 of the 92400 refugees relocated over 25 countries (Canadian Press, 2019). Toronto, Vancouver, and Montreal continue to be the place of residence for over half of all immigrants and recent immigrants to Canada; however, in recent years, more immigrants are choosing to live in the Prairie and Atlantic provinces.

Multiculturalism and Diversity Legislation in Canada

Multiculturalism is a belief that "all citizens maintain their identities, take pride in their ancestry and have a sense of belonging" (Government of Canada, 2019a). *Multiculturalism* also "refers to the public policy of managing **cultural diversity** in a multiethnic society, emphasizing tolerance and respect for cultural diversity" (Srivastava, 2007, p. 323). Over the years, laws have been passed to protect the rights of all Canadians and support diversity and multiculturalism. The *Official Languages Act* (1969) declared English and French as Canada's official languages and equality of status. One of the key principles was that all Canadians have the right to communicate and receive services from federal institutions in either language. In 1988, the Act was updated as a result of the *Canadian Charter of Rights and Freedoms*, to also include the support and development of English and French linguistic minority communities and advance the equality of status and use of the English and French languages within Canadian society (Government of Canada, 2009). As Canada continues to increases in cultural diversity, there will need to be consideration of how people who speak languages other than English and French also receive services.

The *Canadian Charter of Rights and Freedoms Act* (1982) protects the basic rights and freedoms that are essential to maintaining Canada as a free and democratic society. The Charter upholds multiculturalism and protects the rights of Indigenous people in Canada (Government of Canada, 2019b). The *Canadian Human Rights Act* (1985) ensures that Canadians have the right to be treated fairly in the workplace, free from discrimination on the basis of gender, race, ethnicity, religion, age, sexual orientation, gender identity or expression, marital status, family status, genetic characteristics, disability or conviction for an offence for which a pardon has been granted or a record has been suspended (Government of Canada, 2020). **Discrimination** is defined as an action or decision that treats a person or a group badly for reasons such as their race, age, or disability (Canadian Human Rights Commission, n.d.). Canada was the first country in the world to adopt a multiculturalism policy, in 1971, that led to the *Canadian Multiculturalism Act* (1988). This Act recognizes multiculturalism as an invaluable resource in the shaping of Canada's future. Through this Act, all Canadians are enabled to preserve, enhance and share their cultural heritage and enhance the use of languages other than English and French. The Act states that all individuals receive equal treatment and protection while respecting and valuing diversity (Government of Canada, 2019b).

COMPLEXITY OF CULTURE

Traditionally, culture has been examined with the assumption that people from a particular group share common traits, practices, languages. and attributes such as ethnicity, race, and religion (Vandenberg, 2010; Varcoe & Browne, 2015). **Ethnicity** is defined as a group of people who share common ancestry, culture, language, and religion (Astle et al., 2019). **Race** is based on biological, physical characteristics such as skin colour, eye shape, and hair texture (Varcoe & Brown). Often, *race* and *ethnicity* are used interchangeably, yet they are very different.

Cultural sensitivity is a term that has been used to describe awareness of a person's culture and being tolerant and sensitive to the person's differences. Cultural sensitivity involves knowledge and respect of cultural differences and values, understanding the importance of the person's values and beliefs, and adapting care for people of other cultures (Foronda, 2008). An example of this is when cultural inventories and generalizations describe the different norms, behaviours, and values and beliefs of a cultural group.

While cultural inventories and generalizations are intended to foster cultural sensitivity and a better understanding of persons and their culture, in reality, no one group has uniformly common characteristics. Most people may have some characteristics of the cultural group but do not follow or have all the practices outlined in the cultural description. This type of information can lead to stereotypes and discrimination. Cultural sensitivity also can overlook important aspects of a person's life and context (Varcoe & Browne, 2015). Simulation Exercise 7.1 begins your own critical self-reflection and awareness of your cultural contexts and of how generalizing about a person's culture, values, and beliefs is limited in helping to understand the multiple contexts that influence a person's health experience. Cultural sensitivity can also be perceived as the dominant majority group being tolerant and accepting of a group of "others" with less power.

Diversity is term with different interpretations. Diversity has been linked to multiculturalism, cultural sensitivity, and being aware of cultural differences among a group of people, such as their values and beliefs, country of birth, language, religion, customs, and group affiliations (Foronda et al., 2016; Edmunds & Samuels-Dennis, 2015). A more comprehensive way to explore diversity includes examining "values and belief systems, social group membership, social power, social class, social injustice, oppression, health disparities, different conceptualizations of sickness and health; healthcare demands, linguistic differences, multiple viewpoints, heterogeneity of attitudes, material privilege, various ideas, customs, lifestyles, taboo, and different ethnicities, religion, or group affiliation" (Foronda et al., 2016, p. 212).

SIMULATION EXERCISE 7.1   **Cultural Sensitivity**

Purpose

To begin to develop self-reflection and awareness of your own cultural contexts and the categorizing of a person's culture by outlining common characteristics and generalizations for a cultural group

Procedure

1. Select the country or countries that you associate with and reflect how the culture influences your values, beliefs, and attitudes.
2. Compare your own values, beliefs, and attitudes with others you know from the same cultural background. How are they similar and different?

3. Give examples of stereotyping and labelling.

Discussion

1. Discuss in groups of three to four students your own reflection of values, beliefs, and attitudes based on your cultural background.
2. What surprised you about your own reflection and how it differed from others who have the same cultural background?
3. How can assumptions of cultural common characteristics influence nursing practice?

Considering a person's culture solely based on ethnicity, race or nationality is inadequate and can lead to stereotyping, false assumptions, and failure to recognize the person's individual culture and needs (Doane & Varcoe, 2015). As nurses, we cannot make assumptions that every person in a cultural group has the same values and beliefs based on nationality, race, or ethnicity. Understanding culture in this way is limiting. No two persons share the identical cultural context. Individuals have their own values and beliefs, traditions, languages, ethical and moral perspectives, and individual historical, political, and socioeconomic experiences (Almutairi et al., 2017). Individuals also often associate with multiple group cultures beyond ethnicities, nationalities, and places of birth and are influenced by diverse experiences and values and beliefs that can change over time.

Case Example: Mary Dion

Mary Dion was born in Montreal, Quebec, and became a nurse. Based on traditional ways of examining culture, you may assume Mary Dion is a francophone—her first language is French and she grew up in a French-Canadian home, following the Catholic religion. In fact, Mary Dion was born in Montreal to immigrant parents. Her father, who was Polish, met her mother in England following World War II. They immigrated to Canada in the 1950s and settled in Montreal. Her parents spoke only English at home. Mary grew up in an English suburb of Montreal and celebrated, British, Polish, French, and Canadian traditions. While she was raised in the Catholic religion, she no longer practises any defined religion. Mary learned how to speak French only so that she could

practise nursing in Quebec. Mary's maiden name was Kowalski, but when she married in 1980, she assumed her husband's last name, Dion; he was also raised as an English Quebecer, even though his last name has French origins.

Mary and her family moved to Toronto in the 1990s. When she began practising as a nurse, her colleagues assumed she was French, based on her last name and that she came from Quebec. She experienced some people making comments to her such as, "Why don't you have a 'French accent'?." Over time, Mary and her family assumed more of the ways of living in Ontario, yet many of Mary's values and beliefs are based on growing up in Montreal. Her children, growing up in Ontario, have no understanding of what it means to be an anglophone in Montreal or be raised in the Catholic religion. When Mary visits Montreal, she is viewed as being from Ontario, and when she is in Ontario, she is viewed as being a Quebecer. Mary believes she is both.

MULTIPLE CONTEXTS OF CULTURE

Viewing culture in the traditional way, based on religion, nationality, ethnicity, and race, minimizes the complexity within every culture (Blanchet Garneau & Pepin, 2015). Canada prides itself in being multicultural. The *Multicultural Act* (1988) states that there is cultural freedom and cultural opportunity for everyone. However, many Canadians have difficulty finding employment, housing, and nutrition and face barriers to accessing health care (Varcoe & Browne, 2015). When looking at culture in

Canada, there continue to be racism, marginalization, and health inequities within vulnerable populations, based on race, gender orientation, and socioeconomic factors (CNA, 2018; Simpson, et al., 2011). **Racism** is defined as a prejudice or discrimination directed against a person or people on the basis of their membership in a racial or ethnic group, while **marginalization** is a term used to describe the treatment of a person, group, or concept as insignificant or peripheral. To **racialize** is to categorize or divide a person or people according to their race. Multiple, interrelated contexts (consciously and simply by existing, such as the colour of your skin) influence who each person is. Examining the contexts that make up a person and the complexity of the way they interact is necessary in practising culturally safe, relational nursing practice (Astle et al., 2019; Doane & Varcoe, 2015). The person's historical, sociopolitical, material/economic, physical, and linguistic/discursive contexts are all interrelated and can be used to explore and understand a person's culture (Doane & Varcoe). See (Fig. 7.1). Table 7.1 outlines topics within each context that you can explore to gain a better understanding of the influence of context on the person, family, and community.

Historical Context

History is always exerting an influence on individuals and communities. Canada was built on colonization and

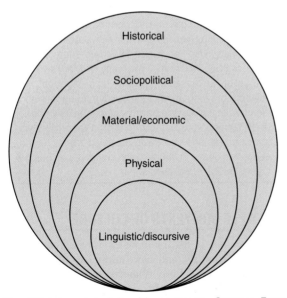

Fig. 7.1 Interrelated health contexts. Source: From Doane, G. H., & Varcoe, C. (2015). *How to nurse: Relationship inquiry with individuals and families in changing health and health care contexts* (p. 152). Wolters Kluwer.

TABLE 7.1   Areas to Examine Related to Cultural Contexts

Historical Context
- Explore the influence of history on the individual, family, and community.
- Follow the lead of the individual and family to learn what is important in relation to their history.
- Examine how history influences the present situation.
- Questions to ask the person and family:
  - What do you think led to this health experience?
  - Is there anything related to your culture that can help me care for you?
  - Have you and your family experienced a similar situation in the past? How did you address it?

Sociopolitical Contexts
- Examine what role power plays in this situation.
- Explore the sociopolitical barriers (a person's race, ethnicity, culture, political and spiritual beliefs, social or marital status, gender, gender identity, gender expression, sexual orientation, age, health status, place of origin, lifestyle, mental or physical ability, socioeconomic status, or any other attribute) to health and health care in this situation.
- Critically reflect on how access to health care is being influenced by sociopolitical contexts.

Material/Economic Contexts
- Examine the communities' material/economic contexts:
  - What are the economic demographics of individuals and families in the community?
  - What key historical events have shaped the economic realities at national, regional, and local levels?
  - How is health within the community influenced by material and economic contexts?
- At the individual and family level explore:
  - How is the individual and family's health influenced by their ability to access material resources?
  - How does the individual and family's health influence their ability to access material resources?

Physical Contexts
- Critically reflect and explore:
  - What are the key environmental issues on health within the community?
  - How do these issues influence the health of members in the community?
  - Do individuals and their families have other patterns of health than those in the community?
  - How does the place of work ensure or not ensure health and well-being?
  - How can the place of work improve on promoting health and well-being?

(Continued)

TABLE 7.1 Areas to Examine Related to Cultural Contexts—cont'd.

Linguistic/Discursive Contexts

- Examine within health care organizations:
  - What are the stereotypes and labels being used to describe persons or health problems?
  - Who or what is viewed as an issue?
  - What language and practices are being used to discourage people from accessing or not accessing health care?
- Examine at the individual and family level:
  - What labels, stereotypes, or other language are being used that is likely harmful to others?
  - How will I respond to these practices? Will I participate? Will I passively resist or advocate for change?

Adapted from Doane, G. H., & Varcoe, C. (2015). *How to nurse: Relationship inquiry with individuals and families in changing health and health care contexts.* Wolters Kluwer.

colonialism. Colonialism occurs when a foreign power rules over a nation and attempts to impose their values and beliefs on the people. In Canada, colonialism occurred when both the British and French came to Canada, developed institutions and policies by European and Euro-American governments. Christian-European languages, values, and beliefs were imposed on Indigenous peoples, with the intent of suppressing their ways of being, languages, and ways of governing, oppressing their identity and assimilating them into the Christian-European norms. (Doane & Varcoe, 2015; Barton & Foster Boucher, 2019; Wasekeesikaw & Parent, 2015).

The *Truth and Reconciliation Commission* (TRC) was established in 2008 to address the legacy of residential schools and advance the process of Canadian reconciliation against Indigenous people. The TRC (2015) made 94 calls to action in the areas of legacy and reconciliation. Calls to Action 18–24 are associated with health and include the following: recognizing and providing the health care rights of Indigenous people; improving health outcomes; recognizing, respecting, and addressing distinct health needs; recognizing the value of Indigenous healing practices and using them in caring for Indigenous people; and providing

⟫ DEVELOPING AN EVIDENCE-INFORMED PRACTICE

Purpose

The purpose of this paper is to examine the support needs of new parents who are refugees to Canada from Sudan and Zimbabwe and identify support preferences that can increase mental health in refugee parents and children

Method

A multimethods participatory research design was used with new parents, individually interviewed, from Zimbabwe (n = 36) and Sudan (n = 36), having children ranging from 4 months to 5 years, born in Canada. The parents also completed standardized measures on social support resources and support-seeking as a coping strategy. Four group interviews (n = 30) were then done with refugee new parents to compare, contrast, and elaborate on the findings from the individual interviews, and two group interviews (n = 30) were conducted with service providers (n = 15) and policy influencers (n = 15) working in communities in Alberta, with refugees from African countries.

Findings

Participants expressed feelings of isolation and loneliness, being separated from family and cultural supports. They also described lacking support during pregnancy, birth, and the postpartum period and having limited contact and interactions with people from similar cultural contexts. The findings indicated that new parents who are refugees need support in accessing services and overcoming barriers involving language, navigating complex systems, and limited financial resources. The participants also described support preferences that included emotional and information support from their cultural community and culturally sensitive service providers.

Implications for Nursing Practice

The study examines support systems and intervention preferences of new parents who are refugees from Sudan and Zimbabwe. The findings can inform health care providers in diverse settings and program and policy development in designing culturally appropriate practices, programs, and policies to support new parents from diverse cultures who are refugees.

From Stewart, M. et al. (2016). Social support needs of Sudanese and Zimbabwean refugee new parents in Canada. *International Journal of Migration, Health and Social Care, 13*(2), 234–252.

cultural competency and skills-based education to all health care providers and students in conflict resolution, human rights, and anti-racism (TRC, 2015). Chapter 8 will explore in depth how to engage with humility through authentic interpersonal communication in partnership with people who are Indigenous.

As a result of colonialism, a person's culture is often viewed in comparison to the dominant group. In Canada, the dominant culture is seen as people originating from England and France who have white skin colour (Hilario et al., 2018). Multiculturalism is based on diversity and tolerance of multiple cultures, but this approach can lead to *racialization*, where people who are non-White are characterized by their race. As a result, negative sociopolitical and economic effects can occur, with social inequities and determinants of health not being considered as part of a person's culture (Doane & Varcoe, 2015; Varcoe & Browne, 2015). Common phrases are used that foster this belief—for example, the term **visible minority**, which indicates that people are being compared to the perceived dominant group of people in Canada who are White, with white skin colour, and are not Indigenous. Statutory holidays in Canada such as Christmas and Easter are in recognition of celebrations from the dominant cultures in Canada of the Christian faith. Those who are of other faiths, such as Hindus who celebrate Diwali, or Muslims observing Eid, have to take vacation days from work to celebrate their holidays. Canadians also have statutory holidays such as Victoria Day, declared a holiday by the government of Canada in 1845 to celebrate Queen Victoria of England (Government of Canada, 2018a), while those who are Indigenous must take a vacation day to celebrate National Indigenous Peoples Day.

Your history and the histories of the people you care for are important as they influence how each individual views the world and how they are viewed. To learn more about a person's history, you can ask questions exploring what is important to the person and family in relation to their history that influences their health needs (Doane & Varcoe, 2015).

Case Example

Rodnita is a Canadian whose skin colour is black. While she now graduates from university with her nursing undergraduate degree, she realizes that no matter what she achieves in her life, she will continue to be judged and assumptions will continue to be made because of the colour of her skin.

Sociopolitical Contexts

Social determinants of health, such as where a person is born, grows up, lives, and works, as well as their economic status, education, sexual orientation, and social inclusion, are influenced by social and political factors that can influence access to health care (CNA, 2013). Chinn & Falk-Rafael (2015) describe how all human relationships are influenced by the use of power. Power can create collective strength and individual well-being, or it can be adversarial, with power being exerted over another. Power is often based on a person or group of people being perceived as having privilege and "power over" another. The dominating groups have values and beliefs that are expected to be followed by "others." Individuals can be considered "ethnic others" by the dominant group and seen as different, which can lead to marginalization, discrimination, and a pressure to assume the practices of the dominant culture by abandoning their own ethnic origins and identities (Van Laer & Janssens, 2014). **Acculturation** describes how immigrants from a different culture learn and choose to adapt to the behaviour and norms of a new culture that holds different expectations. This can be a complicated process because it includes embracing new social and hierarchal relationships, consistent with an unfamiliar cultural context (Page, 2005). Becoming acculturated creates stress due to the competing pressures of reconciling a familiar cultural identity with the need to adopt new customs essential to functioning effectively in the adopted culture (Marsiglia & Booth, 2015). A hybrid sense of self can develop, where the person tries to have sameness with whichever audience they are with. They attempt to adapt to the expectations of the dominant culture yet hold on to their own culture and identity when they are with people who have a similar culture (Van Laer & Janssens, 2014).

Individuals from the dominant culture are often unaware that they are engaging in "othering." For example, the person who is admitted for abdominal pain who is wearing a hijab is described as "the Muslim in Room 2" rather than describing the person with their name. Simulation Exercise 7.2 starts your exploration of your own positions of power and how they may influence your practice, by examining your personal and cultural history, values, and beliefs, in their political, social, and historical contexts.

Nurses need to be aware of the power differences that exist within health care. Health care providers can be viewed as having power over the person in making decisions about their health care without looking at the complexity of who the person is. There are multiple sociopolitical factors influencing people accessing health care and following through with prescribed treatments. They often cannot afford what they are being told to do and are fearful of being judged, stigmatized, discriminated against, or treated poorly, based on their socioeconomic factors such as lifestyle, sexual orientation, race, and economic status. Box 7.1 describes challenges people who are transgender experience when seeking health care.

SIMULATION EXERCISE 7.2 Social Positions and Power

Purpose

To begin to develop self-reflection and awareness of you own social positions and power contexts. Examine your attitudes, values, beliefs, assumptions, and experiences of advantage and disadvantage that have shaped the way you understand the world and in relation to others. This exercise focuses on your positions of power by examining which powerful (dominant) and less powerful groups you belong to. Examples can include education, language, skin, colour, roles, socioeconomic status, gender, religion, diversity, sexual orientation, race, and so on. Depending on your cultural contexts, these groups can be considered either powerful or less powerful.

Procedure

Answer the following:

1. What three dominant groups do you belong to?

2. What three less powerful groups do you associate with?

3. How do they relate to your own values and beliefs towards yourself and others?

4. How do these groups of power and less power influence your opportunities and challenges in life?

Discussion

1. Share your answers in groups of three to four students.

2. What surprised you in your discussion? Why?

3. Were there some sources of power that were viewed as dominant for some and less powerful for others? Why do think this was occurring?

4. How will your understanding of positions of power influence caring for persons from diverse cultures?

Adapted from Varcoe, C., & Browne A. J. (2015). Culture and cultural safety: Beyond cultural inventories. In D. Gregory, C. Raymond-Seniuk, L. Patrick et al. (Eds.), *Fundamentals Perspectives on the Art and Science of Canadian Nursing* (p. 224). Wolters Kluwer.

BOX 7.1 Health Issues in People With a Transgender Cultural Context

The term *transgender* is used for persons who express their gender in ways that are different from their established assigned gender at birth, as being male or female (Baldwin et al., 2018; Merryfeather & Bruce, 2014). *Transgender* is an umbrella term that includes individuals who are trans women, trans men, and people who are gender queer, gender fluid, nonbinary, gender nonconforming, two-spirited, gender retired, transsexual, intersex, cross-dressers, drag queens, and drag kings (Kellet & Fitton, 2017). People who are transgender can experience higher levels of poor physical and mental health, HIV and other sexually transmitted infections, drug and alcohol use, self-harm, suicide, homelessness, poverty, and underemployment (Baldwin et al., 2018). When individuals who are transgender try to access health care, they frequently experience discrimination and stigma. In a study done in Ontario, research findings indicated that of the respondents (n = 433), 21% avoided going to emergency departments as they believed being trans would have a negative impact on their care, and 52% indicated they had negative experiences when they had gone to the emergency departments in the gender they feel themselves to be (Kellett & Fitton). Another study's findings identified that people who are transgender had positive health experiences when health care providers used inclusive language and treated identity disclosure as routine. Negative experiences resulted from misgendering (using the pronoun "him" or "her" based on their gender at birth rather the gender they express), when health care providers were unfamiliar with people who are transgender and their health issues, and from transphobic practices (Baldwin et al., 2018).

When caring for people, it is important to be aware of the power dynamics and how they are influencing the relationship and the care being provided. With person-centred care, discussed in Chapter 5, the nurse and other health care providers work with the person and family as equal partners and focus on health issues alongside the person's values, cultural context, family, diversity, social circumstances, and lifestyles (Hafskjold et al., 2015; Kuluski et al., 2016). As a nurse, your interactions with persons can acknowledge who they are as a person and what is important to them. You can also ask, "What name would you like to be called and what pronouns would you prefer being used?" This will also assist in decreasing the person's fear of being judged and discriminated against. As nurses, it is also important to be self-aware of your own values and beliefs, and conscious and unconscious biases, to question how they are influencing your perceptions of the people you are caring for and how you are communicating with them.

Material/Economic Context

Material and economic contexts are interrelated to historical and sociopolitical cultural contexts (Varcoe & Browne, 2015). Links have been made between health outcomes and the way wealth and power are distributed in economies (CNA, 2013). For those with low levels of income and education, who live in inadequate housing with limited access to health care, social supports are more likely to have poorer physical and mental health outcomes than for those living in better circumstances (CNA, 2012). A report on the key health inequalities in Canada found that there were overall significant health inequalities among people who are Indigenous, sexual and racial minorities, and immigrants; people living with functional limitations; and people experiencing inequalities of socioeconomic status such as income, education level, and employment and occupation status (Government of Canada, 2018b).

In 2018, 12.7% of Canadians reported housing that was unaffordable, with shelter costs being more than 30% of before-tax household income, in need of major repairs or unsuitable for the size of people in the household or they could not afford a suitable or adequate home in their community (Statistics Canada, 2020). In 2014, 11.2% of Canadians aged 12 years and older reported not receiving health care when they felt they needed to. In 2017–2018, 8.7% of Canadian households reported being moderately to severely food insecure as they did not have enough money to purchase or access a sufficient amount and variety of food to live a healthy lifestyle (Statistics Canada).

If you were to look at the culture of a person and food preferences through the traditional lens of broad assumptions related to the race and ethnicity of the person, you might assume that the person was eating a certain diet because of cultural and dietary influences. If you looked at the person's context and culture together, you might discover the food they are eating is also influenced by what they can afford, availability, and what is viewed as acceptable within the environment they live in (Doane & Varcoe, 2015). For example, you are assessing Xi Luu, a 40-year-old woman who is a single mother with three children. Ms. Luu and her family eat rice with every meal. You might assume they do so because of her Chinese culture, yet upon speaking with her, you discover it's because she cannot afford other nutritional food. You might also assume that rice is a large part of Tim Yu's diet as he is from a Korean culture. However, upon asking him about his food preferences, he says he prefers food more traditionally found in Canada rather than the food his parents eat. These example demonstrates how you must consider both the context and culture of the person. As the nurse, you also have to be aware of your own food biases and what you consider to be healthy,

ethically acceptable (e.g., vegetarian vegan versus eating meat), and your own dietary preferences.

Physical Context

Physical environments affect health. The world is globally connected, with economic, climate, and ecological challenges such as global warming; pollution; and occupational environments that influence the health, welfare, and physical and emotional well-being of all. Environment changes influence the development of respiratory and cardiovascular illness, cancer, mental health issues, increased occupational health hazards, intestinal disorders, and viruses (Government of Canada, 2019c).

The effect of people's physical context on health became very apparent in 2020, when the COVID-19 virus pandemic had a global health impact and needed to be addressed collectively by individuals, communities, countries, and globally. Where a person lived during the pandemic highlighted vulnerabilities to COVID-19. To explore social inequities in COVID-19 deaths in Canada, an analysis of COVID-19 death rates from January to August 2020 was done, with the focus on factors such as residence in large cities, income, dwelling type, household type, and household size (Government of Canada, 2021). Key findings demonstrated significant inequalities in COVID-19, with higher death rates for those living in large cities, apartments, lower income neighbourhoods, and neighbourhoods with more people who are a visible minority, recently immigrated to Canada, and speak neither English nor French (Government of Canada, 2021).

Access to vaccines also varies from one country to another. In 2021, the *Washington Post* identified the world as split into countries that have access to vaccines and those that do not, with 45% of all vaccine doses administered to just 16% of the world's population in high-income countries (Mirza & Rauhala, 2021). It has been estimated that the world's 92 poorest countries will reach only 60% of their populations being vaccinated by 2023 or later.

Where a person lives influences their health. For example, the type of work (e.g., farming, mining, office work, service industry), resources (environmental, such as water or access to health care), and lifestyles (sedentary lifestyle versus very active one) can all influence a person's health (Bradford et al., 2016; White et al., 2012). Nurses need to be aware of how the physical context and culture influence their own well-being and health, alongside the people in need of care.

Linguistic/Discursive Contexts

Within our multicultural country, there are people who do not speak the languages of English or French. Words and nonverbal messages can have different meaning and

BOX 7.2 Guidelines for Using Interpreters in Health Care

Whenever possible, the translator should not be a family member.

Ask the person when possible, if a male or female interpreter is preferred.

Orient the translator to the goals of the clinical interview and expected confidentiality.

Look directly at the person when either you or the person is speaking.

Ask the translator to clarify anything that is not understood by either you or the person.

Speak slowly and use short sentences. After each completed statement, pause for translation.

Following the session, debrief with the interpreter on their observations and if there is anything health care providers should be aware of.

be misinterpreted. de Moissac and Bowen (2019) describe that, when there is a language barrier, quality of care related to appropriateness, continuity, person-centred services, and safety differ in those who speak the dominant language and those who do not. Language barriers have also been found to influence the quality of chronic disease management, end-of-life care and pain management. Where available, the use of interpreter services are recommended to better communicate and understand the person's needs. Interpretive services are more readily available in diverse, urban settings compared to rural areas that may be less diverse. Box 7.2 provides guidelines for the use of interpreters in health interviews.

Whenever possible, it is best not to use as interpreters family members, children, friends, or persons who work in the health care setting if they are not trained to be interpreters. They may not be familiar with medical terminology and may unintentionally or intentionally misrepresent the meaning of the translated message. Technology such as Google Translate or other translation Internet sites are being used more often, although they should be used with caution, for a variety of reasons: they are not always available; they may not be appropriate for the person's needs, such as in an emergency situation; words have different interpretations depending on a persons' cultural contexts; and for doing mental health assessments (de Moissac and Bowen, 2019).

Communication and the way it is used by health care providers is related to the context of culture. There is the likelihood that persons can be stereotyped or labelled based on their race, class, religion, age, gender, income, or

sexual orientation. Think of times when you have heard or referred to a person as being "difficult," "demanding," "cooperative," or "high risk," based on their cultural context, individual characteristics, gender, and behaviours, or as a result of association with certain social groups (Varcoe & Browne, 2015).

Case Example

A woman who is Black was experiencing right lower abdominal pain, fever, and nausea and vomiting. Concerned she had appendicitis, she went to the emergency department in the hospital where she worked. She spent 6 hours in emergency, informing the health care providers that her pain was getting worse and she felt increasingly unwell. She did not ask for pain medication as she didn't want to mask any symptoms and her nonverbal behaviours did not indicate she was in pain. After 6 hours, she was discharged home, after being told it was probably a flu or food poisoning. She returned to the emergency department 6 hours later in debilitating pain and was diagnosed with a perforated (ruptured) appendix, requiring emergency surgery and a lengthy hospital stay. Once she recovered, she asked her surgeon why no one listened to her on her first emergency visit. She was told that "because she didn't ask for any pain medication, and didn't indicate nonverbally that she was in pain, the health care team made the assumption that her symptoms were not serious."

Nurses can be the change agent, increasing awareness of stereotyping and labelling based on culture. This change can occur through self-awareness of your own assumptions and language being used, not using this type of language, and helping others increase their awareness of language and how it can influence the care being provided. For example, instead of labelling a person who frequently returns to the urgent care clinic as a "frequent flyer," the nurse can assess and advocate for understanding why the person continues to return to the clinic. When the nurse hears a person is "demanding," they can ask, "What do you think is making the person demanding?"

In summary, through exploring the person and family's contexts, examining historical, sociopolitical, material/economic, physical, and linguistic/discursive contexts, the nurse can have a better understanding of the person's unique culture and how their experiences influence their health care needs. Examining the different contexts can also inform your practice and conscious and unconscious biases and identify inequities related to the people you care for. Provincial and territorial standards and the

---

TABLE 7.2   Canadian Nurses Association (2017) Code of Ethics Related to Cultural Context in Nursing Practice

- Nurses work with persons receiving care to explore the range of health care choices available to them, recognizing that some have limited choices because of social, economic, geographic, or other factors that lead to inequities.
- Nurses are sensitive to the inherent power differentials between care providers and persons receiving care. They do not misuse that power to influence decision making.
- In health care decision making, in treatment and in care, nurses work with persons receiving care to take into account their values, customs, and spiritual beliefs as well as their social and economic circumstances, without judgement or bias.
- Nurses do not discriminate on the basis of a person's race, ethnicity, culture, political and spiritual beliefs, social or marital status, gender, gender identity, gender expression, sexual orientation, age, health status, place of origin, lifestyle, mental or physical ability, socioeconomic status, or any other attribute.
- Nurses respect the special history and interests of Indigenous peoples as articulated in the Truth and Reconciliation Commission of Canada's *Calls to Action* (2012).
- Nurses recognize that vulnerable groups in society are systemically disadvantaged (which leads to diminished health and well-being) and advocate to improve their quality of life while taking action to overcome barriers to health care.
- Nurses recognize the significance of social determinants of health and advocate for policies and programs that address them (e.g., safe housing, supervised consumption sites).
- Nurses maintain an awareness of major health concerns, such as poverty, inadequate shelter, food insecurity, and violence, while working for social justice (individually and with others) and advocating for laws, policies, and procedures that bring about equity.
- Nurses make fair decisions about the allocation of resources under their control, based on the needs of persons receiving care. They advocate for fair treatment and fair distribution of resources.

Adapted from Canadian Nurses Association. (2017). *Code of ethics for registered nurses.* https://www.cna-aiic.ca/~/media/cna/page-content/pdf-en/code-of-ethics-2017-edition-secure-interactive.

CNA (2017) Code of Ethics outline the importance of providing quality compassionate care, dignity, and respect for all through a cultural context. See Table 7.2 for ethical responsibilities outlined in the Code of Ethics related to providing cultural context through promoting justice, human rights, equity, fairness, and the public good in nursing practice.

APPLICATION OF CULTURAL CONTEXTS IN NURSING PRACTICE

Nursing Theories on Culture

Examining culture through a theoretical lens began with Dr. Madeleine Leininger, a nurse anthropologist. She developed the first major theory-based approach, Transcultural Nursing Theory in the 1950s that was published in 1991, to describe the importance of culture in health care from a nursing perspective (Astle et al., 2019). The theory was based on the belief that nurses must have knowledge about diverse cultures to provide care that recognizes the person and their cultural background and context. While the theory was developed prior to the focus on person-centred care, it captures the importance of focusing on the person's

values, beliefs, and attitudes related to their context and culture. The Sunrise Model based on Leininger's work has been used in nursing to promote culturally competent care with people from diverse cultures (Astle et al., 2019).

In Canada, Dr. Rani Srivastava (2007) built on Leininger's work, focusing on power to explore culture in relation to racism and inequity. Her model encourages nurses to examine the power dynamics and histories of persons and how this influences their cultural context and the care that is needed. Dr. Joan Anderson emphasized that culture is a dynamic process involving the person's political, social, historical, and economic contexts. She advocates for nurses to take a lead in addressing inequitable policies, practices, and power relations in health care. Dr. Diana Gustafson also focuses on the need for nurses to transform social practices and relations that reinforce the social practices and relations of the dominant culture (Varcoe & Browne, 2015).

As discussed, culture is much more complex than belonging to a group with values, beliefs, and attitudes related to race, ethnicity, and nationality. Doane and Varcoe (2015) define culture as a "dynamic relational process of selectively responding to and integrating particular historical, social, political, economic, physical and linguistic structures and processes. Culture is relationally determined and contextual. These responses are expressed in multiple ways, including values, beliefs, attitudes and practices" (p. 139). With culture being relational, nurses are encouraged to explore beyond a person being a member of a cultural group. Instead, nurses alongside the person should focus on examining the interplay of their values, beliefs, attitudes, and practices as well at their multiple contexts to identify what is important to them and their family's health care needs (Doane & Varcoe).

Relational Practice

Relational practice is a way for the nurse to care for a person, encompassing their diverse cultural contexts. **Relational practice** is defined as being "guided by conscious participation with clients using a number of relational skills including listening, questioning, empathy, mutuality, reciprocity, self-observation, reflection and sensitivity to emotional contexts" (College of Nurses of Ontario, 2018, p.11). Relational practice requires a commitment to caring and compassionate nursing practice with clinical competencies of a strong knowledge base; the ability to observe, be curious, and authentic; and explore and analyze information to guide clinical judgement, decision making, and practice. Using relational practice builds on the strengths of the person. Without bias, and being aware of the multiple contexts influencing who the person is and their health experience, the nurse responds to and with the person in a way that is meaningful to them (Doane & Varcoe, 2007; Doane & Varcoe, 2015).

As discussed in Chapter 1, systems theory focuses on the complexity of interrelationships and interdependencies within the health care system. Relational practice is facilitated by relational inquiry that provides care through navigating within the relationships and complexities of the person, nurse, health care providers, and the health care system. The nurse needs to explore how the person, situations, contexts, environment, and processes are all interacting and integrally connected (Doane & Varcoe, 2007). This is achieved through looking at the intrapersonal, interpersonal, and contextual influences. The *intrapersonal* influences are related to what all the people are experiencing *within* themselves, including yourself, the person, family, and any others engaged in the interaction. The *interpersonal* influences involve then examining what is occurring *among and between* people. How are people acting towards one another? What are they focusing on? What are they ignoring? Are the nonverbal and verbal aspercts of communication congruent with one another? *Contextually*, the nurse then considers what is going on *around* the people in relation to their multiple contexts (historical, sociopolitical, economic, physical, etc.). By focusing on the intrapersonal,

interpersonal, and contextual influences, you are intentionally focusing on the details within the interrelationships and interdependencies. This relational consciousness makes you aware of the relational complexities of what is happening, the ongoing interactions within and among those involved, and the contexts. You can then intentionally choose how best to respond to the complexities and interactions (Doane & Varcoe, 2015). Simulation Exercise 7.3 provides an opportunity to begin to apply relational practice.

Reflexivity

Reflexivity is a reflective practice described as the ability to understand and question your own contexts, attitudes, values, beliefs, assumptions, and experiences of advantage and disadvantage that have shaped the way you understand the world and in relation to others (Landy et al., 2016; Verdonk, 2015). It is important to examine how your own personal and cultural history and contexts influence your practice.

Reflexivity is essential to relational inquiry and involves nurses looking at both what they are doing and how they are doing it (Doane & Varcoe, 2007). *Intrapersonally*, it is important to pay attention to what is going on within yourself, in being aware of what you are doing, feeling, and thinking in the moment and how your own contexts influence this. *Interpersonally*, you need to be aware of and critically analyze how you are relating to others and how they relate with you. *Contextually*, you are aware of your surroundings and what is happening that is influencing the situation (Doane & Varcoe, 2015). Simulation Exercise 7.4 examines how to begin using reflexivity in increasing self-awareness and critical self-reflection.

Critical **self-reflection** is a process of linking past, present, and future experiences. This process involves integrating the values, beliefs, attitudes, and emotions you felt during an experience to understand and examine the experience through multiple perspectives. This will help you recognize how the experience could be understood in different ways, identify the lessons learned; and identify how your behaviours could be changed in the future as the result of the reflective practice (Aronson, 2011). Critical reflection also moves beyond self-reflection to focus on the application of critical theory in examining social and systemic forces (yours and those of others) that were involved in the experience to increase awareness of the social, cultural, economic, and political forces at work (Ng et al., 2015). By doing reflective practice, you will become more aware of your own thoughts and actions and how they influence how you relate with others. Rather than viewing reflective practice as irrelevant, see it as something that should occur on a continual basis, not only as a student but throughout your career as a nurse (Song & Stewart, 2012). Learning how to do reflective practice is a way to challenge one's own

SIMULATION EXERCISE 7.3 Relational Practice

Purpose

To increase your ability to apply relational practice

Procedure

1. Think of a nursing or life situation that bothered you, and where you felt unsettled, uncomfortable, or disturbed by what occurred. Examine the situation, assigning responsibility to what each of the individuals did to make the situation uncomfortable.
2. Now examine the same situation using relational inquiry.
   - What intrapersonal elements occurred? What were you feeling and doing during the interaction that contributed to the situation?
   - What interpersonal elements were taking place? How were the people involved relating to each other? What were they focusing on and what were they ignoring? What nonverbal communication was occurring?
   - What was the context of the situation? What priorities did the different people have? What power and system influences were in play?
3. How does your understanding of the situation differ between the two different ways of examining the same situation? What questions arise?
4. When you look at the situation through the relational inquiry lens, does your understanding of the situation and what could have been done change?

Discussion

1. Discuss your reflections with another classmate about what you learned and how your understanding of the situation changed when using relational inquiry.
2. How do you see applying relational inquiry in your nursing practice to understand people's cultural contexts?

Adapted from: Doane, G. H., & Varcoe, C. (2015). How to nurse: Relationship inquiry with individuals and families in changing health and health care contexts (p. 11). Wolters Kluwer.

SIMULATION EXERCISE 7.4 Practising Reflexivity

Purpose

To begin to develop reflexivity (intrapersonally, interpersonally, and contextually), self-awareness, and critical self-reflection

Procedure

Answer the following questions:

1. Personal Self-Awareness (Intrapersonally)
   - What are my own historical, sociopolitical, material/economic, physical, and linguistic contexts?
   - How do these influence my identity, values and beliefs, attitudes, and behaviours?
   - How are my contexts influencing the way I relate to others?
2. Professional Self-Awareness (Interpersonally)
   - How do I relate to others from different cultures?
   - What stereotypes do I attach to others and what am I assuming about them and why? What knowledge supports and challenges my assumptions?
   - What contexts may be influencing how others relate to me?
3. Contextual Self-Awareness
   - What are the values and principles of the organization related to diversity and culture?
   - How does the organization address unique and dynamic cultural identities of persons and communities being served?
   - What power or system contexts influence providing culturally safe health care?

Discussion

1. Explore each of these areas and write down your reflections.
2. Share your reflections in a group of three to four students.
3. Identify common themes.
4. Did your answers based on your own contexts differ from those of your classmates?
5. Discuss as a group how reflexivity can inform your nursing practice and how you see applying it in your practice.

Adapted from: Astle, Barton, Johnson, et al. (2019). Global health. In P.A. Potter, A. G. Perry, J. C. Ross-Jerr, et al. (Eds.), *Canadian Fundamentals of Nursing* (6th ed.) [E-reader edition]. Elsevier; Doane, G. H., & Varcoe, C. (2015). *How to nurse: Relationship inquiry with individuals and families in changing health and health care contexts.* Wolters Kluwer.

assumptions, build new knowledge, care for others, and learn ways to navigate the changing and complex health care environments that you will be practising in (Ng et al.).

CULTURAL SAFETY

Providing culturally safe care to persons, families, and communities is a progression that involves both cultural competence and cultural humility.

Cultural Competence

Cultural competence is defined as a "set of attitudes, skills, behaviours, and policies enabling individuals and organizations to establish effective interpersonal relationships that supersede cultural differences" (Nguyen et al., 2020, p. 2). Cultural competence acknowledges culture as being fluid; changing and diversity exists with all (Danso, 2016). Cultural competence is also defined as a "process by which individuals and systems respond respectfully and effectively to people of all cultures, languages, classes, races, ethnic backgrounds, religions, spiritual traditions, immigration status and other diversity" (Danso). Included in cultural competence is the importance of nurses self-reflecting about their own cultural values and beliefs and being aware of how this influences their nursing care (CNA, 2018). This involves an ongoing process of critical reflection and action, which the nurse then uses to provide safe, congruent, and effective care in a partnership with the person, family, and community, taking into account their contexts and the influences of power (Blanchet Garneau & Pepin, 2015).

While cultural competence is important, it is not sufficient on its own when working in partnerships with diverse populations. The belief of having cultural competence can lead nurses to believe they have the knowledge and skill to care for a person, family, and community without critical self-reflection and exploring unique characteristics, context, and group differences of the people they care for (Nguyen et al., 2020).

Cultural Humility

In order to provide cultural safety, cultural humility is needed alongside cultural competence. **Cultural humility** is an ongoing lifelong commitment to having the humility to learn from the person and the critical-self-reflection to identify and address biases, prejudices, attitudes, and behaviours in addressing power imbalances within the relationship (Foronda et al., 2016; Nguyen et al., 2020). When cultural humility occurs, mutual empowerment, partnerships, respect, trust, optimal care, and lifelong learning exist. Cultural humility is a lifelong process, where competence is never achieved as internal and external factors influencing caring for people are continually changing (Nguyen et al.).

Cultural humility is made up of having attributes of openness; self-awareness; egoless, supportive interactions; and self-reflection and critique (Foronda et al., 2016). Openness is having an open mind in exploring new ideas with the people you are caring for and not assuming knowledge of a person based on their culture. Self-awareness is being aware of one's own strengths, limitations, values and beliefs, behaviours, and how you appear to others. We all have an ego, but to have cultural humility, the nurse must be humble and view persons as equals. A nurse is egoless when power imbalances do not exist and the nurse and person are working together in an equal partnership. Supportive interactions occur when there is sharing, the person feels supported, and the nurse is actively engaged in the interaction. Self-reflection and critique is the last attribute of cultural humility, where the nurse engages in self-questioning, critiquing actions taken, and discovery. In summary, cultural humility is described as ongoing self-reflection, learning and discovery, mutual understanding, and respect between the nurse and the person, family, and community (Foronda et al., 2016; Nguyen et al., 2020).

Cultural Safety

Cultural safety is a term first used in New Zealand, in recognition of the impact of colonialism on the Maori peoples and the need to move beyond cultural sensitivity in providing better health care (Browne et al. 2009; Varcoe & Browne, 2015). In Canada, this concept is now used to include all people, in recognition that cultures are dynamic, depending on power relations and individual contexts (Doane & Varcoe, 2015). Cultural safety focuses on power imbalances, inequitable social relationships and social justice. Box 7.3 describes social justice (CNA, 2018). In promoting cultural safety to meet the health needs of persons, families, and communities, the nurse acknowledges, respects, and supports their unique cultural identity.

The central principles of cultural safety are as follows:
- Culture is dynamic and rooted within and changing in response to historical, economic, political, and social contexts.
- Instead of viewing a person through a lens based on a generalized description of culture-specific values, beliefs, and activities and what members of a group should think and do, it is important to focus on the person or group's needs and how they are actually perceived and treated.
- Social, economic, and political positions of groups influence health and health care.
- Individual and organizational discrimination in health care can result in health risks for persons and specific groups seeking care. This occurs when persons perceive health care providers who hold power and engage with

them in a way that feels demeaning, diminished, or disempowering. An example of this is the increasing level of people developing diabetes mellitus, with a higher incidence occurring in Indigenous peoples. This is a result of colonialism; racial discrimination; social inequities in relation to education, employment, and housing; access to affordable nutritional food and health care; and a lack of trust and confidence in the Canadian government and health care system with Indigenous peoples (Leung, 2016).

- Critical reflexivity is necessary in reflecting on how your own personal values and beliefs and cultural history influence your interactions and nursing practice. You need to also be aware of not imposing your own values and beliefs on a person based on your history.
- Promoting cultural safety requires you to recognize, respect, and nurture the unique and dynamic cultural identities of the persons you care for. Your nursing care should then safely meet people's needs, expectations, and rights, given their own unique contexts (Doane & Varcoe; Varcoe & Browne, 2015). Box 7.4 is a poem by nurse poet Dr. J. Reich (2015), on the importance of providing cultural safety.

Applying Cultural Safety in Practice

The nurse acknowledges that every person has a unique culture, based on their multiple contexts. There are two sets of mnemonics, "the 3 Ds" and "the 3 Rs" that can assist you in providing culturally safe practice. "The 3 Ds" remind nurses to be aware of behaviours that could be perceived as demeaning, devaluing, or disempowering. The 3 "Rs" of revise, respect, and the rights of the person represent the words in promoting cultural safety. These words remind you to revise or change the situation by being self-aware and recognizing cultural differences, while respecting and promoting the rights of the person, family, and community (Richardson et al., 2016).

Applying cultural safety in practice also requires continually challenging your own assumptions, stereotypes, and labelling. Rather than assuming knowledge of a person based on their culture, you need to be open-minded and respectful in inquiring about the person's contexts. This requires you to be actively listening in a nonjudgemental way to better understand the persons you are caring for. The case example about Simon Gull describes how making assumptions, not actively listening, and stereotyping persons from a cultural group can result in negative health outcomes.

Case Example

Simon Gull lives and works in Toronto and is Indigenous. He has been feeling unwell with nausea, always being thirsty, increased fatigue, and frequently having to urinate. As his symptoms worsen, he decides to seek out medical attention at an emergency department at a downtown Toronto hospital. When the triage nurse assesses him, he finds

Mr. Gull confused, slurring his speech, and with his breath smelling like alcohol. The nurse makes the assumption that Mr. Gull has alcohol intoxication because he is Indigenous and puts him in a room to sleep it off. Another nurse checks on Mr. Gull a few hours later and finds him unresponsive. Blood work is ordered, and the lab results indicate Mr. Gull has diabetic ketoacidosis, not alcohol intoxication.

You will need to anticipate in which circumstances you will have difficulty remaining nonjudgemental and identify how you will address these experiences. For example, you may believe that abusing drugs is morally wrong. How then will you care for a person with an opioid addiction? Using reflexivity activities can help you better understand why you are feeling the way you are and how to provide culturally safe nursing care.

When people say they are feeling unsafe and discriminated against, it is important to listen to their concerns. In these situations, instead of becoming defensive, actively listen to what the person is saying and feeling. If people are feeling not valued and discriminated against, then that is their experience, and it is important to explore why they are feeling this way. When you are feeling uncomfortable and don't know what to say, or feel you have said the wrong thing, be honest with others. Most people will understand when your intentions are good (Varcoe & Browne, 2015).

To address cultural safety with colleagues and within your organization, you will need to find ways to challenge stereotypes, generalizations, labelling and discriminatory organizational practices. This will increase awareness and role modelling of cultural safety and being respectful of the person regardless of their culture.

Another way to increase awareness of cultural safety is to have increased knowledge and understanding of greater social and political contexts. For example, judgements are made that a person being homeless and asking for spare change is lazy, should just get a job, and get off the streets. Increased understanding of their contexts, such as being abused at home, and being discriminated against based on sexual orientation, race, mental health issues, and poverty could all be contributing to the person being homeless. When you hear judgemental comments, you can raise awareness of the larger issues that could be contributing factors.

At the organizational level, you can advocate for culturally safe practices through getting to know the interprofessional team and their roles in providing culturally safe practices. If you notice that there are a number of people who speak a certain language, you can advocate for creating resources with common phrases that can assist communicating with them and accessing interpreter services where possible (Varcoe & Browne, 2015). Simulation Exercise 7.5 provides an opportunity to apply cultural safety in caring for a person.

Conflict With One's Conscience

As a nurse, you will care for people whose behaviours, values, and beliefs you don't agree with. The CNA (2017) Code

---

SIMULATION EXERCISE 7.5 Applying Cultural Safety

Purpose
To begin to learn how to incorporate cultural safety into your nursing practice

Procedure
1. Assess a classmate's multiple cultural contexts (historical, sociopolitical, material/economic, physical environment and linguistic/discursive), to better understand their culture and what is important to them.
2. Conduct the interview using relational practice in being aware of the intrapersonal, interpersonal, and contextual influences while you do the interview. What were these influences?
3. As you are conducting the interview, be aware of how you are applying the principles of cultural competence and humility.
4. Following the interview, stop and reflect on how you felt during the interview. Write down your reflections.
   • How did your own multiple cultural contexts influence the way you conducted the interview?

• What were the intrapersonal and interpersonal influences on the interview?
• What would you do differently the next time?

5. As the person being interviewed, write down your own reflections.
   • How did you feel being interviewed, regarding being aware of the intrapersonal, interpersonal, and contextual influences?
   • How did your own values and beliefs and contexts influence your answers?

Discussion
1. For the interviewer, debrief with your classmate on what information you observed and assessed from the interview.
2. For the interviewee, describe how you felt during the interview based on your own reflections.
3. Describe what you both learned from your critical self-reflections.
4. Ask for feedback on how you conducted the interview and suggestions on how to improve.

BOX 7.5   CNA's Conscientious Objections

"If nursing care is requested that is in conflict with the nurse's moral beliefs and values but in keeping with professional practice, the nurse provides safe, compassionate, competent and ethical care until alternative care arrangements are in place to meet the person's needs or desires. But nothing in the Criminal Code compels an individual to provide or assist in providing medical assistance in dying. If nurses can anticipate a conflict with their conscience, they notify their employers or person receiving care (if the nurse is self-employed) in advance so alternative arrangements can be made" (CNA, 2017, p. 35).

of Ethics and provincial and territorial nursing standards identify that nurses provide care for all persons. The CNA Code of Ethics state that "nurses do not discriminate on the basis of a person's race, ethnicity, culture, political, and spiritual beliefs, social or marital status, gender, gender identity, gender expression, sexual orientation, age, health status, place of origin, lifestyle, mental or physical ability, socio-economic status, or any other attribute" (p.15). If you are caring for a person with whom you have a conflict of conscience, you cannot abandon caring for the person until someone else can take over caring for the person. A conflict of conscience can occur when a nurse is opposed to certain procedures and practices in health care and would have difficulty willingly participating in activities that others find morally acceptable (CNA, 2017). Examples of when this might occur would be situations such as suicide attempts, abortion, blood transfusions, refusal of treatment, being transgender, and medical assistance in dying. Box 7.5 describes *conscientious objection*, outlined in the CNA Code of Ethics. If you find yourself in this type of situation, you will need to notify your supervisor and request being removed from providing care. When making decisions around conflict of conscience, you need to ensure your conflict is not based on prejudice, fear, or convenience (CNA, 2017).

SUMMARY

This chapter explores the complexity of communication in providing culturally safe nursing practice. Canada prides itself in being multicultural. Traditionally, culture has been examined with the assumption that people from a particular group share common traits, practices, languages, and attributes such as ethnicity, race, and religion. Considering a person's culture solely based on ethnicity, race or nationality is inadequate and can lead to stereotyping, false assumptions, and failure to recognize the person's individual culture and needs. No two persons share the identical cultural context. Persons from different cultures have their own values and beliefs, traditions, languages, ethical and moral perspectives, and historical, political, and socioeconomic experiences (Almutairi et al., 2017). Individuals also often associate with multiple groups and are influenced by diverse experiences, values, and beliefs that can change over time.

A comprehensive definition of *culture* is described as a dynamic relational process of selectively responding to and integrating particular historical, social, political, economic, physical, and linguistic contexts. Examining the contexts that make up a person and the complexity of the way they interact and are interrelated are necessary to understand a person's culture and provide culturally safe relational nursing practice.

Relational practice is a way for the nurse to care for a person encompassing their diverse contexts of culture. This is achieved through exploring the *intrapersonal*, *interpersonal*, and *contextual* influences on the health care experience. *Reflexivity* is essential to relational practice. Reflexivity includes looking at both what you are doing and how you are doing it; your ability to understand and question your own contexts, attitudes, values, beliefs, assumptions; and experiences of advantage and disadvantage. All these aspects influence the way you understand the world and influence how you relate to others and they relate to you.

Applying *cultural safety* practice requires continually challenging your own assumptions, stereotypes, and labelling. Rather than assuming knowledge of a person based on their cultural contexts, you need to be open-minded and respectful in inquiring about the person's contexts while recognizing that contexts are always changing. This requires you to be actively listening in a nonjudgemental way. Cultural safety moves beyond *cultural sensitivity* to meet the health needs of persons, families, and communities, by acknowledging, respecting, and supporting their unique cultural identity through practising cultural competence and humility. *Cultural competence* acknowledges culture as being fluid, changing and diversity exists within all of us. *Cultural humility* is an ongoing, lifelong commitment to having the humility to learn from the person and the critical self-reflection to identify and address biases, prejudices, attitudes, and behaviours in addressing power imbalances within the relationship. As Canada continues to grow as a diverse nation, nurses play an integral and vital role in providing quality compassionate care, dignity, and respect for all, through culturally safe nursing practice.

👤 ETHICAL DILEMMA

What Would You Do?

You are working on a general medicine floor and told by the nurse in charge that you will be getting an admission from the emergency department. The admission is Ms. Carter, 29 years of age, who is being admitted for observation following a car accident. You learn from the report that she has an alcohol addiction and was driving under the influence of alcohol. She drove through a red light and crashed into the side of a car at high speed, resulting in a family of four (two mothers and their two children) being injured. You are told one mother and a child are in grave condition, while the other mother and child have fractured bones, but their injuries are not life threatening. When you hear the admission report, you are angry at how a family and four people's lives are changed, possibly forever, because Ms. Carter chose to drive while under the influence of alcohol. You do not want to provide nursing care to Ms. Carter. What would your next steps be?

QUESTIONS FOR REVIEW AND DISCUSSION

1. How will you incorporate cultural competence and humility into your nursing practice?
2. Identify what approaches you can use to challenge your colleagues when they use language that stereotypes, labels or generalizes or makes assumptions about a person's culture.
3. What are the different roles in the interprofessional team and how do they contribute to providing culturally safe practice?

REFERENCES

Almutairi, A. F., Adlan, A. A., & Nasim, M. (2017). Perceptions of the critical cultural competence in Canada. *BMC Nursing, 16*, 47. https://bmcnurs.biomedcentral.com/track/pdf/10.1186/s12912-017-0242-2.

Aronson, L. (2011). Twelve tips for teaching reflection at all levels of medical education. *Medical Teacher, 33*, 200–205.

Astle, B. J., Barton, S. S., Johnson, L. et al. (2019). Global health. In P. A. Potter, A. G. Perry, J. C. Ross-Jerr, et al. (Eds.), *Canadian Fundamentals of Nursing* (6th ed.) [E-reader edition]. Elsevier.

Baldwin, A., Dodge, B., Schick, V. R. et al. (2018). Transgender and genderqueer individuals' experiences with health care providers: What's working, what's not, and where do we go from here? *Journal of Health Care for the Poor and Underserved, 29*(4), 1300–1318. https://muse.jhu.edu/article/708243.

Barton, S. S. & Foster Boucher, C. (2019). Indigenous Health. In P. A. Potter, A. G. Perry, J. C. Ross-Jerr, et al. (Eds.), *Canadian Fundamentals of Nursing* (6th ed.) [E-reader edition]. Elsevier.

Blanchet Garneau, A. & Pepin, J. (2015). Cultural competence: A constructivist definition. *Journal of Transcultural Nursing, 26*(1), 9–15. https://doi.org/10.1177/1043659614541294.

Bradford, L. E. A., Bharadwaj, L. A., Okpalauwaekwe, U. et al. (2016). Drinking water quality in Indigenous communities in Canada and health outcomes: A scoping review. *International Journal of Circumpolar Health, 75*(1). https://www.tandfonline.com/doi/pdf/10.3402/ijch.v75.32336?needAccess=true.

Browne, A. J., Varcoe, C., Smye, V. et al. (2009). Cultural safety and the challenges of translating critically oriented knowledge in practice. *Nursing Philosophy, 10*, 167–179.

Canadian Nurses Association. (2009). *Social Justice in Practice.* https://www.cna-aiic.ca/~/media/cna/page-content/pdf-en/ethics_in_practice_april_2009_e.pdf.

Canadian Nurses Association. (2010). *Social Justice...a means to an end, an end in itself.* https://www.cna-aiic.ca/~/media/cna/page-content/pdf-en/social_justice_2010_e.pdf.

Canadian Nurses Association. (2012). *National Expert Commission: A nursing call to action.* https://www.cna-aiic.ca/~/media/cna/files/en/nec_report_e.pdf.

Canadian Nurses Association. (2013). *Position statement: Social determinants of health.* https://www.cna-aiic.ca/-/media/cna/page-content/pdf-en/social_determinants_of_health_e_nov2013.pdf?la=en&hash=5309AE489ED7E37C5BE6BC2843889093D0618F37.

Canadian Nurses Association. (2017). Code of ethics for registered nurses. https://www.cna-aiic.ca/~/media/cna/page-content/pdf-en/code-of-ethics-2017-edition-secure-interactive.

Canadian Nurses Association. (2018). *Position statement: Promoting cultural competence in nursing.* https://www.cna-aiic.ca/-/media/cna/page-content/pdf-en/position_statement_promoting_cultural_competence_in_nursing.pdf?la=en&hash=4B394DAE5C2138E7F6134D59E505DCB059754BA9.

Canadian Press. (2019). Canada welcomed more refugees than any other nation in 2018, UN report says. (June 19, 2019). *Global News.* https://globalnews.ca/news/5408395/canada-refugee-statistics-united-nations/.

Chinn, P. L., & Falk-Rafael, A. (2015). Peace and power: A theory of emancipatory group process. *Journal of Nursing Scholarship, 47*(1), 62–69. https://doi.org/10.1111/jnu.12101.

College of Nurses of Ontario. (2018). *Entry-to-practice competencies for registered nurses.* https://www.cno.org/globalassets/docs/reg/41037-entry-to-practice-competencies-2020.pdf.

Danso, R. (2016). Cultural competence and cultural humility: A critical reflection on key cultural diversity concepts. *Journal of Social Work, (0)*, 1–21. https://doi.org/10.1177/1468017316654341.

de Moissac, D., & Bowen, S. (2019). Impact of language barriers on quality of care and patient safety for official language minority francophones in Canada. *Journal of*

Patient Experience, 6(1). https://journals.sagepub.com/doi/pdf/10.1177/2374373518769008.

Doane, G. H., & Varcoe, C. (2007). Relational practice and nursing obligations. *Advances in Nursing Science, 30*(3), 192–205.

Doane, G. H., & Varcoe, C. (2015). *How to nurse: Relationship inquiry with individuals and families in changing health and health care contexts.* Wolters Kluwer.

Douglas, M., Rosenkoetter, M., Pacquiao, D. et al. (2014). Guidelines for implementing culturally competent nursing. *Journal of Transcultural Nursing, 25*(2), 109–121.

Edmunds, K. A., & Samuels-Dennis, J. (2015). Immigrant Canadians. In D. Gregory, C. Raymond-Seniuk, L. Patrick, et al. (Eds.), *Fundamentals Perspectives on the Art and Science of Canadian Nursing* (pp. 1003–1026). Wolters Kluwer.

Foronda, C. L. (2008). A concept analysis of cultural sensitivity. *Journal of Transcultural Nursing, 19*(3), 207–212.

Foronda, C., Baptiste, D. L., Reinholdt, M. M. et al. (2016). Cultural humility: A concept analysis. *Journal of Transcultural Nursing, 27*(3), 210–217. https://doi.org/10.1177/1043659615592677.

Government of Canada. (2009). *40 years of the Official Language Act.* https://www.canada.ca/en/news/archive/2009/09/40-years-official-languages-act.html.

Government of Canada. (2018a). *Victoria Day.* https://www.canada.ca/en/canadian-heritage/services/important-commemorative-days/victoria-day.html.

Government of Canada. (2018b). *Key health inequalities in Canada: A national portrait. Executive summary.* https://www.canada.ca/en/public-health/services/publications/science-research-data/key-health-inequalities-canada-national-portrait-executive-summary.html.

Government of Canada. (2019a). *Multiculturalism.* https://www.canada.ca/en/services/culture/canadian-identity-society/multiculturalism.html.

Government of Canada. (2019b). *Department of Justice: Learn about the Charter.* https://www.justice.gc.ca/eng/csj-sjc/rfc-dlc/ccrf-ccdl/learn-apprend.html.

Government of Canada. (2019c). *Climate change and health: Health effects.* https://www.canada.ca/en/health-canada/services/climate-change-health.html.

Government of Canada. (2020). *Justice laws website: Canadian Human Rights Act.* https://laws-lois.justice.gc.ca/eng/acts/h-6/page-1.html#h-256795.

Government of Canada. (2021). *Social Inequalities in COVID-19 deaths in Canada.* https://health-infobase.canada.ca/covid-19/inequalities-deaths/index.html.

Hafskjold, L., Sundler, A. J., Homstrom, I. K. et al. (2015). A cross-sectional study on person-centred communication in the care of older people: The COMHOME study protocol. *BMJ Open, 5*(4). https://bmjopen.bmj.com/content/5/4/e007864.long.

Hilario, C. T., Browne, A. J., & McFadden, A. (2018). The influence of democratic racism in nursing inquiry. *Nursing Inquiry, 25*(1). https://doi.org/10.1111/nin.12213.

Kellet, P., & Fitton, C. (2017). Supporting transvisibility and gender diversity in nursing practice and education: Embracing cultural

safety. *Nursing Forum, 24*(e12146), 1–7. https://doi.org/10.1111/nin.12146.

Kuluski, K., Peckham, A., Williams, A. P. et al. (2016). What gets in the way of person-centred care for people with multimorbidity? Lessons from Ontario, Canada. *Healthcare Quarterly, 19*(2), 17–23. https://www.longwoods.com/content/24694.

Landy, R., Cameron, C., Au, A. et al. (2016). Educational strategies to enhance reflexivity among clinicians and health professional students: A scoping study. *Forum: Qualitative Social Research, 17*(3), Article 14.

Leung, L. (2016). Diabetes mellitus and the Aboriginal diabetic initiative in Canada: An update review. *Journal of Family medicine and primary care, 5*(2), 259–265. https://doi.org/10.4103/2249-4863.192362.

Marsiglia, F., & Booth, J. (2015). Cultural adaptation of interventions in real practice settings. *Research on Social Work Practice, 25*(4), 423–432.

Merryfeather, L., & Bruce, A. (2014). The invisibility of gender diversity: Understanding transgender and transsexuality in nursing literature. *Nursing Forum, 49*(2), 110–123.

Mirza, A., & Rauhala, E. (2021, April 22). Here's just how unequal the global coronavirus vaccine rollout has been. The Washington Post. https://www.washingtonpost.com/world/interactive/2021/coronavirus-vaccine-inequality-global/.

Ng, S. L., Kinsella, E. A., Friesen, F., et al. (2015). Reclaiming a theoretical orientation to reflection in medical education research: A critical narrative review. *Medical Education, 49*(5), 461–475.

Nguyen, P. V., Naleppa, M., & Lopez, Y. (2020). Cultural competence and cultural humility: A complete practice. *Journal of Ethnic & Cultural Diversity in Social Work, 30*(3), 273–281. https://doi.org/10.1080/15313204.2020.1753617.

Page, J. B. (2005). The concept of culture: A core issue in health disparities. *Journal of Urban Health, 82*(2 Suppl. 3), iii35–iii43.

Registered Nurses' Association of Ontario. (2007). *Embracing cultural diversity in health care: Developing cultural competence.* https://rnao.ca/bpg/guidelines/embracing-cultural-diversity-health-care-developing-cultural-competence.

Reich, J. (2015). *Until we do our part.* Unpublished poem.

Richardson, A., Yarwood, J., & Richardson, S. (2016). Expressions of cultural safety in public health nursing practice. *Nursing Inquiry, 24*(e12171). https://doi.org/10.1111/nin.12171.

Simpson, J. S., James, C. E., & Mack, J. (2011). Multiculturalism, colonialism and racialization: Conceptual starting points. *The Review of Education, Pedagogy, and Cultural Studies, 33*, 285–305. https://doi.org/10.1080/10714413.2011.597637.

Song, P., & Stewart, R. (2012). Reflective writing in medical education. *Medical Teacher, 34*, 955–956.

Srivastava, R. H. (2007). *The health care professional's guide to clinical cultural competence.* Elsevier.

Statistics Canada. (2017a). *Ethnic and cultural origins of Canadians: Portrait of a rich heritage.* https://www12.statcan.gc.ca/census-recensement/2016/as-sa/98-200-x/2016016/98-200-x2016016-eng.cfm.

Statistics Canada. (2017b). *Immigration and ethnocultural diversity: Key results from 2016 census.* https://www150.statcan.gc.ca/n1/daily-quotidien/171025/dq171025b-eng.htm.

Statistics Canada. (2019). *Annual demographic estimates: Canada, provinces and territories, 2019.* https://www150.statcan.gc.ca/n1/pub/91-215-x/91-215-x2019001-eng.htm.

Statistics Canada. (2020). *Dimensions of poverty hub.* https://www.statcan.gc.ca/eng/topics-start/poverty.

Stewart, M., Kushner, K. E., Dennis, C. L., et al. (2016). Social support needs of Sudanese and Zimbabwean refugee new parents in Canada. *International Journal of Migration, Health and Social Care, 13*(2), 234–252. https://doi.org/10.1108/IJMHSC-07-2014-0028.

Truth and Reconciliation Commission of Canada. (2015). *Calls to action.* http://trc.ca/assets/pdf/Calls_to_Action_English2.pdf.

Vandenberg, H. E. R. (2010). Culture theorizing past and present trends and challenges. *Nursing Philosophy, 11,* 238–249.

Van Laer, K., & Janssens, M. (2014). Between the devil and the deep blue sea: Exploring the hybrid identity narratives of ethnic minority professionals. *Scandinavian Journal of Management, 30,* 186–196.

Varcoe, C., & Browne, A. J. (2015). Culture and cultural safety: Beyond cultural inventories. In D. Gregory, C. Raymond-Seniuk, L. Patrick, et al. (Eds.), *Fundamentals Perspectives on the Art and Science of Canadian Nursing* (pp. 216–231). Wolters Kluwer.

Verdonk, P. (2015). When I say…..reflexivity. *Medical Education, 49,* 147–148.

Wasekeesikaw, F. H., & Parent, M. (2015). Aboriginal people and nursing. In D. Gregory, C. Raymond-Seniuk, L. Patrick, et al. (Eds.), *Fundamentals Perspectives on the Art and Science of Canadian Nursing* (pp. 216–231). Wolters Kluwer.

White, J. P., Murphy, L., & Spence, N. (2012). Water and Indigenous peoples: Canada's paradox. *International Indigenous Policy Journal, 3*(3). https://ir.lib.uwo.ca/iipj/vol3/iss3/3/.

8

Engaging With Humility: Authentic Interpersonal Communication in Partnership
With Indigenous Peoples

Sheila Blackstock

OBJECTIVES

At the end of the chapter, the reader will be able to:

1. Understand and apply critical elements of a decolonizing approach to interrelating with Indigenous peoples.
2. Understand the importance of learning and enacting protocol(s) as a foundation to engagement with Indigenous peoples.
3. Situate themselves authentically to create a culturally appropriate space for others to engage in a therapeutic conversation.
4. Co-create relationally by engaging cultural safety, cultural competence, and humility through holistic communication with individuals and communities.
5. Understand the interrelatedness of Indigenous ways of knowing and being within relational interactions.
6. Understand the importance of protocol(s) in the co-creation of person-centred goals in nursing care planning with Indigenous peoples.
7. Recognize relevant documents related to professional communication with Indigenous peoples and interprofessional and paraprofessional teams: Canadian Indigenous Nurses Association (CINA) and Canadian Nurses Association (CNA) professional practice standards; Community Health Nurses of Canada (CHNC) professional practice model and standards of practice (Community Health Nurses of Canada, 2019); and Canadian Nurses Association *Code of Ethics for Registered Nurses* (Canadian Nurses Association, 2017).

The purpose of this chapter is to strengthen the interpersonal communication with Indigenous people through insights and practical applications to develop your awareness of self and others that will enable authentic engagement with Indigenous peoples. Cultural safety and humility are approaches, practices, and relational ways of being that are foundational to this chapter. Cultural safety is enacted when nurses consider the historical and social contexts as well as structural and interpersonal power imbalances that shape health and health care services. Cultural humility is a stance of being open to the cultures of other individuals and communities. It is important for nurses to understand that cultural safety, cultural competence, and humility are an evolving process informed by our experiences as well as an ongoing understanding of Indigenous knowledge, traditions, languages, and ceremonies. (This topic is discussed in more detail in Chapter 7). For the purposes of this chapter, the term *Indigenous* is used to refer to First Nations, Métis, Inuit, and urban Indigenous peoples in Canada. Concepts discussed in this chapter are depicted within the diagram shown in Fig. 8.1, Engaging with humility.

The diagram in Fig. 8.1 is circular, representing the importance of each concept playing a key role and reflecting how wisdom is shared through sharing circles: the wooden rim forms the shape of a drum on which the hide is affixed and sewn on in the back with sinew. (*Sinew* is a long tendon harvested from moose, elk, or deer that is cleaned and dried. Once the tendon is dry, it is manually stretched and

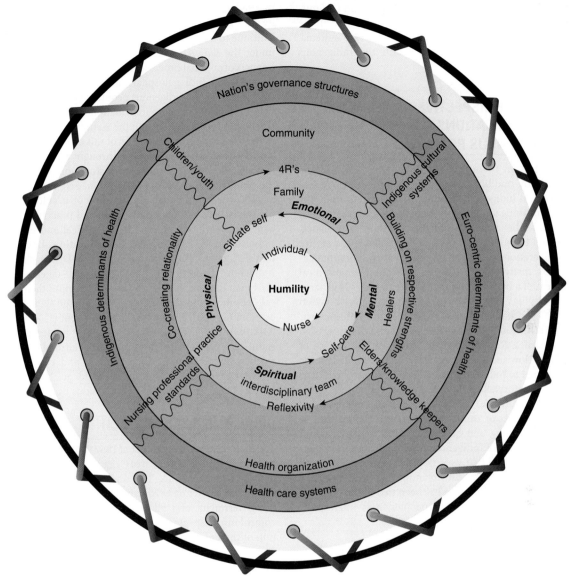

Fig. 8.1 Engaging with humility. Art concept source: Dr. Sheila Blackstock. (2021). Gitxsan First Nation.

pulled to remove the hair and make the fibre longer and thinner; this process takes a great deal of time and strength. The resulting product can be used to sew hides onto the rims of drums, buckskin for clothing, or shelter.) The face of the drum is where communication is symbolized and is relayed through oral tradition, our own stories, songs, and the sound of our voices sharing our experiences and those of our relations. The cross ties in the diagram represent the sinew of the drum demonstrating how children and youth, Elders and Knowledge Keepers, Indigenous cultural

systems, and nursing professional practice standards intersect and are related to one another and together each bring strength. At the core of the circle is the individual and the nurse, interacting in a reciprocal manner, situating themselves through introductions, protocols, and engaging with humility. Around the nurse and the individual are spiritual, physical, emotional, and mental health, all working and depending on each other to achieve holistic health and honouring the four directions: north, south, east, and west. Moving outward, the next circle represents intra and interprofessional collaborative teams, family and community members working together but each dependent on the Indigenous determinants of health, health care systems, and Eurocentric determinants of health and Indigenous governance structures.

HISTORICAL PERSPECTIVES ON COMMUNICATIONS AND INDIGENOUS PEOPLES

Communication in Indigenous culture is rooted in the land, culture, traditions, and Indigenous governance systems. Within Indigenous communities, communication is holistic, meaning it is not only verbal and nonverbal; it also encompasses behaviours, protocols, ceremony, governance, songs, and the passing on of traditional names and stories from generation to generation. Historically, communication took many shapes, such as indicating geographical land areas of a nation through territory markers (e.g., large rocks, carvings in trees), relaying information between neighbouring nations and communities through messengers, and the tradition, language, songs, and practices used in ceremonies. Reading signs in nature on the surface of the land, below and above, and all creatures situated on the land, are tied to Indigenous teachings, through verbal (e.g., oral history, storytelling, songs) and nonverbal (e.g., gathering practices, dance) communications. Sharing teachings of the behaviours of animals, plants, trees, the patterns of weather in the sky, and how that relates to water are all important aspects of Indigenous teachings for preservation of land and survival that were traditionally communicated and passed on to the youth in Indigenous communities. Importantly, communication has been tied to the land and is fundamental to Indigenous peoples; it is intertwined with historical communication processes.

Colonial Impacts on Communication

Oral communication is an important tenet of oral history within Indigenous communities. Oral communications were severed within Indigenous communities through the impacts of colonial processes such as the use of residential schools, wherein children were removed from their homes and forbidden to speak their language, practise traditional songs, and have communication with their families. In addition, nonverbal communication was impacted since Indigenous peoples could not practise traditional ceremonies and songs, where the dancers relay the story through their movements, wearing traditional regalia and sequencing use of traditional medicines. The impact of colonial processes continues today as a result of Section 91.24 of the *Constitution Act*, 1867. This act states

that federal Parliament has the constitutional responsibility for "Indians and Lands reserved for Indians" and has continue to administer and manage Indian lands and assets under the *Indian Act* since the 1870s (Miller, 1989). The impacts of colonial processes such as residential schools, the Sixties Scoop, Indian hospitals, and intergenerational effects continue today as Indigenous peoples begin to reclaim self-determination. For more information on intergenerational trauma, Indian hospitals, and the Sixties Scoop, please refer to the Web Resources at the end of this chapter.

Self-determination occurs through reclaiming land, language, cultural traditions, oral history, songs, and healing the nations as a result of colonization. Self-determination occurs when individuals and groups of a culture define their existence through their traditional practices, knowledge, ceremonies, language, laws, political and economic rights, and ways of being. The United Nations Declaration on the Rights of Indigenous Peoples (UNDRIP) states that Indigenous peoples have the right to self-determination. This guarantees the right to freely determine their political condition and the right to freely pursue their form of economic, social, and cultural development (U.N. General Assembly, 2007). Thus, it is important for nurses to understand the role of self-determination given that they must work with individuals, their families, and communities, through therapeutic communication to positively impact health and social outcomes of Indigenous peoples.

DECOLONIZING APPROACH

The *British North America Act* of 1867 (the *Constitution Act*) gave the federal government of Canada control of Indigenous peoples and their lands. This was followed nine years later by the *Indian Act* of 1876, which extinguished Indigenous self-government and allowed the federal government to control most aspects of Indigenous life. The original intention of the *Indian Act* was to assimilate Indigenous peoples into a Eurocentric society, through policies that eliminated social, economic, language, cultural, and political distinctness. Métis people and Inuit were not covered under this act. These colonizing policies led to the creation of residential school systems, the Sixties Scoop, Indian hospitals, and Indigenous peoples being moved onto reserves, away from their homes. Although residential schools and Indian hospitals are no longer in existence, the *Indian Act* remains in place, and colonizing effects continue, through intergenerational effects, racism, and many other types of inequities.

Decolonization is an approach to undo colonialism. It requires non-Indigenous individuals, governments, institutions, and organizations to create space and support for Indigenous peoples to reclaim and restore their culture, land, language, relationships, and health. "Power, dominance, and control are rebalanced and returned to Indigenous peoples, and Indigenous ways of knowing and doing are perceived, presented, and practised as equal to Western ways of knowing and doing (Attas, n.d.). The UNDRIP (U.N. General Assembly, 2007) was established as a universal framework of minimum standards for the survival, dignity, and well-being of Indigenous peoples of the world and elaborates on existing human rights and standards and fundamental freedoms as they apply to the specific situation of Indigenous peoples." It is the most comprehensive international instrument on the rights of Indigenous peoples.

Canada has endorsed and implemented the principles of the UNDRIP (U.N. General Assembly, 2007). In terms of nursing practice and communication, the UNDRIP has relevance given that it is the fundamental declaration of rights of Indigenous peoples guiding nursing care and practice to ensure cultural safety, deliverance of equitable services, and working in partnership with Indigenous peoples to positively impact holistic health outcomes.

The Canadian Indigenous Nurses Association (CINA) was founded in 1975 by a group of nurses to identify and contact other nurses of Indigenous ancestry. Since then, the association has expanded its role and plays many international, national, and provincial and territorial roles in guiding professional nursing practice, informing curriculum development, and engaging in research, based on partnerships with communities. In addition, the National Collaborating Centre for Indigenous Health (NCCIH) is a resource to support First Nations, Inuit, and Métis public health equity through knowledge exchange and translation. There are many resources available to expand your knowledge and understanding, to improve your nursing practice with Indigenous peoples.

INDIGENOUS DETERMINANTS OF HEALTH

Oral traditions and cultural practices are being reclaimed as Indigenous communities work through the impacts of colonization through healing and learning their traditional languages and cultural practices. Elders teach the traditions and cultural practices residential school survivors and this learning is passed on to youth in the community. Self-determination is achieved in part through reclamation of physical land and the associated environmental elements. Reclaiming the territorial land and the environment that nations inhabited prior to colonization is critical to an Indigenous and Inuit population health approach (Richmond & Ross, 2009). Richmond and Ross identified Indigenous determinants of health as a result of a narrative analysis of interviews with 26 community health representatives (CHRs) from First Nation, Inuit, Métis, and rural and urban communities across Canada. They identified six critical determinants: balance, life control, education, material resources, social resources, and environmental /cultural connections (Richmond & Ross, 2009). (See Box 8.1.)

Acknowledging the importance of Indigenous determinants of health through self-determination is a key factor in achieving co-created nursing interventions that reflect person-centred approaches. As described in the Developing an Evidence-Informed Practice box, the importance of person-centred approaches with cultural awareness of nurse and physician providers (n = 263) was found to be a key factor in improving health outcomes of Indigenous peoples in Canada with diabetes (Bhattacharyya et al., 2011). The Truth and Reconciliation Commission (TRC) of Canada final report includes the Calls to Action report (2015), a call to Canadians to begin a process of reconciliation between Indigenous and non-Indigenous peoples to address the

---

BOX 8.1 Six Critical Indigenous Determinants of Health

1. Balance: Balance is a reflection of the maintenance of holistic health, through mental, physical, emotional, and spiritual elements. Any imbalance in holistic health leads to poor health.
2. Life control: Life control reflects the ability of an individual to care for themselves through maintenance of a healthy life and management of illness or disease.
3. Education: Education is a vital determinant to one's economic status and overall well-being.
4. Material resources: Material resources refer to income from work.
5. Social resources: Social resources are the breadth and depth of social ties to rely on others in times of need.
6. Environmental and cultural connections: Environment and cultural connections reflect people's abilities to access environmental resources for the purposes of cultural practices and Indigenous ways of being. Cultural practices and language are threaded through the identity and traditions of Indigenous peoples as well as their community identities that are attributes to spiritual, emotional, physical, and mental well-being. Cultural and language are Indigenous social determinants of health that are essential for improving health outcomes, through traditional structures and governance, cohesion, and quality of life.

National Collaborating Centre for Indigenous Health. (2016). *Social determinants of health: Culture and language as social determinants of First Nations, Inuit and Métis health.* https://www.ccnsa-nccah.ca/docs/determinants/FS-CultureLanguage-SDOH-FNMI-EN.pdf.

⟫ DEVELOPING AN EVIDENCE-INFORMED PRACTICE

Purpose

Compared with the general population, there are disproportionately higher global rates of type 2 diabetes and associated complications in Indigenous peoples. This is particularly true of First Nations peoples in Canada. It is therefore essential to conduct research into the unique barriers health care providers face when working on reserve in First Nations communities, so that they can develop effective quality improvement strategies (Bhattacharyya et al., 2011).

Method

This study was conducted in two phases, the first consisting of interviews and focus groups and the second consisting of a survey. Phase I interviews were held with 24 health care providers in the Sioux Lookout Zone in northwestern Ontario. In Phase 2, the researchers developed a survey based on the qualitative work from Phase 1, as part of a larger project, the Canadian First Nations Diabetes Clinical Management and Epidemiologic (CIRCLE) study. The survey was completed by 244 health care providers, in 19 First Nations communities in 7 Canadian provinces. Of the 19 participating communities, 4 were non-isolated, 6 were semi-isolated, and 9 were isolated; populations in these communities ranged from 500 to 10,000 people. The basis of the interviews, focus groups, and survey was to explore barriers to providing optimal diabetes care in First Nations communities.

Findings

Key findings at the patient, provider, and systemic level were revealed from the interviews and focus group discussions. Across the three isolation levels, results from the survey indicated that health care providers perceived patient factors as having the largest impact on care. They also found that physicians were significantly less likely than community health representatives to rank patient–provider communication as having a large impact.

Application to Your Practice

The researchers concluded that the highest impact strategy for improving diabetes care was to address patient factors such as helping patients seek preventative care and adopt a healthy lifestyle. Patient–provider communication links good communication with improved health outcomes (Stewart, 1995); barriers to effective patient–provider education stem from social and cultural differences between patients and providers. These include a provider's lack of understanding of the history of Indigenous peoples and the negative intergenerational impacts seen today (e.g., poverty, poor housing, high unemployment). It is important for nurses and other health providers to learn effective communication skills and educate themselves about the history of Indigenous peoples, intergenerational impacts, the importance of trust building, and knowing how to make time for effective communication, all of which may positively impact patient outcomes.

Adapted from Bhattacharyya, O., Rasooly, I. R., Estey, E. et al. (2011). Challenges to the provision of diabetes care in first nations communities: Results from a national survey of healthcare providers in Canada. *BMC Health Services Research, 11*(283), 1–10; Stewart, M. A. (1995). Effective physician–patient communication and health outcomes: A review. *CMAJ, 152*(9), 1423–1433.

ongoing effects of intergenerational trauma stemming from the legacy of residential school systems. As professionals, nurses have a moral and ethical obligation to advocate for unjust inequities through constructive disruption of systemic and structural racism embedded in communication systems, policies, and interactions with First Nations, Inuit, and Métis peoples. The UNDRIP (U.N. General Assembly, 2007) is a foundational resource to guide you in your nursing practice and policy development. For more information, refer to the Web Resources at the end of this chapter.

REFLECTION AND REFLEXIVITY

In nursing practice, a **reflection** is used to examine our interpretations of events that happened, our role, and the role of others. This reflection process is a valuable tool to examine our nursing practice for strengths and areas of improvements. **Reflexivity** is a process where we consider how that process of interpretation was achieved. When we practise reflexivity, we find strategies to question our own attitudes, biases, prejudices, habitual actions, and thought processes (Freshwater & Rolfe, 2001). Thus, as nurses, we examine how our values align with organizational structures, power imbalances, and diversity. It is through the process of continual self-examination that you become aware of the limits of your knowledge and understand how your behaviour plays into organizational practices and why those practices may marginalize groups or exclude individuals (Freshwater & Rolfe). (See Case Example: Student Nurse). Reflexivity, combined with cultural safety and humility in nursing practice, can assist us in identifying our professional practice goals and strengthening our relational practice (Doane & Varcoe, 2015) with Indigenous and non-Indigenous peoples. (Try Simulation Exercise 8.1).

SIMULATION EXERCISE 8.1 Reflection and Reflexivity Exercise

Purpose

To practise using reflection and reflexivity lenses to consider what may be done differently

Procedure

You can choose to do this activity using Case Example: Student Nurse in this chapter or a scenario from your own practice, with a partner or in a sharing circle format. Think about a situation or nursing scenario that you either experienced as a student nurse or witnessed in a health care setting that still has you thinking that "something could have been done differently" (Cinel & Blackstock, 2014). If you were the student nurse in the scenario, perhaps you would do or say something differently now, given the knowledge and experience you have acquired. If you are in the role of a nurse in practice or a nurse researcher, you may have encountered a dilemma; in that case, what could have been done differently? It may be that you would have sought out an advocate, given the inherent power differentials at play when you are a student practising on a ward or in a community.

Reflective Analysis and Discussion

1. Using a reflection lens, think about what happened. Share your scenario with a peer and discuss the following:
   What was my role?
   What was the role of others?
2. In a larger group, using a sharing circle, share your scenario and responses to the questions. (See Box 8.2).
   Now, thinking about the same scenario, use a reflexivity lens to think about your approach to the scenario. Explore your attitudes, biases, prejudices, habitual actions, and thought processes that may have influenced your interpretation of the events that led to your actions.

3. In this step, consider the following questions:
   What knowledge would have been helpful in the scenario?
   What organizational policies and procedures or processes facilitated or were barriers to working through the scenario? Did any of these organizational policies and procedures or processes marginalize or exclude people?
4. How do these findings align with your nursing values, professional practice standards* (e.g., Community Health Nurses of Canada ([CHNC], 2019), Canadian Nurses of Canada *Code of Ethics for Registered Nurses* (CNA, 2017)? What professional practice standards* (CHNC, 2019) or Code of Ethics (CNA, 2017) are not being upheld? What needs to change?
   *Access your provincial or territorial regulatory nursing professional practice standards, and review for this exercise.

Share your thoughts and responses to the questions with a peer or within your sharing circle. Did you notice a difference between using reflection or reflexivity lens? If so, what was the difference?

You will find that using reflexivity allows for you to get closer to the issues at play in the scenario. Through this process, you can inform how you approach similar scenarios and how you determine where, what, and how to increase your knowledge or skill in an area as a part of your profession practice. In addition, you can identify areas that need to be addressed in the organization because they may perpetuate structural racism and marginalize vulnerable people. You can use this process as a part of your everyday practice and to inform your self-assessment of your professional practice to set goals to address areas in which you need more knowledge.

Case Example: Student Nurse

Sumitra is a student nurse on a surgical ward, receiving a morning report from the registered nurse who describes an Indigenous person post-operative day 1, who underwent an abdominal hysterectomy. The nurse rolls her eyes as she begins to give Sumitra report and states, "Oh yes, this one … this is where I spent most of my night, dealing with this one." Sumitra feels shocked and is not sure what to do with the description. She fears what her day might look like, based on this comment. The nurse goes on to say that although the person has been receiving patient-controlled analgesia and in fact had a stat dose/bolus of narcotic for pain during the night, "The person still moaned all night!" The nurse goes on to say that the other people couldn't sleep because all the family members kept coming in and out all night too. "At one point they were singing and playing a drum—quietly, but still, it was weird."

The foundation for this chapter is built on acknowledgement of Indigenous self-determination in engagement with individuals, families, and community members. In this manner, you are led through engaging with humility within interactions with Indigenous peoples, beginning with the exploration and understanding of Indigenous ways of knowing and being, situating self in the importance of introductions within protocols. Table 8.1 outlines the concepts and approaches referred to in this chapter that capture engaging with humility.

INDIGENOUS WAYS OF KNOWING AND BEING

Indigenous ways of knowing reflect sacred entities of stories, history, lands, water, sky, spiritual beliefs, and systems of Indigenous peoples. This knowledge about these entities is shared and passed on to generations through processes of experiential learning, listening, viewing, sensing, and observing. Indigenous ways of knowing serve as guides for establishing relations among entities (Martin & Mirraboopa, 2003). Ways of being are the rights and responsibilities to carry out with all living things, country, self, and others (Martin & Mirraboopa). Indigenous peoples enact ways of knowing and being all at once through their ceremonies, culture, language, engagement with others, and holistic health and healing. Indigenous ways of knowing and being in the context of

TABLE 8.1 **Co-creating Relationality Through Engaging With Humility**		
Indigenous Approach	**Nursing Approach**	**Co-Creating Approach**
• Protocols • Time invested to ensure protocols, sharing, and respect of Elders and ceremonies • Sacred teachings of being and engaging with others • Lessons shared when the recipient is ready • Sharing • Use all our senses for goodness, sharing, caring, listening, and appreciating essences	• Task-based focus • High job demands and time pressures • Top-down approach • Written, verbal, and nonverbal communication • Linear two-way conversations	• Creating a safe environment • Introductions • Allow the person to self-identify whether they practise traditional cultural ways as a part of their health and healing
Indigenous Experience	**Nursing Experiences**	**Co-Creating Experiences**
• Intergenerational trauma and colonial effects • People disconnected from family as a result of being transferred from a rural to a regional health centre • Mixed experiences with health care/hospital services	• Cultural safety and humility training • Learning local Indigenous protocols • Wanting to demonstrate reconciliation • Working within health care organization policies and procedures	• Using trauma-informed practices • Engaging with Indigenous liaison workers • Connecting with the person's supports in their community [paraprofessionals/professionals] • Working through divergent perspectives toward mutual understanding
Indigenous Medicines & Practices	**Nursing/Western Medicines**	**Person-Centred Holistic Health**
• Traditional medicines, herbs, food as medicines • Health is tied to land, medicines, ceremonies, traditional foods • Talking circles: each person has equal importance • Holistic health • Culture, ceremony in medicine gathering • Medicine women and men • Elders • Knowledge Keepers	• Western-based medicines • Nursing knowledge and skills • Interdisciplinary teams • Medical coverage/health care benefits • Health care services	• Nurse: Two-eyed seeing approach. The best of Western health practices with Indigenous ways of knowing and being • Person: Their perspective on health • Interprofessional collaborative teams • Gathering in a sacred space within the health care organization • Working together to make discharge planning goals based on relevant health care coverage and services when the person is being discharged to home community.

holistic health are framed in a First Nations Wholistic Policy and Planning Model (Assembly of First Nations, 2013). A health model informs conceptualization of Indigenous health. The model acknowledges the disproportionate acute and chronic health issues compared to most Canadians and builds on the medicine wheel approach; it includes environmental health, sustainable development and cultural and social elements as key tenets to reframe health inequity among Indigenous peoples (see Fig. 8.2).

The Medicine Wheel

The sacred medicine wheel teachings have origins in Ojibwa teachings. The medicine wheel is a ceremonial, sacred, holistic symbol and healing tool based on the number four. Overall, when an individual is in good health, they are said to have balance in mind, body, and spirit and live in harmony with Mother Earth. Thus, when an individual is ill, they are considered to have an imbalance in one or more of these areas. Elders drew a circle in the earth to explain the four elements of the circle and related concept of Indigenous teachings:

- Four directions: north, east, south, and west
- Holistic health: mind, body, spirit, and harmony with Mother Earth
- The changing seasons: early spring, spring, summer, early fall, fall, and winter
- Stage of life: childhood, adolescence, adulthood, and old age
- Races: red, white, black, and yellow, which, for some, stand for the human races; for others, they represent the four directions or the seasons
- The four elements: water, air, fire, and earth
- The four sacred medicines: tobacco, cedar, sage, and sweetgrass

Indigenous ways of knowing and health are the foundation of learning for future nurses and other health care providers to learn to engage with humility through practising reflexively.

THE 4 RS, PROTOCOL, AND SITUATING SELF

The 4Rs

The 4 Rs of respect, reciprocity, responsibility, and relevance (Kirkness, 2002) guide us in culturally safe and appropriate interactions with Indigenous peoples. According to the TRC Calls to Action, "… reconciliation is about establishing and maintaining a mutually respectful relationship between Aboriginal and non-Aboriginal peoples in this country" (TRC, 2015, p. 6). A key aspect of the TRC Calls to Action report is to call upon Canadians to take action and change behaviours to support and build upon this mutual respect. Non-Indigenous people have an opportunity to learn about how to be an **ally/enacting allyship** to plan and deliver culturally safe care to Indigenous peoples, which requires social action, strength, courage, humility, and a support network. Cultural safety consists of examining historical and political factors to ensure the advancement of cultural safety. As a health care provider, if you witness racism or stereotyping, you can act as an ally by addressing the behaviours and actions. People may be acting on implicit biases and may not be aware of their actions. Intervene with an advocate, nursing faculty member, or manager. Choose an appropriate setting to have a conversation and challenge the stereotypes. Report culturally unsafe care and encounters to management, and debrief with a peer and nursing faculty member.

Referring to the 4 Rs (Kirkness, 2002) is an active way that settlers and First Nations' allies can be advocates and work with Indigenous peoples to decolonize their nursing practices. A detailed discussion of the 4Rs follows.

Respect

Respect is conveyed through an understanding and demonstration of regard and value of cultural knowledge, traditions, values, and activities relevant to each Indigenous community (Kirkness, 2002). Respect is a concept that seems abstract and yet is conveyed as a result of key relational factors of "presencing" (Doane & Varcoe, 2015), based on a foundation of attending to cultural integrity. *Presencing* is a process between the nurse and the person receiving care that is based on the nurse devoting deliberate attention to awareness of the other's shared experiences of humanity; presencing results in the growth of both the nurse and the person in the interaction (Doane & Varcoe, 2015). Learning about the intergenerational impacts of colonialism and contrasting them with your experiences growing up in your family helps to understand how we all may have unconscious biases and behaviours. If you recognize and understand the negative emotions that arise when confronting these topics, then you can critically exercise cultural safety and humility (discussed in Chapter 7). As noted previously, when you address our biases and use reflexivity, you can authentically engage in interpersonal interactions. You can become actively involved in Indigenous events that honour residential school survivors through orange shirt day activities (e.g., see https://news.umanitoba.ca/2018-orange-shirt-day/), Have a Heart Day activities to advocate for equitable funding for First Nations children and Jordan's Principle (see https://fncaringsociety.com/have-a-heart), and learning about Indigenous nursing and resources from sources such as the CINA website, at https://indigenousnurses.ca.

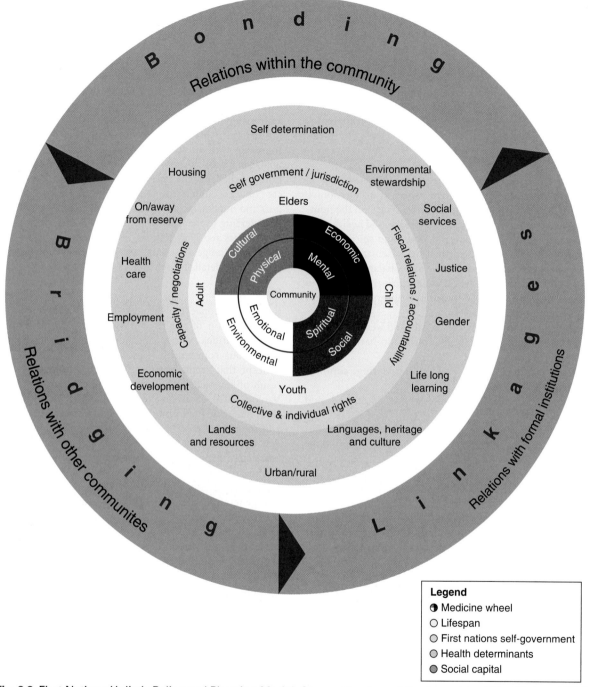

Fig. 8.2 First Nations Holistic Policy and Planning Model. Source: Courtesy of the Assembly of First Nations (2013).

Reciprocity

Reciprocity means there is mutual benefit from an interpersonal interaction, where both individuals are learning from each other, giving and receiving information (Kirkness, 2002). Reciprocity in a nurse–person interaction can occur through nonverbal and verbal communication with Indigenous peoples. For example, reciprocity can be achieved through creating and ensuring a safe place for traditional cultural practices, policies that welcome family member(s) as a support person(s), language translator, and Indigenous navigators. Creating and ensuring a safe place is achieved through presenting yourself in an open manner and co-creating an approach with the person as well as through providing a quiet area, big enough to enable the person and their family to gather. In some hospitals and health care agencies there are designated cultural rooms that have been set up to welcome cultural practices such as smudging. **Smudging** is the practice of burning select medicines and herbs (e.g., sage, cedar, tobacco). The smoke from the burning of the medicines is either cupped in the hands or fanned with a sacred feather to wash it over areas of the body. Smudging is said to assist with cleansing the mind, spirit, heart, and body by washing away negative energy, and it readies people for holistic health and healing.

Through the practice of introducing yourself, as you will learn in this chapter, you enact protocol and convey reciprocity. In community health nursing, when students are practising in the community, reciprocity might be conveyed and enacted through hosting an appreciation luncheon for Elders in the community. Another example of reciprocity could be meeting with the key people involved in nursing practice placements and asking what is needed in the community. When students are in a local community practising nursing, the practice placement coordinator could meet with the community in advance to discuss what types of projects or programs are needed by the community for nursing students to develop. In addition, subsequent cohorts could also develop a health promotion program for the agencies during their community health nursing placement. In this manner, the community identifies issues of local significance that health promotion or prevention programs can be developed to address, and this would be a way of giving back to the community. Reciprocity is important in nursing research, where the Indigenous community decides what research is relevant to their community, what knowledge is shared, and who owns the knowledge, while the researcher demonstrates reciprocity through authentic interpersonal interaction guided by Indigenous ethical research protocols. Research ethics boards determined by local Indigenous research ethics boards are an important part of self-determination in research by Indigenous communities (Nuu-chah-nulth Tribal Council Research Ethics Committee, 2008).

Responsibility

The fourth R represents responsibility for active participation in the conversations around reconciliation and Indigenous events and activities, which, when appropriate, can represent a step toward reconciliation (Kirkness, 2002). Indigenous Elders say that you learn more from an individual based on how they carry themselves within their families, to other individuals, and to their local community. Responsibility can be enacted through involvement with local Indigenous communities in events and activities and through organizing reconciliation activities as allies. In your nursing practice, you can make a choice to advocate for and address unjust situations and scenarios to demonstrate cultural safety and humility.

For more information, see the discussion on the 4 Rs on the Alaska Native Knowledge Network: http://www.ankn.uaf.edu/IEW/winhec/FourRs2ndEd.html.

Relevance

Relevance refers to behaviours and actions that occur when respect is embedded within our learning of local Indigenous protocols, acknowledgement of local land and territories, application of cultural safety and humility in nursing practice, and advocating for dismantling of structural racism embedded within organizational structures and policies (Kirkness, 2002). Acknowledgement of territory is a sign of both respect and relevance as Indigenous world views are based on deep connections with the land and Indigenous determinants of health. Land is foundational to protocols, acknowledgement of territory, ceremonies, and traditions and practices. You can start to learn the local Indigenous history from a respected Indigenous Elder or Knowledge Keeper. An **Elder** is a respected older community member known for their knowledge of language, culture, ceremonies, and traditions specific to their nation. The person is named an Elder through the traditional systems and they are not determined an Elder merely based on advancing age. A **Knowledge Keeper** is a respected community members known for their developing knowledge of language, culture, ceremonies, and traditions specific to their nation. They are typically being groomed and mentored by Elders in the community to demonstrate and apply protocols in respectful engagement with other Indigenous and non-Indigenous peoples.

Learn to acknowledge the traditional Indigenous territory that you live in, and learn, guided by an Elder, how to pronounce and understand the meaning of the words in the acknowledgement.

In British Columbia, the BC Assembly of First Nations has created an interactive map to trace the different Indigenous communities across BC and help people learn more about their unique identities. The map takes you to an information page about the local language spoken, governance structure, geographical areas of the nation, treaties, and so on. You can identify the Indigenous community through this link: https://www.bcafn.ca/first-nations-bs/interactive-map.

It is helpful to approach the local band office and ask to speak with a representative to guide you on the protocols of the area, language, traditions, and ceremonies. If you have the honour of being invited to an Indigenous event or if you can attend because it is open to the public, take the time to participate and introduce yourself, using proper protocols, as noted below. In time, you can learn some of the local language and customs, as guided by a local Elder. You can also search for the local language, once you know what it is, through the software, First Voices, at this site: https://www.firstvoices.com/content/get-started; you can download the app on your phone. With First Voices, you can learn general greetings and practise them with a local Indigenous person. The most important thing you can do is to show interest, to let the local Indigenous peoples know what you do not know, and you can humbly ask for guidance on protocols in engaging with people from their community and how to support them in the acute care or community health nursing settings.

Protocols and Territory Acknowledgement

Protocol is a sequence of culturally appropriate behaviours that acknowledge the traditional ways of knowing and being inherent and expected in respectful interactions with Indigenous peoples. Protocols beginning with acknowledgement of the territory can also involve presenting a gift that is meaningful to the Indigenous community (e.g., giving tobacco, a blanket). To determine the relevance of the gift offering to the local Indigenous peoples in the local territory, it is best to contact a respected Elder or Knowledge Keeper from the community for guidance; this person will clarify who to contact, how to respectfully engage, and what are the protocols of engagement.

Case Example: Protocol and Territory Acknowledgement

A community health nurse arranges to meet with an Elder from the community to learn the protocol(s) and territorial acknowledgement of the community in advance of a health workshop. The nurse also asks whether the Elder has any dietary restrictions (e.g., diabetic diet, allergies) or preferences (e.g., traditional foods) to make sure appropriate foods and beverages are offered at the workshop for the Elder. The Elder offers to do a prayer to start off the workshop, and the nurse finds out an appropriate honorarium to give to the Elder, arranges transportation of the Elder to and from the workshop, and buys a small gift in advance of the workshop. The Elder guides the community health nurse in learning the territorial acknowledgement, and they talk about how the prayer will start, introductions, any direction on protocols for blessings of traditional local foods for a luncheon, and the order in which people should be invited to eat. The Elder also requests the nurse to ensure that someone is available to assist or serve the Elders.

Foundational to protocols is engaging with humility and respect. Given the importance of oral communication and the interrelationships of acknowledging land, culture, and ceremonies to the nations, introductions are used as a part of protocols to relay lineage and cultural location so that connections can be made on cultural, social, and relational grounds. In some scenarios, a gift may be presented that represents the nation and people. Whenever possible, the traditional language to introduce oneself is used.

Situating Self Authentically

Situating self authentically is embedded in the protocol of introducing yourself in your traditional language and sharing your family lineage and the Indigenous community that you come from. Then you would translate what you said into English and explain the meaning to your audience. This process allows for transparency of who you are and where you come from and gives people a sense of your culture. Through sharing your family lineage, those who are meeting you can understand the family connections to each other, the lands, the waters, and Mother Earth. Simulation Exercise 8.2 provides practice introducing yourself authentically.

Case Example: Situating Self Authentically

My name is Sheila Blackstock. I am of Gitxsan descent on my father's side, and on my mother's side, of mixed European and Russian origins. My grandmother was from the Frog clan. My formative years were spent living in northern rural communities of British Columbia. In the summer months, our family journeyed back to our community in the Gitxsan Territories to gather fish and berries and be with family. I am learning more about my Gitxsan heritage—the language, customs, protocols, and clan system governance.

SIMULATION EXERCISE 8.2 Introduction of Self-Learning Activity

Purpose

To discover ways to introduce yourself and convey information about your unique cultural background

Procedure

Considering the significance of oral communication within Indigenous cultures in Canada, it is important that you learn to introduce yourself as a part of the protocol engagement. Students can work in groups or individually and present back to the group.

Think about your heritage, culture, and upbringing. How would you convey this information to someone you have not met before as a form of introduction? You'll need to take this time to acknowledge that your reflection of family, upbringing, and culture will be different from those of others as this makes you unique! You can also use your own language to introduce yourself (if English is not your first language) and then translate what you have conveyed into English. You can use these details to incorporate into your introduction:

- Your name
- Family heritage
- Cultural background

Reflective Analysis and Discussion

Think about what you have learned about yourself, your family and culture, and your upbringing and discuss what you have discovered with your peers. Are you able to easily convey information when introducing yourself? What did you learn about your peers and their unique backgrounds?

Elders say the first thing that newcomers to a community can learn and practise is the importance of learning protocols, which are demonstrated through the 4 Rs (Kirkness, 2002). As a new nurse to Indigenous communities or urban Indigenous agencies, you must learn and understand who the respected Elders and Knowledge Keepers are and arrange a meeting to begin to learn the local Indigenous culture, protocols, and practices. Knowledge Keepers can be of any age; this is in contrast with Elders, who are older and typically have a long family lineage in the community, as recognized by their traditional name given to them as well as by their role within the community. You can reach out to local Indigenous governance councils to request a meeting. Taking these steps indicates interest and, more importantly, a desire to engage in an authentic manner. Once you meet with the local Elder or Knowledge Keeper (or both), you can be guided on the protocols when meeting with community members, how to create a safe space for Indigenous peoples when providing nursing care to co-create nursing interventions, plans of care, and discharge teaching.

Sharing Circles

The experiences of sharing circles are a result of working with Indigenous peoples and learning from Elders in First Nations, Inuit, and Métis communities. **Sharing circles** are a part of Indigenous cultures and are used in many different forms for different purposes. (See Box 8.2.) The format shared here is meant to create an educational environment in which student nurses can learn about sharing circles, the principles, and some of the protocols respected and enacted in the circle. Community health nurses in Indigenous communities use sharing circles for activities such as health promotion and prevention, support, and interdisciplinary teaching and debriefing exercises. The person hosting the Elder or Knowledge Keeper would meet with them prior to the sharing circle, following protocols, discussing the following: how they want the circle to proceed, any preferences for how the circle is arranged, whether to keep an area in the middle available for medicines or a spiritual bundle, the topics being discussed, and whether a support person (e.g., counsellor, Elder or Knowledge Keeper) should be available as some circles can evoke an emotive response. The nurse should ensure that the Elder or Knowledge Keeper has a comfortable chair, some water, tea or coffee, and a snack nearby, as discussed prior to the circle. The nurse should also ensure that other supplies (e.g., tissues, blankets), are available for the Elder or Knowledge Keeper and participants. In sharing circles in which an Elder or Knowledge Keeper is present, as a sign of respect, the nurse clarifies with the Elder or Knowledge Keeper whether they would like to co-facilitate with the nurse. If so, the Elder or Knowledge Keeper leads the participants. It is important that local representation (e.g., Elder or Knowledge Keeper) of the nation the circle is being held in are present and that that territory's protocols and traditions are followed. These details are as follows.

The physical layout of the sharing circle is structured so that participants are seated comfortably, facing inwards to each other, with boxes of tissues within reach to share in case people are feeling emotional. A circle is representative of the medicine wheel, adapted from North American influences. Each person in the circle is equal, and each person's voice and perspective matters, to share or be present and listen—everyone's.

The Elder or Knowledge Keeper—or in some scenarios, a designated facilitator—may co-lead with the Elder or Knowledge Keeper or lead on their own. The person who leads

BOX 8.2   Sharing Circles and Circle Talks

The experiences of sharing circles are a result of working with Indigenous peoples and learning from Elders while being in First Nations communities. Sharing circles are a part of many Indigenous cultures and are used in many different forms for different purposes. The format shared here is meant for an educational environment, to teach student nurses about sharing circles and their principles along with some of the protocols that are respected and enacted in the circle. Sharing circles are used by community health nurses working in Indigenous communities for the purposes of activities such as health promotion and prevention, support, and interdisciplinary teaching and debriefing exercises.

Protocol, Preparation, Planning and Process

- As the person hosting the Elder or Knowledge Keeper, meet with them prior to the sharing circle, following protocols.
- Ask what type of honorarium is required (e.g., monies, traditional medicine, gift certificate or gift card).
- Discuss with the Elder or Knowledge Keeper how they want the circle to proceed, any preferences in how the circle is arranged, whether an area in the middle should be left available for medicines or a spiritual bundle, the discussion topics, availability of a support person (e.g., counsellor, Elder or Knowledge Keeper) as some circles can evoke an emotive response.

- Advertise your circle talk through the local newspaper, online resources, radio or television news, and posters in the clinic. Ensure that you indicate the topic, which professional or paraprofessional team members will be in attendance (e.g., nurse, Elder or Knowledge Keeper), whether childcare is provided, and what will be offered—for example, food, coffee and tea, and prizes.
- Ensure that the Elder or Knowledge Keeper has a comfortable chair, some water, tea or coffee, and a snack nearby, as discussed prior to the circle.
- Ensure that supplies are available for the Elder or Knowledge Keep and participants—for example, tissues, blankets, snacks, and beverages.

---

the circle typically asks participants if they would like to participate in a cleansing, through smudging or cleansing with a cedar bough, prior to starting the circle sharing. (See the Web Resources at the end of this chapter for more information.)

In each nation, the protocol(s) vary—for example, in some nations, the direction for talking and sharing in the circle might be clockwise and in other nations, counterclockwise. Cleansing of participants may be done using a moist cedar bough instead of smudging. Smudging medicines vary according to the nation and its traditions. Starting with a smudge or cleansing rids participants of any negative energies and allows for the circle to start off in a good way. In addition, the Elder or Knowledge Keeper conducts a circle prayer with the participants. This person may ask participants to join hands during the prayer. Usually, you stand facing toward the inner circle, adjoining your hands with the people beside you, in the following manner. Your right palm faces upward, adjoining to the person to your right, and your left palm faces downward, adjoining to the person to your left. This method of adjoining hands allows the energy from the prayer, participants, and ancestors to flow in a circular pattern. If it is your first time being in the prayer, the Elder or Knowledge Keeper may say the prayer first in their traditional language, perhaps sing a song as well, and then they will translate what they said in the prayer into English. You can cast your eyes downward to the centre of the circle, while the Elder or Knowledge Keeper sings and says the prayer. In some cases, when you go to a conference or gathering and an Elder may rise to say a blessing or prayer, it is customary for all the participants to rise, unless otherwise directed.

General guidelines for the circle are as follows:

- What is shared in the circle stays in the circle unless there is a danger to self or others.
- If a talking stick or stone is used, the person holding the stick or stone talks and everyone else listens.
- There is no cross talking; only the person with the talking stick or stone speaks. If you have a response to something someone has said, you can respond when you are holding the stick or stone or in a subsequent round.
- It is customary to keep both feet on the ground, to keep you grounded while seated.
- If you must leave the circle for any reason, stand, back up, and exit the circle by going either clockwise or counterclockwise, depending on the local nations' protocol(s) and through the opening. When returning to the circle, enter through the opening and again, go in the direction of the nation (i.e., clockwise or counterclockwise) back to your seat.
- If a participant becomes emotional during the circle, other participants can support them by offering them tissues or by moving around the circle per the protocol, to stand behind them and breathe deeply and slowly. This process is said to support the participant to release emotive energy and breathe in positive energy.
- When the talking circle comes to a close, the Elder or Knowledge Keeper does a closing prayer.

ENGAGING WITH INDIGENOUS COMMUNITIES

It is important to learn the structure and interrelationships of clan governance and communication, and this learning will bring meaning to you as a nurse working with Indigenous people. Importantly, learning, understanding, and demonstrating protocol(s) as a nurse working with Indigenous peoples and community members is foundational to creating a culturally safe environment. A brief overview of current Indigenous governance systems as a result of colonial processes and the ongoing journey to self-governance is provided below. (See the following sections on Indigenous Governance.) When developing care plans and discharge teaching, it is important to realize the impacts of colonization, which have foundational relevance to communication and to understanding the multiple health care systems and potential barriers to health care. Review the interweaving of individuals, families, and community and each of their roles that combine to strengthen communication with Indigenous peoples.

Clan Systems and Communication

Indigenous Governance

Historically, Indigenous governance systems are based on culture, ceremony, and clan systems. Each Indigenous community has different systems, so as a nurse working in or near an Indigenous community, it is important for you to learn about the culture and governance systems of that community. For example, in my community, the **clan** system is the governance structure within houses. In each house, the clan has chief and house representatives of sister and brother clans. Important decisions are made during **potlach** ceremonies that are used in the governing structure, culture, and spiritual First Nations traditions, as well as other important cultural events based on the traditional systems of governance. Traditional governance is conducted using ceremonies, when a community member from a clan dies, they are honoured through a potlach ceremony. All the clans come to the ceremony with monetary gifts to cover the costs associated with the funeral as well as food as both an offering and gift to those attending the ceremonies. These ways of supporting the family through financial and other gifts are an important feature of traditional systems of governance related to communication of sister or brother clans in times of health care crisis. Nurses and health care team members in the hospital caring for Indigenous peoples may also find other Indigenous community members from brother or sister clans tasked with supporting the family and the person during their stay at the hospital and later when the person is discharged.

Individuals, Families, and Community

When Indigenous peoples are in your care, it is important to get to know them as individuals. Although the intergenerational effects of residential schools continue today, you cannot assume that all Indigenous peoples went to residential school or practise traditional cultures and language. For example, you may care for an Indigenous person who went to residential school and continues to practise the Catholic faith. As nurses, we are often rushing as a result of time pressures to finish nursing tasks, at times experiencing compassion fatigue and dealing with competing priorities; this rushing means we may not allow time or space in conversations for responses. Do your best in providing nursing care to allow for a **safe place/space** by introducing yourself and others providing care on your team, letting the person know where the cultural spaces are within your organization so they and their families can practise cultural traditions.

In the hospital setting, there is often an Indigenous patient navigator who is a local Indigenous person hired to be an advocate, facilitate communication, and support individuals and their families. This role is particularly helpful to both the person and the hospital staff so that person-centred care is supported. Importantly, the Indigenous navigator works with the person and their family members to create a welcoming space for visiting, in which they can ask questions of the health care team. If there is an Indigenous navigator in the health care organization you work in, tell people you provide care for who that person is and how they can support the person and their family members.

Responsibilities of Sister or Brother Clans

As noted previously, traditional Indigenous systems of governance are interrelated to supporting community members, particularly when they are hospitalized or undergoing treatments and nursing care. Thus, nurses may observe sister or brother clans visiting the person and providing support to both the person and their family members. This is experienced as several visitors often coming in groups or coordinating a round-the-clock schedule of visitors to support the person and family members. This does not mean that the nurse needs to disclose confidential information; it merely means that if the nurse and interdisciplinary team are aware of the importance of the network of support then they can create a safe place for cultural practices and traditional support of the person. If possible, a room that allows for a comfortable area for the visitors and the person is recommended.

COMMUNICATION BARRIERS

Oral storytelling is a tradition within Indigenous cultures based on conveying meaning through lessons, language, ceremonies, traditions, and governance structures.

Indigenous language is being taught and revitalized in communities as an important part of healing amidst the intergenerational traumas of residential school, the Sixties Scoop, the closing of Indian hospitals (see the Web Resources at the end of this chapter), and years of colonial practices. (See Box 8.3.) Building respectful care relationships begins with the nurse practising cultural safety, enacting the 4 Rs (Kirkness, 2002), and creating a safe environment for the person and family members. Begin with introducing yourself as you practised earlier in this chapter. Communication can be facilitated by and through creating a respectful environment, where the person and family feel comfortable and safe to talk with the interdisciplinary team. Indigenous navigators, where available, meet with the person and educate staff on cultural protocols, provide translator services, and support family members. If there is not an Indigenous navigator within the health care organization, health care providers can contact the local Indigenous health centres for guidance on resources available and appropriate protocols. Facilitating a time and place for family to gather, and ensuring the person has family support systems to receive important information regarding their care, are essential to facilitate **discharge planning**. Indigenous peoples may be taking Western medicines along with traditional medicines and herbs as preventative and curative measures. Importantly, facilitating communication can support traditional practices while the person is in hospital and provide quiet spaces such as spiritual rooms for smudging.

Two-Eyed Seeing Approach

A two-eyed seeing approach values viewing the world using one eye grounded in Indigenous world views while the other eye is grounded in Eurocentric ones (Bartlett et al., 2012). A two-eyed seeing approach combines traditional Eurocentric medical and nursing knowledge and practices with Indigenous ways of knowing and being. Indigenous nursing practice experiences within Indigenous communities use two-eyed seeing in nursing to deliver health care services (Blackstock, 2017, 2018). This means that nurses are practising cultural safety, humility, and protocols (see Case Example: Two-Eyed Seeing Approach).

Case Example: Two-Eyed Seeing Approach

Scenario

Rupinder is a student nurse who has been placed in an Indigenous urban agency to work with the agency to develop culturally appropriate information posters and pamphlets on diabetes. The agency's mandate is to serve the local Indigenous peoples, using an interdisciplinary team of community health nurses, Elders, peer support workers, social workers, and nurse practitioners. The educational resources will be used by the community health nurse in monthly talking circles focused on supporting individuals with diabetes.

Two-Eyed Seeing Approach

Rupinder meets with the community health nurse and the Elder working at the agency, and they agree that he should attend a talking circle to understand some of the issues and barriers that the individuals are dealing with as they live with diabetes. In preparation, Rupinder learns the protocol of introductions and the talking circle processes. He also meets with the Elder to understand the local Indigenous traditional medicines and treatments used to treat diabetes. In addition, he reviews the incidence and prevalence of diabetes in the community, reviewing the agency's data and contrasting it with the medical health officer's annual report for the territory. In this manner, he is learning the Indigenous protocols and traditional medicines used to treat diabetes (using one eye to view the Indigenous ways of being), acknowledging how he is situated (by introducing himself and his cultural background), and applying knowledge from his nursing training (using the other eye for Eurocentric knowledge of science, nutrition, health, and healing) to gather information from the individuals living with diabetes to find out what educational resources, training, and support are needed.

Rupinder attends the monthly talking circle and learns from the individuals with diabetes the educational resources and support they require. He uses an interprofessional approach (described; see Interprofessional Collaboration) to develop a draft of the necessary resources. He uses evidence-informed resources on diabetes (i.e., the best of Eurocentric ways of knowing, with one eye), and meeting with the community health nurse, peer support workers, and the Elder to ensure that culturally appropriate images, words, language, and use of traditional medicines are also addressed in the resources (i.e., Indigenous ways of knowing and being with the other eye). He returns to the talking circle and shares the draft of the resources with the talking circle group to obtain feedback and changes from the group members through a collaborative process. The resources are finalized and brought back to the talking circle for final review. Once everyone agrees with the resources, they are brought to the interprofessional team for review and processes on usage.

BOX 8.3 Indigenous Languages: Reclaiming Indigenous Language

"Our languages are central to our ceremonies, our relationships to our lands, the animals, to each other, our understandings, of our worlds, including the natural world, our stories and our laws." —National Chief Perry Bellegarde, Opening Remarks to the Federal-Provincial-Territorial Ministers Responsible for Culture and Heritage, Orford, Québec. August 22, 2017. https://www.afn.ca/category/policy-sectors/languages-and-culture/.

First Nations people have advocated for many years for a legislated commitment from the federal government respecting Indigenous languages. In 2016, Statistics Canada reported that, for about 40 Indigenous languages, there are 500 or fewer speakers. In 2016, the *Indigenous Languages Act*, S.C. 2019, c. 23, received Royal Assent on June 21, 2019. Section 5 outlines the purposes of the Act:

5 The purposes of this Act are to

(a) support and promote the use of Indigenous languages, including Indigenous sign languages;

(b) support the efforts of Indigenous peoples to reclaim, revitalize, maintain and strengthen Indigenous languages, including their efforts to

(i) assess the status of distinct Indigenous languages,

(ii) plan initiatives and activities for restoring and maintaining fluency in Indigenous languages,

(iii) create technological tools, educational materials and permanent records of Indigenous languages, including audio and video recordings of fluent speakers of the languages and written materials such as dictionaries, lexicons and grammars of the languages, for the purposes of, among other things, the maintenance and transmission of the languages,

(iv) support Indigenous language learning and cultural activities—including language nest, mentorship and immersion programs—to increase the number of new speakers of Indigenous languages,

(v) support entities specialized in Indigenous languages, and

(vi) undertake research or studies in respect of Indigenous languages;

(c) establish a framework to facilitate the effective exercise of the rights of Indigenous peoples that relate to Indigenous languages, including by way of agreements or arrangements referred to in sections 8 and 9;

(d) establish measures to facilitate the provision of adequate, sustainable and long-term funding for the reclamation, revitalization, maintenance and strengthening of Indigenous languages;

(e) facilitate cooperation with provincial and territorial governments, Indigenous governments and other Indigenous governing bodies, Indigenous organizations and other entities in a manner consistent with the rights of Indigenous peoples and the powers and jurisdictions of Indigenous governing bodies and of the provinces and territories;

(e.1) facilitate meaningful opportunities for Indigenous governments and other Indigenous governing bodies and Indigenous organizations to collaborate in policy development related to the implementation of this Act;

(f) respond to the Truth and Reconciliation Commission of Canada's Calls to Action numbers 13 to 15; and

(g) contribute to the implementation of the United Nations Declaration on the Rights of Indigenous Peoples as it relates to Indigenous languages.

The Assembly of First Nations prepared *A Guide to An Act respecting Indigenous languages: A Tool for First Nations Language Revitalization* to assist those who are ready to start or are already involved in language revitalization. Language revitalization programs are offered at several universities in Canada.

Communities are actively documenting languages, and organizations like First Voice (https://firstvoicenl.ca/) and the First Peoples' Cultural Council (fpcc.ca) work to support Indigenous languages. In Atlantic Canada, there are 36 government-funded programs to support language recovery and revitalizations. Individual efforts are also underway. In Nova Scotia, Tom and Carol Ann Johnson from the Eskasoni First Nation Mi'kmaq community worked with producers of the television series *Vikings* to produce authentic translation and pronunciation of the Mi'kmaq language for the series.

Sources: Indigenous Languages Act, S.C. 2019, C. 23. https://laws-lois.justice.gc.ca/eng/acts/I-7.85/page-1.html; Assembly of First Nations. (2019). *Languages and culture.* https://www.afn.ca/policy-sectors/languages-and-culture/; Assembly of First Nations. (2019). An Act respecting Indigenous languages: A tool for First Nations language revitalization. https://www.afn.ca/wp-content/uploads/2020/04/Respecting_Languages_Report_ENG.pdf; Rice, K. (2020). Indigenous Language Revitalization in Canada. https://www.thecanadianencyclopedia.ca/en/article/indigenous-language-revitalization-in-canada; Kelloway, B. (2021). Mi'kmaq couple bring their language to hit TV show Vikings. https://www.cbc.ca/news/canada/nova-scotia/cape-breton-couple-mi-kmaq-language-1.5951646.

INTERPROFESSIONAL COLLABORATION

Interprofessional collaboration is a process of developing and maintaining effective interprofessional working relationships with learners, practitioners, people and their families, and communities to facilitate optimal holistic health outcomes. The participants within an interdisciplinary collaborative team vary depending on the organizational context, the type of professionals and paraprofessionals (e.g., Elders and Knowledge Keepers, peer support people) available and the health care services being provided by the agency. Nursing students are taught to work with interdisciplinary teams in health care organizations using a Eurocentric/medical model approach to health care delivery. However, there is a gap for Indigenous peoples and their families when they are discharged from hospitals, often into the care of interprofessional collaborative teams in their communities. In Indigenous communities, elements of collaboration include respect, trust, shared decision making, and partnerships among professionals, paraprofessionals, medicine people, and Elders. Interdisciplinary collaborative practice models have been used to prepare nursing students to practise in Indigenous communities (Blackstock, 2017, 2018) engaging with paraprofessionals, interdisciplinary team members, and Knowledge Keepers.

When nurses practise as part of interdisciplinary collaborative teams within Indigenous community health services, they work with Elders, Knowledge Keepers, social workers, health care assistants, nurses, doctors, and often peer community mentors and leaders. Thus, when nurses are preparing discharge planning, teaching, and setting up home care resources, they need to arrange transfer of care and communicate with the interprofessional collaborative team within the Indigenous community. If existing information is within the agency on transfer of care, nurses, social workers, and managers will direct you to the information. If the agency does not have existing resources, then begin with a conversation with the individual in your care to clarify the health services they typically use in their community. Connect with the health services and then fill in any gaps in services with other resources. Further, nurses must contact the health care providers in the person's community to coordinate ongoing care rather than having the person appear without the receiving authority knowing about the person's health and nursing care needs. To obtain up-to-date information, consult the Government of Canada's Crown-Indigenous Relations and Northern Affairs Canada (CIRNAC) and Indigenous Services Canada (ISC) about the benefits and rights for Indigenous peoples and explanation of status, non-status, Inuit, and Métis peoples (see the Web Resources at the end of this chapter).

HEALTH TRANSFER, TRIPARTITE HEALTH SERVICES, AND COMMUNICATION CHALLENGES

Historic landmark events in Indigenous health governance have many implications for which health care services are governed, developed, and delivered. For example, in British Columbia, since the signing of the Tripartite First Nations Health Plan (First Nations Leadership Council and British Columbia, 2007) and the British Columbia Tripartite Framework Agreement on First Nations Health Governance, in 2011, Tripartite Partners (Health Canada, BC Ministry of Health, and BC First Nations) continue to work to develop a new First Nations health governance structure to improve health outcomes for BC First Nations Communities. Currently, Indigenous health care services can be provided through either First Nations and Inuit health services, for communities that have undergone or are in the midst of health transfer. This means that an Indigenous person may have different types of health care coverage, access to health care services, and, depending on two factors. First, in addition to their employer's health care benefits, they may have additional health coverage and benefits if they have First Nations status coverage. Second, their access to health care services depends on whether they live on or off reserve or in the urban setting. For health care providers and nurses providing teaching and discharge planning, it is important to be informed and aware of the aforementioned factors to ensure that people in their care have the resources, support, medical and extended health care coverage, financial resources, and access to appropriate services in their communities and homes. In addition, when working with people living in urban settings, the nurse can coordinate resources and services to customize discharge planning that is realistic and relevant to the individual.

ENGAGING WITH HUMILITY

Table 8.1 outlines the important concepts you have learned through the readings and activities in this chapter. The goal for this table is to provide you with insights on how the Indigenous approach varies from the nursing approach and how, together, you can co-create relationality through engagement with Indigenous peoples and their family members and support systems. "**Relationality** is a philosophy that describes the interconnections between all of creation and kinship consists of family, community, and all extended human and more-than-human relations" (Campbell et al., 2020, p. 8).

⚖ ETHICAL DILEMMA
What Would You Do?

Abigail is a second-year student nurse working on an acute care ward with her nursing faculty member for a clinical rotation. She arrives to the floor the day before clinical to find out who has been assigned to her so she can prepare for the following day. She finds out that one of the people she will be looking after is an Indigenous person who was transferred to the hospital from their home community 500 kilometres away. While she is reviewing the person's chart and medication administration records, she is interrupted by a care aide and nurse coming back from their coffee break. They ask Abigail, "Do you have that person assigned to you tomorrow?" and she responds "yes." The care aide says, "Thank goodness, that Indian is so demanding with all the family coming and going, asking questions all day!" The nurse adds, "They've asked us to rearrange our care so they can do some drum song thing—such a hassle!" Abigail is in shock. She says, "I'm sorry, I'm not sure I heard you correctly—could you please repeat what you said?" The nurse and care aide repeat their statements, adding some body movements, pretending to drum and sing into a microphone.

1. What ethical principle is being violated in this situation?
2. What message do the care aide's and nurse's behaviours convey?
3. How would you react in this situation, and what steps would you take to address the situation?

SUMMARY

This chapter is meant to be a guide to facilitate communication with Indigenous peoples and communities. It begins with you—your cultural desire and humility in using a decolonizing approach to nursing care. Engage in cultural safety training and practice, be an ally, learn about Indigenous culture in general and that of the local Indigenous communities where you live and work. Practise the 4Rs and be an advocate within your health care organization to create change and dismantle racism in it many forms.

QUESTIONS FOR REVIEW AND DISCUSSION

1. Given what you have learned about engaging with humility, how will you practise these skills in nursing practice?

2. Discuss similarities and differences between interprofessional and paraprofessional teams and how they collaborate when working within Indigenous communities.
3. What health topics would lend themselves well to using a sharing circle format, and what steps would you take as a student nurse or nurse to plan, develop, and deliver the session(s)?
4. How do you plan to develop your cultural knowledge of local Indigenous peoples to inform your cultural safety practices as a nurse?
5. What are the Indigenous health agencies in your area? What services do they offer?

REFERENCES

Assembly of First Nations. (2013). *First Nations wholistic policy and planning: A transitional discussion document on the social determinants of health.* https://citeseerx.ist.psu.edu/viewdoc/download?doi=10.1.1.476.9397&rep=rep1&type=pdf.

Attas, R. (n.d.). *What is decolonization? What is Indigenization?* Queen's University Centre for Teaching and Learning. https://www.queensu.ca/ctl/teaching-support/decolonizing-and-indigenizing/what-decolonizationindigenization.

Bartlett, C., Marshall, M., & Marshall, A. (2012). Two-eyed seeing and other lessons learned within a co-learning journey of bringing together Indigenous and mainstream knowledges and ways of knowing. *Journal of Environmental Studies and Sciences, 2,* 331–340.

Bhattacharyya, O. K., Rasooly, I. R., Naqshbandi, M., et al. (2011). Challenges to the provision of diabetes care in first nations communities: Results from a national survey of health care providers in Canada. *BMC Health Services Research, 11*(283), 1–10. https://doi.org/10.1186/1472-6963-11-283.

Blackstock, S. (2017). Shifting the academic lens: Development of an interdisciplinary Indigenous health course. *Journal of Education and Practice, 7*(1), 11–16. https://doi.org/10.5430/jnep.v7n1p11.

Blackstock, S. (2018). Otsin: Sharing the spirit—Development of an Indigenous rural nursing practice course. *Journal of Education and Practice, 8*(12), 29–35.

Canadian Nurses Association. (2017). *Code of Ethics for Registered Nurses.* https://www.cna-aiic.ca/-/media/can/page-content/pdf-en/code-of-ethics-2017-edition-secure-interactive.pdf?la=en&hash=09C348308C44912AF216656BFA31E33519756387.

Campbell, E., Austin, A., Bax-Campbell, M., et al. (2020). Indigenous relationality and kinship and the professionalization of a health workforce. *Turtle Island Journal of Indigenous Health, 1*(1), 8–13. https://doi.org/10.33137/tijih.v1i1.34016.

Cinel, J., & Blackstock, S. (2014). *Bias paper: Course assignment from relational practice III.* Kamloops, British Columbia, Canada: Thompson Rivers University, School of Nursing.

Community Health Nurses of Canada. (2019). *2019 Canadian Community Health Nursing Professional Practice Model &*

Standards of Practice. https://www.chnc.ca/en/standards-of-practice.

Doane, G. H., & Varcoe, C. (2015). *How to nurse: Relational inquiry with individuals and families in changing health and health care contexts* (1st ed.). Wolters Kluwer/Lippincott Williams & Wilkins.

Freshwater, D., & Rolfe, G. (2001). Critical reflexivity: A politically and ethically engaged research method for nursing. *Nursing Times Research, 6*(1), 526–537.

Kirkness. V. J. (2002). *Transforming the landscape of aboriginal higher education: Respect, relevance, reciprocity, responsibility.* University of British Columbia. https://open.library.ubc.ca/clRcle/collections/ubclibraryand archives/67246/items/1.0103053.

Martin, K., & Mirraboopa, B. (2003). Ways of knowing, being and doing: A theoretical framework and methods for indigenous and indigenist research. *Journal of Australian Studies, 27*(76), 203–214.

Miller, J. R. (1989). *Skyscrapers hide the heavens: A history of Indian-White relations in Canada* (1st ed.). University of Toronto Press.

Nuu-chah-nulth Tribal Council Research Ethics Committee. (2008). *Protocols & principles for conducting research in a Nuu-chah-nulth context.* https://icwrn.uvic.ca/wp-content/uploads/2013/08/NTC-Protocols-and-Principles.pdf.

Richmond, C. A. M., & Ross, N. A. (2009). The determinants of First Nation and Inuit health: A critical population health approach. *Health Place, 15,* 403–411.

Truth and Reconciliation Commission of Canada. (2015). *Truth and Reconciliation Commission of Canada: Calls to Action.* https://www2.gov.bc.ca/assets/gov/british-columbians-our-governments/indigenous-people/aboriginal-peoples-documents/calls_to_action_english2.pdf.

United Nations General Assembly. (2007). United Nations Declaration on the Rights of Indigenous Peoples: Resolution/adopted by the General Assembly. https://www.refworld.org/docid/471355a82.html.

WEBSITE/RESOURCES LIST

A Brief Look at Indian Hospitals in Canada https://www.ictinc.ca/blog/a-brief-look-at-indian-hospitals-in-canada-0.

Birth of a Family: I Feel Ripped Off https://www.cbc.ca/player/play/1046773315947.

Canadian Indigenous Nurses Association https://indigenousnurses.ca.

Crown-Indigenous Relations and Northern Affairs Canada https://www.canada.ca/en/crown-indigenous-relations-northern-affairs.html.

How to Smudge: Burning Sage https://www.youtube.com/watch?v=6fIMumk2cnA&list=PLeyJPHbRnGaZFu8_xxuXPlYG-j-9cogsx&index=45&t=0s.

Indigenous Languages—Learning and Teaching Resources https://www.noslangues-ourlanguages.gc.ca/en/ressources-resources/autochtones-aboriginals/apprentissage-learning-eng.

Indigenous Services Canada https://www.canada.ca/en/indigenous-services-canada.html.

Mistreated: The legacy of segregated hospitals haunts Indigenous survivors https://www.cbc.ca/news2/interactives/sh/jTCWPYgkNH/mistreated/.

National Collaborating Centre for Indigenous Health (NCCIH) https://www.nccih.ca/en/.

Raising Reconciliation: Inter-Generational Trauma https://calgary-journal-podcasts.simplecast.com/episodes/740a22fe.

The Sixties Scoop Explained https://www.cbc.ca/cbcdocspov/features/the-sixties-scoop-explained.

United Nations Declaration on the Rights of Indigenous Peoples https://www.un.org/esa/socdev/unpfii/documents/DRIPS_en.pdf.

9

Communicating in Groups

Claire Mallette

Originating US Chapter by *Elizabeth C. Arnold*

OBJECTIVES

At the end of the chapter, the reader will be able to:
1. Define group communication in health care.
2. Identify the characteristics of small group communication in contemporary health care.
3. Describe the phases of small group development.
4. Discuss theory-based concepts of group dynamics.
5. Apply group concepts in therapeutic groups.
6. Compare and contrast different types of therapeutic groups.
7. Apply concepts of group dynamics to work groups.
8. Discuss differences in small group communication and team communication.

In clinical practice, group communication formats are used extensively as a major means of communication for clinical knowledge sharing and decision making. Group communication provides unique opportunities for students to learn how to express and defend their ideas in task, project, and discussion groups. In group settings, each participant brings their own personal perspective and draws from distinctive experiences of other members. Knowledge sharing is not the only advantage of group interaction. Group membership can create productive relationships with other group members that might not occur otherwise.

This chapter focuses on small group communication in contemporary health care. The chapter identifies theory-based concepts related to small group dynamics and processes and describes group role functions as a foundation for interactive applications in clinical and work groups. The chapter concludes with a discussion of applications for clinical and work groups.

BASIC CONCEPTS

Rothwell (2013) defines a *group* as "a human communication system composed of three or more individuals, interacting for the achievement of some common goal(s) who influence and are influenced by each other" (p. 36). Unlike communication between two people, there are multiple inputs and responses to each conversational segment in a group format.

Group relationships are interdependent. Each group member's contribution has an influence on the behaviour and responses of other group members. In this way, group communication shares a key characteristic with system and team concepts (see Chapters 1 and 24). However, while a team is a group, a group is not a team. Over time, a group culture emerges, supported by stories and metaphors about the group and how it functions.

Primary and Secondary Groups

"Membership in groups is inevitable and universal" (Johnson & Johnson, 2017, p. 2). Groups are categorized as primary or secondary. *Primary groups* are characterized by an informal structure and close personal relationships. Group membership in primary groups is automatic (e.g., in a family) or voluntarily chosen because of a strong common interest (e.g., in a friendship). There are no previously determined end dates. Primary groups have an important influence on self-identity and the development of socialization skills.

Secondary groups represent time-limited group relationships with an established beginning and end. Group size is determined by its goals and functions. In contrast with primary groups, secondary groups have a prescribed formal structure, usually a designated leader, and specific goals (Forsyth, 2018). When the group completes its task or achieves its goals, the group ends.

People join secondary groups to meet established goals, to develop knowledge and skills, or because it is required by the larger community system to which the individuals belong. Formal work groups, which are critical to the accomplishment of predetermined organizational goals, are also classified as secondary groups, as are therapy and support groups. Other group formats with a work-related rather than friendship basis include social action, specific task, clinical teams, and education groups.

Beebe and Masterson (2014) suggest that systems theory explains how a group as a system relates to smaller individual systems within it and to the larger organizational systems of which the group is a part. Simulation Exercise 9.1 presents the role that group communication plays in a person's life.

Group Communication in Health Care

Intraprofessional (multiple members of the same profession) and interprofessional (a team of different health providers) health care teams functioning within a larger health care system setting, work groups, and counselling and therapy groups all rely on aspects of group communication to achieve designated goals in health care settings. Multiple informational inputs available in small groups are an invaluable input resource in professional clinical education.

Nurses are increasingly involved in task forces and committees to help strengthen health systems and improve clinical outcomes within the profession, on interprofessional health care teams, and within the larger community (Yang et al., 2012). In the community, nurses come together with other health providers and concerned citizens to advocate for clinical approaches that address specific and global health needs in the community. Examples include citizen advisory groups to advocate for the needs of older people and people with mental health disorders, drug addictions, homelessness, and disabilities.

In your nursing program, group communication provides a central means of communicating with other students and health providers within and between clinical settings. As you work with other students in small group formats to complete educational projects or engage in related reflective analysis discussions of simulated and experiential clinical scenarios, you are using group communication skills. Intra- and interprofessional education and practice collaborations, now a global initiative in health care, use small group communication as a fundamental form of interaction (see Chapter 24).

The Canadian Nurses Association [CNA] (2017) Code of Ethics and all provinces and territories' professional standards identify the importance of collaborating and promoting intra- and interprofessional person-centred care. The CNA (2020) states that, "Intra-professional collaboration is a relational, respectful process among nursing colleagues that allows for the effective use of the knowledge, skills and talents of all nursing designations to establish and achieve optimal client and health system outcomes (Nova Scotia College of Nurses, 2019; Nurses Association of New Brunswick & Association of New Brunswick Licensed Practical Nurses, 2015)" (p. 1). The College of Registered Nurses of Manitoba (2019) describes interprofessional collaborative care as "when multiple providers from different professions provide comprehensive services by working with clients, their support networks, care providers, and communities to deliver the highest quality of care across all settings (p.1).

Working in groups in intra- and interprofessional collaborations requires respect, trust, shared decision

---

SIMULATION EXERCISE 9.1   Groups in Everyday Life

Purpose

To help students gain an appreciation of the role group communication plays in their lives

Procedure

1. Write down all the groups in which you have been a participant (e.g., family, interest groups, sports teams, community, religious, work, and social groups).
2. Identify which are primary groups and which are secondary groups. How are or were they different?
3. Describe the influence that membership in each of these groups had on the person you are today.
4. Identify the ways in which membership in different groups are or were of value in your life.

Discussion

1. How similar or dissimilar were your answers from those of your classmates?
2. What factors account for differences in the quantity and quality of your group memberships?
3. How similar were the ways in which membership enhanced your self-esteem?
4. If your answers were dissimilar, what makes membership in groups such a complex experience?
5. Could different people get different things out of very similar group experiences?
6. What implications does this exercise have for your nursing practice?

making and partnerships. The National Interprofessional Competency Framework describes competencies that can guide education and collaborative practices for health care students in a variety of health care settings. For intra- and interprofessional communication and collaboration to be effective, the teams need to address conflicting perspectives and reach acceptable compromises (Canadian Interprofessional Health Collaborative [CIHC], 2010).

Group learning formats use group communication concepts and simulated group experiences to help students develop critical thinking about coordinated intra- and interprofessional clinical approaches in clinical settings. Clinical simulations prepare students experientially to work together in simulated situations similar to those they will encounter in actual practice. Students share information, question and negotiate with one another, and also communicate with standardized people in simulated clinical scenarios. They begin to experientially understand the practices, processes, and concerns of their own and other disciplines in a system-based therapeutic approach to person-centred care. Reflective analysis group discussions on their individual roles and team functioning are critical components of intra- and interdisciplinary team learning processes (CIHC, 2010; CNA, 2020; Michaelsen & Sweet, 2011).

CHARACTERISTICS OF SMALL GROUP COMMUNICATION THERAPY

Group Purpose

The group purpose provides the rationale for a group's existence (Powles, 2007). Purpose provides direction for group decisions and influences the type of communication and activities required to meet group goals. For example, the purpose of an intra- or interprofessional (or both) health team would be to deliver quality health care to people; the purpose of group therapy would be to improve the interpersonal functioning of individual members. In a work group, the purpose would support a better solution to implementation of a specific work-related issue, such as wait times, transfer processes, or introduction of a new program or process. The purposes of different group types are presented in Table 9.1.

Group Goals

Group goals define expected outcomes in a process group or describe a defined work outcome in a task group, indicating goal achievement. Goals serve as benchmarks for successful achievement. In health care teams and work groups, the match should be between group members' expertise and skills, interests, goal requirements, and meeting the needs of people, families, and communities. Matching group

TABLE 9.1   Therapeutic Group Type and Purpose

Group Type	Purpose
Therapy	Reality testing, encouraging personal growth, inspiring hope, strengthening personal resources, developing interpersonal skills
Support	Giving and receiving practical information and advice, supporting coping skills, promoting self-esteem, enhancing problem-solving skills, encouraging autonomy, strengthening hope and resiliency
Activity	Getting people in touch with their bodies, releasing energy, enhancing self-esteem, encouraging cooperation, stimulating spontaneous interaction, supporting creativity
Health education	Learning new knowledge, promoting skill development, providing support and feedback, supporting development of competency, promoting discussion of important health-related issues

goals with member needs and characteristics is essential in counselling and therapeutic groups.

General group goals should be of interest to the group members. Group members need to understand and commit to achieving group goals. Goals need to be achievable, measurable, and within the capabilities of group membership. A good match energizes a group; members develop commitment and interest because they perceive the group as having value. A common acronym used to guide the development of group goals is SMART, which stands for specific, measurable, achievable, realistic, and timely (McShane et al., 2015). Table 9.2 outlines each characteristic of SMART goals.

Group Size

Group purpose dictates group size. There is no one size that fits all groups. One factor to take into consideration is the role of the group. A general rule is that the group needs to be large enough to accomplish the group goal and provide the necessary knowledge, skills, and perspectives to successfully achieve the goals of the group yet small enough to maintain efficient coordination and meaningful contributions from each member (McShane et al., 2015). Regardless

TABLE 9.2   SMART Goal Characteristics

SMART Goal	Characteristics
Specific	Specific goals identify what needs to be achieved. They are detailed, focused, and clearly stated.
Measurable	Goals need to be measurable to identify whether the goal was achieved. The goal needs to be quantifiable in order to measure how much and how well the goal was realized.
Achievable	Ideally, goals need to be challenging but not so difficult that they are not attainable.
Realistic/**R**elevant	The goal must be meaningful and important in relation to what needs to be achieved.
Time-limited	The goal needs to have a specific time line and deadline for when it must be accomplished.

Adapted from the College of Nurses of Ontario. (2019). *Developing SMART learning goals*, p.3. https://www.cno.org/globalassets/docs/qa/2019/smart-goals-2019.pdf; McShane, S. L., Steen, S. L., & Tasa, K. (2015). *Canadian organizational behaviour* (9th ed.), p. 125. McGraw-Hill Ryerson.

of group size, the group should be large enough to interact and influence one another and be mutually accountable to group functioning.

The group role will influence the group size. For example, education-focused groups can vary in size, with groups learning psychomotor skills in a simulation centre having 10 or more members, depending on the activity. Membership on intra- and interprofessional teams varies, depending in part on the person's health care needs. Typically, group members reflect the essential number of health care providers needed to coordinate and share responsibility for people's health care needs. Person-centred therapeutic groups usually consist of six to eight members. With fewer than five members, deep sharing tends to be limited. If one or more members are absent, group interaction can become intense and uncomfortable for the remaining members.

Group Member Composition

Careful selection of group members should be based on the purpose and goals of the group, functional similarity, commitment to identified goals, and basic knowledge of how

group communication processes enable goal achievement. A person's capacity to derive benefit from the group and to contribute to group goals is a critical requirement for health-related person-centred groups, such as group therapy. In health care–related work (task) groups, group member composition depends on the purpose and goals of the group. In groups that involve complex issues and the need for innovative solutions, a more diverse group is preferable.

Selection of group members can be selected based on functional similarity. *Functional similarity* is defined as choosing the group members who are similar enough—intellectually, emotionally, and experientially—to interact with one another in a meaningful way to accomplish the group goal. In work (task) groups, functional similarity consists of choosing members with complementary experiential knowledge or skill sets, plus the interest, commitment, and essential skills to contribute to group goals. This type of functional match can produce a higher level of group performance in establishing norms of the group and implementing the task more quickly than a group with more diverse members (Civettini, 2007).

In group therapy groups, a group member who is different from the other members can be at a disadvantage from an acceptance perspective. For example, a single adolescent boy placed in a group of similar-aged girls can be marginalized simply because of personal characteristics beyond that individual member's control. In a different group, with members having similar characteristics, the treatment outcomes might be quite different.

Interpersonal compatibility among group members is desirable as this can enhance task interdependence and the desire to work together as a group. On the other hand, differences in outlook and opinion can enrich group conversation if not extreme. Group members from different backgrounds have diverse life experiences, which can help group members consider alternative viewpoints. Working through differences to achieve consensus makes the group process a richer experience and the outcome will reflect a broader consensus. Simulation Exercise 9.2 provides an opportunity to explore the concept of functional similarity.

Group Norms

Group norms refer to the unwritten behavioural rules of conduct expected of group members. Norms provide needed predictability for effective group functioning and make the group safe for its members. There are two types of norms: universal and group specific.

Universal norms are explicit behavioural standards, which must be present in all groups to achieve effective outcomes. Examples include confidentiality, regular attendance, and using the group as the forum for discussion rather than individual discussion with members outside of

---

SIMULATION EXERCISE 9.2 **Exploring Functional Similarity**

Purpose
To provide an experiential understanding of functional similarity

Procedure
1. Break the class up into groups of four to six people.
2. One person per group should take notes on the discussion.
3. Identify two characteristics or experiences that all members of your group have in common other than that you are in the same class.
4. Identify two things that are unique to each person in your group (e.g., only child, never moved from the area, born in another country, unique skill or life experience).

5. Each person should elaborate on both the common and different experiences.

Discussion
1. What was the effect of finding common ground with other group members?
2. In what ways did finding out about the uniqueness of each person's experience add to the discussion?
3. Did anything in the discussion of either the commonalities or differences in experience stimulate further group discussion?
4. How could you use what you have learned in this exercise in your clinical practice?

SIMULATION EXERCISE 9.3 **Identifying Norms**

Purpose
To help identify norms operating in groups

Procedure
1. Divide a piece of paper into three columns.
2. In the first column, write the norms you think exist in your class or work group. In the second column, write the norms you think exist in your family. Examples of norms might be as follows: no one gets angry, decisions are made by consensus, assertive behaviours are valued, missed sessions and lateness are not tolerated.
3. Share your norms with the group, first related to the school or work group and then to the family. Place this

collective information from sharing of each other's group norms in the third column.

Discussion
1. What were some of the differences in existing norms for school, work, and family?
2. What surprised you in the similarities and differences?
3. Were there any universal norms on either of your lists?
4. Was there more or less consistency in overall student responses about class and work group norms and family norms? If so, what would account for it?

---

the group (Burlingame et al., 2006). Unless group members in process groups believe that personal information will not be shared outside the group setting (confidentiality), trust will not develop. Regular attendance at group meetings is critical to group stability and goal achievement. Even if a member is a perfect fit with group goals, they must also fully commit to regular attendance and full participation for the group to function well.

Group-specific norms are constructed by group members. They represent the shared beliefs, values, and unspoken operational rules governing group functions (Rothwell, 2013). Norms help define member interactions. They are often implicit. Examples include the group's norms of respect, participation by all, level of tolerance for lateness, use of humour, or confrontation, and talking directly to group members when there is an issue rather than about

them to others. Simulation Exercise 9.3 can help you develop a deeper understanding of group norms.

Group Role Positions

A person's role in the group corresponds with the status, power, and internal image that other members in the group hold for that member. Group members assume, or are ascribed, roles that influence their communication and the responses of others in the group. They usually have trouble breaking away from roles they have been cast in, despite their best efforts. For example, in group therapy, people will look to the "supportive" group member for advice, even when that person lacks expertise or personally needs the group's support. That identified "supportive" member may suffer because they do not always receive the support they need. Other times, group members project a role position onto a particular group member that represents a hidden agenda or an unresolved issue for the group as a whole. Unconscious biases about people with different cultural contexts from your own can also influence how a person is perceived in the group. You need to be self-aware of your own biases, values and beliefs, and cultural contexts described in Chapter 7 that influence how you view members of the group. Projection is largely unconscious, but it can be destructive to group functioning (Moreno, 2007). For example, if the group as a whole seems to place blame, marginalize, ignore, defer to, or consistently idealize one of its members, this group projection can compromise the group's effectiveness because of an unrealistic focus on one group member. Simulation Exercise 9.4 considers group role-position expectations.

Group Dynamics

Group dynamics is a term used to describe the communication processes and behaviours that occur during the life of the group (Forsyth, 2018). These underlying forces represent a complex blend of individual and group characteristics that interact with each other to achieve the group purpose. Bernard et al. (2008) categorized the primary forces operating in groups as individual dynamics (member variables), interpersonal dynamics (group communication variables), and the dynamics of the group as a whole, related to purpose, norms, and so on. The group leader is charged with integrating these multiple variables into a workable group process (Fig. 9.1). Group work can enhance member confidence, interpersonal skills, and cultural awareness (Forehand et al., 2016).

Group Process

Group process refers to the structural development of small group relationships. Tuckman and Jensen (1977) describe the five-phase model of small group development (forming, storming, norming, performing, and adjourning). This model has become the most commonly and widely used framework for the structural development and relationship process of small groups such as in work and therapeutic groups (Fig. 9.2). The model also serves the purpose of providing a framework for identifying

---

SIMULATION EXERCISE 9.4 Headbands: Group Role Expectations

Purpose
To experience the pressures of role expectations on group performance

Procedure
1. Break the class up into groups of six members.
2. Make up labels or headbands in a way that each group member cannot see their own label, but the other members can see it easily.
3. Each label or headband is lettered with directions on how the other members should respond to the role, for example:
   - Comedian: laugh at me
   - Expert: ask my advice
   - Insignificant: ignore me
   - Loser: pity me
   - Boss: obey me
   - Helpless: support me
   - Blocker: disagree with everything being said

4. Provide a topic for discussion (e.g., why the members chose nursing, social justice) or have the group decide on a topic. Instruct each member to interact with the others in a way that is natural. Do not role-play; be yourself. React to each member who speaks by following the instructions on the speaker's label or headband. Don't tell each another what their labels say, but simply to react to them.
5. After about 10 minutes, the facilitator halts the activity and directs each member to guess what their label was and then to take it off and read it.

Discussion
Initiate a discussion about how each member felt by the reactions of group members to their statements. Possible questions include the following:
1. What were some of the problems of trying to be yourself under conditions of group role pressure?
2. How did it feel to be consistently misinterpreted by the group—to have them laugh when you were trying to be serious or ignore you when you were trying to make a point?
3. Did you find yourself changing your behaviour in reaction to the way the group treated you—withdrawing when they ignored you, acting confident when they treated you with respect, giving orders when they deferred to you?
4. How can this experience inform how you will respond to group members in the future?

Modified from Pfeiffer, J., & Jones, J. (1977). *A handbook of structured experiences for human relations training* (Vol VI). University Associate Publishers.

and exploring key issues of group dynamics (Bonebright, 2010). The five phases of group development describe the process beginning from when individuals come together to form a group until the group achieves its goals and adjourns. Groups do not spend the same amount of time or energy in each phase. They may also not go through the phases sequentially and they may return to a phase, such as when new members are introduced into the group or the role of the group changes (Jhangiani & Tarry, 2014).

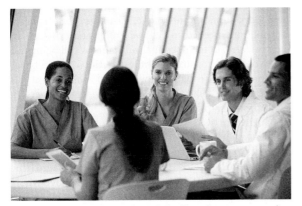

Fig. 9.1 Group dynamics describe the communication processes and behaviours that occur during the life of a group. Source: iStock.com/LumiNola.

Today's complex and dynamic environments influence how groups go through the phases.

Forming

The forming phase begins when members come together as a group. Members may enter group relationships as strangers to one another. The leader orients the group to the group's purpose and asks members to introduce themselves. The information each person shares about themselves should be brief and relate to personal data relevant to achieving the group's purpose.

During the forming phase, the leader introduces universal norms (group ground rules) for attendance, participation, and confidentiality. Getting to know one another, finding common threads in personal or professional experience, and acceptance of group goals and tasks are initial group tasks. Members have a basic need for acceptance, so communication is more tentative than it will be later, when members know and trust one another.

Storming

The storming phase focuses on power and control issues. Members use testing behaviours around boundaries, communication styles, and personal reactions with other members and the leader. Conflict amongst group members can occur in this phase. Conflict occurs within any human relationship and is explored in Chapter 14. Characteristic

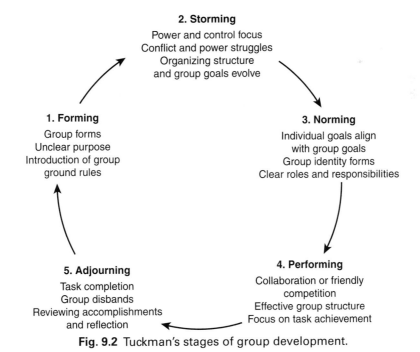

Fig. 9.2 Tuckman's stages of group development.

behaviours may include disagreement with the group format, topics for discussion, the best ways to achieve group goals, and comparisons of member contributions. Setting group goals evolves from a brainstorming discussion in which members generate alternative concerns that the group might persue. The next step is to choose the most promising issues to focus on as top priorities that the group feels it can address. Although the storming phase is uncomfortable, successful resolution leads to the development of group-specific norms.

Norming

In the norming phase, individual goals become aligned with group goals. Group-specific norms help create a supportive group climate characterized by dependable fellowship and purpose. These norms make the group "safe," and members begin to experience the cohesiveness of the group as "their group." The group holds its members accountable and challenges individual members who fail to adhere to expected norms.

Brainstorming consists of the group members thinking of as many ideas as possible related to meeting the group's goals and resolving an identified issue. Criticism of any ideas or statements of judgement is not permitted in the early stages of brainstorming. Later, the group members begin to prioritize which potential solutions are the most workable. When using brainstorming, it is important to be aware that the first few ideas can cause participants to limit their ideas to those ones or not listen to others ideas. It is important for the facilitator to ensure that all the ideas are described by participants and considered (McShane et al., 2015).

Cohesiveness is defined as the relational bonds that link members of a group to one another and to the group as a whole. A sense of interconnection is the basis for group identity. It is an essential characteristic of optimum group productivity. It develops when all group members accept group-specific behavioural standards as operational norms for the group and view the group as a united whole. Sources of cohesiveness include shared goals, working through and solving problems, and the nature of group interaction.

Performing

Most of a group's work gets accomplished in the performing phase. This phase of group development is characterized by interdependence, acceptance of each member as a person of value, and the development of group cohesion. Members feel loyal to the group and engaged in its work. They are comfortable taking risks and are invested enough in one another and the group process to offer constructive comments without fearing criticism from other members.

Adjourning

Tuckman introduced the adjourning phase at a later date, as a final phase of group development (Tuckman & Jensen, 1977). This phase is characterized by reviewing what has been accomplished, reflecting on the meaning of the group's work together, creating deliverables, and making plans to move on in different directions.

Group Role Functions

Functional roles differ from the positional roles that group members assume. Group roles relate to the type of member contributions needed to achieve group goals. Benne and Sheats (1948), in their seminal work that is still being used today, describe constructive role functions as the behaviours members use to move toward goal achievement (task functions) and behaviours designed to ensure personal satisfaction (maintenance functions).

Balance between task and maintenance functions increases group productivity. When task functions predominate, member satisfaction decreases, and a collaborative atmosphere is diminished. When maintenance functions override task functions, members have trouble reaching goals. Members do not confront controversial issues, so the creative tension needed for successful group accomplishment is compromised. Task and maintenance role functions found in successful small groups are listed in Box 9.1.

Benne and Sheats (1948) also identified nonfunctional role functions. Self-roles are roles a person unconsciously uses to meet self-needs at the expense of other members' needs, group values, and goal achievement. Self-roles, identified in Table 9.3, detract from the group's work and compromise goal achievement by taking time away from group issues and creating discomfort among group members.

APPLICATIONS TO HEALTH-RELATED GROUPS

In clinical settings, a health-related group purpose and goals dictate group structure, membership, and format. For example, a group of people recently diagnosed with diabetes would have an educational purpose. A group for parents with critically ill children would have a family support design, while a therapy group would have restorative healing functions. Activity groups are used therapeutically with children and people with mental health issues who have difficulty fully expressing themselves verbally. In an education group, exploration of personal feelings would be limited and related to the topic under discussion. In a therapy group, such probing would be encouraged.

BOX 9.1 Task and Maintenance Functions in Group Dynamics

Task Functions: Behaviours Relevant to the Attainment of Group Goals

- **Initiating:** Identifies tasks or goals; defines group problem; suggests relevant strategies for solving problem
- **Seeking information or opinion:** Requests facts from other members; asks other members for opinions; seeks suggestions or ideas for task accomplishment
- **Giving information or opinion:** Offers facts to other members; provides useful information about group concerns
- **Clarifying, elaborating:** Interprets ideas or suggestions placed before group; paraphrases key ideas; defines terms; adds information
- **Summarizing:** Pulls related ideas together; restates key ideas; offers a group solution or suggestion for other members to accept or reject
- **Consensus taking:** Checks to see whether group has reached a conclusion; asks group to test a possible decision.

Maintenance Functions: Behaviours That Help the Group Maintain Harmonious Working Relationships

- **Harmonizing:** Attempts to reconcile disagreements; helps members reduce conflict and explore differences in a constructive manner.
- **Gatekeeping:** Helps keep communication channels open; points out commonalties in remarks; suggests approaches that permit greater sharing.
- **Encouraging:** Indicates by words and body language unconditional acceptance of others; agrees with contributions of other group members; is warm, friendly, and responsive to other group members.
- **Compromising:** Admits mistakes; offers a concession when appropriate; modifies position in the interest of group cohesion.
- **Setting standards:** Calls for the group to reassess or confirm implicit and explicit group norms when appropriate.

Note: Every group needs both types of functions and needs to work out a satisfactory balance of task and maintenance activity.

Modified from Rogers, C. (1972). The process of the basic encounter group. In R. Diedrich & H. A. Dye (Eds.), *Group procedures: Purposes, processes and outcomes.* Houghton Mifflin.

TABLE 9.3 Nonfunctional Self-Roles

Role	Characteristics
Aggressor	Criticizes or blames others, personally attacks other members, uses sarcasm and hostility in interactions
Blocker	Instantly rejects ideas or argues an idea, cites tangential ideas and opinions, obstructs decision making
Joker	Disrupts work of the group by constantly joking and refusing to take group tasks seriously
Avoider	Whispers to others, daydreams, doodles, acts indifferent and passive
Self-confessor	Uses the group to express personal views and feelings unrelated to group tasks
Recognition	Seeks attention by excessive talking, tries to gain leader's favour, expressing extreme ideas or demonstrating strange behaviours

Modified from Benne, K. D., & Sheats, P. (1948). Functional roles of group members. *Journal of Social Issues, 4*(2), 41–49.

Group Membership

Therapeutic and support groups are categorized as closed or open groups, and as having homogeneous or heterogeneous membership (Corey & Corey, 2013). Closed therapeutic groups have a selected membership with an expectation of regular attendance for an extended time period. Group members may be added, but their inclusion depends on a match with group-defined criteria. Most psychotherapy groups fall into this category. Open groups do not have a defined membership. Most community support groups are open groups. Individuals come and go depending on their needs. One week, the group might consist of two or three members and the next week, 15 members. Some groups, such as Alcoholics Anonymous, have open meetings that anyone can attend and "closed" meetings that only members who misuse alcohol can attend.

Having a homogeneous or heterogeneous membership identifies member characteristics. *Homogeneous* groups share common characteristics—for example, diagnosis (e.g., breast cancer support group) or personal attribute (e.g., gender, age). Twelve-step programs for alcohol or drug addiction, eating disorders, and gender-specific consciousness-raising groups are examples of homogeneous groups. Psychoeducation (e.g., groups for people with mental health issues) groups often have a homogeneous membership related to a particular illness.

Heterogeneous groups represent a wider diversity of member characteristics and personal issues. Members vary in age, gender, and psychodynamics (unconscious and conscious mental and emotional forces that make up personality and motivation). Most psychotherapy and insight-oriented personal growth groups have a heterogeneous membership. Psychotherapy aims to improve an individual's well-being and mental health. Psychotherapy groups focus on specific issues such as depression, social anxiety, chronic pain, esteem issues, and grieving.

Creating the Group Environment

Privacy and freedom from interruption are key considerations in selecting an appropriate location. A sign on the door indicating that the group is in session is essential for privacy. Seating should be comfortable and arranged in a circle so that each member has face-to-face contact with all other members. Being able to see facial expressions and respond to several individuals at one time is essential to effective group communication. Often, group members choose the same seats in therapy groups. When a member is absent, that seat is left vacant.

Therapy groups usually meet weekly, at a set time. Support groups meet at regular intervals, more often monthly. Educational groups meet for a predetermined number of sessions and then disband. Unlike individual sessions, which can be convened spontaneously in emergency situations, therapeutic groups meet only at designated times. Most therapeutic and support groups meet for 60 to 90 minutes on a regular basis, with established, agreed-on meeting times. Groups that begin and end on time foster trust and predictability.

GROUP LEADERSHIP

Group leadership is based on two assumptions: (1) group leaders have a significant influence on group process; and (2) most issues in groups can be avoided or reworked productively if the leader is aware of and responsive to the needs of individual group members, including the needs of the leader (Corey & Corey, 2013).

Effective leadership requires adequate knowledge of the topic, preparation, professional attitudes and behaviour, responsible selection of members, and an evidence-informed approach. Personal characteristics demonstrated by effective group leaders include commitment to the group purpose; self-awareness of personal biases and interpersonal limitations, careful preparation of the group, and an accepting attitude toward group members. Knowledge of group dynamics, training, and supervision are additional

requirements for leaders of psychotherapy groups. Health education group leaders need to have expertise about the topic to be discussed.

Throughout the group's life, the group leader models an attitude of caring, objectivity, and integrity. Effective leaders are good listeners; they can adapt their leadership style to fit the changing needs of the group. They respectfully support the reliability of group members as equal partners in meeting group goals. Successful leaders trust the group process enough to know that group members can work through conflict and difficult situations. The bonds that build between group members are real. Leaders know that even mistakes can be temporary setbacks and can be used for discussion to promote group member growth (Rubel & Kline, 2008).

INFORMAL GROUP LEADERS

Informal power is given to members who best clarify the needs of the other group members or who move the group toward goal achievement. Informal leaders develop within the group because they have a good grasp of the situational demands of the task at hand. They are not always the group members making the most statements. Some individuals, due to the force of their personalities, knowledge, or experience, will emerge as informal leaders within the group.

Ideally, group leadership is a shared function of all group members, with many opportunities for different informal leaders to divide up responsibility for achieving group goals.

Emergent informal leaders become the voice of the group. Their comments are equated with those of the designated leader. Emergent leaders are more willing to take an active role in making a recommendation and generally move the group task forward.

Case Example

Sahid is a powerful informal leader in a job search support group. Although he makes few comments, he has an excellent understanding of and sensitivity to the needs of individual members. When these are violated, Sahid speaks up, and the group listens.

Co-Leadership

Co-leadership represents a form of shared leadership found primarily in therapy and support groups. It is desirable for several reasons. The co-leader adds another perspective related to processing group dynamics. Co-leaders can provide a wider variety of responses and viewpoints that can be helpful to group members. When one leader is being challenged, it can increase the other leader's confidence, knowing that an opportunity to process the session afterward is available.

Respecting and valuing each other, with sensitivity to a co-leader's style of communication, is characteristic of effective co-leadership (Corey & Corey, 2013). Problems can arise when co-leaders have different theoretical orientations or are competitive with each other. Needing to pursue solo interpretations rather than explore or support the meaning of a co-leader's interventions is distracting to the group. Yalom and Leszcz (2005) state, "You are far better off leading a solo group with good supervision than being locked into an incompatible co-therapy relationship" (p. 447).

Co-leaders should spend sufficient preparation time together prior to meeting with a therapy group to ensure personal compatibility and come to consensus regarding an understanding of the group purpose. Co-leaders need to process group dynamics together, preferably after each meeting. Processing group dynamics allows leaders to consider different meanings and evaluate what happened in the group session and what might need to be addressed to productively move the group ahead.

APPLICATIONS

Therapeutic Groups

Group communication is more complex than individual conversations because each member brings a different set of perspectives, perception of reality, communication style, and personal agenda to the group. It can also be a more powerful communication method. Counselman (2008) refers to the power of a group as being able to resonate with a member's experience, change behaviours, and strengthen emotions as being unparalleled. "Group demonstrates that there truly are multiple realities" (p. 270).

A major difference between group and individual communication is that the leader relates to the group as a whole instead of with only one person. The leader joins member responses and themes together and points to conversational differences as providing broader information. Instead of immediately responding to individual members, group leaders highlight different options by engaging additional group responses.

Making important connections among multiple realities offers different possibilities to individual people to learn about and test out new interpersonal communication skills. Table 9.4 displays therapeutic factors found in therapeutic group formats.

Pregroup Interview

Adequate preparation of group members in pregroup interviews enhances the effectiveness of therapeutic groups (Yalom & Leszcz, 2005). A pregroup interview makes the transition into the group easier as group members have an initial connection with the leader and an opportunity to ask questions before committing to the group. Reservations held by either the leader or potential group member are handled beforehand. The description of the group and its members should be short and simple as this information will be repeated in initial meetings.

Forming Phase

How well leaders initially prepare themselves and group members has a direct impact on building the trust needed within the group (Corey & Corey, 2013). The forming phase in therapeutic groups focuses on helping people establish trust in the group and with one another. Communication is tentative. Members are asked to introduce themselves and share a little of their background or reason for coming to the group. An introductory prompt such as, "What would you most like to get out of this group?" helps members link personal goals to group goals.

In the first session, the leader introduces group goals. Clear group goals are particularly important to provide a frame for the group in its initial session. Even if the members know one another, it is helpful to ask each group member to introduce themselves and tell what they would like to get out of the experience. The leader clarifies how the group will be conducted and what the group can expect from the leader and from each other, regarding group goals. Orienting statements may need to be restated in subsequent early sessions, especially if there is a lot of anxiety in the group.

The leader also introduces universal behavioural norms such as confidentiality, regular attendance, and mutual respect (Corey & Corey, 2013). Confidentiality is harder to implement with group formats because members are not held to the same professional ethical standards as the group leader. However, for the integrity of the group, all members need to commit to confidentiality as a universal group norm (Lasky & Riva, 2006).

Storming Phase

The storming phase focuses on the differences among group members rather than the commonalities. It is usually characterized by some disagreements among group members. This is normal behaviour as group members feel more comfortable with expressing authentic opinions. The leader plays an important facilitative role in the storming phase by accepting differences in member perceptions as being expected and growth producing. By affirming genuine but different strengths in individual members, leaders model handling conflict with productive outcomes. Linking constructive themes while identifying the nature

TABLE 9.4   Therapeutic Factors in Groups

Installation of hope	Occurs when members see others who have overcome problems and are successfully managing their lives
Universality	Sharing common situations validates member experience, decreases sense of isolation: "Maybe I am not the only one with this issue."
Imparting information	New shared information is a resource for individual members and stimulates further discussion and the learning of new skills.
Imitative behaviour	Members learn new behaviours through observation and the modelling of desired actions and gain confidence in trying them—e.g., managing conflict, receiving constructive criticism.
Socialization	Group provides a safe learning environment in which to take interpersonal risks and try new behaviours
Interpersonal learning	Group acts as a social microcosm; focus is on members learning about how they interact and getting constructive feedback and support from others
Cohesiveness	Sense of "we"-ness. Emphasizes personal bonds and commitment to the group. Members feel acceptance and trust from others. Cohesiveness serves as the foundation for all curative factors.
Catharsis	Expression of emotion that leads to receiving support and acceptance from other group members
Corrective recapitulation of primary family	Allows for recognition and handling of transference issues in therapy groups. This helps group members avoid repeating destructive interaction patterns in the "here and now."
Altruism	Providing help and support to other group members enhances personal self-esteem.
Existential factors	Highlights primary responsibility for taking charge of one's life and the consequences of their actions, creating a meaningful existence

Adapted from Yalom, I., & Leszcz, M. (2005). *The theory and practice of group psychotherapy* (5th ed.). Basic Books.

of the disagreement is an effective modelling strategy. These discussions are important. However, if members test boundaries through discriminatory or sexually provocative statements, flattery, or insulting remarks, the leader should step in immediately and promptly set limits. Refer to the work of the group as being of the highest priority, and respectfully ask the person to align remarks with the group purpose. Working through conflicts allows members to take stands on their personal preferences without being defensive and to compromise when needed. Conflict issues in groups inform what is important to group members and how individual members handle difficult emotions. Resolution leads to the development of cohesion.

Norming Phase

Once initial conflict is resolved in the storming phase, the group moves into the norming phase. Tasks in the norming phase centre on the development of the implicit group-developed rules governing their group behaviours. Group-specific norms develop spontaneously through group-member interactions. They represent the group's shared expectations of its members. For example, lateness may not be tolerated. The group leader encourages member contributions and emphasizes cooperation in recognizing each person's talents and contributions related to group goals. Successful short-term groups focus on here-and-now interactions, giving practical feedback, sharing personal thoughts and feelings, and listening to one another (Corey & Corey, 2013).

Cohesion begins to develop as a sharing of feelings deepens the trust in the group as a safe place. *Cohesion* describes the emotional bonds members have for one another, and underscores the level of member commitment to the group (Yalom & Leszcz, 2005). Research suggests that cohesive groups experience more personal satisfaction with goal achievement and that members of such groups are more likely to join other group relationships. In a cohesive group, members demonstrate a sense of common purpose, a caring commitment to one another, collaborative problem solving, a sense of feeling personally valued, and a team spirit (Powles, 2007). Teams with higher cohesion tend to perform better than teams with lower cohesion (McShane et al., 2015). See Box 9.2 for communication principles that facilitate cohesiveness.

BOX 9.2   Communication Principles to Facilitate Cohesiveness

- Group tasks should be within the membership's range of ability and expertise.
- Comments and responses should be non-evaluative, focused on behaviours rather than on personal characteristics.
- The leader should identify group accomplishments and acknowledge member contributions.
- The leader should be empathetic and assist members in giving effective feedback.
- The leader should help group members view and work through creative tension as being a valuable part of goal achievement.

Performing Phase

The performing phase is similar to the working phase in individual relationships; members focus on problem solving and developing new behaviours. It is during this phase that the group's serious work takes centre stage. The group leader is responsible for keeping the group on task to accomplish group goals. Group members are responsible for working with the group leader(s) to maintain a supportive group-work environment. If group members seem to be moving off track, foreward movement can be restored through asking open-ended questions or verbally observing group processes. Modelling respect, empathy, inclusivity, appropriate self-disclosure, and ethical standards helps ensure a supportive group climate. Working together and participating in another person's personal growth allows members to experience one another's personal strengths and the collective caring of the group. Of all the possible interactions in a group, individual members report feeling affirmed and respected by other group members as being most valuable.

Because members function interdependently, they are able to work through disagreements and difficult issues in ways that are acceptable to each individual and the group. Effective group leaders trust group members to develop their own solutions, but they call attention to important group dynamics when needed. This can be introduced with a simple statement, such as, "I wonder what is going on here right now" (Rubel & Kline, 2008). Feedback should be descriptive and specific to the immediate discussion. As with other types of constructive feedback, the feedback should focus only on modifiable behaviours. Think about how you can word your message so that it helps a member better understand the impact of a behaviour, make sense of an experience, and grow from the experience.

Monopolizing

Monopolizing is a negative form of power communication used to advance a personal agenda without considering the needs of others. It may not be intentional but rather a member's way of handling anxiety. When one member monopolizes the conversation, there are several ways the leader can respond. Acknowledging this person's contribution and broadening the input with a short, open-ended question, such as, "Has anyone else had a similar experience?" can redirect the attention to the larger group. Looking in the direction of other group members as the statements are made encourages alternative member responses. If a member continues to monopolize the conversation, the leader can respectfully acknowledge the person's comment and refocus the issue within the group directly. "I appreciate your thoughts, but I think it would be important to hear from other people as well. What do you think about this, Farzana?" or "We don't have much time left; I wonder if anyone else has a comment or something they need to talk about."

Adjourning Phase

The final phase of group development—termination or adjournment—ideally occurs when the group members have achieved desired outcomes. The termination phase is about task completion and disengagement. The leader encourages the group members to express their feelings about one another with the requirement that any concerns the group may have about an individual member or suggestions for future growth be stated in a constructive way. The leader should present their comments last and then close the group with a summary of goal achievement. By waiting until the group ends to share closing comments, the leader has an opportunity to soften or clarify previous comments and connect cognitive and feeling elements that need to be addressed. The leader needs to remind members that the norm of confidentiality continues after the group ends (Mangione et al., 2007). Referrals are handled on an individual, as-needed basis. Simulation Exercise 9.5 considers group closure issues.

TYPES OF THERAPEUTIC GROUPS

The group provides a microcosm of social dynamics in the larger world. Individuals tend to act in groups as they do in real life. Through group participation, people can learn how others respond to them in a safe learning environment. A group dynamic that allows member to feel supported and accepted can help reduce stigma and isolation (Centre for Addiction and Mental Health [CAMH], 2020). The group also provides an opportunity for individual members to practice new and different interpersonal skills (interpersonal learning).

The term *therapeutic*, as it applies to group relationships, refers to more than treatment of emotional and behavioural disorders. In today's health care arena, short-term groups

SIMULATION EXERCISE 9.5   Group Closure Activities

Purpose

To develop closure skills in small-group communication

Procedure

1. Focus your attention on the group member next to you and think about what you like about the person, how you see them in the group, and what you might wish for for that person as a member of the group.

2. After five minutes, your instructor will ask you to tell the person next to you to use the three themes in making a statement about the person. For example, "The thing I most like about you in the group is . . ."; "To me, you represent the _____ in the group"; and so on.

3. When all of the group members have had a turn, start the discussion.

Discussion

1. How did you feel telling someone about your response to them in the group?

2. What did it feel like being the group member receiving the message?

3. What did you learn about yourself from doing this exercise?

4. What implications does this exercise have for future interactions in group relationships?

---

are designed for a wide range of different populations as a first-line therapeutic intervention to either address issues or prevent them (Corey & Corey, 2013). Therapeutic groups offer a structured format that encourages people to experience their natural healing potential (instillation of hope) and achieve higher levels of functioning. Other group members provide ideas and reinforce individual group members' strength.

Therapeutic groups provide reality testing. People under stress lose perspective. For example, other group members can gently challenge cognitive distortions carried over from previous damaging relationships such as the impact of family dynamics and harmful childhood experiences. Within the safety of the group, the member can learn new behaviours rather the unhelpful patterns learned as a child, while receiving support through validation and empathy. Because of the nature of a therapy group, group members can say things to the person that friends and relatives are afraid or unable to say—and they are able to do so in a compassionate, constructive way. It becomes difficult for a troubled member to deny or turn aside the constructive observations and suggestions of five to six people who know and care about the member.

Inpatient Therapy Groups

Therapy groups in inpatient settings are designed to stabilize the person's behaviour enough for them to functionally transition back into the community. Here-and-now group interaction is the primary vehicle of treatment (Beiling et al., 2009). Since hospitalizations are brief, people attend focused therapy groups on a daily basis. The goal of inpatient therapy is to increase the person's awareness of themselves through interactions with group members who provide feedback about their behaviour, assist with their interpersonal social skills, and help them feel less isolated

(Koukourikos & Pasmatzi, 2014). When situations cannot be changed, psychotherapy groups help the person attend to this reality and move on with their lives by empowering and supporting their efforts to make constructive behavioural changes. The value of a short-term process group is an immediate interaction.

Deering (2014) suggests allowing a theme to emerge and then using it to stimulate interaction about possible ways to handle difficult issues. A hidden benefit of group therapy is the opportunity to experience giving and receiving help from others. Helping others is important, especially for people with low self-esteem, who feel they have little to offer others.

Leading Groups for People With Psychosis

Staff nurses are sometimes called upon to lead or co-lead unit-based group psychotherapy on inpatient units (Clarke et al., 1998). Other times, staff nurses participate in community group meetings comprised mostly of people with psychosis who may see, hear, or believe things that are not real. Because the demands of leadership can be so intense in these types of therapy groups, co-leadership is recommended.

Co-therapists can share the group-process interventions, model healthy behaviours, offset negative **transference** (transferring feelings to the therapist) from group members, and provide useful feedback to each other. Every group session should be processed immediately after its completion.

A directive, but flexible, leadership approach works best with people who have psychosis. Active encouragement of group comments related to relevant concrete topics of potential interest facilitates communication. This strategy is more effective than asking people to share their feelings. For example, the leader could ask the group to discuss how to handle a simple behaviour in a more productive way. This type of discussion allows people to feel more successful with their contributions. Full attention on the speaker and offering praise for their efforts and contributions are useful. Other members can be encouraged to provide feedback, and the group can choose the best solution.

Before the group begins, the leader should remind individual members that the group is about to take place. Some people may want to leave the group before it ends. If the leader views this action as a sign of anxiety, they can gently encourage the person to remain for the duration of the group.

A primary goal in working with people with psychosis is to respect each person as a unique human being with a potentially valuable contribution. Although their needs are disguised as symptoms, you can help people "decode" a psychotic message by uncovering the underlying theme and translating it into understandable language. Or the leader might ask, "I wonder if anyone in the group can help us understand better what Li-Ju is trying to say." Keep in mind how difficult it is for the person to tolerate close interaction and how necessary it is for the person to interact with others if they are to succeed in the outside environment.

Therapeutic Groups in Long-Term Settings

Therapeutic groups in long-term settings offer opportunities for socially isolated individuals to engage with others. Common types of such groups include reminiscence, reality orientation, remotivation groups, resocialization groups, and therapeutic activity groups.

Reminiscence Groups

Reminiscence groups focus on life review and pleasurable memories (Stinson, 2009). They are not designed as insight groups but rather to provide a supportive, ego-enhancing experience. Each group member is expected to share a few memories about a specific weekly group focus (e.g., holidays, first day of school, family photos, songs, favourite foods, pets). The leader encourages discussion. Depending on the cognitive abilities of the group members, the leader will need to be more or less directive. Sessions are held on a weekly basis and meet for an hour.

Reality Orientation Groups

Used with people with confusion, *reality orientation groups* help people maintain contact with the environment and reduce confusion about time, place, and person. Reality orientation groups are usually held each day for 30 minutes. Nurses can use everyday props, such as a calendar, a clock, and pictures of the seasons to stimulate interest. The group should not be seen as an isolated activity; what occurs in the group should be reinforced throughout the

24-hour period. For example, on one unit, nurses placed pictures of the residents in earlier times on the doors to their bedrooms.

Remotivation Groups

Remotivation groups are designed to stimulate thinking about activities required for everyday life. Originally developed by Dorothy Hoskins Smith for use with people with a mental health history, remotivation groups represent an effort to reach the unwounded areas of the person's personality (i.e., those areas and interests that have remained healthy). Remotivation groups focus on tapping into strengths through discussions of realistic scenarios that stimulate and build confidence. They are successfully used in long-term settings, for substance use prevention, with people who have mental health issues, and in combination with recreational therapy (Dyer & Stotts, 2005). Group members focus on a defined, everyday topic, such as the way plants or trees grow, or they might consist of poetry readings or art appreciation. Visual props engage the participants and stimulate more responses.

Resocialization Groups

Resocialization groups are used with older people with confusion, whose cognition may be too limited to allow them to benefit from a remotivation group but who still need companionship and involvement with others. Resocialization groups focus on providing a simple social setting for people to experience basic social skills again—for example, eating a small meal together. Although the senses and cognitive abilities may diminish in older people, basic needs for companionship, interpersonal relationships, and a place where one is accepted and understood remain the same throughout the life span. Improvement of social skills contributes to improved self-esteem.

Therapeutic Activity Groups

Activity groups offer people a variety of self-expressive opportunities, through creative activity rather than through words. They are particularly useful with children and early adolescents (Aronson, 2004). The nurse functions as the group leader, or as a support to other disciplines in encouraging group members' participation. Activity groups include the following types:

- *Occupational therapy* groups allow participants to work on individual projects or to participate with others in learning life skills. Examples are cooking, artwork, making ceramics, and activities of daily living groups. Tasks are selected for their therapeutic value and in response to participants' interests. Life skills groups use a problem-solving approach to help participants successfully negotiate interpersonal situations.

- *Recreational therapy groups* offer opportunities for participants to engage in leisure activities that release energy. This also provides a social format for learning interpersonal skills as some people never learned how to build needed leisure activities into their lives.
- *Exercise or movement therapy groups* allow participants to engage in structured exercise. The nurse models the exercise behaviours, either with or without accompanying music, and encourages participant engagement. This type of group works well with those who have mental health issues and with older people.
- *Art therapy groups* encourage participants to reveal feelings through drawing or painting. It is used in different ways. Participants are able to reveal feelings through expression of colour and abstract forms when they have trouble putting their feelings into words. The art can be the focus of discussion. Children and adolescents may engage in a combined group effort to make a mural.
- *Poetry and bibliotherapy groups* select readings of interest and invite participants to respond to literary works. Reading circles have been found to have significant results in increasing well-being in participants (Pettersson, 2018). Reported results include a decrease in negative emotions by more positive feelings. Art therapy has also been found to promote problem solving and increase compassion, empathy, self-awareness, and getting in touch with their personal creativity (Pehrsson & McMillen, 2007).

Self-Help and Support Groups

Self-help and support groups provide emotional and practical support to people and their families experiencing a health issue, ill health of a family member, or crises. Held mostly in the community, peer support groups are led informally by group members rather than professionals, although often a health provider acts as an adviser. Criteria for membership is having a particular health condition (e.g., cancer, multiple sclerosis) or being a support person (family member of a person with Alzheimer's disease). Self-help groups are voluntary groups, led by consumers and designed to provide peer support for individuals and their families struggling with health issues. Support groups have an informational function in addition to social support (Percy et al., 2009). Nurses are encouraged to learn about support group networks in their communities. Simulation Exercise 9.6 offers an opportunity to learn about them.

Self-help groups are often associated with hospitals, clinics, and national health organizations. They provide a place for people with health care issues to interact with others experiencing similar physical or emotional challenges.

Educational Groups

Community health agencies sponsor educational groups to provide important knowledge about lifestyle changes needed to promote health and prevent illness. For example, family education groups provide families with the

---

SIMULATION EXERCISE 9.6   Learning About Support Groups

Purpose
To provide direct information about support groups in the community

Procedure
1. Assess the social media site for a support group in your community. (Ideally, students will choose different support groups so a variety of groups are shared.)
2. What information did you learn from the website? Was the information easy to find?
3. Directly contact the support group.
4. Identify yourself as a nursing student, and indicate that you are looking at community support groups. Ask for information about the group (e.g., the time and frequency of meetings, purpose and focus of the group, how a person joins the group, who sponsors the group, issues the group might discuss, and cost, if any).
5. Write a two-paragraph report, including the information you gathered, and describe your experience in

searching on the website and asking for the support group information.

Discussion
1. Examine the different information you learned from the social media site and by speaking to someone. Which one was more helpful and why?
2. How did you feel (e.g., anxious, scared) contacting the support group? Did these feelings change once you had finished your discussion?
3. How easy was it for you to obtain information?
4. Were you surprised by any of the informants' answers?
5. If you were a person interested in the group, would the information you obtained inform your decision to join the support group? If not, what else would be important to you?
6. What did you learn from doing this exercise that might be useful in your nursing practice?

knowledge and skills they need to care for a loved one with a health issue such as dementia.

Educational groups are time-limited group applications (e.g., the group might be held for four 1-hour sessions over a 2-week period or as an 2-hour, 8-week seminar). Examples of primary prevention groups are those for help with coping with a chronic illness, childbirth education, parenting, caring for older parents, and stress reduction.

Groups offered after a health crisis such as in myocardial infarction or cerebral vascular accident can offer the person and families effective ways to carry out the therapeutic medical treatment plan, ways to address emotional issues associated with the disease, and rehabilitation information. A typical sequence would be to provide information about the following:

- The disease and how the medical treatment plan works to return to an optimal level of health
- A description of prescribed medications, including purpose, dosage, timing, side effects, and what to do when the person does not take the medication as prescribed
- The rehabilitation plan, and ways to address the emotional issues related to the disease process
- Follow-up appointments, tests, and procedures

Providing written instructions and materials to be read between sessions helps if the educational group is to last more than one session. Take-home activities to be reviewed between sessions can also be beneficial to assess understanding of the information presented during the session and time for the person and family to think about other questions and concerns they may have. Allowing sufficient time for questions and encouraging an open, informal discussion of the topic mobilizes participant energy to share concerns and fears that might not otherwise come to light.

Discussion Groups

Functional elements found in effective discussion groups are found in Table 9.5.

Careful preparation, formulation of relevant questions, and use of feedback ensure that personal learning needs are met in discussion groups. Discussion group topics often include prepared information and group-generated material, which is then discussed in the group. Before the end of each meeting, the leader or a group member should summarize the major themes developed from the content material.

Equal group participation should be a group expectation. Although the level of participation is never quite equal, discussion groups in which only a few members actively participate are disheartening to group members and limited in learning potential. *Social loafing* is when individual group members fail to do their part of the work or skip or come late to group project meetings, and it can be frustrating for other group members (Aggarwal & O'Brien, 2008).

TABLE 9.5   Elements of Successful Discussion Groups

Element	Rationale
Careful preparation	Thoughtful agenda and assignments establish a direction for the discussion and the expected contribution of each member.
Informed participants	Each member should come prepared so that all members are communicating with relatively the same level of information, and each is able to contribute equally.
Shared leadership	Each member is responsible for contributing to the discussion; evidence of members not actively participating is effectively addressed.
Good listening skills	Concentrates on the material, listens to content. Challenges, anticipates, and weighs the evidence; listens between the lines to emotions about the topic
Relevant questions	Focused questions keep the discussion moving toward the meeting objectives.
Useful feedback	Thoughtful feedback maintains the momentum of the discussion by reflecting different perspectives of topics raised and confirming or questioning others' views.

Because the primary purpose of a discussion group is to promote the learning of all group members, members are charged with the responsibility of contributing their ideas and encouraging the participation of more silent members. As an individual group member, make it a practice to make at least one relevant contribution to the discussion in each group session and encourage another group member to participate. This practice will help you develop ease with group discussion, which is one of the most important skills you can develop as a nursing professional.

Cooperation, not competition, needs to be developed as a conscious group norm for all discussion groups. Strategies can include allowing more room for more quiet members by asking for their thoughts or opinions. Sometimes, when verbal participants keep quiet, these group members begin to speak. An invitation, said in a nonthreatening manner and without pressure, can invite the impressions of others—for example, saying, "I wonder what your experience of . . . has been." Simulation Exercise 9.7 provides an opportunity to explore potential group participation issues.

PROFESSIONAL TASK AND WORK GROUPS

Unlike therapeutic groups, task and work groups do not emphasize personal behavioural change as a primary focus (Gladding, 2011). Instead, organizations use work groups to identify problems, plan and implement change, and engage in strategies to more effectively communicate with one another. Groups allow health providers, staff, and involved stakeholders to more quickly develop and implement new evidence-informed initiatives. Work groups (e.g., standing committees, ad hoc task forces, and quality circles) accomplish a wide range of tasks related to organizational goals. Involvement of stakeholders helps ensure the needed buy-in for recommendation acceptance.

SIMULATION EXERCISE 9.7 Addressing Participation Issues in Professional Discussion Groups

Purpose

To provide an opportunity to develop response strategies in difficult group participation issues

Procedure

A class has been assigned a group project for which all participants will receive a common group grade. Develop a group understanding of the feelings experienced in each of the following situations and a way to respond to each. Consider the possible consequences of your intervention in each case.

1. Gavin tells the group that he is working full time and will be unable to make many group meetings. There are so many class requirements that he is not sure he can put much effort into the project, although he would like to help and the project interests him.
2. Nelab is very outspoken in the group. She expresses her opinion about the choice of the group project and is willing to make the necessary contacts. No one challenges her or suggests another project. At the next meeting, she informs the group that the project is all set up and she has made all the arrangements.
3. Mia promises she will have her part of the project completed by a certain date. The date comes, and Mia does not have her part completed.

Discussion

1. Break up into groups of three to four students.
2. What are some actions the participants can take to ensure the group moves forward and successfully completes the project on time?
3. Identify what you would actually say to each participant described above, and then role-play saying it to each other.
4. What group norms could have been established at the beginning to prevent issues like this from occurring?
5. How can you use this exercise as a way of understanding and responding effectively in group projects?

⟫ DEVELOPING AN EVIDENCE-INFORMED PRACTICE

Purpose

The purpose of this study was to explore the impact of interprofessional team composition on team dynamics, related to conflict and open-mindedness. Using a cross-sectional correlational design, survey data from 218 team members of 47 interprofessional teams in an acute care setting were analyzed to investigate two moderated mediation pathways.

Results

Study results demonstrated a significant relationship between interprofessional composition, and affective conflict for teams rated highly for individualized professional identification. Findings also indicated that professional diversity can have a dysfunctional effect on debate and open-mindedness.

Practice Implications

Study results indicate the need to develop a shared group identity with reinforcement of shared values related to person care, as a means of improving interprofessional team communication dynamics.

Mitchell, R., Parker, V., Giles, M. et al. (2014). The ABC of health care team dynamics: Understanding complex affective, behavioural, and cognitive dynamics in interprofessional teams. *Health Care Management Review, 39*(1), 1–9.

Work groups are an embedded part of a larger organizational system, operating within a smaller, work-related political culture. The small group operates as an adaptive open system (Beebe & Masterson, 2014; Tubbs, 2011). All aspects of group work should incorporate the values, norms, general mission, and philosophy of the larger work system. Group strategies, group activities, and methods of evaluation should be congruent with the philosophy and goals of the larger organizational system to achieve maximum success (Mathieu et al., 2008).

Work groups are concerned with content and process. The content (task) is predetermined by organizational parameters or the group's purpose. Effective group leaders need to have a strong working knowledge of task expectations and their relationship to existing tasks. Having sufficient available resources in terms of time, information, member expertise, resources, and appropriate funding where necessary, is essential to achieving successful outcomes. Group membership should reflect stakeholders and key informants with the different knowledge and skill set expertise needed to accomplish group goals. Essential member matching with task requirements includes matching with the following:

- Group goals
- Identified expectations for group achievement
- Capacity for ensuring deliverables
- Availability

Task groups usually take place within specified time frames and need consistent administrative support to flourish. Table 9.6 lists characteristics of effective versus ineffective task groups.

Leadership Styles

Effective **leadership** develops from leader characteristics, situational features, and members working together. The types of leadership styles found in groups are authoritarian, democratic, transformational, and laissez-faire. Leaders demonstrating an **authoritarian leadership** style take full responsibility for group direction and control group interaction. Authoritarian leadership styles work best when the group needs a strong structure to function and there is limited time to reach a decision. **Democratic leadership** is a form of participatory leadership, which involves members in active discussion and shared decision making (Rothwell, 2013). Democratic leaders are goal-directed but flexible. They offer members a functional structure while preserving individual member autonomy. Group members feel ownership of group solutions. Transformational leadership is similar to democratic leadership in that the leader is inspirational and focuses on motivating the group members to achieve a high level of performance in achieving group goals, through collaboration, creativity, and raising

TABLE 9.6 Characteristics of Effective and Ineffective Work Groups

Effective Groups	Ineffective Groups
Goals are clearly identified and collaboratively developed.	Goals are vague or imposed on the group without discussion.
Open, goal-directed communication of feelings and ideas is encouraged.	Communication is guarded; feelings are not always given attention.
Power is equally shared and rotates among members, depending on ability and group needs.	Power resides in the leader or is delegated with little regard to member needs; it is not shared.
Decision making is flexible and adapted to group needs.	Decision making occurs with little or no consultation. Consensus is expected rather than negotiated based on data.
Controversy is viewed as healthy because it builds member involvement and creates stronger solutions.	Controversy and open conflict are not tolerated.
There is a healthy balance between task and maintenance role functioning.	There is a one-sided focus on task or maintenance role functions to the exclusion of the complementary function.
Individual contributions are acknowledged and respected. Diversity is encouraged.	Individual resources are not used. Conformity and being an "organizational person" is rewarded; diversity is not respected.
Interpersonal effectiveness, innovation, and problem-solving adequacy are evident.	Problem-solving abilities, morale, and interpersonal effectiveness are low and undervalued.

questions (Gaudine & Lamb, 2015). **Laissez-faire leadership** is more "hands off" in that the group leader allows group members to decide on how to complete the task within the defined time frame. This type of leadership has been criticized because the leader is seen as disengaged, leading to role confusion and decreased productivity. However, laissez-faire leadership can be effective with groups who are experts in their fields and independent and creative in using their resourcefulness to accomplish group goals.

Another way to look at leadership styles in professional group life is by using a situational framework (Blanchard et al., 2013). This format requires group leaders to match their leadership style to the situation and the maturity of the group members. A situational leadership style can be particularly adaptive in organizational group life when a new project is the object of group focus. The situational leader varies the amount of direction and support to a group based on the complexity of the task and the followers' experience and confidence with achieving task or group goals.

Group maturity involves two forms of maturity: job maturity and psychological maturity related to the work. Job maturity refers to the level of group members' knowledge, work abilities, and skills, which are often consistent with job experience. Psychological job maturity refers to the group members' feelings of confidence, willingness, and motivation. The capacity and readiness of situational maturity play a role in the type of preferred leadership style necessary to accomplish goals. A basic assumption about leadership is that it should be flexible and adapted to group needs.

Effective leaders adapt to the amount of structure required by changes in the group's maturity in working together. As the group matures, leaders turn more of the responsibility for the group's productivity over to its members. Decision making is collaborative. The leader seeks member input, acts as a discussion facilitator, and seeks consensus.

Leader and Member Responsibilities

Leadership tasks in work groups include the following:
- Forming the group structure
- Clarifying the group's tasks and goals (providing background data and material if needed)
- Group facilitation to ensure active participation of group members in accomplishment of tasks
- Motivation and establishing a positive atmosphere
- Overseeing group processes, and supporting individual group members where needed
- Ensuring the group stays focused on achieving the group goals and meeting established deadlines
- Administrative roles such as establishing meeting dates, agendas, and how minutes will be taken

Group members should take responsibility for coming prepared to meetings, demonstrating respect for other members' ideas, and taking an active participatory role in the development of viable solutions. Affirming the

contributions of team members helps build cohesion and investment in ensuring productive outcomes.

Task Groups

Pregroup Tasks

Successful work groups do not just happen. Before the group starts, participants should have a clear idea of what the group task commitment will entail in terms of time, effort, and knowledge—and be willing to commit to the task. Selected group members should have the experience, and enough in common, to engage in meaningful communication, relevant knowledge of the issues or expertise needed for resolution, a willingness to make a contribution to the group solution, and the ability to complete the task.

Effective Group Planning

Effective planning should be considered a major focus of and reason for participating in work groups. Successful outcomes reflect the responsible engagement of group members and careful planning. Berger (2014) defines planning as "a process that produces a plan or plans as its product" and suggests focusing on the processes in planning by these actions:
- Assessing the situation
- Deciding what goal or goals to pursue
- Creating or retrieving plans
- Executing them (p. 91)

Group communication is a thoughtful endeavor. The group leader should come to each meeting prepared with a clear agenda and an overview of key issues and member concerns. Inviting members to submit agenda items and involving others in developing an agenda stimulates interest and commitment. The plan is more likely to become about how to accomplish "our project" rather than a doing a set of tasks. Nothing is more compelling than enthusiasm backed by facts and a willingness to work together with others to make something important happen. The outcome is also usually better because it is the result of input from all group members.

Structural Group Development

Forming Phase

Even if members are known to one another, it is useful to have each person give a brief introduction that includes their reason for being part of the work group. The leader should explain the group's purpose and structural components (e.g., time, place, and commitment) and ask for commitment of the group members. Member responsibilities should be outlined clearly, with time for questions. A task group with vague or poorly understood goals or structure can create confusion, boredom or frustration, leading to power struggles and inadequate task resolution.

Storming Phase

The storming phase is marked by conflict amongst team members as their personalities emerge, offering divergent opinions and ideas, during which members may try to influence or control how the task will be achieved. Competition for team roles, resistance to change, and lack of understanding of the group purpose and goals can also occur. The leader's role should focus on supporting the group in resolving the interpersonal conflict, and creating an environment that is supportive and in which it is safe to express different points of view. The leader can also assist members to begin establishing norms of appropriate expectations and behaviours to accomplish the task.

Norming Phase

To be successful, group norms should support accomplishment of stated goals. Norms are the informal rules and expectations of each other in the group. They are used to guide and facilitate team behaviours that are important to group process and how members interact with one another. Norms are established when the team is forming by clearly establishing acceptable group behaviours such as being respectful, accountable for contributing to the group goal,

and prepared, and by attending meetings. The leader guides the discussion of the creation of norms for the group.

Performing Phase

Most of the group's work to meet the team goals gets accomplished in the performing phase. Leader interventions should focus on supporting the team through encouragement, and providing knowledge and feedback when necessary, using well-defined communications.

Brainstorming

Brainstorming is a commonly employed strategy used to generate solutions during the performing phase. Guidelines for brainstorming include the following:
- Entertaining all ideas without criticism or critique
- Testing the more-promising ideas for relevance
- Exploring the consequences of each potential solution
- Identifying human and instrumental resources, including availability and feasibility
- Achieving agreement about the best-possible solutions.
Simulation Exercise 9.8 provides an opportunity to experience brainstorming.

Groupthink

Extreme cohesiveness can result in negative group phenomena, referred to as **groupthink**. Originally defined by Janis

---

SIMULATION EXERCISE 9.8 Brainstorming: Selecting Alternative Strategies

Purpose
To help students use a brainstorming process for considering and prioritizing alternative options

Procedure
You have two exams and one paper due this week. You need to do groceries and get some food. Work is asking you to come in for an extra shift. Your significant other is complaining that you are ignoring them. Because of all the work you have been doing, you have not had time to call your parents and they are not happy with you. Your laundry is overflowing on the floor and you have no clean clothes to wear. Several of your friends have decided to go to a movie and dinner and want you to go along. How can you handle it all?

1. Give yourself approximately 5 minutes to write down all the ideas that come to mind for handling these multiple responsibilities. Use single words or phrases to express your ideas. Do not eliminate any possibilities, even if they seem farfetched.

2. In groups of three or four students, choose someone to write down all the strategies. Each person then shares all their ideas.
3. Once all the ideas are written down, discuss the relevant pros and cons of each one.
4. Select the three most promising ideas.
5. Develop several small, concrete, achievable actions to implement these ideas.
6. Share the small group findings with the class group.

Discussion
1. In what ways were the solutions you chose similar or dissimilar to those of your peers?
2. Were any of your ideas or ways of achieving alternative solutions surprising to you or to others in your group?
3. What did you think about the process and the final three most promising ideas?
4. If you are working as a nurse with a person you are providing care for, what could you take from doing this exercise to generate possible solutions to seemingly impossible situations?

(1982), this interpersonal situation represents "a mode of thinking that people engage in when they are deeply involved in a cohesive in-group, when the members' strivings for unanimity override their motivation to realistically appraise alternative courses of action" (p. 9). Symptoms of groupthink occur when the approval of other group members becomes so important that it overrides a reasonable decision-making process or presents a group outcome that group members fundamentally do not agree with but agree with for the sake of harmony. Realistic evaluation of issues does not occur because group members minimize the conflict in an effort to reach consensus. Warning signs of groupthink are listed in Box 9.3. Groupthink can create dissatisfaction with goal achievement and produce unworkable solutions. Fig. 9.3 displays the characteristics of groupthink.

BOX 9.3   Warning Signs of Groupthink

1. Illusion of invulnerability and overconfidence
2. Collective rationalization that disregards warnings
3. Belief in inherent morality of the decision
4. Stereotyped or negative views of people outside of the group
5. Direct pressure on dissenters to not express their concerns
6. Self-censorship—individual members with doubts do not express them
7. Illusion of unanimity in which majority view is held to be unanimous
8. Self-appointed "mind guards" within the group who withhold data that would be problematic or contradictory to the groupthink activities

Adapted from Janis, I. (1982). Groupthink: Psychological studies of policy decisions and fiascoes (2nd ed.). Houghton Mifflin.

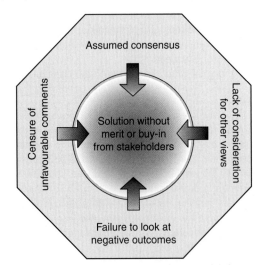

Fig. 9.3 Characteristics of groupthink.

Norms that diminish the potential impact of groupthink allow members to do the following:
- Hold different opinions from other group members
- Seek fresh information and outside opinions
- Create openness and group debate by bringing forward new ideas

Adjourning Phase

Termination in work groups takes place when the group task is accomplished or at a designated ending time established earlier in the group's life. As the group moves toward its close, the leader should summarize the work of the group, allow time for processing the level of goal achievement, and identify any need for follow-up. Task groups typically disband once their goal is achieved. They should not simply move on into a never-ending commitment without negotiation and the agreement of participants to continue with another assignment.

Groups Versus Teams

Teams and groups have certain characteristics in common, but there also are some clear differences. Team communication occurs as a continuous communication thread, with multiple levels of formal and informal working arrangements (see Chapter 24). The development and implementation of collaborative, multiskilled, intra- and interprofessional teams are a key priority in providing safe, quality, person-centred care.

Forsyth (2018) maintains that while teams are fundamentally groups having similar characteristics of interdependence, structure, and ways of interacting, there are notable differences. A health care team differs from a group in distinctive ways. First and foremost, it acts as a single coordinated unit of intra- and interprofessional providers. Team members have complementary knowledge, skills and management responsibilities related to person care as their deliverable goal. They share accountability for goal achievement as an intra- or interprofessional team (or both) (Beebe & Masterson, 2014).

On an ongoing team with no defined end, members are expected to develop shared meanings related to defined health goals, achieve consensus and constructively manage conflict, coordinate their actions, and offer interpersonal support to one another. Implementation takes place through actions related to specified health goals. Communication takes place through electronic channels and face-to-face communication (see Chapter 24 for details on team communication).

The involved person and family are considered part of the health team. Team roles, functions, and provider contributions are interconnected and reinforce each other in completing the work of the team, whose goal is to achieve desired clinical outcomes. Discussion in team meetings focuses on collaborative problem solving and decision making, always with the goal of achieving effective coordination and implementation of quality person-centred care.

Group member composition is different for intra- and interprofessional health care teams than for task or other types of work groups. The team brings together people with individual knowledge, skills, and abilities to function as a clinical unit, with collaborative specialized tasks related to common person-centred health goals. The number of members varies, and team composition needs to reflect specific health-related goals.

SUMMARY

This chapter looks at the ways in which a group experience enhances people's abilities to meet therapeutic self-care demands, provides meaning, and is personally affirming. The rationale for providing a group experience for people is described. Group dynamics include individual member commitment, functional similarity, and leadership style. Group concepts related to group dynamics consist of purpose, norms, cohesiveness, roles, and role functions.

Tuckman's phases of group development—forming, storming, norming, performing, and adjourning—are discussed. In the forming phase of group relationships, the basic need is for acceptance. The storming phase focuses on issues of power and control in groups. Behavioural standards are formed in the norming phase that will guide the group toward goal accomplishment, when the group becomes a safe environment in which to work and express feelings. Most of the group's work is accomplished during the performing phase. In health-related therapeutic groups, feelings of warmth, caring, and intimacy follow; members feel affirmed and valued. In professional task and work groups, the group works to accomplish the group task in the performing phase. Finally, when the group task is completed to the satisfaction of the individual members, or of the group as a whole, the group enters an adjourning (termination) phase.

Different types of groups found in health-related therapeutic groups include therapy, support, educational, and discussion focus groups. Professional task and work groups are used to identify problems and issues, plan and implement change to improve person-centred care, and meet organizational goals. Intra- and interprofessional teams have many similar communication characteristics as small working groups. Clear differences exist in that team communication occurs on multiple levels of formal and informal relationships. The team works as a single coordinated unit of intra- or interprofessional providers with the specific goal of providing optimal person-centred care and will be discussed in Chapter 24.

ETHICAL DILEMMA
What Would You Do?

Mrs. Murphy is 39 years old and has been admitted to the psychiatric unit in the manic phase of her bipolar disorder. She wants to participate in group therapy but is disruptive when she is in the group. The group gets angry with her monopolization of their time. She says she has just as much right as any other group member to talk if she chooses. How do you balance Mrs. Murphy's rights with those of the group? Should she be excluded from the group if her behaviour is not under her control, even though she can benefit from being in the group? How would you handle this situation from an ethical perspective?

DISCUSSION QUESTIONS

1. How would you describe the differences between a working task group and a collaborative intra- or interprofessional health care team?
2. How do active listening strategies differ in group communication versus communication between two people?
3. What do you see as potential ethical issues in group communication formats?
4. As the group leader, what facilitation and engagement processes would you use in developing the norms with group members?

REFERENCES

Aggarwal, P., & O'Brien, C. L. (2008). Social loafing on group projects: Structural antecedents and effects on student satisfaction. *Journal of Marketing Education, 30*(3), 255–264.

Aronson, S. (2004). Where the wild things are: The power and challenge of adolescent group work. *The Mount Sinai Journal of Medicine, New York, 71*(3), 174–180.

Beebe, S., & Masterson, J. (2014). *Communicating in small groups: Principles and practices* (11th ed.). Pearson.

Beiling, P., McCabe, R., & Antony, M. (2009). *Cognitive-behavioural therapy in groups.* Guilford Press.

Benne, K. D., & Sheats, P. (1948). Functional roles of group members. *Journal of Social Issues, 4*(2), 41–49.

Berger, C. (2014). Planning theory of communication: Goal attainment through communicative action. In D. Braithwait & P. Schrodt (Eds.), *Engaging theories in interpersonal communication: Multiple perspectives* (2nd ed.). Sage Publications.

Bernard, H., Birlingame, G., Flores, P. et al. (2008). Clinical practice guidelines for group psychotherapy. *International Journal of Group Psychotherapy, 58*(4), 455–542.

Blanchard, K., Zigarmi, P., & Zigarmi, D. (2013). *Leadership and the one minute manager updated.* Harper Collins.

Bonebright, D. A. (2010). 40 years of storming: A historical review of Tuckman's model of small group development. *Human Resource Development International, 13*(1), 111–120. https://www.tandfonline.com/doi/abs/10.1080/13678861003589099.

Burlingame, G., Strauss, B., Joyce, A. et al. (2006). *Core battery—revised.* American Group Psychotherapy Association.

Canadian Interprofessional Health Collaborative [CIHC]. (2010). *A national interprofessional competency framework.* http://ipcontherun.ca/wp-content/uploads/2014/06/National-Framework.pdf.

Canadian Nurses Association. (2017). *Code of ethics for registered nurses.* https://www.cna-aiic.ca/~/media/cna/page-content/pdf-en/code-of-ethics-2017-edition-secure-interactive.

Canadian Nurses Association. (2020). *Position Statement: Intra-Professional Collaboration.* https://www.cna-aiic.ca/-/media/cna/page-content/pdf-en/cna-position-statement_intra-professionalcollaboration.pdf?la=en&hash=1158AB98CC407AB4C815A79F9CC3DDEA1960B9A6.

Centre for Addiction and Mental Health. (2020). *Group therapy.* https://www.camh.ca/en/health-info/mental-illness-and-addiction-index/group-therapy.

Civettini, N. H. W. (2007). Similarity and group performance. *Social Psychology Quarterly, 70*(3), 262–271.

Clarke, D., Adamoski, E., & Joyce, B. (1998). In-person group psychotherapy: The role of the staff nurse. *Journal of Psychosocial Nursing and Mental Health Services, 36*(5), 22–26.

College of Registered Nurses of Manitoba. (2019). *Interprofessional Collaborative Care.* https://www.crnm.mb.ca/uploads/document/document_file_261.pdf?t=1561125779.

Corey, M., & Corey, B. (2013). *Groups: Process and practice* (9th ed.). Brooks/Cole.

Counselman, E. (2008). Reader's forum: Why study group therapy? *International Journal of Group Psychotherapy, 58*(2), 265–272.

Deering, C. G. (2014). Process-oriented groups: Alive and well? *International Journal of Group Psychotherapy, 64*(2), 164–179.

Dyer, J., & Stotts, M. (2005). *Handbook of Remotivation Therapy.* The Haworth Clinical Practice Press.

Forehand, J., Leigh, K., Farrel, R. et al. (2016). Social dynamics in group work. *Teaching and Learning in Nursing, 11*, 62–66.

Forsyth, D. (2018). *Group dynamics* (6th ed.). Wadsworth Cengage Learning.

Gaudine, A., & Lamb, M. (2015). *Nursing leadership and management: Working in Canadian health care organizations.* Pearson.

Gladding, S. (2011). *Groups: A counseling specialty* (6th ed.). Merrill.

Janis, I. (1982). *Groupthink: Psychological studies of policy decisions and fiascoes* (2nd ed.). Houghton Mifflin.

Jhangiani, R., & Tarry, H. (2014). *Understanding social groups. Principles of social psychology.* https://opentextbc.ca/socialpsychology/chapter/understanding-social-groups/.

Johnson, D., & Johnson, F. (2017). *Joining together: Group theory and group skills* (12th ed). Pearson Education Limited.

Koukourikos, K., & Pasmatzi, E. (2014). Group therapy in psychotic inpatients. *Health Science Journal, 8*(3), 400–408.

Lasky, G., & Riva, M. (2006). Confidentiality and privileged communication in group psychotherapy. *International Journal of Group Psychotherapy, 56*(4), 455–476.

Mangione, L., Forti, R., & Iacuzzi, C. (2007). Ethics and endings in group psychotherapy: Saying good-bye and saying it well. *International Journal of Group Psychotherapy, 57*(1), 25–40.

Mathieu, J., Maynard, T., Rapp, T. et al. (2008). Team effectiveness: A review of recent advancements and a glimpse into the future. *Journal of Management, 34*, 410–476.

McShane, S. L., Steen, S. L., & Tasa, K. (2015). *Canadian organizational behaviour* (9th ed.). McGraw-Hill Ryerson.

Michaelsen, L.K., & Sweet, M. (2011). *Team-based learning: Small group learning's next big step. New directions in teaching and learning.* https://doi.org/10.1002/tl.467.

Moreno, K. J. (2007). Scapegoating in group psychotherapy. *International Journal of Group Psychotherapy, 57*(1), 93–104.

Nova Scotia College of Nurses. (2019). *Effective utilization of RNs and LPNs.* https://cdn1.nscn.ca/sites/default/files/documents/resources/EffectiveUtilization.pdf.

Nurses Association of New Brunswick & Association of New Brunswick Licensed Practical Nurses. (2015). *Guidelines for intraprofessional collaboration. Registered nurses and licensed practical nurses working together.* http://www.nanb.nb.ca/media/resource/NANBGuidelinesIntraprofessionalCollaborationRNsandLPNsWorkingTogether-E-2015-10.pdf.

Pehrsson, D.E., & McMillen, P. (2007). Bibliotherapy: Overview and implications for counselors. *American Counseling Association,* (ACAPCD-02). https://www.counseling.org/resources/library/ACA%20Digests/ACAPCD-02.pdf.

Percy, C., Gibbs, T., Potter, L. et al. (2009). Nurse-led peer support group: Experiences of women with polycystic ovary syndrome. *Journal of Advanced Nursing, 65*(10), 2046–2055.

Pettersson, C. (2018). Psychological well-being, improved self-confidence, and social capacity: Bibliotherapy from a user perspective. *Journal of Poetry Therapy, 31*(2), 124–134. https://www.tandfonline.com/doi/full/10.1080/08893675.2018.1448955.

Rothwell, D. (2013). *In mixed company.* Wadsworth Cengage Learning.

Powles, W. (2007). Reader's forum: Reflections on "what is a group?" *International Journal of Group Psychotherapy, 57*(1), 105–113.

Rubel, D., & Kline, W. (2008). An exploratory study of expert group leadership. *The Journal for Specialists in Group Work, 3*(2), 138–160.

Stinson, C. (2009). Structured group reminiscence: An intervention for older adults. *Journal of Continuing Education in Nursing, 40*(11), 521–528.

Tubbs, S. (2011). *A systems approach to small group interaction* (11th ed.). McGraw Hill.

Tuckman, B., & Jensen, M. (1977). Stages of small-group development revisited. *Group & Organization Management, 2*(4), 419–427.

Yalom, I., & Leszcz, M. (2005). *The theory and practice of group psychotherapy* (5th ed.). Basic Books.

Yang, K., Woomer, G., & Matthews, J. (2012). Collaborative learning among undergraduate students in community health nursing. *Nurse Education in Practice, 12*(2), 72–76.

10

Self-Concept in Professional Interpersonal Relationships

Claire Mallette

Originating US Chapter by *Eileen O'Brien*

OBJECTIVES

At the end of this chapter, the reader will be able to:
1. Define self-concept.
2. Describe the features and characteristics of self-concept.
3. Identify theoretical frameworks explaining self-concept.
4. Identify health concerns related to self-concept issues.
5. Apply the nursing process in caring for people with self-esteem health issues.
6. Use therapeutic communication and interventions related to self-concept issues.
7. Recognize and apply therapeutic communications that meet a person's spiritual needs in health care.

This chapter focuses on self-concept as a key dynamic in communication, therapeutic relationships, and strategies to enhance self-concept in adapting to one's environment. The chapter identifies basic concepts and frameworks related to the development of self-concept and describes its impact on individual development. The Application section discusses communication strategies that nurses can use with people to enhance positive self-concepts and empowering of healthy behaviours.

BASIC CONCEPTS

Definition

Self-concept is defined as the totality of each person's beliefs about their inner self. It represents an integration of each individual's cultural contexts, environment, gender roles, cultural and racial identity, spiritual beliefs and values, child development, education, basic personality traits, and cumulative life experiences.

This multidimensional construct mirrors an integration of individual's personal beliefs, values, attitudes, and behaviours. The self-concept has physical, emotional, social, and spiritual dimensions linked to functional well-being and health behaviours. It also incorporates feedback from others. How people perceive us helps to create or reinforce our self-perceptions.

Constructing the self-concept requires a cultural context foundation (Shweder et al., 2006). As discussed in Chapter 7, a person's culture is complex as it is a dynamic relational process of selectively responding to and integrating particular historical, social, political, economic, physical, and linguistic contexts. Examining the contexts that make up a person and the complexity of their interactions are necessary to understand how they influence a person's self-concept.

Closely intertwined with self-concept is self-esteem, defined as a person's personal sense of worth and well-being. The terms *self-image*, *self-concept*, and *self-perception* are often used interchangeably to refer to the way individuals view and assess themselves. The amount of self-esteem a person has is related to multiple factors related to childhood development and life experiences.

An important feature of self-concept involves self-clarity, which is described as the extent to which a person clearly and confidently knows who they are; self-clarity remains consistent over time and is intertwined with healthy identify development (Baumeister & Vohs, 2007).

This relates to the individual's **self-efficacy**, which is described as the person's beliefs about their ability and capacity to accomplish a task and to deal with the challenges of life. Self-efficacy plays a major part in determining whether the person will be successful in what they strive to achieve. This feature of the self-concept helps people to address control issues and cope with the many aspects of life. Some psychologists rate self-efficacy above talent in achieving success (Bandura, 1997).

A healthy self-concept including the above features, regardless of culture, reflects attitudes, emotions, and values that are realistic, congruent with each other, and consistent with a meaningful purpose in life. Fig. 10.1 identifies characteristics of a healthy self-concept. Each of these features is discussed further in the applications.

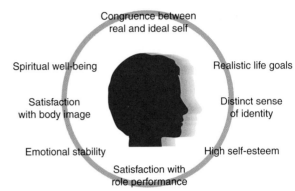

Fig. 10.1 Characteristics of a healthy self-concept

always form a unified consistent whole and that contradictions are bound to be encountered throughout life (Schachter, 2005). Nevertheless, choices congruent with the self-concept feel true, whereas those that are not consistent with one's personally determined self-concept create cognitive dissonance (inconsistent thoughts, beliefs, or attitudes), doubt, uncertainty, and anxiety (Cooper, 2007). Thus, the clarity of self-concept becomes muddled.

Significance of Self-Concept in Health Care

A strong sense of self has been described as a protective factor in coping with chronic illness (Mussato et al., 2014). When people experience a major health disruption, it alters the way they think, feel, value their sense of self, and communicate with others.

Features and Functions of Self-Concept

Cunha and Goncalves (2009) refer to the self as an open system—fluid and dynamic. A person's self-concept consists of various coexisting self-images. Different aspects of the self-concept become visible, depending on the situation (Prescott, 2006). For example, a student might struggle with English literature but excel in a mathematics course on differential equations. Which is the true self, or are both valid?

Self-concept helps people to make sense of their past and present; it helps them to communicate across varied situations and to imagine what they are capable of becoming—physically, emotionally, intellectually, socially, and spiritually—in relation to others in the future.

Over the course of a lifetime, self-concept changes and develops in complexity. Hunter (2008) noted, "As one ages, the 'self' develops and becomes a more and more unique entity formed by personal experiences and personally developed values and beliefs" (p. 318). Simulation Exercise 10.1 provides an opportunity for you to practise self-awareness by examining your self-concept.

Self-Fulfilling Prophecies

Possible selves is a term used to explain the future-oriented component of self-concept. Personal wishes and desires are

---

Case Example

I once interviewed a person with advanced cancer. Tears came to his eyes as he told me about how he had had to leave his job, could not run around with his grandchildren, could not do the things he loved—not like he used to, not anymore. A single diagnosis had inflicted such profound devastation. Note the pervasive impact on self-concept—it affects work, family, parental role, and social activities.

Self-concept reflects a person's personal reality, particularly in close relationships, careers, communication patterns, and life choices. Classically, adolescence was seen as the time of life during which individuals confronted the "self" developmentally. However, postmodern identity theory challenges the idea that these varied aspects of the self do not

---

SIMULATION EXERCISE 10.1   **Simulation Exercise: Who Am I?**

Purpose

To help students understand some of the self-concepts they hold about themselves

Procedure

1. Spend 10–15 minutes reflecting on how you would have defined yourself during high school and how you would define yourself today.
2. What has changed in your sense of self, and if there were changes, why did they occur?
3. Using only five one-word descriptors, describe yourself today. There are no right or wrong answers.
4. Pick the one descriptor that you believe defines yourself best.
5. In groups of four to six students, share your results.

Discussion

1. Were you surprised with the changes from your earlier descriptors as a teen?
2. Were you surprised with any of your choices as current descriptors?
3. How hard was it to pick the one best descriptor out of the five?
4. How did you describe yourself? Could your self-descriptors be categorized or prioritized in describing your overall self-concept?
5. What did you learn about the process of examining your self-concept from doing this exercise? What situational factors seemed to impact your descriptor choice?
6. How could you use this information in professional interpersonal relationships with people you care fo?

Beheshtifar, M., (2012). Role of self-concept in organizations. *European Journal of Economics, Finance and Administrative Sciences, 44*(44), 159–164. https://www.researchgate.net/publication/281175780_Role_of_Self-Concept_in_Organizations.

---

valuable influences in goal setting and motivation, when they lead to realistic actions. For example, a nursing student might think, "I can see myself becoming vice-president of nursing." Such thoughts help the novice nurse work harder to achieve professional goals. Negative possible selves can also become a self-fulfilling prophecy (Markus & Nurius, 1986). For example, Tyler receives a performance evaluation indicating a need for improved self-confidence. Seeing this criticism as a negative commentary on his "self" he fulfills the attribution by performing awkwardly when he is being assessed in the clinical area.

Development of Self-Concept and Self-Esteem

Self-concept represents an interaction between the life experiences and challenges that occur and the individual's response to them. Consider the differences in the life experience and socialization of a child born to parents with white skin colour and are university educated, with professional roles, versus a child born into poverty with parents who are both immigrants, who have black skin colour, and are both working in minimum wage–paying jobs to provide for their children. What implications do you see for the development of each child's self-concept? Life experiences, social status, significant relationships, and opportunities influence how people define themselves throughout life. Interactions in the family environment were previously considered the primary source in the development of self-esteem (Robson, 1988). However, several studies have challenged this traditional view, demonstrating that genetic factors also play a significant role in the development of self-esteem (Kendler & Gardner, 1998; Kamakura et al.,

2001; Neiss et al., 2002). The external social context into which a child is born and personal caretaking relationships contribute as well to shaping the resulting self-concept.

Social environment plays an important role in shaping and supporting one's personal self-concept. Current research supports the idea that a nurturing home environment, participation in activities and interest groups, academic success, religious and spiritual affiliation, professional opportunities, praise for successful accomplishments, and supportive mentors tend to encourage the development of a positive self-concept (Arnett, 2013). Factors such as poverty, a chaotic upbringing, loss of a parent, poor educational opportunities, and adverse life events contribute to the development of a negative self-concept.

There are individuals, though, who experience unfortunate social circumstances yet develop a dynamic self-concept as a reaction to their circumstances, creating a resiliency to the impact of negativity. They are often interested in improving their environment and serve as role models to others about what is possible against all odds. Others with more fortunate life circumstances may develop negative self-concepts or overinflated positive self-concepts with little grounding in reality. At times these individuals may be at risk for having difficulty accepting negative events in life. This further illustrates how understanding an individual's self-concept without making assumptions assists nurses in their therapeutic relationships and in caring for people during health events. When life presents individuals with unpredictable trauma or devastation, nurses can play a critical role in helping people to reframe a potentially incapacitating sense of self into one that includes more hope and broader options. In an effort to enhance **resilience**, nurses can help people revisit personal strengths, consider new possibilities, incorporate new information, and seek out appropriate resources as a basis for making sound clinical decisions for themselves and taking constructive actions. Sometimes, a nurse's "supportive presence" can give a person energy and reason to hope (Adler et al., 2014).

Self-Concept in Interpersonal Relationships

Self-concept is formed in relation to others (Guerrero et al., 2017). When two people communicate, each person's perceptions are influenced by their own self-concept and level of self-esteem. The factors presented in Chapter 5, Fig. 5.2 can implicitly influence interpersonal interactions. A person's cultural contexts will also influence their self-concept clarity and self-esteem.

Language is influential in forming perceptions of the self and others and reflects society's values. Self-concept can easily be influenced by communication; therefore, it is vital for nurses to be self-aware and sensitive to the impact of language in interactions, as discussed in Chapters 5, 6, and 7. **Microaggressions** involve communicating subtle and often unintentional discrimination pertaining to self-concepts of race, ethnicity, gender, sexual orientation, or any other cultural contexts. This type of communication can be viewed as influencing self-concept through marginalized communication. Sue (2010) clarifies that "microaggressions are used in three forms: microassault, microinsult, and microinvalidation."

Sue (2010) describes a **microassault** as an explicit negative verbal or nonverbal communication that marginalizes an individual through criticism, racial stereotyping, or purposeful prejudicial actions. For example, stereotyping people who are Indigenous as people who misuse alcohol or following a person who has black skin colour throughout a store. This kind of racial stereotyping would clearly influence a person's self-concept and can block communication.

Microinsults are verbal, nonverbal, and environmental communications that convey rudeness and insensitivity and put down a person's culture or identity. For example, during the nutritional assessment of a person with diabetes, a nurse comments that "All people with diabetes cheat on their diet." This not only demeans the person's efforts to control their glucose levels but also reduces their identity to a diagnosis.

Microinvalidations are communications that discount or invalidate a person's values, culture, or lifestyle (Sue, 2010). For example, asking a person who has brown skin what country they are from can imply that they don't belong to the dominant group in Canada of being White, with white skin colour.

Although these nurse–person communications may seem harmless, they clearly communicate an expectation or labelling that can lead to increased levels of anger and mistrust and loss of self-esteem.

It is critical for nurses to develop self-awareness. Attribution theory (Malle, 2011) holds that nurses' responses can compromise interaction with people by unintentionally limiting a person's sense of self-esteem. Therapeutic communication requires a well-defined, straightforward, unbiased approach, which allows nurses to more authentically connect with people.

Cultural Identity

A person's cultural identity is positively or negatively related to a clear self-concept and self-esteem (Usborne & Taylor, 2010). Individuals also often associate with multiple groups and are influenced by diverse experiences and values and beliefs that can change over time. An understanding of the complexity of culture can help nurses to frame supportive interventions in ways that support a person's cultural contexts and self-concept (see Chapter 7). For example, the cultural context of a person's ethnicity and race can influence self-concept. The 2016 census showed that 20.8% of people of colour in Canada are low-income, compared to 12.2% of nonracialized people (Statistics Canada, 2019). In 2017, hate crimes motivated by hatred of race or ethnicity represented 43% of all hate crimes, followed by those targeting religion (41%). Crimes motivated by hatred of sexual orientation accounted for 10% of hate crimes, with other factors such as language, disability, and age accounting for 6% (Armstrong, 2019).

Gender

Gender refers to "socially constructed roles and behaviours that occur in a historical and cultural context and that vary across societies and over time" (Leerdam et al., 2014, p. 53). Self-perceptions regarding gender evolve from socially learned behaviours that are constructed by dominant cultures. Despite progressive feminist changes, subtle gender differences for women are still evidenced in examples such as social expectations, career options, pay differentials, and primary caregiver responsibilities. Gender differences also exist in how people are treated, what is important to them, and how people are socialized to respond to verbal and nonverbal cues in communication.

This social construction has limitations. Many individuals do not fit into traditional gender categories and genuinely do not feel related to the socially constructed gender roles of society. Transgender people face discrimination, transphobic practices, and stigma within societies that may hold rigid boundaries around the constructs of sex and gender (discussed in Chapter 7). Nurses working with people need to approach gender identity as distinct from biology and recognize the individual's chosen gender identity in their language and communication. An example of this is including a question in nursing assessments such as, "What name and pronouns would you prefer being used?"

Case Example

Morgan is a trans man who frequently experiences discrimination, stigma, and invisibility in his chosen identity. One area of negative experiences is when he seeks out health care. Morgan tells the nurse that while he has physical characteristics of a woman, his chosen sexual identity is a trans man. Health care providers often do not acknowledge his chosen sexual identity and see and treat him as a woman. Nurses, instead, need to be supportive of the person's right for self-determination in their chosen sexual identity, through providing safe, compassionate, and culturally safe care.

Theoretical Frameworks

Self-Concept Frameworks

Self-concept has been explored in many ways since the beginning of theorizing about the self by Socrates and Plato (Marsh et al., 2012). The self is a central construct in theories of personality. These theories argue that our self-concept develops from and is influenced by social interactions with others. Sullivan (1953) described **self-concept** as a self-system that people develop to (1) present a consistent image of self, (2) protect themselves against feelings of anxiety, and (3) maintain their interpersonal security.

Humanism (Rogers, 1959) defines the *self* as "an organized, fluid, but consistent conceptual pattern of perceptions of characteristics and relationships or the 'I' and the 'me' together with values attached to these concepts" (p. 498). When the "actual self" (who we believe we are) and the "ideal self" (how a person would ideally like to be) are similar, the person is likely to have a positive self-concept and self-esteem. Rogers equated having a coherent, well-integrated self-concept with being mentally healthy and well adjusted (Diehl & Hay, 2007).

Posthumanism casts doubt on who is the person and their self-concept within the technological unconsciousness and nonconsciousness of our modern world (Callus & Herbrechter, 2012). The theory of posthumanism reflects on the effects of the influence of technology, biotechnology, and the sociopolitical, cultural, and environmental influences on who the person is and is in the process of becoming. The person and their self-concept cannot be explored without taking these influences and interrelationships into account (Callus & Herbrechter).

For example, a cardiac pacemaker controls abnormal heart rhythms and ensures the heart beats at a normal rate. The person who has a pacemaker relies on it to continue to live with quality of life. The technology of the pacemaker becomes part of who the person is and influences their self-concept. Thus, using a posthuman framework, the person implanted with this technological device no longer retains the classical understanding of what a human is and enters the identity realm of cybernetics. With the inclusion of the pacemaker as part of the person's being, they could be considered a cyborg.

Cognitive approaches (Fattore et al., 2017) state that a child is born without a concept of self and must learn to differentiate the self from others in the intimate sphere of family, in friendships, and in cultural practices. This requires relating to others and having vast interaction in the environment.

Behaviourists believe that early childhood interactions foster self-concepts of a "good me" (resulting from reward and approval experiences), a "bad me" (resulting from punishment and disapproval experiences), and a "not me" (resulting from anxiety-producing experiences that are dissociated by the person as not being a part of their self-concept). These influences continue through adulthood and influence a person's responses to life. Through therapeutic relationships, the nurse can help people develop a different, more positive sense of self.

George Mead applies a sociological approach to the study of self-concept. The self-concept affects and is influenced by how people experience themselves in relation to others (Elliott, 2013). Mead's model emphasizes the influence of culture, moral norms, and language in framing self-concepts through interpersonal interactions (symbolic interactionism).

Uri Bronfenbrenner developed a systems theory on human development based on bioecology, where a person influences and is influenced by the environment (Rosa & Tudge, 2013). Bronfenbrenner's theory describes the interactions of development occurring within a microsystem, mesosystem, exosystem, and macrosystem that change over time, described as the chronosystem. The microsystem includes the personal relationships with family, peers, teachers, and caregivers. How these groups interact influence the child's development. The mesosystem is described as interrelationships between the microsystem environments and other systems where the child interacts, such as day care, community activities, and school. The exosystem influences are the systems that influence the micro and mesosystem interactions—for example, access to health care, employment, and the community where they live. The macrosystem consists of the larger sociological and ecological systems that influence a person's development and include political, environmental, and socioeconomic systems, laws, and cultural contexts. The chronosystem recognizes that these systems can change over time and influence the child's development (Mordoch, 2015).

Erikson's Theory of Psychosocial Development

Erik Erikson's (1968, 1982) theory of psychosocial self-development is a well-known model. His theory originates from his work as a therapist, and it has stimulated a wealth of research and application. Central to his framework is the concept of identity formation. He believed that "identity formation neither begins nor ends with adolescence: it is a lifelong development" (Erikson, 1959, p. 122). Personality develops as a person responds to evolving developmental challenges (psychosocial crises) during the life cycle. As individuals pass through higher stages of ego development, with mastery of each developmental task, a personal sense of identity evolves. This is most obvious during adolescence, when teens experiment with different roles as they seek to establish a strong, comfortable personal identity. This development is not linear, nor does it occur across physical, emotional, and social development in the same sequential order. This is seen in the physically mature adolescent who may behave in a less mature fashion, socially and emotionally.

The first four stages of Erikson's model serve as building blocks for his central developmental task of establishing a healthy ego identity (identity versus identity diffusion). Erikson's stages of ego development are outlined in Table 10.1.

Erikson believed that stage development is never final. Reworking of developmental stages can occur at any time during the life span. Erikson's model can help nurses to analyze the age-appropriateness of behaviour from an ego development perspective. For example, a teenager giving birth is still coping with issues of self-identity rather than generativity. Simulation Exercise 10.2 focuses on applying Erikson's concepts to people's situations.

APPLICATIONS

Role of Self-Concept in Person-Centred Relationships

This Applications section identifies strategies to strengthen self-concept, self-efficacy, and self-esteem in health care relationships and communication. It is important to initiate caring relationships with the understanding that each person is unique, with strengths, values, cultural contexts, and concerns related to life experience. What health providers say, how they say it, and what they do matter in establishing relationships that are supportive of people's identities and person-centred care (Drench et al., 2011).

Self-concept is an essential starting point for understanding people's behaviours related to coping, engagement in meaningful activities, and improved mood (van Tuyl et al., 2014). Self-concept variables can act as facilitators or barriers to a person's efforts to engage in healthier lifestyle

TABLE 10.1   Erikson's Stages of Psychosocial Development, Clinical Behaviour Guidelines, and Stressors

Stage of Personality Guidelines	Ego Strength or Virtue	Clinical Behaviour Guidelines	Stressors
Trust versus mistrust	Hope	Appropriate attachment behaviours Ability to ask for assistance with an expectation of receiving it Ability to give and receive information related to self and health Ability to share opinions and experiences easily Ability to differentiate between how much one can trust and how much one must distrust	Unfamiliar environment or routines Inconsistency in care Pain Lack of information Unmet needs (e.g., having to wait 20 minutes for a bedpan or pain injection) Losses at critical times or accumulated loss Significant or sudden loss of physical function (e.g., a person with a broken hip being afraid to walk)

(Continued)

TABLE 10.1   Erikson's Stages of Psychosocial Development, Clinical Behaviour Guidelines, and Stressors—cont'd.

Stage of Personality Guidelines	Ego Strength or Virtue	Clinical Behaviour Guidelines	Stressors
Autonomy versus shame and doubt	Willpower	Ability to express opinions freely and to disagree tactfully Ability to delay gratification Ability to accept reasonable treatment plans and hospital regulations Ability to regulate one's behaviours (overcompliance, noncompliance, suggest disruptions) Ability to make age-appropriate decisions	Overemphasis on unfair or rigid regulation (e.g., putting to bed people in nursing homes at 7 p.m.) Cultural emphasis on guilt and shaming as a way of controlling behaviour Limited opportunity to make choices in a hospital setting Limited allowance made for individuality
Initiative versus guilt	Purpose	Ability to develop realistic goals and to initiate actions to meet them Ability to make mistakes without undue embarrassment Ability to have curiosity about health care Ability to work for goals Ability to develop constructive dreams and plans	Significant or sudden change in life pattern that interferes with role Loss of a mentor, particularly in adolescence or with a new job Lack of opportunity to participate in planning of care Overinvolved parenting that does not allow for experimentation Hypercritical authority figures No opportunity for play
Industry vs. inferiority	Competence	Work is perceived as meaningful and satisfying Appropriate satisfaction with balance in lifestyle pattern, including leisure activities Ability to work with others, including staff Ability to complete tasks and self-care activities in line with capabilities Ability to express personal strengths and limitations realistically	Limited opportunity to learn and master tasks Illness, circumstance, or condition that compromises or obliterates one's usual activities Lack of cultural support or opportunity for training
Identity vs. identity diffusion	Fidelity	Ability to establish friendships with peers Realistic assertion of independence and dependence needs Demonstration of overall satisfaction with self-image, including physical characteristics, personality, and role in life	Lack of opportunity Overprotective, neglectful, or inconsistent parenting Sudden or significant change in appearance, health, or status Lack of same-sex role models
Identity vs. isolation	Fidelity	Ability to express and act on personal values Congruence of self-perception with nurse's observation and perception of significant others	Lack of opportunity to interact with others Lack of guidance about socially proactive behaviours Loss of significant others Loss of memory Impaired hearing

(Continued)

TABLE 10.1   Erikson's Stages of Psychosocial Development, Clinical Behaviour Guidelines, and Stressors—cont'd.

Stage of Personality Guidelines	Ego Strength or Virtue	Clinical Behaviour Guidelines	Stressors
Intimacy vs. isolation	Love	Ability to enter into strong reciprocal interpersonal relationships Ability to identify a readily available support system Ability to feel the caring of others Ability to act harmoniously with family and friends	Competition Communication that includes a hidden agenda Projection of images and expectations onto another person Lack of privacy Loss of significant others at critical points of development
Generativity vs. stagnation and self-absorption	Caring	Demonstration of age-appropriate activities Development of a realistic assessment of personal contributions to society Development of ways to maximize productivity Appropriate care of whatever one has created Demonstration of a concern for others and a willingness to share ideas and knowledge Evidence of a healthy balance among work, family, and self-demands	Aging parents, separately or concurrently with adolescent children Terminated or layoff in career "Me generation" attitude Inability or lack of opportunity to function in a previous manner Children leaving home Forced retirement
Integrity vs. despair	Wisdom	Expression of satisfaction with personal lifestyle Acceptance of growing limitations while maintaining maximum productivity Expression of acceptance of certitude of death, as well as satisfaction with one's contributions to life Lack of opportunity	Rigid lifestyle Loss of significant other Loss of physical, intellectual, and emotional faculties Loss of previously satisfying work and family roles

---

SIMULATION EXERCISE 10.2   Simulation Exercise: Erikson's Stages of Psychosocial Development

Purpose

To help students apply Erikson's stages of psychosocial development to situations with people they care for.

Procedure

This exercise may be done in class or as a homework exercise, with the results shared in class.

To apply your knowledge of Erikson's stages of psychosocial development, identify the psychosocial crisis or crises each of the following people might be experiencing:

1. A 14-year-old single adolescent having her first child

SIMULATION EXERCISE 10.2   Simulation Exercise: Erikson's Stages of Psychosocial Development—cont'd.

2. A 50-year-old executive "let go" (fired) from his job after 18 years of employment
3. A 40-year-old who has had a stroke and is paralyzed on the left side
4. A 50-year-old woman caring for her 80-year-old mother who has Alzheimer's disease

Discussion
1. What criteria did you use to determine the most relevant psychosocial stage for each situation?
2. What conclusions can you draw from doing this exercise that would influence how you would respond to each of these people?

DEVELOPING AN EVIDENCE-INFORMED PRACTICE

This study used a group comparison on self-report questionnaires to examine the multidimensional self-concept, global self-esteem, and psychological adjustment of an age- and gender-matched study sample of 41 individuals with traumatic brain injury (TBI) compared with 41 control participants. Three self-report questionnaires (Rosenberg Self-Esteem Scale, Tennessee Self-Concept Scale, and the Hospital Anxiety and Depression Scale) were administered to all study subjects.

Results: People with TBI showed significantly lower means of global self-esteem and self-concept on the Rosenberg Self-Esteem and Tennessee Self-Concept scales. Subjects with TBI rated themselves lower on self-dimensions related to social, family, academic and work, and personal self-concept as compared with controls. They also reported higher mean levels on the Hospital Anxiety and Depression Scales.

Application to Your Clinical Practice: Recognition of self-concept and self-esteem as potential issues for people with TBI with negative emotional consequences may be an important underlying dynamic with these people. Strategies to enhance self-esteem and strengthen self-concept should be components of effective care for people with TBI.

Modified from Ponsford, J., Kelly, A., & Couchman, G. (2014). Self-concept and self-esteem after acquired brain injury: A control group comparison. *Brain Injury, 28*(2), 146–154.

---

behaviours and the self-management of chronic conditions (see also Chapter 11).

The development of a person's self-concept is complex and can be influenced by many factors, such as a person's body image and how they perceive themselves. Their self-identity also contributes to their overall self-concept and is based on their values and beliefs, cultural contexts, characteristics and abilities, relationships with others, and place in the world. A person's self-efficacy in completing what is expected of them and their ability to enact different roles in society, such as in relationships and employment, both influence self-concept. An illness or injury can lead to a significant change in a person's ability to successfully achieve these expectations, which can lead to changes in their self-concept. These factors and their influence on self-concept with nursing applications will be discussed in greater detail in the following sections.

Health Patterns Related to Self-Concept

Gordon (2007) identifies related functional health patterns as self-perception, self-concept, and value–belief patterns. Injury, illness, and treatments can challenge these functional health patterns regardless of specific health issues. As a person's perception of self-concept is disturbed, perception of the future becomes uncertain and unpredictable (Ellis-Hill & Horn, 2000).

Body Image Issues

Body image involves people's perceptions, thoughts, and behaviours associated with their appearance (Bolton et al., 2010). Perception of one's body image changes throughout life, influenced by the appraisals of others, cultural and social factors, and physical changes resulting from aging, illness, injury, and even treatment effects. For example, the potential for impotence and incontinence with prostate surgery can, secondary to treatment, create a body image issue for men; some women may gain weight as a result of aging and being post-menopausal (Harrington, 2011). These body image changes may have further implications for nurses' assessment of self-esteem issues.

Body image refers to how people perceive their physical characteristics, not how they realistically appear to others. A critical dimension of body image is self-esteem—the value people place on their appearance, or biological or functional intactness (Slatman, 2011). For example, individuals with an eating disorder may see themselves as "fat" despite being dangerously underweight. Ideal body image reflects sociocultural norms and popular media portrayals. Research consistently finds that physical appearance is strongly related to overall self-esteem (Harter, 2006); therefore nurses need to be cognizant of people's perceptions of physical changes.

Cultures differ in their value of specific physical characteristics. Sociocultural theories of body image suggest that body dissatisfaction results from a person's inability to meet unrealistic societal ideals. There is also increasing evidence of the important role that appearance and attractiveness appear to play on social media networks. Any changes in physical appearance or function can challenge self-concept (Arnett, 2013; Dropkin, 1999; Vandenbosch & Eggermont, 2016).

Permanent and even temporary changes in appearance influence attributions that others may make and how individuals perceive these responses. Discrimination can be subtle or overt, and the experience of a distorted body image can be longlasting. In a study of overweight adolescents, a primary theme that emerged was "a forever knowing of self as overweight" (Smith & Perkins, 2008, p. 391), even after the study participants lost significant weight in later years.

Less overt body image disturbances—for example, infertility, loss of bladder function, and loss of energy from radiation treatments—can affect the person's self-concept and require therapeutic care. Chronic pain or intermittent symptoms can also undermine a person's self-identity and self-confidence. People with these issues or conditions with fluctuating symptoms, such as inflammatory bowel disease, can experience similar feelings of vulnerability and insecurity related to body image, without validation from others.

Nursing Strategies

The *meaning* of body image is highly individual. Some people frame a potentially negative body image as a positive feature of their identities. Examples include Terry Fox, whose right leg had been amputated above the knee as a result of a malignant tumour and who began a cross-Canada run for cancer, and Rick Hansen, who had paraplegia following an accident at 15 years of age and who has raised $200 million for spinal cord injury–related programs. Others let a physical deviation become their defining feature. People with the same health condition can have different body image issues (Bolton et al., 2010). Assessment should take the following into account:

- Negative communications about the body
- Preoccupation with or no mention of changes in body structure and function following medical interventions
- Reluctance to look at or touch a changed body structure

- Social isolation and loss of interest in friends and work after a change in body structure, appearance, or function
- Expressed concerns or fears about changes

Person-centred assessment includes the person's strengths, expressed needs and goals, the nature and accessibility of the person's support system, and the perception of the impact the changes have on lifestyle. Frequently, deficits are magnified and compensatory personal resources are overlooked. Nurses can use a strengths-based approach by drawing on supportive family and friends, autonomy efforts, persistence, life skills, talents, spiritual beliefs, and hope. Simply listening to the person's response to changes in health can provide insight into its effect on self-concept.

Case Example

The Honourable Chantal Petitclerc, who is a senator of Canada, received the Lou Marsh Trophy for Canadian Athlete of the Year and is a decorated Olympic, athlete inducted into the Canadian Paralympic Hall of Fame. At the age of 13, she lost the use of her legs in a farm accident. She went on to learn how to swim as she was unable to participate in other gym activities. She credits learning how to swim as making her stronger, live more independently in a wheelchair, and discover her competitive drive. She then moved on to wheelchair racing and has 14 gold, 5 silver, and 2 bronze medals, from Paralympic games from 1992 to 2008. Senator Petitclerc strives to build a more inclusive society and is quoted as saying, "Excellence doesn't happen accidently. It's true; we can't choose what happens to us in life. However, as an individual or a country, we can always choose the attitude we will have to face life's challenges." (Freeborn, 2016; Senate of Canada, n.d.).

Nurses can model acceptance for people experiencing an altered body image. Acceptance is a process, and people need time to reconcile body image issues. Open-ended questions about what the person expects, and helping them identify social supports, can facilitate acceptance. Talking with others who have similar changes can provide credible, practical advice. For example, a "Canadian Breast Cancer Network" volunteer visits with a person who had a mastectomy and provides referrals to support groups that can assist the person's self-concept needs.

Personal Identity

Identity is described as an intrapersonal psychological process consisting of a person's beliefs and values, characteristics and abilities, relationships with others, how they fit into the world, and personal growth potential (Arnett, 2013;

Karademas et al., 2008). The identity develops and changes over time in relation to stage of life, situations, and experiences. There are multiple dimensions to personal identity, just as there are in self-concept: gender and sexual identities, social role identity (parent, student, widow, etc.), cultural contexts such as economic contextual identity, spirituality, and so forth. Each component affects a person's world view, sense of self, and communication patterns with others.

Individuals pass through each life stage as outlined by Erikson; our perceptions of personal identity change to reflect who we are in the present moment, physically, psychologically, contextually, and spiritually. Jung (1960) contends that "The afternoon of life is just as full of meaning as the morning; only its meaning and purpose are different" (p. 138). Prior to midlife, the energy focus is outward; in midlife, the focus changes to a more selective inner reflection, thoughtful choices, and a more authentic reordering of priorities.

When a major or sudden change in health status forces a reappraisal of personal identity, its impact on a person can be swift, life-altering, and compelling.

Case Example

"When I got up at last . . . and had learned to walk again, one day I went to a long mirror to look at myself, and I went alone. I didn't want anyone . . . to know how I felt when I saw myself for the first time. But here was no noise, no outcry; I didn't scream with rage when I saw myself. I just felt numb. That person in the mirror couldn't be me. I felt inside like a healthy, ordinary, lucky person—oh, not like the ONE in the mirror! Yet when I turned my face to the mirror there were my own eyes looking back, hot with shame . . . when I did not cry or make any sound, it became impossible that I should speak of it to anyone, and the confusion and the panic of my discovery were locked inside me then and there, to be faced alone, for a very long time to come" (Goffman, 1963).

In this passage, note the speaker's expression of aloneness and reluctance to share the impact of bodily changes on personal identity.

Other individuals, with cognitive impairment, experience more complicated but shared alterations in identity. Sensory images enter the brain, but the neural cognitive connections people use to interpret meaning cannot occur. Lake (2014) speaks of dementia as a disorder that "slowly diminishes personhood and devastates the relationships that personhood enables" (p. 5). People with dementia lose their ability to set realistic goals, implement coherent patterns of behaviour, maintain stable emotional

responses, communicate clearly, and control basic elements of their lives. As the disease progresses, they may no longer recognize significant others, lose their sense of personal identity, experience hallucinations and paranoia, and demonstrate fluctuating awareness of the self. As one caregiver described it, "There are two deaths with Alzheimer's disease—the death of self and the actual death" (Capps, 2008). Interestingly, however, in a study of adults with dementia, Fazio and Mitchell (2009) found that these people could identify themselves in photographs taken with an instant camera, despite forgetting the photo had been taken minutes earlier. This finding suggests a persistence of self even when memory is significantly impaired.

Application to Clinical Practice

Since self-narrative may be effective in maintaining the self in people with Alzheimer's disease (AD), if begun in the preliminary stages of AD, caring for them should include time for the sharing of narrative information that will allow the person to continue to share memories and their self-representations with others. One therapeutic intervention is listening to stories and narratives that may be repeated and changed over time, but the activity supports the social self.

Nursing Strategies

Changes in self-perception occur with change in health status. Heijmans et al. (2004) suggest that in addition to accepting an illness and learning new self-management skills, many people have to adapt to an altered social identity and renegotiate relationships. This activity involves a degree of emotional discomfort because things are not the same for the person or for those with whom the person interacts. Renegotiating relationships can be difficult and anxiety-producing, and the person often needs the nurse's support in determining how to respond.

Case Example

Renard is a registered nurse working in a busy surgery centre. Returning to work after a hospitalization for major depression, he finds he has been relieved of his position as charge nurse. Other staff are highly protective of him. He is carefully watched to ensure that he is not going to relapse, and he is given simpler tasks to avoid causing stress. Renard cannot understand why his coworkers don't see him as the same person he was before. Although his depression is in remission, Renard has been "labelled" and he feels he is experiencing the stigma of mental health disorders in the eyes of his coworkers. His colleagues' efforts are well intentioned, but they have a negative effect on Renard's's sense of personal identity.

▶▶ DEVELOPING AN EVIDENCED-INFORMED PRACTICE

Research into the initial stages of Alzheimer's disease (AD), with the scope of developing some sort of "salvage therapy" is rather scarce.

Purpose: The purpose of this study was to extend knowledge about how subjects with a probable AD diagnosis or in a medium-low phase of the disorder maintain the continuity of self.

Method: This research was done from a psycholinguistic point of view, with the goal of identifying how people with Alzheimer's disease maintain the self through narrative.

Results: The structure of the narrative and the subsequent analysis of the transcribed material demonstrated the need to give shape to people's stories. The analysis of this particular segment of the initial phase of the disease, and how the disease progressively worsens, seemed useful in helping to understand how the person's psyche reacts to the diagnosis and how the person reorganizes their self-representation. Finally, it seemed useful in helping to understand if and in which way the subjects' identity begins to deteriorate. Self-narrative may be effective in maintaining the self in people with AD if it is begun in the preliminary stages of the disease.

Toffle, M. E., & Quattropani, M. C. (2015). The self in the Alzheimer's patient as revealed through psycholinguistic-story based analysis. 6th world conference on psychology counseling and guidance. *Society Behavioral Science,* 205, 361–372.

Blazer (2008) suggests that developing self-perceptions of achieving personal health and well-being may be as important as objective data for predicting health outcomes over time. Nurses can help people reestablish a more positive self-identity by encouraging the person and family to engage in open-ended questions in mutual discovery, related to the following:

- What is this person coping with in relation to self-identity?
- What is this person able to do in their current circumstances?
- What is needed to support this person in reconnecting with the person they are capable of being?

Including a significant family member in this discussion can be helpful. Family may not anticipate or have an awareness of a change in personal identity, as often the focus of return to health is more physically defined. Benner (2003) advocates exploring what matters to the person and emphasizing a person's strengths as a basis for developing and enhancing creative meaning. This strengths-based approach creates a climate where the person *can* improve their situation and create new possibilities for enhancing personal identity during illness. Even the smallest positive movement can increase the person's changed personal identity. Box 10.1 describes person-centred interventions to enhance personal identity.

Perception

Perception is a process through which we interpret sensory information and whereby a person transforms sensory data into connected personalized understanding. According to self-perception theory, we interpret our own actions in the same way as we interpret others' actions, and our actions are often socially influenced and not produced of our own free will, as we might expect (Bem, 1972).

Consider the image in Fig. 10.2. Depending on whether you focus on the background or the form, you can draw different conclusions. Which image do you see—a vase or two figures looking at each other? Any shift of focus, whether self-imposed or directed by others, can transform what you see as a perceptual image. Perceptions are subjective, made up of how information is filtered through memories that feel familiar, have already been experienced, or are similar enough to anticipate their meaning (Gottlieb & Gottlieb, 2013).

The same possibility applies to life situations. Helping people to refocus their attention in thinking about difficult circumstances, or using a new perspective, can alter meaning and suggest different options. Perceptions differ because individuals develop mindsets that alter information in

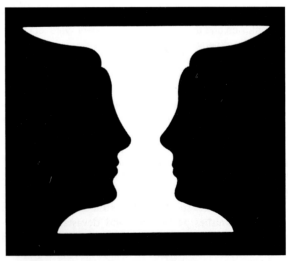

Fig. 10.2 The figure-ground phenomenon

BOX 10.1 Person-Centred Interventions to Enhance Personal Identity: Perceptions and Cognition

- Explain to newly admitted people their clinical environment, person rights, and expected care routine.
- Actively listen and facilitate the person's "story" of the present health care experience, including concerns about coping, impact on self and others, and hopes for the future.
- Remember that each person is unique. Respect and tailor responses to support individual differences in personality, identity, responses, intellect, values, culture, and understanding of medical processes.
- Encourage as much input from the person as an integral member of the health care team.
- Provide information as it emerges about changes in treatment, personnel, discharge, and aftercare. Include family members whenever possible and desired, particularly when giving difficult news.
- Explain treatment procedures, including rationale, and allow appropriate amount of time for questions and discussion.
- Encourage family members to bring in familiar objects, pictures, or a calendar, particularly if the person is in the hospital or care facility for an extended period.
- Encourage as much independence and self-direction as possible.
- Avoid sensory overload and repeat instructions if the person appears anxious.
- Use perceptual checks to ensure you and the person have the same understanding of important material.
- Encourage older people to maintain an active, engaged lifestyle in line with their interests, capabilities, and values.

personal ways. People with delirium or psychoactive drug reactions experience global perceptual distortions, whereas those with mental health issues can experience personalized perceptual distortions (the individual perceives differently from others). Distorted perceptions influence interpretation of communication, whether sending, receiving, or interpreting verbal messages and nonverbal behaviours. Simple perceptual distortions can be challenged with compassionate questioning and sometimes targeted humour. Validation of perceptual data is needed because the nurse and the person may not be processing the same reality.

Case Example

Mariam Pereira is a 70-year-old widow with arthritis, who is overweight and has failing eyesight. While being admitted for a minor surgical procedure, a bunion removal on her right foot, Ms. Pereira tells the nurse she does not know why she is putting herself through all of this. Nothing can be done for her because she is too old and it won't make a difference in her quality of life.

- *Nurse:* As I understand it, you came in today for removal of your bunions. Can you tell me more about your health issue as you see it? *(Asking for this information separates the current situation from an overall assessment of quality of life.)*
- *Ms. Pereira:* Well, I've been having trouble walking, and I can't do some of the things I like to do that involve a lot of walking. I also have to buy "clunky" shoes that make me look like an old woman.

- *Nurse:* So you're not willing to be an old woman yet? *(Taking the person's statement and challenging the cognitive distortion presented in her initial comments with humour allows the person to view her statement differently.)*
- *Ms. Pereira* (laughing): Right, there are a lot of things I want to do before I'm ready for a nursing home.

Questioning perceptions and active listening by the nurse help a person make sense of perceptual data in a more conscious way, and the person feels heard. A cognitive appraisal of personal identity in the face of health issues can contribute to an improved health condition and an enhanced sense of well-being. Keeping communication simple, delivering straightforward messages with compassion, and making interactions participatory with a back-and-forth dialogue assist the nurse to understand and better address the person's needs based on their perceptions.

Cognition

Cognition represents the thinking processes people use in making sense of the world. What people *think* about their perceptions connects perceptions with associated feelings and meanings and directly influences clinical outcomes. According to Beck and Beck (2011), incorrect perceptions of a situation can stimulate automatic negative thoughts that may not be realistic. Our mind can convince us of something that isn't true—for example, believing you have the "worst luck in the world" can lead you to believe everything will go wrong. Referred to as cognitive distortions, automatic thoughts about self-constructed realities create negative feelings, which can have a powerful impact on communication and behaviour.

Conscious, reality-based thought processes are essential to acquiring and sustaining an accurate interpretation of self. Nurses can use supportive strategies to assist people to examine cognitive distortions so that they are better able to develop realistic solutions to address health issues. Examples of these strategies are outlined in the following paragraphs; they can help people to reappraise their thinking, making it more conducive to effective functioning. Fig. 10.3 demonstrates the link between perceptions and behaviours.

Supportive Nursing Strategies

Cognitive behavioural approaches, originally developed by Aaron Beck, focus on encouraging people to reflect on difficult situations from a broader perspective. Beck refers to cognitive distortions as "thinking errors" where the person perceives reality inaccurately. Reflection on a variety of explanations provides people with more options to realistically interpret the meaning of their perceptions. Cognitive approaches help people identify, reflect on, and challenge negative automatic thinking processes instead of accepting them as reality. Common cognitive distortions are identified in Box 10.2. Modelling cues to behaviour and coaching people to challenge cognitive distortions with positive **self-talk** and mindfulness are helpful. Feedback and social support are powerful antidotes to cognitive distortions.

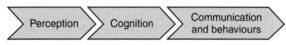

Fig. 10.3 Cognitive reappraisal

Self-Esteem

Self-esteem is defined as the *emotional* value a person places on their self-concept and worth as a person. Self-esteem also involves feelings of self-acceptance and self-respect (Orth & Robins, 2014). People who view themselves as worthwhile and of value have high self-esteem. They challenge negative beliefs that are unproductive or that interfere with successful functioning. With a positive attitude about self, an individual is more likely to view life as the perception of a glass half full rather than half empty. People with low self-esteem do not value themselves and do not feel valued by others.

Baumeister et al. (2007) reviewed how self-esteem can have a strong relationship with happiness. Their findings indicated there appeared to be a strong association between high self-esteem and greater happiness, based on perceptions of life and relationships. Since then, well-designed longitudinal studies have examined prospective effects of self-esteem on life outcomes. The results of these studies support the belief that self-esteem is predictive of a person's success and well-being in important life events such as relationships, employment, physical and mental health, and education (Orth & Robins, 2014). Individuals with high self-esteem have been found to experience more happiness, optimism, and motivation than those with low self-esteem and also less depression and anxiety, and fewer negative moods (Neff, 2011). Low self-esteem has been associated with depression. Using data from a 23-year longitudinal study (n = 1 527), the findings indicated that individuals who entered adolescence with low self-esteem or declined further during the adolescent years (or both) were more likely to demonstrate symptoms of depression as adults (Steiger et al., 2014).

Verbal and nonverbal behaviours presenting as frustration, inadequacy, anxiety, anger, or apathy suggest low self-esteem. This pattern tends to be defensive in relationships

---

BOX 10.2   Examples of Cognitive Distortions

1. "All or nothing" thinking—the situation is all good or all bad; a person is trustworthy or untrustworthy
2. Overgeneralizing—an incident happening once is treated as if it happens all the time; picking out a single detail and dwelling on it
3. Mind reading and fortune telling—deciding a person does not like you without checking it out; assuming a bad outcome with no evidence to support it
4. Personalizing—seeing yourself as flawed instead of separating the situation as something you played a role in but did not cause
5. Acting on "should" and "ought to"—deciding in your mind what is someone else's responsibility without perceptual checks; trying to meet another's expectations without regard for whether it makes sense to do so
6. "Awfulizing"—assuming the worst, that every situation has a catastrophic interpretation and anticipated outcome

and seeks constant reassurance from others because of self-doubt. Instead of taking constructive actions that could raise self-esteem, people worry about what issues they cannot control and see life's challenges as problems rather than opportunities. Table 10.2 identifies behaviours associated with high versus low self-esteem.

Self-esteem has been shown to change over time. Research indicates that self-esteem tends to increase from adolescence to middle adulthood, peak at approximately age 50 to 60 years, and then declines as a person grows older (Orth & Robins, 2014). Over the course of adulthood, individuals increasingly occupy positions of power and

status, which might promote feelings of self-worth. Many life span theorists have suggested that in midlife, people are concerned with trying to figure out how they want to spend their later years and what is important to them personally (Erikson, 1985).

Self-esteem declines in old age. The few studies of self-esteem in old age suggest that self-esteem begins to decline around 70 years of age. This decline may be due to the many physical and emotional changes that occur in old age, including changes in work (e.g., retirement), relationships (e.g., the loss of a spouse), and physical functioning (e.g., health issues) as well as a decline in socioeconomic status. This may also reflect a shift toward a more modest, humble, balanced view of the self in old age (Erikson, 1985).

The experience of success or failure can also cause fluctuations in self-esteem (Crocker et al., 2006). Sources of situational challenges include loss of a job; loss of an important relationship; and negative changes in one's appearance, role, or status. Longstanding issues of verbal or physical abuse, neglect, chronic illness, codependency, and criticism by significant others can result in lowered self-esteem. Illness, injury, and other health issues also challenge a person's self-esteem. Findings from a sizable number of research studies demonstrate an association with changes in health status, functional abilities, and emotional issues, and lowering of self-esteem (Vartanian, 2009; Vickery et al., 2008). Simulation Exercise 10.3 assists you in examining what is important to you and how it is related to your self-esteem.

TABLE 10.2 Behaviours Associated With High Versus Low Self-Esteem

People With High Self-Esteem	People With Low Self-Esteem
Expect people to value them	Expect people to be critical of them
Are active self-agents	Are passive or obstructive self-agents
Have positive perceptions of their skills, appearance, sexuality, and behaviours	Have negative perceptions of their skills, appearance, sexuality, and behaviours
Perform equally well when being observed as when not being observed	Perform less well when being observed
Are nondefensive and assertive in response to criticism	Are defensive and passive in response to criticism
Can accept compliments easily	Have difficulty accepting compliments
Evaluate their performance realistically	Have unrealistic expectations about their performance
Are relatively comfortable relating to authority figures	Are uncomfortable relating to authority figures
Express general satisfaction with life	Are dissatisfied with their lot in life
Have a strong social support system	Have a weak social support system
Have a primary internal locus of control	Rely on an external locus of control

Case Example

Elina was diagnosed with advanced metastatic breast cancer. All her life, Elina had been a take-charge person, with confidence and high self-esteem and self-concept. She was proud of her coping strategies for addressing life stressors. Rachel was also diagnosed with a similar advanced metastatic breast cancer. She has low self-esteem and self-concept and struggles with self-confidence, anxiety, and coping with life stressors. Elina and Rachel both have the same type of mastectomy surgery. Following the surgery, while both women were coping with their changed body image, Elina had lower levels of anxiety and depression compared to Rachel.

Reed's (2014) middle-range theory of self-transcendence can help people to expand their boundaries as a resource in difficult times. The theory encompasses the following four components:

- Intrapersonal (toward greater awareness of one's philosophy, values, and dreams)

SIMULATION EXERCISE 10.3   What Matters to Me?

Purpose
To help students understand the relationship between self-concepts and what is valued

Procedure
This exercise may be done as a homework exercise and shared with your small group.
- Spend 10–15 minutes reflecting about the three activities, roles, or responsibilities you value most in your life. (There are no right or wrong answers.)
- Now prioritize them and identify the one that you value the most. (This is never easy.)

- In one to two paragraphs, explain why the top contender is most important to you.
- In groups of four to six students, share your results.

Discussion
1. Were you surprised by any of your choices or what you perceived as being most important to you?
2. In what ways do your choices affirm self-concept and self-esteem?
3. What are the implications of doing this exercise for when you are helping people understand what they value and how this reflects self-esteem?

SIMULATION EXERCISE 10.4   Social Support

Purpose
To help students understand the role of social support in significant encounters

Procedure
1. Describe a "special" interpersonal situation that led to change, gave you direction, or had deep meaning for you.
2. Identify the person or people who helped make the situation meaningful for you.

3. Describe the actions taken by the people or person just identified that made the situation memorable.

Discussion
1. What did you learn about yourself from doing this exercise?
2. What do you see as the role of social support in making memories?
3. How might you use this information in your practice?

- Interpersonal (to relate to others and one's environment)
- Temporal (to integrate one's past and future in a way that has meaning for the present)
- Transpersonal (to connect with dimensions beyond the typically discernible world) (p. 111)

Self-esteem can also be enhanced through social support. Rebuilding relationships with family, friends, and teachers, as well as participation in social activities, can promote the process of achieving self-esteem. Simulation Exercise 10.4 introduces the role of social support in building self-esteem.

Nurses can help people sort out and clarify the beliefs and emotions that get in the way of an awareness of their intrinsic value and strengths. Note how the person describes achievements. Does the person devalue accomplishments, project blame for problems onto others, minimize personal failures, or make self-critical remarks? Does the person express shame or guilt? Does the person seem hesitant to try new things or situations or express anxiety about coping with events? Observe defensive behaviours. Poor hygiene, self-destructive behaviours, hypersensitivity to criticism, a need for constant reassurance, and the inability to accept compliments are behaviours that can be associated with low self-esteem.

Self-Esteem and Social Media

It is estimated that over 3 billion people report that they are actively using social media sites and that it has become an important part of their daily life (Saiphoo et al., 2020). Research has indicated that making social comparisons to content posted on social media sites can contribute to either an increase or decrease in self-esteem, based on such activities as the number of "likes" received for posts. There is conflicting evidence on self-esteem, with some research findings indicating frequent use is related to low self-esteem while other study findings indicate the opposite, with frequent use being associated with higher self-esteem (Saiphoo et al.).

The Internet and social media sites are also becoming more of an area of research in examining how they influence the development of self-concept and self-esteem in adolescents. Adolescence is a critical time for the development of a clear sense of self-concept. Social media sites provide the platform for trying out different presentations of themselves and how others respond to them. In one study, it was found that adolescents who had a less stable sense of self were more likely to present themselves on their site as their idealized self versus their actual self. Those adolescents with a stronger self-concept indicated posting their self-presentation online as similar to their offline self-presentation (Fullwood et al., 2016).

Social comparison theory indicates that self-esteem influences the tendency to compare oneself with others. Social media can contribute to a constant comparison to others and negative influence on self-esteem. Negative experiences with social media are related to feeling inadequate about life and appearance, fear of missing out, depression and anxiety, and self-absorption (Abel et al., 2016; HelpGuide, 2020). It is important for nurses to be aware of the potential negative effects of social media on a person's self-concept, self-esteem, and well-being. As part of your health assessment, you can ask about the person's use of social media and how it makes them feel (Warrender & Milne, 2020).

Therapeutic Strategies

When people have low self-esteem and low self-worth, beliefs that no one really cares can take over their emotions. By understanding these underlying feelings as a threat to self-esteem (e.g., fear, distress about an anticipated loss, and lack of power in an unfamiliar situation), nurses can facilitate opportunities for the person to share their concerns and feelings. The nurse might identify a legitimate feeling by saying, "It must be frustrating to feel that your questions go unanswered" and then asking, "How can I help you?"

Nurses also help people increase self-esteem by being psychologically present to the person's thoughts and concerns. The process of engaging with another person who offers a different perspective and who demonstrates control in responding to events can enhance self-esteem.

The implicit message the nurse conveys with personal presence and interest, information, and a guided exploration of the problem is twofold. The first is confirmation of the person—"You are unique, you are important, and I will stay with you through this uncomfortable period."

The second is the introduction of the possibility of hope—"There may be some alternatives you haven't thought of that can help you cope with this problem. Would you ever consider . . .?" Once a person starts to take control over their responses to events, a higher level of well-being can result. It is important to remember, as the nurse, to not minimize the energy required to change. As clear as the pathway to hope may be, the nurse needs to understand that it is not a simple road for the person.

Using a strengths-based approach offers the person some control. It is helpful to say, for example, "The thing that impresses me about you is . . ." or "What I notice is that although your body is weaker from your disease, it seems as if your spirit remains strong. Would you say this is true?" You could also ask how the person has coped in the past in difficult times and whether they could use those coping strategies in the present situation. Such questions help the person focus on positive strengths. Behaviours suggestive of enhanced self-esteem include the following:

- Taking an active role in planning and implementing self-care
- Verbalizing personal psychosocial (psychological, emotional, social, and spiritual) strengths
- Expressing feelings of satisfaction with self and ways of handling life events

Self-Efficacy

Self-efficacy is "the belief in one's capabilities to organize and execute the courses of action required to manage prospective situations" (Bandura, 2007). In other words, self-efficacy is a person's belief in their ability to succeed in a particular situation. People who believe that they can make changes and take control over their situation value their abilities to succeed. They are less likely to have self-doubts or focus on personal deficiencies when difficulties arise. Research indicates that there is a relationship with higher levels of self-efficacy supporting successful self-management strategies (Marks et al., 2005; Simpson & Jones, 2013). **Self-management** can be defined as the tasks and strategies that an individual carries out to live well with chronic health conditions. These include increasing confidence to cope with the medical treatments, the change in roles, and managing the emotions associated with managing the chronic condition (British Columbia Ministry of Health, 2011).

Support of self-efficacy is critical to helping people with mental health issues live successfully in the community (Suzuki et al., 2011). Self-efficacy improves motivation and helps people sustain their efforts in self-management activities.

Self-management support should include specific problem-solving skills and processes that people need to cope. Breaking difficult tasks down into achievable steps and completing them reinforces self-efficacy. It helps to explain why each step is important for the next and remind people of their progress toward a successful outcome.

Identify people's strengths. Skills training in areas where people have areas of development while also focusing on their strengths and persistence can encourage them to take their next steps. Work with the person to use solutions and resources that are affordable and that the person believes are achievable. For example, exercise may become an acceptable option if the person knows of free or low-cost exercise programs for seniors living in the community.

It is also important to ask the person what they believe is needed to help them continue to succeed in their self-management activities (Health Council of Canada, 2012). Encourage significant others in the person's life to give support and approval. Families appreciate receiving specific suggestions and opportunities to give appropriate support.

Self-help and support groups can also support self-management activities. Discovering that others with similar issues have found ways to cope encourages people and reinforces self-efficacy that they too can achieve similar success. The understanding, social support, and reciprocal learning found in these groups can provide opportunities for valuable information sharing and role modelling (Humphreys, 2004).

Role Performance

Role performance requires self-efficacy with links to self-concept. Johnson et al. (2012) suggest that professional identity can be conceptualized as a "logical consequence of self-identity" (p. 562). How effectively people are able to function within expected roles influences their value within society and affects personal self-esteem.

Role performance and associated role relationships matter to people, as evidenced in symptoms of depression, feelings of emptiness, and even suicide, when a significant personal or professional role ceases to exist.

Case Example

"My values in life have changed completely. It was incredibly difficult to realize following my heart attack that as a 52-year-old man, I felt 'worthless.' I had been the strong one at work and in my family. I was the person everybody relied on. Suddenly, it was I who had to ask others for help. I'm prone to cardiovascular disease and I know that one day I will probably have another heart attack. The next time it will in all likelihood be worse than this time" (Raholm, 2008).

Nurses need to be sensitive to the changes in role relationships that illness and injury produce for self, family, and relationships. An individual's social role can rapidly transform from independent self-sufficiency to vulnerability and dependence on others. New role behaviours may be uncomfortable and anxiety-producing. Asking open-ended and focused questions about the person's relationships across family, work, and social groups is a useful strategy for assessing role change. Box 10.3 presents suggestions that can be integrated into your assessments related to role relationships.

Preconceived ideas of role disruption for a person who becomes ill or disabled occur more commonly when the illness will be a chronic condition, or seriously role-disruptive.

BOX 10.3 Sample Assessment Questions Related to Role Relationships

Family
1. "Who do you see in your family as being supportive of you?" or "Who can you rely on to help you through any changes?"
2. "Who do you see in your family as being most affected by your illness (condition)?" or "Who do you think will need to adjust more than any other family member?"
3. "What changes do you anticipate as a result of your illness (condition) in the way you function in your family?" or "Will your health change how things get done in the family?"

Work
1. "What are some of the concerns you have about your job at this time?"
2. "Who do you see in your work situation as being supportive of you?"

Social
1. "How has your illness affected the way people who are important to you treat you?"
2. "Is there anyone outside of family you turn to for support?"
3. "If (name)_____ is not available to you, who else might you be able to call on for support?"

Walker (2010) notes that when people have to leave paid employment because of a chronic illness, it affects self-concept, because many people's social and personal identities are tied to their work roles. Nurses can coach people about how to present themselves when they return to work. They can help people learn how to respond to subtle and not-so-subtle discriminatory actions associated with others' lack of understanding of the person's health situation.

Spiritual Aspects of Personal Identity

When health fails or circumstances seem beyond control, it is often the person's spiritual self-concept that sustains a sense of self and helps to maintain a more balanced equilibrium. Spirituality, religion, medicine, and health care have been interrelated throughout time. In highly developed countries, such as in the West (including Canada), these systems of healing are no longer interrelated in the same way, but in other countries, they continue to influence one another (Koenig, 2012). Spirituality and religion are recognized as important factors in coping with disease and life events and in maintaining quality of life (Nita, 2019). Numerous studies indicate that spirituality and religion can positively influence addressing life experiences such as coping with stress, mental and physical health, formation of social relationships, conflict, life satisfaction, work attitudes, and development of values (Dein et al., 2012; Nita, 2019).

The terms *spirituality* and *religion* are often used interchangeably, but there are differences, with multiple definitions for both. *Religion* can be defined as "an organized system, or set of beliefs, that provides answers to questions about life through sacred texts, rituals and practices" (Chaze et al., 2015, p. 88). Religions usually have rules about life and death; interacting with others; and praying to a divine, heavenly or higher power being. Examples are God, Allah, HaShem, Brahman, Buddha, and Dao (Koenig, 2012).

Spirituality can be experienced within or outside a formalized religion and community, or individually (Dein et al., 2012). Spirituality is closely linked to a person's world view, providing a foundation for a personal belief system about the nature of a higher power, moral-ethical conduct, and reality. The Canadian Nurses Association [CNA] (2010) defines **spirituality** as "whatever or whoever gives ultimate meaning and purpose in one's life, that invites particular ways of being in the world in relation to others, oneself and the universe" (p.1).

Spirituality and religion can assist people in answering vital questions about what it is to be human, which life experiences have depth and value, and what are the imaginative possibilities of being.

Over the course of a lifetime, spiritual and religious beliefs change, deepen, or are challenged by life events. Spiritual aspects of self-concept can be expressed through the following:

1. Membership in a specific religious faith community
2. Mindfulness, meditation, or other personalized lifeways and practices
3. Cultural and family beliefs about forgiveness, justice, human rights, and social justice
4. Crises or existential situations that stimulate a search for purpose, meaning, and values beyond the self

The CNA Code of Ethics for Registered Nurses (2017) and their position statement on spirituality, health, and nursing practice (2010) identify the following:

- Nurses in their professional capacity relate to all people receiving care, with respect.
- In health care decision making, in treatment, and in care, nurses work with people receiving care to take into account their values, customs, and spiritual beliefs as well as their social and economic circumstances, without judgement or bias.
- Sensitivity to and respect for diversity in spiritual beliefs, support or spiritual preferences, and attention to spiritual needs, are recognized by CNA as required competencies.
- When providing care, nurses do not discriminate on the basis of an individual's spiritual beliefs.

As Canada is a multicultural country, many immigrants come from other countries, for example, countries in East and Southeast Asia, where religion and spirituality are important parts of their self-concept and their health and healing. Christianity remains the largest self-identified religious group in Canada, but its percentage is declining. The number of Canadians self-identifying as Muslim, Hindu, Buddhist, and Sikh is steadily and significantly increasing; the number of Canadians identifying as having no religious affiliation is also steadily increasing (Statistics Canada, 2013).

The importance and recognition of spirituality and religion within health care systems is often minimal or invisible. This lack of recognition is as a result of the focus on the biomedical health issues, and of health care providers being reluctant or unsure of how to incorporate spirituality into their practice based on their own values and beliefs, and lack of education on how this can be implemented (Chaze et al., 2015). It is important to be self-aware of your own values and beliefs related to religion and spirituality. Box 10.4 asks questions for self-reflection to begin to develop a greater awareness of how to better care for people's spiritual needs.

Spiritual dimensions encompass people's spiritual beliefs; cultural practices; religious affiliation and level of participation; personal spiritual practices such as prayer, mindfulness, or meditation; feeling connected to a higher power; and the subjective importance of these practices and beliefs in a person's life (Blazer, 2012).

Assessment should take account of these aspects of people's religious and spiritual practices:

- Willingness to talk about personal spirituality or beliefs
- Belief in a personal god or higher power

BOX 10.4 Self-Reflective Questions Related to Incorporating Spiritual Care Into Your Practice

1. What concerns and fears do you have in relation to providing spiritual care in your practice?
2. What can you do or who can you speak to in helping you examine and better understand these fears and concerns?
3. Who could be a mentor for you when it comes to becoming better at incorporating spiritual care in your nursing practice? What practices do they do that make you believe they would be a good mentor?
4. What can you learn from the people you care for in relation to spiritual care?

Adapted from Scott Barrs, K., Clarke Arnault, V., & McDonald, M. S. (2015). Spirituality and Nursing: Presence and Promise. In D. Gregory, C. Raymond-Seniuk, L. Patrick, et al. (Eds.), *Fundamentals Perspectives on the Art and Science of Canadian Nursing.* (p. 1069). Wolters Kluwer.

- Relevance of specific cultural or religious practices to the individual
- Changes in religious practices or beliefs
- Areas of specific spiritual concern initiated by the illness—for example, is there an afterlife?
- Extent to which health issues, injury, or disability has had an effect on the person's spiritual beliefs
- Sources of hope and support
- Desire for visitation from a spiritual leader who can support their religious and spiritual needs

A person's spiritual and religious needs may be obvious, with a defined philosophical understanding of life and one's place in it and firmly anchored in positive relationships, with a defined religious leader such as a rabbi in the Jewish faith, an imam in the Muslim religion, or a priest or minister in Christianity religions. Spiritual needs and beliefs can provide comfort and peace or evidence of conflict or anger toward a higher power, such as their god punishing or abandoning them in times of a health crisis. Alternatively, a spiritual sense of self can be expressed as a disavowal of a spiritual identity or allegiance to religious beliefs.

Identifying a person's current spiritual beliefs and practices is important, as is inquiry about their religious, spiritual, or cultural rituals. Spiritual rituals and practices can be used to promote hope and support and relieve anxiety for a person. Inquire about current spiritual practices by asking, "Are there any spiritual practices that are particularly important to you now?" In addition, people who have never committed to a strong sense of religion previously may seek religious support in times of crisis (Baldacchino & Draper, 2001). If a person makes a comment, for example, "It is the Lord's way" you might follow up with a question such as, "It seems like religion is very important in your life. Can you tell me more?" Spiritual assessment information and the person's spiritual needs should be met and appropriately documented.

Spiritual well-being can be demonstrated in the face of adversity, in compassion for self and others, and in a sense of inner peace. Nurses see this in a person's will to live or the complete serenity of some individuals in the face of life's most adverse circumstances. Useful assessment questions might consist of, "What do you see as your primary sources of strength at the present time?"; "In the past, what have been sources of strength for you in difficult times?"; "Are there any spiritual or religious values and beliefs that can assist you at this time?"

Case Example

Adeela was diagnosed with breast cancer and given a planned treatment regime, including chemotherapy and radiation. During her second session with chemotherapy, she commented to the nurse, "I can't handle any more of this. Allah has tested me enough and it's time to just stop and let the disease kill me." The nurse recognized the feelings of despair and commented, "You have four more sessions and I can only imagine how difficult having breast cancer must be for you. Can you tell me more about how you are feeling?" Note that even when people's behaviours appear to be supportive of lifesaving efforts, the self can remain conflicted and hopeless.

Simulation Exercise 10.5 focuses on spiritual responses to distress. Spirituality can be a powerful resource in families and it is important to incorporate questions about the

---

SIMULATION EXERCISE 10.5   Responding to Issues of Spiritual Distress

Purpose
To help students understand responses in times of spiritual distress

Procedure
Review the following case situations and develop an appropriate response to each.
1. Mary is 16 years old and has just found out she has a sexually transmitted infection. Her family belongs to a Christian church in which sex before marriage is not permitted. Mary feels guilty about her current status and sees it as "God punishing me for having sex before marriage."
2. Kema is married to an abusive, husband who misuses alcohol. She reads the Quran daily during Ramadan and prays for her husband's healing. She feels that Allah will turn the marriage around if she continues to pray for

changes in her husband's attitude. "Praised be Allah . . . guide us to the right path," she implores.
3. Ari tells the nurse, "I feel that God has let me down. I was taught that those who follow the law or do good are rewarded, while those who don't are punished. I have been a good rabbi, husband, father, and son. Now the doctors tell me I'm going to die and I am 50 years old and I feel abandoned by my God."

Discussion
1. Share your answers with others in your group. Did you have to explore spiritual beliefs beyond your own?
2. Give and get feedback on the usefulness of your responses.
3. In what ways can you use this new knowledge in your nursing care?

family's spirituality if they are involved in supporting the person. Tanyi (2006) suggests nurses can incorporate spiritual assessment with the family, using questions such as the following:

- What gives the family meaning in their daily routines?
- What gives the family strength to deal with stress or crisis?
- How does the family describe their relationship with a higher power such as God, Allah, or Brahma, or any other spiritual beliefs?
- What spiritual rituals, practices, or resources do the family use for support?
- Are there any conflicts between family members related to spiritual views?
- If so, what might be the impact on the current health situation?

Nursing Strategies. The compassionate presence of the nurse in the nurse–person relationship is the most important tool the nurse has in helping the person explore spiritual and existential concerns (Carson & Koenig, 2008). Providing opportunities for people to be self-reflective helps them sustain their beliefs, values, and spiritual sense of self in the face of hardship and tragedy. Gordon and Mitchell (2004) wrote, "Spiritual care is usually provided in a one-to-one relationship, is completely person-centred, and makes no assumptions about personal conviction or life orientation" (p. 646).

Providing privacy and quiet times for spiritual activities is important. Most health care organizations have designated spaces of nonspecific tradition or religion, formerly called "chapels." They are welcoming spaces, open to people of all faiths, spiritualties, and cultural traditions that are politically and spiritually appropriate in all societies of religious and spiritual diversity and uncertainty (Reimer-Kirkham et al., 2011). These spaces, sometimes called "sacred spaces," provide a place for anyone to come to sit, reflect, talk, pray, or simply gather their thoughts (Nita, 2019).

Another important component of nursing care is helping people address their spiritual identity by providing time for spiritual practices and referral to spiritual leaders—for example, or a Elder or Knowledge Keeper for a person who is Indigenous. Elders and Knowledge Keepers are respected and honoured for their sacred knowledge of traditional teachings through the medicine wheel, with the alignment and interaction between the physical, emotional, mental, and spiritual realities. Advocating for the person's spiritual practice is also important in relation to dietary restrictions, mindfulness settings, holy day activities, meditating or praying, and end-of-life cultural practices. For example, a person who is hospitalized and practises the Muslim faith may want to be cared for by a nurse of the same gender.

Prayer and Meditation. Praying with a person, even when the person is of a different faith, can be a soothing intervention. A spiritual care–based therapeutic relationship requires a personal perception of the nurse's own spirituality, which influences the degree to which the person's spiritual needs are perceived (Vlasblom et al., 2011; Wu & Lin, 2011). There should be some evidence from the person's conversation that praying or reading a holy book with a person would be a desired support. According to some researchers (Daaleman et al., 2008; Sulmasy, 2006), spiritual support can be effectively provided through indirect means, such as protecting people's dignity, helping people find meaning in their suffering, offering presence (sitting with people and their families), and talking about what is important to them.

Supporting Spirituality. Addressing spirituality is important in order to unify scientific knowledge, in practice, with an expression of human sensitivity and a deep awareness of the human being (Veloza-Gómez et al., 2017). The self-concept is a dynamic construct, composed of many features, capable of developing new paths to help answer such question as, "Who am I?" and "What is important to me in this situation or phase of life?" As a professional nurse, you will have many opportunities to help people answer these questions.

SUMMARY

This chapter focuses on the self-concept as a key variable in the nurse–person relationship. *Self-concept* refers to an acquired group of thoughts, feelings, attitudes, and beliefs that individuals have about the nature and organization of their personality. Self-concept develops through the interaction between experiences with the environment and personal characteristics.

Aspects of self-concept discussed in the chapter include body image, personal identity, role performance, self-esteem, self-efficacy, self-clarity, and spirituality. Disturbances in body image refer to issues related to changes in appearance and physical functions, both overt and hidden. Personal identity is constructed through cognitive processes of perception and cognition. Serious illnesses such as dementia and mental health issues such as psychosis can threaten a person's sense of personal identity. Self-esteem is associated with the emotional aspect of self-concept and reflects the value a person places on their personal self-concept and their place in the world. Self-efficacy pertains to individuals' sense of control to make changes in the face of challenges to self-clarity, which relates to the stability of the defined self. Self-esteem hopefulness, and spirituality have been shown to be positively related to health-related quality of life. Assessment of spiritual needs and corresponding spiritual care is an important part of your nursing practice in providing compassionate, quality care. Understanding these elements of self-concept and the critical role they play in quality of life and coping with life issues are key to working effectively with people of all ages. It is a core variable to consider in therapeutic communication, nurse–person relationships, and interventions.

🕵 ETHICAL DILEMMA
What Would You Do?

Jimmy is a 68-year-old man with diabetes; he was brought to the emergency room in kidney failure. The doctor has indicated that Jimmy needs to agree to dialysis, but Jimmy refuses, saying "This only prolongs the final result." He refuses to listen to any long-term plan of care, and his wife is confused about options beyond dialysis. As the nurse caring for this person, what would you do?

QUESTIONS FOR REVIEW AND DISCUSSION

1. What role do the various social media networks play in the development and validation of a person's self-esteem and self-concept?
2. In what ways are spirituality and world view connected in defining self-concept?
3. Drawing on your experience, what are some specific ways in which you can help another person develop a stronger sense of self?
4. Describe a personal exchange with a person or an observed clinical encounter with another provider in which you felt that you learned something important about the value of the health provider's presence in promoting self-esteem.

REFERENCES

Abel, J. P., Buff, C. L., & Burr, S. A. (2016). Social media and the fear of missing out: Scale development and assessment. *Journal of Business & Economics Research, 14*(1), 33–43. https://clutejournals.com/index.php/JBER/article/view/9554/9632.

Adler, R., Rosenfeld, L., & Proctor, R. (2014). *Interplay: The process of interpersonal communication.* Oxford University Press.

Armstrong, A. (2019). *Police-reported hate crime in Canada, 2017.* https://www150.statcan.gc.ca/n1/pub/85-002-x/2019001/article/00008-eng.htm.

Arnett, J. (2013). *Adolescence and Emerging Adulthood* (5th ed.). Pearson Publishing Co.

Baldacchino, D., & Draper, P. (2001). Spiritual coping strategies: A review of the literature. *Journal of Advanced Nursing, 34*(6), 833–841.

Bandura, A. (1997). Self-efficacy. *The exercise of control.* W.H. Freeman and Company.

Bandura, A. (2007). Self-efficacy in health functioning. In S. Ayers (Ed.), *Cambridge handbook of psychology, health and medicine.* (2nd ed.) (pp. 191–193). Cambridge University Press.

Baumeister, R.F., & Vohs, K.D. (2007). *Encyclopedia of Social Psychology.* https://doi.org/10.4135/9781412956253.n477.

Beck, J., & Beck, A. (2011). *Cognitive conceptualization. Cognitive behavior therapy* (pp. 29–46). Guilford Press.

Bem, D. J. (1972). Self-perception theory. *Advances in Experimental Social Psychology, 6,* 1–62.

Benner, P. (2003). Reflecting on what we care about. *American Journal of Critical Care, 12*(2), 165–166.

Blazer, D. (2008). How do you feel about . . .? Health outcomes late in life and self-perceptions of health and well-being. *Gerontologist, 48*(4), 415–422.

Blazer, D. (2012). Religion/spirituality and depression: What can we learn from empirical studies? *American Journal of Psychiatry, 169,* 10–12.

Bolton, M. A., Lobben, I., & Stern, T. A. (2010). The impact of body image on patient care. *Primary Care Companion to the Journal of Clinical Psychiatry, 12*(2).

British Columbia Ministry of Health. (2011). *Self-management support: A health care intervention.* https://www.selfmanagementbc.ca/uploads/What%20is%20Self-Management/PDF/Self-Management%20Support%20A%20health%20care%20intervention%202011.pdf.

Callus, I., & Herbrechter, S. (2012). Introduction: Posthumanist subjectivities, or, coming after the subject. *Subjectivity, 5*(3), 241–264.

Canadian Nurses Association. (2010). *Position statement: Spirituality, health and nursing practice.* https://www.cna-aiic.ca/~/media/cna/page-content/pdf-en/ps111_spirituality_2010_e.pdf?la=en.

Canadian Nurses Association. (2017). *Code of ethics for registered nurses.* https://www.cna-aiic.ca/~/media/cna/page-content/pdf-en/code-of-ethics-2017-edition-secure-interactive.

Capps, D. (2008). Alzheimer's disease and the loss of self. *Journal of Pastoral Care and Counseling, 62*(1–2), 19–28.

Carson, V., & Koenig, H. (2008). *Spiritual dimensions of nursing practice* (revised ed.). Templeton Press.

Chaze, F., Thomson, M. S., George, U. et al. (2015). Role of cultural beliefs, religion, and spirituality in mental health and/or service utilization among immigrants in Canada: A scoping review. *Canadian Journal of Community Mental Health, 34*(3), 87–101. 10.7870/cjcmh-2015-015.

Cooper, J. (2007). *Cognitive dissonance: 50 years of a classic theory.* Sage Publications.

Crocker, J., Brook, A. T., & Niiya, Y. (2006). The pursuit of self-esteem: Contingencies of self-worth and self-regulation. *Journal of Personality, 74*(6), 1749–1771.

Cunha, C., & Goncalves, M. (2009). Commentary: Accessing the experience of a dialogical self: Some needs and concerns. *Culture Psychology, 15*(3), 120–133.

Daaleman, T., Usher, B. M., Williams, S. et al. (2008). An exploratory study of spiritual care at the end of life. *Annals of Family Medicine, 6*(5), 406–411.

Dein, S., Cook, C. C. H., & Koenig, H. (2012). Religion, spirituality and mental health: Current controversies and future directions. *The Journal of Nervous and Mental Disease*, 200(10), 852–855.

Diehl, M., & Hay, E. (2007). Contextualized self-representations in adulthood. *Journal of Personality*, 75(6), 1255–1283.

Drench, M., Noonan, A., Sharby, N. et al. (2011). *Psychosocial aspects of health care* (3rd ed.). Prentice Hall.

Dropkin, M. J. (1999). Body image and quality of life after head and neck cancer surgery. *Cancer Practice*, 7, 309–313.

Elliott, A. (2013). *Concepts of the self*. Polity Press.

Ellis-Hill, C., & Horn, S. (2000). Change in identity and self-concept: A new theoretical approach to recovery following a stroke. *Clinical Rehabilitation*, 14(3), 279–287.

Erikson, E. (1959). *Identity and the life cycle: Selected papers*. International Universities Press.

Erikson, E. (1968). *Identity: Youth and crisis*. Norton.

Erikson, E. (1982). *The life cycle completed: A review*. Norton.

Erikson, E. H. (1985). *The Life Cycle Completed*. Norton.

Fattore, T., Mason, A. J., & Watson, E. (2017). Self, identity and well-being. *Children's Well-Being: Indicators and Research*, 14, 116.

Fazio, S., & Mitchell, D. (2009). Persistence of self in individuals with Alzheimer's disease. *Dementia*, 8, 39–59.

Freeborn, J., (2016). *Chantal Petitclerc*. The Canadian Encyclopedia. https://www.thecanadianencyclopedia.ca/en/article/chantal-petitclerc.

Fullwood, C., James, B. M., & Chen-Wilson, C. H. (2016). Self-concept clarity and online self-presentation in adolescents. *Cyberpsychology, Behavior, and Social Networking*, 1–6. 10.1089/cyber.2015.0623.

Goffman, E. (1963). *Stigma and social identity. Stigma: Notes on the management of spoiled identity*. Prentice Hall.

Gordon, M. (2007). Self-perception-self-concept pattern: *Manual of Nursing Diagnoses* (11th ed.). Bartlett Jones.

Gordon, T., & Mitchell, D. (2004). A competency model for the assessment and delivery of spiritual care. *Palliative Medicine*, 18(7), 646–651.

Gottlieb, L.N. & Gottlieb, B. (2013). *Strengths-based nursing care: Health and healing for person and family*. Springer Publishing Company.

Guerrero, L., Anderson, P., & Afifi, W. (2017). *Close encounters: Communication in relationships* (4th ed.). Sage Publications.

Harrington, J. (2011). Implications of treatment on body image and quality of life. *Seminars in Oncology Nursing*, 27(4), 290–299.

Harter, S. (2006). The self. In N. Eisenberg (Ed.), *Handbook of child psychology* (pp. 505–571). Wiley.

Health Council of Canada. (2012). *Self-management support for Canadians with chronic health conditions*. https://www.selfmanagementbc.ca/uploads/HCC_SelfManagementReport_FA.pdf.

Heijmans, M., Rijken, M., Foets, M. et al. (2004). The stress of being chronically ill: From disease-specific to task-specific aspects. *Journal of Behavioral Medicine*, 27, 255–271.

HelpGuide. (2020). Social media and mental health. https://www.helpguide.org/articles/mental-health/social-media-and-mental-health.htm#.

Humphreys, K. (2004). *Circles of recovery: Self-help organizations for addictions*. Cambridge University Press.

Hunter, E. (2008). Beyond death: Inheriting the past and giving to the future, transmitting the legacy of one's self. *Omega*, 56(40), 313–329.

Johnson, M., Cowin, L. S., Wilson, I. et al. (2012). Professional identity and nursing: Contemporary theoretical developments and future research challenges. *International Nursing Review*, 59(4), 562–569.

Jung, C. G. (1960). *Collected works. The psychogenesis of mental disease* (Vol. 3). Pantheon.

Kamakura, T., Ando, J., & Ono, Y. (2001). Genetic and environmental influences on self-esteem in a Japanese twin sample. *Twin Research*, 4(6), 439–442.

Karademas, E., Bakouli, A., Bastouonis, A. et al. (2008). Illness perceptions, illness-related problems, subjective health and the role of perceived primal threat: Preliminary findings. *Journal of Health Psychology*, 13(8), 1021–1029.

Kendler, K., & Gardner, K. (1998). A population-based twin study of self-esteem and gender. *Psychological Medicine*, 28(6), 1403–1409.

Koenig, H.G. (2012). Religion, spirituality and health: The research and clinical implications. International Scholarly Research Network. 10.5402/2012/278730.

Lake, N. (2014). *The caregivers: A support group's stories of slow loss, courage, and love*. Simon & Schuster, Inc.

Leerdam, L., Rietveld, L., Teunissen, D. et al. (2014). Gender-based education during clerkships: A focus group study. *Advances in Medical Education and Practice*, 26(5), 53–60.

Malle, B. (2011). Attribution theories: How people make sense of behavior. In C. Derck (Ed.), Theories in Social Psychology. (pp. 72–95). Wiley Blackwell Publishing Ltd.

Marks, R., Allegrante, J., & Lorig, K. (2005). A review and synthesis of research evidence for self-efficacy-enhancing interventions for reducing chronic disability. Implications for health education practice (Part II). *Health Promotion Practice*, 6(2), 148–156.

Markus, H., & Nurius, P. (1986). Possible selves. *American Psychologist*, 41, 954–969.

Marsh, H. W., Xu, M., & Martin, A. J. (2012). Self-concept: A synergy of theory, method, and application. In K. R. Harris, S. Graham, & T. Urdan (Eds.), *APA Educational Psychology Handbook: Vol.1. Theories, Constructs and Critical Issues* (pp. 427–458). American Psychological Association.

Mordoch, E. (2015). Fostering a positive self-concept. In D. Gregory, C. Raymond-Seniuk, L. Patrick et al. (Eds.), *Fundamentals perspectives on the art and science of Canadian nursing* (pp. 216–231). Wolters Kluwer.

Mussatto, K., Sawin, K. J., & Schiffman, R. (2014). The importance of self-perceptions to psychosocial adjustment in adolescents with heart disease. *Journal of Pediatric Health Care*, 28(3), 251–261. http://doi.org/10.1016/j.pedhc.2013.05.006.

Neff, K. D. (2011). Self-compassion, self-esteem and well-being. *Social and Personality Psychology Compass*, 5(1), 1–12.

Neiss, M. B., Sedikes, C., & Stevenson, J. (2002). Self-esteem: A behavioral genetic perspective. *European Journal of Personality*, 16, 351–367.

Nita, M. (2019). 'Spirituality' in health studies: Competing spiritualties and the elevated state of mindfulness. *Journal of Religion and Health*, 58, 1605–1618. doi.org/10.1007/s10943-019-00773-2.

Orth, U., & Robins, R. W. (2014). The development of self-esteem. *Association for Psychological Science*, 23(5), 381–387.

Prescott, A. P. (2006). *The concept of self in education, family and sports*. Nova Science Publishers.

Raholm, M. B. (2008). Uncovering the ethics of suffering using a narrative approach. *Nursing Ethics*, 15(1), 62–72.

Reed, P. G. (2014). Theory of self-transcendence. In M. J. Smith & P. R. Liehr (Eds.), *Middle range theory for nursing* (3rd ed., pp. 109–140). Springer.

Reimer-Kirkham, S., Sharma, S., Pesut, B. et al. (2011). Sacred spaces in public places: Religious and spiritual plurality in health care. *Nursing Inquiry*, 19(3), 202–212. 10.1111/j.1440-1800.2011.00571.x.

Robson, P. J. (1988). Self-esteem - A psychiatric view. *The British Journal of Psychiatry*, 153, 6–15.

Rogers, C. (1959). A theory of therapy, personality and interpersonal relationships as developed in the client-centered framework. In S. Koch (Ed.), *Psychology: A study of a science. Vol. 3: Formulations of the person and the social context*. McGraw IIill.

Rosa, E. M., & Tudge, J. (2013). Uri Bronfenbrenner's theory of human development: Its evolution from ecology to bioecology. *Journal of Family Theory & Review*, 5(December 2013), 243–258. 10.1111/jftr.12022.

Saiphoo, A. N., Halevi, L. D., & Vahedi, Z. (2020). Social networking site use and self-esteem: A meta-analytic review. *Personality and Individual Differences*, 153, (2020), 109639.

Schachter, E. (2005). Erikson meets the postmodern: Can classic identity theory rise to the challenge? *Identity*, 5(2), 137–160.

Senate of Canada, (n.d.). *Senator Chantal Peticlerc*. https://sencanada.ca/en/senators/petitclerc-chantal/.

Shweder, R., Goodnow, J., Hatano, R. et al. (2006). The cultural psychology of development: One mind, many mentalities. In W. Damon (Ed.), *Handbook of child psychology* (6th ed.). John Wiley and Sons.

Simpson, E., & Jones, M. C. (2013). An exploration of self-efficacy and self-management in COPD patients. *British Journal of Nursing*, 13(2219), 1105–1109.

Slatman, J. (2011). The meaning of body experience evaluation in oncology. *Health Care Analysis*, 19, 295–311.

Smith, M. J., & Perkins, K. (2008). Attending to the voices of adolescents who are overweight to promote mental health. *Archives of Psychiatric Nursing*, 22(6), 391–393.

Statistics Canada. (2013). 2011 National Household Survey: Immigration, place of birth, citizenship, ethnic origin, visible minorities, language and religion. https://www150.statcan.gc.ca/n1/daily-quotidien/130508/dq130508b-eng.htm.

Statistics Canada. (2019). *Data tables, 2016 Census: Visible Minority, Individual low-income status*. https://www12.statcan.gc.ca/census-recensement/2016/dp-pd/dt-td/Rp-eng.cfm?TABID=2&Lang=E&APATH=3&DETAIL=0&DIM=0&FL=A&FREE=0&GC=0&GID=1341679&GK=0&GRP=1&PID=110531&PRID=10&PTYPE=109445&S=0&SHOWALL=0&SUB=0&Temporal=2017&THEME=120&VID=0&VNAMEE=&VNAMEF=&D1=0&D2=0&D3=0&D4=0&D5=0&D6=0.

Steiger, A. E., Allemand, M., Robins, R. W. et al. (2014). Low and decreasing self-esteem during adolescence predict adult depression two decades later. *Journal of Personality and Social Psychology*, 106(2), 325–338. https://doi.org/10.1037/a0035133.

Sue, D.W. (2010). Microaggressions in everday life: Race, gender and sexual orientation. Wiley.

Sullivan, H. S. (1953). *The interpersonal theory of psychiatry*. Norton.

Sulmasy, D. P. (2006). Spiritual issues in the care of dying patients. *The Journal of the American Medical Association*, 296(11), 1385–1392.

Suzuki, M., Amagai, M., Shibata, F. et al. (2011). Participation related to self-efficacy for social participation of people with mental illness. *Archives of Psychiatric Nursing*, 25(5), 359–365.

Tanyi, R. (2006). Spirituality and family nursing: Spiritual assessment and interventions for families. *Journal of Advanced Nursing*, 53(3), 287–294.

Usborne, E., & Taylor, D. (2010). The role of cultural identity clarity for self-concept, clarity, self-esteem, and subjective well-being. *Personality and Social Psychology Bulletin*, 36(7), 883–897.

van Tuyl, L. H. D., Hewlett, S., Sadlonova, M. et al. (2014). The patient perspective on remission in rheumatoid arthritis: 'You've got limits, but you're back to being you again'. *Annals of the Rheumatic Diseases*, 74(6), 1004–1010.

Vandenbosch, L., & Eggermont, S. (2016). The interrelated roles of mass media and social media in adolescents' development of an objectified self-concept: A longitudinal study. *Communication Research*, 43(8), 1116–1140.

Vartanian, L. (2009). When the body defines the self: Self-concept clarity, internalization, and body image. *Journal of Social Clinical Psychology*, 28(1), 94–126.

Veloza-Gómez, M., Muñoz de Rodríguez, L., Guevara-Armenta, C. et al. (2017). The importance of spiritual care in nursing practice. *Journal of Holistic Nursing*, 35(2), 118–131.

Vickery, C., Sepehri, A., & Evans, C. (2008). Self-esteem in an acute stroke rehabilitation sample: A control group comparison. *Clinical Rehabilitation*, 22, 179–187.

Vlasblom, J. P., Steen, J. V., Knol, D. L. et al. (2011). Effects of a spiritual care training for nurses. *Nurse Education Today*, 31, 790–796.

Walker, C. (2010). Ruptured identities: Leaving work because of chronic illness. *International Journal of Health Services*, 40(4), 629–643.

Warrender, D., & Milne, R. (2020). How use of social media and social comparison affect mental health. *Nursing Times [online]*, 116(3), 56–59. https://www.nursingtimes.net/news/mental-health/how-use-of-social-media-and-social-comparison-affect-mental-health-24-02-2020/.

Wu, L. -F., & Lin, L. -Y. (2011). Exploration of clinical nurses' perceptions of spirituality and spiritual care. *The Journal of Nursing Research*, 19, 250–256.

11

Developing Person-Centred Therapeutic Relationships

Claire Mallette

Originating US Chapter by *Elizabeth C. Arnold*

OBJECTIVES

At the end of this chapter, the reader will be able to:

1. Define a person-centred care (PCC) relationship in health care.
2. Explain the differences between social and therapeutic relationships.
3. Identify theoretical relationship models used in nursing practice.
4. Discuss the core concepts of person-centred relationships in health care.
5. Discuss therapeutic use of self in person-centred relationships.
6. Discuss the main features of each relationship phase.
7. Explain how person-centred communication is embedded in contemporary health care provider relationships.

In Canada and around the world, there has been a shift in health care practices to put the person and family at the centre of care. The World Health Organization [WHO] (2016) developed a *Framework of Integrated People-Centred Health Services* that emphasizes the importance of developing people-centred care to "improve access to care, health and clinical outcomes, better health literacy and self-care, increased satisfaction with care, improved job satisfaction for health workers, improved efficiency of services and reduced overall costs" (p. 2). Across Canada, there have been initiatives to support and enact person-centred care to improve the quality and delivery of health care (Registered Nurses' Association of Ontario [RNAO], 2015). For example, in Alberta, the *Alberta Health Act* (2010) was the outcome of the *Putting People First* report and includes that the Health Charter must recognize that "health is a partnership among individuals, families, communities, health providers, organizations that deliver health services and the Government of Alberta" (Province of Alberta, 2014, p. 6).

Over the past two decades, chronic health conditions have replaced infectious diseases as the leading health care concern (Palmer et al., 2017). In Canada, 44% of adults over 20 years of age have at least 1 of 10 common chronic health conditions, including hypertension, osteoarthritis, osteoporosis, mental health disorders, diabetes, cardiovascular and respiratory diseases, cancer, and conditions causing dementia (Government of Canada, 2019). To facilitate a more effective management of chronic health conditions, person- and family-centred care delivery models are being used. Person-centred care (PCC) supports the principle of offering care with people through including them and their family as essential members of the interprofessional care team. This approach enables and facilitates comprehensiveness, coordination, and continuity of care (Canadian Academy of Health Services, 2017).

Effective PCC relationships are critical in nursing practice and care for the person and family. Whether caring for the person individually or as an interprofessional team member, nurses are in a unique position to gather, provide, and explain essential information throughout a health experience. Nurses are an important professional resource providing ongoing support in the care and compassionate nursing practice that people and their families need when they are feeling vulnerable in health care situations.

With the support of the nurse and interprofessional team, people and their families can learn to self-manage their health challenges and achieve a meaningful life. This chapter explores core concepts and the essential features of PCC relationships.

BASIC CONCEPTS

The importance of person-centred relationships as an essential component of safe, compassionate quality health care delivery cannot be overemphasized. Research indicates that effective PCC relationships are a significant predictor of positive health outcomes (Hibbard, 2017).

Definitions

A person-centred relationship is categorized as a "therapeutic relationship," linked to assisting people to achieve identifiable health goals. The Registered Nurses' Association of Ontario's *Nursing Best Practice Guidelines* [RNAO BPG] (2015) describes a **therapeutic relationship** as integral to PCC. The therapeutic relationship involves knowledge, trust, respect, self-awareness, professional intimacy, empathy, and awareness of power (College of Nurses of Ontario, 2006; Registered Nurses' Association of Ontario, 2015). **Person-centred care (PCC)** relationships represent a subset of professional therapeutic relationships, in which nurses and other health providers engage with people, specifically related to the following:

- Understanding the person's experience of the health issue
- Understanding the person's cultural contexts in relation to their health issues
- Supporting effective self-management of health issues
- Development of healthy lifestyle behaviours to promote health and well-being and prevent or minimize the development of chronic health conditions
- Increased satisfaction with health outcomes and well-being

Person-centredness is based on recognizing the person's knowledge and expertise in managing their health issue. PCC begins with developing a relationship through communication, collaboration, and sharing of information related to decision making on health care and services (RNAO, 2015). The PCC relationship is characterized as a clinical partnership between a person and selected health care providers. A critical dimension of PCC in providing compassionate and coordinated care, based on respect for the person's preferences, values, and needs, is recognizing the person, family and any substitute decision maker as full partners (Dolansky & Moore, 2013).

Professional and personal roles of the nurse are not interchangeable in a PCC relationship. Both roles are relevant to successfully achieving health outcomes, but they complement rather than replace one another. The person receiving care is the best informant about the personalized nature of their health issue and its impact on their life. Current understandings of PCC relationships incorporate the person's needs, values, and preferences in all aspects of care. "Indicators of a strong therapeutic relationship include mutual trust among all parties, coordinated and continuous health care, and the person's perception of feeling respected and cared for" (Street et al., 2009, p. 298). The correlation between therapeutic relationship and person-centredness is portrayed in Fig. 11.1.

The continuum of PCC relationships ranges from those found in acute care to those found in primary care, promoting health and the self-management of health issues. Home and long-term care settings also recognize the importance of PCC. PCC relationships can also take place digitally or through video conferencing. This method became widely used in 2020 as a result of the COVID-19 pandemic, resulting in people now having a new capability to communicate with providers through secure video portals. In some case, people are able to also receive copies of their health records. They can also use technology to communicate directly, make appointments, ask questions, request refills on medications, and report new symptoms. Digital health will be explored further in Chapters 26 and 27.

PCC relationships are time limited and subject to the health issue and other regulatory concerns. A PCC relationship can span a 12-hour shift and it can occur episodically or at regularly scheduled times; it can occur as a single encounter or as an emergency care contact. Longer-term relationships can last over a period of days, weeks, or months, as in an acute mental health care setting or rehabilitation centre. Regardless of the amount of time spent, each PCC relationship can, and should, be meaningful. The relationship typically terminates when identified health goals are achieved or the person is transferred to a different care setting.

Person-Centred Care Relationships

PCC relationships are based on the premise that each person's experience of a health issue, injury, or disease is a total human experience and much more than simply a biomedical process.

"Patient- and family-centered care applies to patients of all ages, and it may be practiced in any health care setting" (Mitchell et al., 2009, p. 543). McCormack and McCance (2010) describe PCC as an "approach to practice established through the formation and fostering of therapeutic relationships between all care providers ... patients and

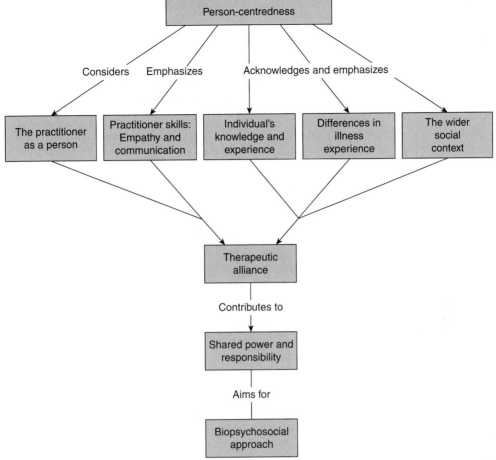

Fig. 11.1 Model of Person-Centredness in Nurse–Person Relationships. From Lhussier, M., Eaton, S., Forster, N. et al. (2015). Care planning for long-term conditions—a concept mapping. *Health Expectations, 18*(5), 605–624.

others significant to them in their lives" (p. 13). What each of these descriptions has in common is an insistence upon the primacy of the person in all aspects of care decision making and health care.

Relational connections in person-centred relationships offer supportive intervention that is holistic, respectful, individualized, and empowering (Morgan & Yoder, 2012). Each relationship is based on the importance of understanding the person as unique, with one or more health issues that may be influencing their life in a meaningful way. In addition to a person's physical and health needs, nurses need to consider each person's cognitive, sociocultural, and emotional contexts, as these influence the person's personalized experience of health issues. Addressing situational, cultural, religious, and family circumstances allows for a more inclusive holistic understanding of the

person's preferences and life goals. This information and knowledge informs nurses in individualizing, supporting, and understanding the fuller dimensions of a person's health issues. Listening to what a person identifies as primary concerns provides stronger information about the person's values and preferences.

Respectful care starts with careful active listening and emphasizes the person's strengths, abilities, wishes, and goals. Respect assumes that people are interested in bettering their health and are active partners in addressing their health concerns. Nurses demonstrate respectful care when they support the person's autonomy and realistic care goals.

PCC is individualized care. Listening to what the person identifies as their main concern provides contextual information about the person's values and preferences within the family and community. Once you have a composite picture of each person, and of what matters to the person and family, it becomes easier to develop a focused care plan based on individual goals and values. Motivation and interest are significant contributors to relevant goal development and continued efforts to achieve personally relevant life and health goals.

A person-centred assessment seeks an integrated understanding of each person's contextual world—including emotional, cultural, and spiritual needs and life issues. The information gathered forms a relational informational platform that is unique to the person and provides a common ground for developing mutually agreed-upon self-management and health-related strategies.

Developing a Person-Centred Care Plan

A PCC plan is designed to encourage autonomy and the development of self-efficacy in all aspects of care. Accurately assessing the person's knowledge base and personal need for information as you search for common ground about each person's life issues and biopsychosocial health needs is critical. Self-efficacy plays an important role in personal motivation (Bandura, 2012). *Self-efficacy* is defined as the confidence that a person holds about personal ability to achieve goals or complete a task. Self-efficacy beliefs affect the quality of human functioning through cognitive, motivational, affective, and decisional processes. Specifically, people's beliefs in their efficacy will influence whether they have confidence in their abilities to achieve the goals they set for themselves.

Self-management can be defined as the tasks and strategies that an individual carries out to live well with chronic health conditions. These include increasing confidence to cope with the medical treatments and the change in roles, managing emotions associated with having a chronic health condition, and achieving the best possible quality of life (British Columbia Ministry of Health, 2011; Canadian Nurses Association [CNA], 2012).

An important person-centred focus of the relationship is on considering options and making choices in partnership with the person and other health team providers. Nurses and other professional health care providers contribute evidence-informed information and professional expertise to the clinical plan. The person provides individualized personal data. Knowledge of a person's coping strategies, strengths, and limitations, plus joint perceptions about symptoms, expectations, and previous life experiences, are significant contextual contributors to a PCC plan. PCC plans ideally revolve around each person's primary reasons for seeking health care, personal and family concerns, and available resources. Shared decision making (SDM), in which people and providers strive to "make health care decisions together," strengthens the person–provider relationship that allows the health relationship to move forward toward successful management of chronic health conditions.

RELATIONAL PROCESSES IN PERSON-CENTRED CARE

Each person being cared for is unique, with their own history. In a professional health relationship, neither the heath care provider nor the person receiving care exists independently of the other. A person-centred relationship seeks to understand the person's emotional, physical, cultural, and spiritual needs for coping with health-related life issues, along with the person's life experiences. What happens within this relationship becomes the shared product of their interactions and its impact on other relationships and personal values—all of which are important to the person and assist in understanding the full picture of a person's health care situation.

Relevant content that emerges in the assessment phase of a PCC relationship becomes the basis for SDM between people and their health care providers. This information influences the specific step progression toward identifying therapeutic goals. Nursing practice requires an evidence-informed foundation, while including an understanding of the full human experience of people in need of health care (Lazenby, 2013).

Once the person and health care providers agree on a workable action plan, an important focus of the care partnership becomes person and family education, compassionate coaching, and informed support of focused self-management strategies. These communication strategies are specifically designed to incorporate the values, preferences, resources of the person as an essential component of care, to whatever extent is possible.

Professional relationships and knowledge transfer are major communication tools used to meet one or more of the following care goals:

- Understanding the person's experience of a health condition
- Helping people to effectively self-manage chronic health issues
- Encouraging people to develop healthy lifestyle behaviours to prevent or minimize the development of chronic health conditions

Collaborative Person-Centred Relationships

Collaborative interprofessional care approaches are embedded in health care teams, rather than single practitioners assuming responsibility for the person-centred health care of people. This paradigm shift is based on the premise that no single health care discipline can provide complete care for a person with today's multiple chronic health care needs (Batalden et al., 2006). Interprofessional PCC practice can positively influence current health issues such as wait times, healthy workplaces, person safety, primary health care, chronic care management, and population health and wellness (CNA, 2011). Interprofessional collaborative relationships bring together the expert knowledge and skills from nursing, medicine, primary care, pharmacy, rehabilitation, psychological care, and social work needed to support desired person-centred outcomes. The relationship aspect develops from mutual respect, trust, and power sharing among all team members, including the person and family, to achieve optimal health outcomes (see also Chapter 24).

The National Interprofessional Competency Framework (Canadian Interprofessional Health Collaborative, 2010) developed for learners and health care providers, describes interprofessional collaboration as a process of developing and maintaining interprofessional effective working relationships with people, families, and communities to achieve optimal health outcomes. Interprofessional education (IPE) prepares learners for collaborative practice and focuses on health care provider students coming together to learn how to become effective interprofessional team members practising collaboratively to provide high quality PCC (Western Health Sciences, n.d.).

Care coordination among multiple care providers is an essential component of interprofessional person-centred relationships (WHO, 2010). Contemporary practice requires that nurses lead, coordinate, and integrate their professional nursing knowledge and skills with those of other health team members (depending on the circumstances), for maximum effectiveness.

Elements of Person-Centred Relationships

Basically, PCC is examining health care from the person perspective of their care and their relationships with the health providers caring for them (Ferguson et al., 2013). A person-centred relationship considers the person first and foremost, with distinctive, personally held values, beliefs, cultural contexts, and life goals. Second, this person with a health issue or disease requires health care and professional support in addressing the health issues. In crisis situations, immediate life-sustaining issues take precedence. However, personal factors, especially those related to the person's dignity and individuality, should still be incorporated into the care provided and the support to the family.

Although nurses continue to have an intimate relationship on many levels with the people they care for, there are an increasing number of people with one or more chronic health conditions such as diabetes, cardiovascular disease, and respiratory disease. These conditions require careful monitoring and personalized focus over significant periods of time, and possibly a lifetime. Self-management of chronic disorder led to the development of the Chronic Care Model, by Dr. Edward Wagner and colleagues (2001). This model proposes "a person-professional partnership, involving collaborative care and self-management education" (Bodenheimer et al., 2002, p. 2469). The six elements of the model include health care organization, decision support, delivery system design, clinical information systems, self-management support, and community resources and policies. This model can assist primary care health teams to be more proactive in health promotion (Canadian Academy of Health Sciences, 2017). The Chronic Care Model is presented in Fig. 11.2 As there is an increased need and focus on health promotion and primary care in Canada, Barr et al. (2003) recommended to expand the community resources component to include guiding health public policy, creative supportive environments, and strengthening of community action to strive to address social determinants of health. They also recommended that the informed activated and engaged person should also include an activated and engaged community. And alongside prepared, proactive practice teams, there should also be prepared, proactive community partners.

A major value of the Chronic Care Model is its integrated effectiveness across multiple care settings. The inclusion of care initiatives across the health continuum helps offset potential gaps in care. In addition to health education and traditional care delivery, nurses work with people and their families to help them develop the self-management skills and strategies they need to address their chronic health conditions and daily lives (Lhussier et al., 2015). Nurses also support and coach people in developing problem-solving skills and other self-management skills to support healthy lifestyle behaviours. Having confidence to self-manage a chronic health condition is consistent with the "quadruple aim," which is an internationally recognized framework for designing and delivering effective health care systems. The four objectives of the quadruple aim are improving the person and caregiver experience, improving the health of populations, reducing health care costs, and improving the work life of health care providers (Government of Ontario, 2019).

Each PCC relationship represents a unique relational encounter that validates the assumption that "a core value of nursing is that the people we serve are uniquely valuable as human beings" (Porter et al., 2011, p. 107). Nurses and the people they care for have different personalities. Their ways of relating with others, and the circumstances surrounding each relationship, differ. What is supportive to one person or family may not be to another.

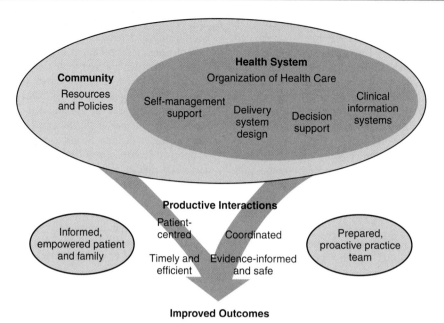

Fig. 11.2 Chronic Care Model (Wagner et al., 1999). From Barr, V. J., Robinson, S., Marin-Link, B. et al. (2003). The expanded chronic care model: An integration of concepts and strategies from population health promotion and chronic care model. *Healthcare Quarterly, 7*(1), 73–82. 10.12927/hcq.2003.16763. https://www.longwoods.com/content/16763.

Caring as a Core Value in Therapeutic Relationships

Caring represents a core foundational value in professional nursing relationships. It is this component of professional relationships that is best remembered by people, families, and nurses. Think about a significant caring relationship you have had with a person, or experienced yourself as a person. What made it special or meaningful to you?

Caring within person-centred relationships is not so much about the words themselves or about specific tasks. Rather, it is about a sustained connection and the meaning that caring connection holds for the recipient(s) (Crowe, 2000). While people will remember the caring connection, professional caring is much more than "being kind." Instead, it is a complex relationship that encompasses knowledge, being present with another, and actions focusing on achieving positive outcomes and well-being. Caring as a key characteristic of professional nursing should be embodied as a visible component of each nurse's relationship, with people and their families and with each other.

Person-Centred Versus Social Relationships

Therapeutic, person-centred relationships share many characteristics with social relationships. All relationships work better when participants are actively engaged, when each participant listens carefully and respects the other as an equal partner. Communication strengths such as authenticity, presence, acceptance, positive regard, empathy, respect, self-awareness, and competence, when deliberately employed, contribute to the success of therapeutic professional relationships.

The differences between social and therapeutic relationships relate to purpose, the type of involvement, and the privacy protections. Social relationships are established and maintained to meet mutual need or friendship purposes. Therapeutic relationships are established for professional, health-related purposes, within a specific time setting. The focus of attention is always on people's health concerns and the actions needed to help them identify and resolve issues related to health and well-being. This is a major distinction between the two types of relationship.

Therapeutic relationships are subject to ethical and legal standards. Unlike social relationships, they are purposefully linked to supporting people in meeting health-related goals. Professional relationships have a defined beginning and ending. There are rules governing the structure, interpersonal behaviours, and topics developed within the relationship. Table 11.1 outlines the differences between social and therapeutic relationships.

TABLE 11.1   Differences Between Helping Relationships and Social Relationships

Helping Relationships	Social Relationships
Health care provider takes responsibility for guiding the relationship and for maintaining appropriate boundaries	Both parties have equal responsibility for contributing to the relationship
Relationship has a specific health-related purpose and goals	Relationship may or may not have a specific purpose or goals
Duration is determined by meeting the professional, health-related needs and goals of the person	Relationship can last a lifetime or terminate spontaneously at any time
Focus of the relationship is on the needs of the person	The needs of both partners can receive equal attention
Relationship is entered into because of a person's health care needs	Relationship is entered into spontaneously for a wide variety of purposes
Members in the relationship are related to the person's health needs, such as family and appropriate health care providers when necessary	Behaviour for both participants is spontaneous; people choose friends
Self-disclosure by the nurse is limited to information that facilitates the health-related relationship; self-disclosure by the person is expected and encouraged	Self-disclosure for both parties in the relationship is expected and encouraged

Theoretical Frameworks

Theoretical frameworks that support the study of person-centred relationships in nursing practice include Peplau's interpersonal nursing theory, Carl Rogers' person-centred theory, and Maslow's hierarchy of needs theory.

Hildegard Peplau's Interpersonal Nursing Theory

Hildegard Peplau's (1997) interpersonal nursing theory is a well-known theory of interpersonal relationships in nursing. She identifies four sequential phases of a nurse–person relationships: pre-interaction, orientation, working phase (problem identification and exploitation), and termination. These phases are an overlapping part of a holistic relationship. Each phase serves to broaden as well as deepen the emotional connection between the nurse and the person receiving care (Reynolds, 1997). Peplau identified six professional roles the nurse can assume during the course of the nurse–person relationship. (See Box 11.1)

Carl Rogers' Person-Centred Model

Carl Rogers' model states that each person has within themselves the capacity to heal if given support and treated with respect and unconditional positive regard, in a caring, authentic, therapeutic relationship. Rogers presents a person-centred approach to the study of therapeutic relationships and the relevant concepts supporting it. He identifies three major provider attributes of person-centred relationships in atherapeutic setting:

- **Authenticity** (being "real" in a relationship, without artificial impressions)

- Trust and respect
- Empathetic understanding

Abraham Maslow's Hierarchy of Needs Theory

The International Council of Nurses (ICN) definition of *nursing* describes nurses' role as autonomous and collaborative in meeting the needs of the person, family, groups, and communities, sick or well, in all settings (ICN, n.d.). Abraham Maslow's (1970) hierarchy of needs theory offers a motivational framework that nurses use to prioritize the person's needs in planning their care. Fig. 11.3 shows Maslow's (1970) model as a pyramid, with need requirements occurring in an ascending fashion, from basic survival needs through to self-actualization.

Maslow defines first-level needs as deficiency needs, meaning that these are fundamental needs required for human survival, and people are motivated when these needs are not met. First-level basic physiological needs include food, drink, shelter, clothing, warmth, sleep, sex, and sensory stimulation. Maslow's second-level, safety and security needs, describe basic physical safety and emotional security—for example, financial safety, freedom from injury, safe neighbourhood, health and well-being, and freedom from abuse.

Satisfaction of basic deficiency needs allows for attention to the fulfillment of growth needs. Love and belonging needs relate to emotionally connecting with, and experiencing, oneself as a part of a family or community. The next level, self-esteem needs, refers to a person's need for recognition and appreciation. A sense of dignity, respect,

---

BOX 11.1   Peplau's Six Nursing Relationship Roles

1. *Stranger* role: Receives the person the same way one meets a stranger in other life situations; provides an accepting climate that builds trust
2. *Resource* role: Answers questions, interprets health data, and gives information
3. *Teaching* role: Gives instructions and provides education; involves analysis and synthesis of the learner experience
4. *Counselling* role: Helps the person understand and integrate the meaning of current life circumstances; provides guidance and encouragement to make essential changes
5. *Surrogate* role: Helps the person clarify domains of dependence, interdependence, and independence; acts on the person's behalf as an advocate
6. *Leadership* role: Helps the person assume maximum responsibility for meeting treatment goals in a mutually satisfying way

---

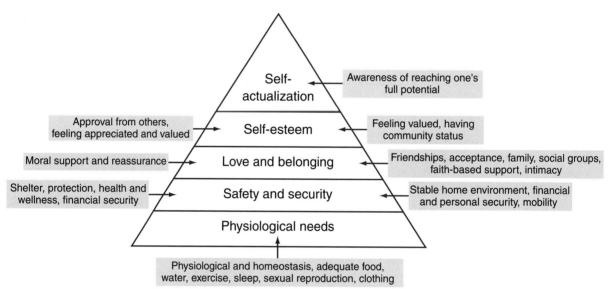

Fig. 11.3 Behavioural examples reflecting Maslow's Need Hierarchy corresponding with Maslow's Hierarchy of Needs

and approval by others for oneself is a symbol of successfully meeting self-esteem needs. Maslow's highest level of need satisfaction, self-actualization, refers to a person's need to achieve their (self-defined) human potential. Self-actualized individuals are not superhuman; they are subject to the same feelings of insecurity that all individuals experience. The difference is that they accept this vulnerability as part of their human condition. Not everyone reaches this developmental stage.

Maslow's five-stage model was expanded in the 1960s and '70s with three stages being added. In the revised model, the bottom four levels are labelled deficiency needs with physiological needs, and safety needs identified as basic needs. Love and belonging and esteem needs are described as psychological needs. The next four levels are labelled as growth needs and include cognitive needs, aesthetic needs, self-actualization, and transcendence. Cognitive needs are knowledge and understanding, curiosity, exploration, and the need for meaning and predictability. Aesthetic needs are related to the appreciation and search for beauty, balance, and so on. Self-actualization needs are the same as in the five-level model. Transcendence needs describe how a person is motivated by values that transcend beyond the personal self, in helping others achieve self-actualization. The five-level model is still widely used with the three additional levels being captured within self-actualization. The revised eight-level model better captures the self-actualization needs and makes them more explicit (McLeod, 2020).

Critiques of the model include that a person's needs often do not occur in a hierarchical order. Some people may fulfill their esteem needs before their safety needs. Hierarchies vary depending on the person. For example, some people may put social status at the top of their personal hierarchy while others may consider personal development and growth the highest level. People have different values that influence what they believe is important (McShane et al., 2015). There are also critiques that the model is based on Western society culture.

Regardless of the limitations of the model, it does provide a holistic perspective. Nurses use Maslow's theory with people and their families to prioritize nursing interventions that best match with the needs and priorities of people in their care. Simulation Exercise 11.1 provides practice using Maslow's model in clinical practice.

APPLICATIONS

The term *person-centred care* (PCC) is not new and describes the emphasis on the role and experience of the person receiving care through bringing their perspectives directly into the planning, delivery, and evaluation of health care (Canadian Patient Safety Institute [CPSI], 2017). PCC represents a significant shift in focus from a disease model to one emphasizing inclusion of the person and family as full partners in planning and implementing meaningful health care. The core concepts include dignity and respect, information sharing, participation, and collaboration to support the person in achieving maximum health and well-being through an action plan tailored to the person's needs, values, and preferences.

SIMULATION EXERCISE 11.1   Understanding Applications of Maslow's Hierarchy of Needs

Purpose
To help students understand the usefulness of Maslow's theory in prioritizing person needs

Procedure
1. Divide the class into small groups (4–6 students), with each group assigned to a step of Maslow's hierarchy.
2. Identify one student as note-taker in each small group of students.
3. Each group then brainstorms examples of different ways a person's needs at each level might be expressed in practice.

4. Identify potential responses from the nurse that might address each need.
5. Share examples with the larger group, and discuss the concept of prioritization of needs, using Maslow's hierarchy.

Discussion and Reflective Analysis
1. In what ways is Maslow's hierarchy helpful to the nurse in prioritizing person needs?
2. What limitations, if any, do you see with the theory?
3. How could you apply Maslow's hierarchy to people in your practice setting?

⟫ DEVELOPING AN EVIDENCE-INFORMED PRACTICE

Purpose: The purpose of this scoping review of the research was to identify the core elements of PCC approaches. Specifically, this review focused on communication, partnership, and health promotion, which were found across PCC models included in this review study.

Method: This scoping review explored articles published since 1990, using Medline, CINAHL, and Embase. The key terms "person-centred or client-centred care" and "framework or model" were used to identify relevant studies.

Findings: This study retrieved 101 articles, of which 19 met inclusion criteria. From these articles, 25 different person-centred frameworks or models were identified. All identified studies incorporated communication, partnership, and health promotion. The authors noted that much empiric evidence was sourced for the most consistently defined component of PCC: "communication" (p. 271).

Application to Your Clinical Practice: This scoping review affirms the importance of communication, partnership, and health promotion as primary components of person-centred approaches in contemporary health care.

Modified from Constand, M. K., MacDermid, J. C., Dal Bello-Hass, V. et al. (2014). Scoping review of person-centered care approaches in health care. *BMC Health Services Research, 14*, 271–281.

The Picker Institute (2017) promotes, provides, and enables the measurement of the perspective and families through surveys examining eight characteristics of care as significant indicators of quality and safety in person-centred relationships. They include the following:

- Respect for the person's values, preferences, and expressed needs
- Coordinated and integrated care
- Clear, high-quality information and education for the person and family
- Physical comfort, including pain management
- Emotional support and alleviation of fear and anxiety
- Involvement of family members and friends, as appropriate
- Continuity, including through care-site transitions
- Access to care (Barry & Edgman-Levitan, 2012, p. 780)

STRUCTURE OF PERSON-CENTRED RELATIONSHIPS

Boundaries

The emotional integrity of the nurse–person relationship depends on maintaining relational boundaries. **Professional boundaries** represent invisible structures imposed by legal, ethical, and professional standards of nursing that respect the rights and privacy of the person and protect the functional integrity of the relationship between the nurse and person. They define how nurses should relate to people in a helping relationship, not as a friend, nor being judgemental, but as a skilled professional partner committed to assisting people to achieve mutually defined health care goals. Professional boundaries outline the parameters of the health care relationship. Examples of professional relationship boundaries include the setting, time, purpose, focus of conversation, and length of contact.

Unlike social relationships, therapeutic relationships incorporate a particular type of communication responsibility and role function throughout the relationship. When people seek health care, they look to their health care providers as skilled, responsible guides to help them achieve optimum health and well-being. The CNA Code of Ethics for Registered Nurses (2017) states that nurses "maintain appropriate professional boundaries and ensure their relationships are always for the benefit of the person. They recognize the potential vulnerability of person receiving care and do not exploit their trust and dependency in a way that might compromise the therapeutic relationship. They do not abuse their relationship for personal or financial gain and do not enter into personal relationships (romantic, sexual or other) with persons receiving care" (p. 13).

Boundary violations take advantage of a person's vulnerability and represent a conflict of interest, capable of compromising the goals of the therapeutic relationship. They can also be subject to ethical and legal constraints.

The nurse, not the person receiving care, is responsible for creating and maintaining professional boundaries. Boundary crossings can lead to boundary violations. Examples of **boundary crossings** include meetings outside of the relationship or disclosing personal intimate details about aspects of the nurse's life that would not be common knowledge (Bruner & Yonge, 2006).

LEVEL OF INVOLVEMENT

Professional behaviours exist on a continuum. To be effective, nurses must maintain an emotional objectivity while remaining human and present to people and their families. The level of involvement on the professional behaviour continuum can fluctuate, depending on person needs. It should never compromise the boundaries of professional behaviour nor minimize the nature of the helping relationship. An important feature of a therapeutic relationship is the nurse's level of involvement, as presented in Fig. 11.4.

The professional level of involvement becomes an issue when a nurse limits involvement to minimum care tasks (under-involvement), or becomes emotionally over-involved in a person's care. Over-involvement can be associated with **countertransference**, which occurs when something in the person activates a nurse's unconscious, unresolved feelings from previous relationships or life events (Scheick, 2011). Over-involvement results in the

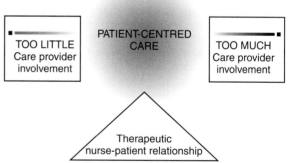

Fig. 11.4 Levels of involvement: A continuum of professional behaviour. From National Council of State Boards of Nursing. (2009). *A nurse's guide to professional boundaries.* NCSBN. https://www.ncsbn.org/ProfessionalBoundaries_Complete.pdf.

nurse's loss of the essential objectivity needed to support the person in meeting health goals. Additionally, over-involvement can compromise one or more of the following: the nurse's obligation to the health care organization, collegial relationships with other health team members, and professional responsibilities and nursing standards.

Warning signs that the nurse is becoming over-involved with a person in their care can include the following:

- Giving extra time and attention to certain people
- Visiting people during off-duty hours
- Doing things for people that they could do for themselves
- Discounting the actions of other professionals
- Keeping secrets with a person
- Believing that they are the only one who understands the person's needs

The opposite of over-involvement is disengagement, which occurs when a nurse emotionally or physically withdraws from having more than a superficial contact with a person. Disengagement can be related to either the person's behaviour or the intensity of suffering. It can be a symptom of burnout or heightened stress for the nurse. For example, an increased number of deaths or high stress levels on a unit can create compassion fatigue, which can lead to disengagement as a self-protective mechanism (Kelly, 2020). Signs of disengagement include withdrawal, limited routine contacts, minimizing the person's suffering, and engaging in defensive or judgemental communication. Regardless of the reason, the outcome of disengagement is that a person feels isolated and sometimes abandoned when care is mechanically delivered, with limited human connection.

Maintaining a Therapeutic Level of Involvement

Maintaining a therapeutic level of involvement is always the responsibility of the professional nurse. To sustain a therapeutic level of professional connection or regain perspective in a relationship, Carmack (1997) suggests that nurses take the following actions:

- Focus on the process of care while acknowledging that the outcome may or may not be within your control
- Focus on the things you can change while acknowledging that there are things over which you have no control
- Be aware and accepting of your professional limits and boundaries
- Monitor your reactions and seek assistance when you feel uncomfortable about any aspect of the relationship
- Balance giving care to a person with taking care of yourself, without feeling compromised

Emotional reactions do occur in clinical situations. Debriefing after a highly emotional event helps nurses resolve and put strong feelings into perspective. Support groups for nurses working in high-acuity nursing situations and for the mentoring of new nurses are recommended. Resilience and self-care strategies are important in addressing the stress of caring for others. As every person is unique, you will need to reflect on self-care strategies that are effective for you. Examples of self-care activities are physical activity (going for a walk, exercise), reading, journal writing, talking to others, mindfulness, and listening to music. Identify what helps you find balance, and then learn to make the time to do it, particularly after a stressful day.

PHASES OF A PERSON-CENTRED RELATIONSHIP

A person-centred relationship consists of three phases: orientation, working, and termination. There is also a short window of time prior to meeting a person for the first time, referred to as the *pre-interaction phase*.

Pre-Interaction Phase

The pre-interaction phase gives you time to think about your own professional goals for the interaction and to address any gaps in your knowledge or potential bias, such that you can work with the person without judgement. It is the only phase of the relationship in which the person is not directly involved. Prior to meeting the person, you should review what is known about them from the available documentation or report. Having a quick overview of a person's status before your first meeting can make a difference in your initial approach. Knowing that the person has had a sleepless night prior to your meeting them, is newly aware of a cancer diagnosis, or is there for a first hospitalization can influence your initial approach. Obstacles are easier to handle when they are anticipated. For example, two young women admitted to the hospital for the delivery of a first baby—one who planned her pregnancy with her partner, the other a teenager who is 16 years of age—may have very different interpersonal needs. Having knowledge of the person's information affords the nurse greater interpersonal sensitivity in approaching each of these people for the first time.

Orientation Phase

Nurses enter a PCC therapeutic relationship in the "stranger" role. The orientation phase shares some characteristics of getting to know someone you have just met in a new relationship. The expectation is that this "introductory" phase will facilitate a level of comfort for the person and development of trust needed to move communication and the relationship to a deeper level.

Creating a comfortable setting where you and the person can sit facing each other at eye level with a comfortable distance between you is essential. The setting should be as private as possible. Assessments and other care interviews should be scheduled at times when the person is alert and not in pain. If a family member is to be involved, seating for that person should be accommodated as a principal contributor to the dialogue.

Establishing Rapport

Establishing rapport is an essential prerequisite for engaging the person and family in PCC. Developing a working relationship with people and their families starts with your first encounter. First impressions count. Start with an introduction of yourself as a professional nurse (or student nurse), including both your first and last name, the time frame you will be working with the person, and your role in caring for the person. After introducing yourself, the next query should be, "How would you preferred to be addressed?

This can be followed by a simple statement like, "I'd like to get to know you better. Can you tell me about what concerns you most at this time?" Listen actively, and ask fewer, rather than more, questions. Simulation Exercise 11.2 provides practice in making introductory statements.

People make sense of things by talking about them. As the person shares their personal story, keep in mind that they may be experiencing a variety of health issues from emotional concerns to cognitive challenges to a full understanding. Your initial response should be to give undivided attention to what the person is saying, use minimum encouragers, and frame any initial comments or open-ended questions in neutral, nonjudgemental language. You can use the suggestions for integrating empathy into listening responses that are presented in Box 11.2.

Each person's health experience is unique, despite similarities in diagnosis or personal characteristics

---

SIMULATION EXERCISE 11.2   Introductions in the Nurse–Person Relationship

Purpose
To provide simulated experience with initial introductions

Procedure
The introductory statement forms the basis for the rest of the relationship. Effective contact with a person helps build an atmosphere of trust and connectedness with the nurse. The following statement is a good example of how one might engage the person in the first encounter:

"Hello, Mr. Okafor. I am Catherine Gagnon, a nursing student. I will be taking care of you on this shift. During the day, I may be asking you some questions about yourself that will help me understand how I can best help you." Role-play the introduction to a new person with one person taking the role of the person; another, the nurse; and a third person, an involved family member, with one or more of the following people:

1. Mrs. Dobish is a 78-year-old woman admitted to the hospital with a diagnosis of diabetes and a question about cognitive impairment.

2. Thomas Charles is a 19-year-old man admitted to the hospital following an auto accident in which he broke both legs and fractured his sternum.
3. Eric Kim is a 53-year-old man who has been admitted to the hospital for tests. The physician believes he may have a renal tumour.
4. Marion Beatty is a 9-year-old girl admitted to the hospital for an appendectomy.
5. Barbara Tangiers is a 78-year-old woman living by herself. She has multiple health problems, including chronic obstructive pulmonary disease and arthritis. This is her first visit.

Discussion and Reflective Analysis
1. In what ways did you have to modify your introductions to meet the needs of the person or circumstances?
2. What were the easiest and hardest parts of doing this exercise?
3. How could you use this experience as a guide in your clinical practice?

BOX 11.2   Guidelines for Effective Initial Assessment Interviews

- Be attentive to the physical and psychological behaviours and communication that express the person's point of view.
- Be self-aware, do self-checks for stereotypes or premature understanding of the person's issues, and set aside personal biases.
- Be open in your listening responses to what you are hearing, and ask for validation frequently.

- Be empathetic to the person's situation, and ask appropriate questions to secure information about any areas or issues you are not clear about.
- Give yourself time to reflect on what the person has said before responding or asking the next question.
- Mirror the person's level of energy and language.
- Be authentic in your responses.

(McCance et al., 2011). Basic understanding of the person's experience should relate to a systematic exploration of the questions, "What is this person's human experience of living with this illness or health issue?" and "How can I, as a health care provider, help this person at this point in time?" The person's preferences and values will become visible as they share their own personal story. Putting a health situation into words places boundaries on it, which enhances the processing of its meaning.

Empathy acts as a human echo in acknowledging that the nurse understands and is interested in the person's perspectives and concerns (Egan, 2014). Guiding principles (e.g., presence, purpose, positive interest, authenticity, active listening, respect for the dignity of the person) strengthen the establishment and healing influence of each therapeutic relationship (McGrath, 2005). Ask for validation of the person's concerns frequently to confirm understanding, especially if you have trouble following the dialogue. This also indicates interest and helps build a common understanding.

Developing a Collaborative Relationship

Engaging the Person

The goal of engaging the person is to take a first step in developing a collaborative working relationship to achieve PCC and health promotion goals. Both the person and the nurse have rights and responsibilities in SDM (shared decision making). Trust is essential to engagement of people and to effective decision making in PCC (Ferguson et al., 2013). A patient or person charter of rights have been developed

as a result of PCC. Charters of rights outline what people can expect when accessing the health care system or services, and when engaging with health care providers. They also often outline people's responsibilities related to accessing care (RNAO, 2015). A sample listing of common person rights and responsibilities is provided in Box 11.3.

Your assessment meeting with the person should have two outcomes. First, the person should emerge from the encounter(s) feeling that the nurse is interested in them as a person separate from their health needs. Second, both the nurse and the person should have a better picture of the person's health needs and issues and a beginning idea of what will be needed to address them.

Collaborative Partnership in Developing Person-Centred Care Goals

An initial integrated assessment strategy allows the nurse and person to jointly and authentically construct the personalized meaning of a health experience into a meaningful whole. The next step in the assessment process is to develop a shared understanding of potential options related to the person's identified needs. PCC goals and action plans of therapeutic relationships usually relate to some or all of the following activities:

- Supporting people and their families to accurately understand the person's personalized experience of a health issue
- Helping people and their families develop practical strategies to effectively self-manage chronic health conditions

---

BOX 11.3   Common Themes in People's Charters of Rights

Person/Patient charters often include the person's rights as follows:

- The right to be treated with respect and dignity
- The right to receive health care without discrimination
- The right to confidentiality and privacy in respect of their health information
- The right to have all their circumstances taken into account in care and wellness planning
- The right to effective communication in order to facilitate their understanding of care and treatment options
- The right to make informed decisions about their care and treatment options, including refusing treatments
- The right to access information in a timely and reasonable manner
- The right to pain and symptom management

- The right to voice their concerns and to receive a timely response

Charters often also include person/patient responsibilities, outlining what people/patients are expected to do:

- Respect the rights of other people/patients and health care providers
- Ensure they understand the information provided by health care providers (e.g., by asking questions, following instructions, and understanding and following their care plan)
- Use health care services appropriately and wisely
- Learn how to access health care services and use them appropriately
- Make healthy choices where possible

Adapted from the Canadian Health Advocates Inc. (2020). *Canadian Patient Rights.* https://canadianhealthadvocatesinc.ca/patient-rights/; Registered Nurses' Association of Ontario. (2015). Clinical Best Practice Guidelines: Person-and Family-Centered Care, (p. 96). https://rnao.ca/sites/rnao-ca/files/FINAL_Web_Version_0.pdf.

- Linking people and families with appropriate health care team providers for relevant information, guidance, and support
- Providing emotional and informational support to help people and their families understand options and make realistic decisions about the best options
- Assisting people and families to cope with, and find meaning in, difficult personal health circumstances
- Helping people discover new directions related to their interests, values, and capabilities
- Helping people access community-based health care resources and rehabilitative services, as needed
- Empowering people with the knowledge and tools they need to be successful advocates in working with their health care team

SHARED DECISION MAKING (SDM)

Shared responsibility for decision making and integrating multiple perspectives in health care management across a continuum of care that extends into the community is or should be a norm in health care delivery. *Shared decision making* refers to an interactive process between health care providers and people they care for, which promotes identifying health issues, exploring options, and providing evidence-informed information so people can participate more actively in care (Epstein & Peters, 2009). Collaborative person-centred planning to address health issues begins with jointly assessing relevant data associated with the health needs, which serves as the basis for SDM between people and their health care providers about realistic, achievable health goals (Elwyn et al., 2012). Assessments should include knowledge and experience with the issues, age, literacy, language, cultural contexts, and access to technology. To educate people about the diagnosis and treatment options, information shared is evidence-informed, including benefits and possible risks (Truglio-Londrigan & Slyer, 2018). Educational materials to assist the person in better understanding the health issues and resources can include written materials, videos, websites, and interactive electronic presentations. A widely used SDM model involves the three steps of ensuring the person understands the available options to manage the health issue, by providing detailed information about the different options and then collaboratively assisting the person explore the options and decide on which one is the best (Lenzen et al., 2018).

SDM is person specific. Coupled with the concept of SDM is the concept of autonomy, in which decisions need to be made about care interventions (Entwistle et al., 2010). The inclusion of people's values and preferences, as well as the reality of the evidence, is essential. Specific opportunities to determine the relevance of the person's priorities in the SDM process include the following:

- Delivering shift reports at the bedside
- Reviewing with people their care plans for the day, early in the shift
- Asking directly about the person's and family members' priorities
- Close collaboration with other health team members to deliver quality care (Jasovsky et al., 2010)

SELF-MANAGEMENT IN PERSON-CENTRED RELATIONSHIPS

People are encouraged to take a prominent role in their own care process, to whatever extent is possible. The desired outcome is to promote the active involvement of the person in developing lifestyle changes consistent with achieving maximum health and well-being. Self-management strategies are designed to enable and strengthen a person's competence and self-efficacy in managing their chronic health conditions. Self-management strategies assists people in achieving the best possible quality of life with their chronic health conditions through having the choice, confidence, and ability to effectively manage their symptoms; treatment; physical, emotional, and social consequences; and lifestyle changes (CNA, 2012).

Respecting and responding to person choices—the essence of PCC—means eliciting, exploring, and questioning choices and helping people create them (Epstein & Peters, 2009). Health counselling has the potential to empower people with the knowledge, skills, and resources to support themselves in maintaining healthy lifestyles, continuing with treatment regimens, and recovering from health challenges.

Self-Management Strategies

People are more motivated when the goals are clear and are important to them. They view the steps needed as being achievable and meaningful. They are not as meaningful if they are not compatible with the person's values or the person does not have the resources or support to achieve or sustain self-management strategies.

Setting Realistic Goals

Exploring a person's interest and motivation for changing behaviours is the starting point. Self-management strategies work best when they are linked to a person's values, cultural contexts, interests, capabilities, and resources. The person has to believe that a goal is both meaningful and achievable. Nurses need to assess the person's and family's ability and motivation to make changes. The following questions can be helpful.

How important is it for you to lose the weight? (Learning about the person's perspective) "Are you interested in learning more about …?

People are expected to be active partners in supporting their own health care processes. PCC health relationships are designed to empower people and their families to assume as much responsibility as possible for the self-management of chronic health conditions. Both nurses and the people they care for have responsibilities to work toward agreed-upon goals. Shared knowledge, negotiation, joint decision-making power, and respect for the capacity of people to actively contribute to their health care to whatever extent is possible are essential components of the PCC partnership (Gallant et al., 2002).

PCC relationships contribute both directly and indirectly to person outcomes, including person self-efficacy, empowerment, and high-quality, evidence-informed SDM that is aligned with people's values and preferences (Reeve et al., 2017). Simulation Exercise 11.3 looks at SDM.

A person-centred partnership honours the person's right to self-determination. It gives the person and family maximum control over health care decisions. The person always has the autonomous right to choose personal goals and courses of action, even if they are at odds with professional recommendations. A collaborative partnership between nurses and the people they care for leads to enhanced self-management, better health care utilization, and improved health outcomes (Hook, 2006). The tasks involved include the following:

- Discussing care management alternatives
- Shared decision making
- Development of realistic action plans

Therapeutic Use of Self

The therapeutic relationship is not simply about what the nurse *does*, but also who the nurse *is* in relation to people and their families. Perhaps the most important tools nurses have at their disposal is their use of self in caring for the whole person, through an optimal connection of nurse and person in a therapeutic relationship.

Authenticity (Realness or Genuineness)

Authenticity is recognized as a precondition for the therapeutic use of self in the nurse–person relationship. Being genuine or authentic is closely aligned with being yourself, based on your values and beliefs, self-awareness, and your actions being congruent with your words. Authenticity is also influenced by a person's cultural contexts (Van den Heever et al., 2015).

Self-awareness is an intrapersonal process that allows nurses to self-reflect on aspects of their personal feelings and beliefs. A common definition of **self-awareness**

SIMULATION EXERCISE 11.3 Shared Decision Making

Purpose

To develop awareness of shared decision making in treatment planning

Procedure

1. Read the following clinical situation.
2. Mr. Jeddore, aged 48 years, is recovering from his second myocardial infarction. After his initial attack, Mr. Jeddore resumed his 10-hour workday, high-stress lifestyle, and usual high-calorie, high-cholesterol diet of favourite fast foods, alcohol, and coffee. He smokes one pack of cigarettes a day and exercises once a week by playing golf. Mr. Jeddore is to be discharged in 2 days. He expresses impatience to return to work but also indicates that he would like to "get his blood pressure down and maybe drop 4.5 kg (10 pounds)."
3. Role-play this situation in dyads, with one student taking the role of the nurse and another student taking the role of Mr. Jeddore.
4. Develop treatment goals with Mr. Jeddore that seem realistic and achievable, considering his preferences, values, and health condition.

5. After the role-playing is completed, discuss some of the issues that would be relevant to Mr. Jeddore's situation and how they might be addressed.
6. What are some realistic ways in which you could engage Mr. Jeddore's interest in changing his behaviour to facilitate a healthier lifestyle?

Discussion and Reflective Analysis

1. As the nurse:
   - What were the easiest and hardest parts of doing this exercise? Why?
   - Discuss whether your own values and beliefs and biases influenced your interaction.
2. As Mr. Jeddore, how did you feel during the interaction? What went well? What areas could have been done differently?
3. What surprised both of you? Why?
4. How can this experience assist you in your clinical practice?

include the nurse's conscious recognition of personal values and beliefs, cultural contexts, thoughts, motivations, strengths, and emotions, and how each can influence their behaviour in the professional relationship (Monat, 2017). This is important in PCC and providing the best nursing practice. For example, in a situation where a nurse realized that the respiratory therapist would be better equipped to explain the process of weaning the person from a ventilator, he arranged for the therapist to provide the explanation while providing his presence and support by staying with the person during the explanation and the weaning process (Levigne & Kautz, 2010).

Self-awareness allows nurses to engage with a person while recognizing their own personal values and beliefs and how they may differ from those of the person needing care. Self-awareness helps identify the interpersonal space and draws the line between the nurse and person, separating the professional and personal realities from one another.

Self-awareness of bias or value conflicts is important to acknowledge because these factors can interfere with the PCC relationship goals. As a nurse, there will be people you care for whose behaviours, values, or beliefs you do not agree with. The CNA (2017) Code of Ethics and provincial and territorial nursing standards identify that nurses provide care for all people. A useful strategy in such situations is to seek further understanding of the person and their cultural contexts that are influencing who they area.

Nurses need to acknowledge over-involvement, avoidance, anger, frustration, or detachment from a person when it occurs.

Case Example

Brian Haggerty is experiencing homelessness and has an opioid addiction. He tells the nurse, "I know you want to help me, but you can't understand my situation. You don't know what it's like out on the streets." Instead of responding defensively or making judgements, the nurse responds, "You're right; I don't know what it's like to be homeless and to have an addiction, but I'd like to know more about your experiences. Can you tell me what it's been like for you?"

With this listening response, the nurse invites him to share his experience. This allows the nurse to learn more about who he is and the cultural contexts that may be influencing him being homeless. The response also conveys the nurse's openness to understand his situation and begin to develop a therapeutic relationship.

Presence

Being "present" in a professional relationship requires a nurse's full attention. Bridges et al. (2013) define *presence* as the "nurse's ability to be 'present' in the relationship, that is to bring aspects of themselves to the relationship," … "to expose themselves fully to the patients and their own experiences, to be open and truthful in their dealings and to be generous in committing to the patient's best interests" (p. 764). Presence involves the nurse's capacity to share the person's experience through active listening, attentiveness, silence, empathy, compassion, and recognition of the person's psychological, psychosocial, and physiological needs (Fahlberg & Roush, 2016; McCormack & McCance, 2006).

McDonough-Means and Kreitzer (2004) describe presence as having two dimensions: "being there" and "being with" (p. S25). Being present with a person enriches the sense of self and the lives of the nurse and person in ways that are unique to each person and situation (Covington, 2003; Hawley & Jensen, 2007).

APPLICATIONS

Although professional relationships in clinical settings share many characteristics with those of social relationships, there are structural and functional distinctions. As discussed previously, Table 11.1 presents the differences between a therapeutic, person-centred relationship and a social relationship. The goal of a therapeutic relationship is ultimately promotion of the person's health and well-being.

Valuing the Person's Experience

The PCC relationship is the unique product of its participants and its context. In today's technological world, it is important to be aware of where your focus is when interacting with people and their families. People and families describe "screen side" interactions, where the health care provider focuses on the technology's screen rather than on them. When technology is used in this way, it can be a barrier in the PCC relationship and communication, with the technology becoming the primary focus of the interaction. It is important to demonstrate during interviews that you value the person as a human being over the technology.

Preparing to Meet the Person and Family

Awareness of your professional goals is important when initiating your first contact. This reflection allows you to select concrete and specific nursing actions that are purposeful and aligned with individualized person needs. For example, a person with a new diagnosis or first hospitalization has different issues from someone with a long history of a chronic health condition, and their self-management concerns are different as well.

The person's specific needs dictate the most appropriate interpersonal setting. In hospital settings, if the door is closed, you need to knock before entering the room. A private space in which the nurse and person can talk without being interrupted is essential. When an assessment interview takes place at the bedside, the door should be closed, or if in a two-bed room, the curtain should be drawn. This area is the person's "space." Each time a nurse is sensitive to the environment in a nurse–person relationship, they model thoughtfulness, respect, and empathy. One-on-one relationships with people with mental health issues commonly take place in a designated private space, away from the person's bedroom. In the person's home, the nurse is always the person's guest and should ask where would be a good place to sit down to talk. If the relationship is to be ongoing—for example, in a health clinic—it is also important to share plans related to time, purpose, and other details with staff. This simple strategy can avoid scheduling conflicts.

Orientation Phase

Peplau's developmental phases parallel the nursing process. The orientation phase correlates with the assessment phase of the nursing process. The identification component of the working phase corresponds to the planning phase, whereas the working phase with the exploitation component of active problem solving parallels with the implementation phase. The final termination phase of the relationship corresponds to the evaluation phase of the nursing process.

Key Concepts

As a nurse, you enter interpersonal relationships with the person not knowing you, and you not knowing the person. Nurses have an advantage as the care environment is familiar to them. This is not necessarily true for people receiving care. Many need not only an introduction to the nurse, but also an orientation to the setting and what to expect in the assessment phase.

You can begin the process of developing trust by providing the person with basic information about yourself (e.g., name and professional status) (Peplau, 1997). This can be a simple introduction: "Good morning, Mrs. Salum., I am Hyacinth Joseph, a registered nurse, and I am going to be your nurse on this shift." Nonverbal supporting behaviours of a handshake (where appropriate), eye contact, and a smile can reinforce your words.

Introductions are important even with people who are confused, have aphasia, are comatose, or are unable to make a coherent response because of mental health issues or dementia. Starting with the first encounter, people begin to assess the trustworthiness of each nurse who cares for them. Sustained attention is probably the single most important indicator of relationship interest.

After introducing yourself, your next query should always be, "How would you prefer to be addressed?"

Clarifying the purpose of the relationship. Clarity of purpose related to identifiable health needs is an essential dimension of the nurse–person relationship. It is difficult to fully participate in *any* working partnership without understanding its purpose and expectations. You should establish basic information about the purpose and nature of the assessment interview, including what information is needed, how the information will be used, how the person wants and can participate in the treatment process, and what the person can expect from the relationship. To understand the importance of orientation information, consider the value of having a clear course outline and expectations for your nursing courses. It can make all the difference in actively engaging your interest.

The length and nature of the relationship dictate the depth of the orientation. A nurse assigned for a shift would provide the person with a different orientation from one given by a nurse who assumes the role of primary care nurse over an extended period. When the relationship is of a longer duration, the nurse should discuss its parameters (e.g., length of sessions, frequency of meetings, and role expectations of the nurse and person). It is important to give the person sufficient orientation information to feel comfortable but not so much that it overloads the initial getting-to-know-you process.

Assessment interview meetings should have two outcomes. First, the person should feel that the nurse is interested in them as a person, apart from their health needs. Second, the person and nurse should emerge from the encounter with a better understanding of the most relevant health issues and know what will happen next. At the end of the contact, the nurse should thank the person for their participation and provide the person with easy ways to access professional help, if needed.

Establishing trust. Carter (2009) defines *trust* as "a relational process, one that is dynamic and fragile, yet involving the deepest needs and vulnerabilities of individuals" (p. 404). People intuitively assess the nurse's trustworthiness through their presence, focused attention, and actions. The person's impression of the nurse's level of interest, knowledge base, and competence are factored into the person's decision to trust and engage actively in the relationship. Compassion, competence, and a willingness to be actively involved get communicated through the nurse's words, tone of voice, nonverbal communication, and actions. Does the nurse seem to know what they are doing? Is the nurse aware and respectful of cultural differences? Confidentiality, sensitivity to person needs, and honesty help to confirm your trustworthiness and to strengthen the relationship. If the person experiences you as someone they can depend on, their sense of vulnerability decreases (Dinc & Gastmans, 2012).

Assessing people's emotional needs in communication. A person's level of trust can fluctuate with illness, age, and the influence of past successful or unsuccessful encounters with others (Carter, 2009). Modifications in your approach make a difference. For example, you would hold a different conversation with an adolescent from one you would hold with an older person. An acutely ill person will need short contacts that are to the point, empathetic, and primarily focus on comfort and care. People with mental health issues may require more time and acceptance to engage in a trusting relationship. For some, the idea of having a professional person—in fact, any person— care about them in any "real way" can be unbelievable. Having awareness of this potential response helps the nurse look beyond the behaviours that some may present with as a response to their fears about helping relationships.

Case Example: Person With Mental Health Issues

Nurse (with eye contact and enough interpersonal space for comfort): "Good morning, Ms. Bauman. My name is Joel Rossi. I will be your nurse today." (Ms. Bauman looks briefly at the nurse and looks away, then gets up and moves away.)

Nurse: "This may not be a good time to talk with you. I will check back with you later. (The nurse needs to be attentive to the nonverbal cues that the person is demonstrating. The introduction coupled with an invitation for later communication respects the person's need for interpersonal space and allows the person to set the pace of the relationship.)

Later, Nurse Rossi notices Ms. Bauman circling around the area he is occupying, but she does not directly approach the nurse. Nurse Rossi smiles encouragingly and repeats nondemanding invitations to Ms. Bauman, which gives her the time and space to become more comfortable.

With purpose and respect, Nurse Rossi engages Ms. Bauman slowly, with a welcoming look and brief verbal contact. Over time, brief meetings that involve an invitation and a statement as to when the nurse will return help reduce the person's anxiety, as indicated in this case example. Some people with mental health issues respond better to shorter, frequent contacts until trust is established.

Participant observation. Peplau describes the role of the nurse in all phases of the relationship as being that of a "participant observer." This means that the nurse simultaneously actively participates in and observes the progress of the relationship as it unfolds. As described in Chapter 7,

reflexivity involves the nurse being aware of what they are doing and how they are doing it, through intrapersonal, interpersonal, and contextual interrelationships. Observations about changes in the person's behaviour, and feedback, help direct subsequent dialogue and actions in the relationship. This self-reflection and self-awareness is critical to the success of the relationship in assessing the person's emerging responses in the relationship (McCarthy & Aquino-Russell, 2009).

Case Example

Terminally ill person (to the nurse): "It's not the dying that bothers me as much as not knowing what is going to happen to me in the process."

Nurse: "It sounds as though you can accept the fact that you are going to die, but you're concerned about what you will have to experience. Tell me more about what worries you."

By linking the emotional context with the content of the person's message, the nurse enters into the person's world and demonstrates a desire to understand the situation from the person's perspective. Nurses need to be aware of the different physical and nonverbal cues that people give with their verbal messages. Noting facial expressions and nonverbal cues with statements like, "You look exhausted" or "You look worried" acknowledges the presence of emotional factors in their nonverbal communication. It is important for the nurse to validate nonverbal cues as they may differ depending on the nurse's and the person's cultural contexts. Simulation Exercise 11.4 is designed to help you critically observe a person's nonverbal cues.

Self-awareness is a critical component of participant observation. Peplau (1997) identifies that nurses must constantly observe their own behaviour, as well as the person's, with self-awareness and total honesty in assessing their behaviours in interactions with the person. In some ways, nurses act as a mirror for the person, reflecting back to them a more complete picture of the human experience of illness and its contextual dimensions.

Self-awareness in therapeutic relationships is a reflective, intrapersonal process. This intrapersonal process helps nurses get in touch with their personal values, cultural contextual biases, feelings, attitudes, motivations, strengths, and limitations—and how these reflections might bias or affect the relationship with people they care for. Critically examining their own behaviours and the impact on the relationship helps nurses create a safe, trustworthy, and caring relationship.

SIMULATION EXERCISE 11.4 Nonverbal Messages

Purpose
To provide practice in validation skills in a nonthreatening environment

Procedure
1. Each student, in turn, tries to communicate the following feelings to other members of the group, without words. The student may choose a feeling written on a piece of paper or may choose one directly from the following list.
2. The other students must guess what nonverbal message the student is trying to enact and then write down the feeling their classmate is trying to convey. Do not share your interpretation until everyone has written down what they thought the nonverbal cue was meant to convey.

Pain	Anxiety	Shock	Disinterest
Anger	Disapproval	Disbelief	Rejection
Sadness	Relief	Disgust	Despair
Confidence	Uncertainty	Acceptance	Tense

Discussion and Reflective Analysis
1. Which emotions were harder to guess from their nonverbal cues? Which ones were easier?
2. Was there more than one interpretation of the emotion?
3. Did your's or others' cultural context influence your/their interpretation of the nonverbal cues?
4. How would you use the information you developed today in your future care of people in your care?

Orientation phase: Where to start with assessment. The person's current health situation is a good starting place for choice of topic. Some fundamental differences such as age and first experience with a medical diagnosis are self-evident from observation and chart review but should be verified for accuracy. Other less obvious differences may emerge as the person tells their story. Framing questions based on your knowledge of developmental and social determinants of health communication is important, even at this stage of the relationship. For example, individual perceptions of personal health needs, values, supportive relationships, cultural contexts, and social concerns of adolescents, parents, older people, and so on are quite different. A person experiencing homelessness may have very different life issues and concerns from those of a person with a similar health condition who lives in appropriate housing.

Sharing information. Open, honest communication and two-way sharing of information are essential for effective SDM and planning. The trust that develops within the relationship is incremental, based on mutual respect for what each person brings to the therapeutic relationship.

It is important to keep in mind that SDM "is shaped by the entire clinical encounter—not just the point where a decision is made—and, even more broadly, by the nature of the patient–provider relationship" (Matthias et al., 2013, p. 176). Therapeutic relationships should directly revolve around the person's needs and preferences.

You can begin to collect information about the person by simply asking why they are seeking treatment at this time. Using questions that follow a logical sequence, when there is something you do not understand, and asking only one question at a time helps a person feel more comfortable. This strategy is also likely to elicit more complete information. You can periodically check in with the person with a simple statement such as, "I wonder if you have any questions so far …," or question like, "Is there anything you would like to add?"

An open, trusting relationship is important to the development of a realistic, committed outcome. The questions you ask should be part of a conversation, not like a cross-examination. Taking time to know the person as a person means understanding the person's thoughts and feelings about the nature of their health issues. How people perceive their health status, their reasons for seeking treatment at this time, and their expectations for health care are critical information. It is important to assess person strengths as these can reinforce the person's decisions and focus attention on potential new initiatives. Their strengths can also be important in choosing and implementing identified treatment goals. Asking about the person's fears and concerns about the impact of the illness or injury on their life and on important relationships should also be included in your assessment. Similarities and differences between the person and family perceptions of illness, and their strengths and treatment preferences, provides relevant supportive information.

Using empathetic responses. Empathetic responses are as critical as the information you provide as they encourage people and families to more fully experience the therapeutic relationship as an equal partnership. Linking your statements such as "I can only imagine how hard this must be for you" or "It must have been quite a shock when this happened" acknowledges that coping with an injury or ongoing chronic health condition process can produce a serious assault to a person's sense of well-being. Most people are very concerned with a significant change in their health.

If there is any reason to suspect the reliability of the person as a historian, interviewing significant others assumes greater importance. For example, if a person has one perception about their self-management and family members have a significantly different awareness, these differences can become a nursing concern if they are not addressed. Differences in expectations can facilitate or hinder the care process. They should be discussed and documented in the person's health record.

Defining the problem(s). Nurses can act as a sounding board, where the person can verbally describe their thoughts, feelings, and concerns to them. The nurse actively listens to what is being said and can then ask questions about parts of the communication that are not understood and help the person to describe their concerns in more specific terms. You can facilitate this process by asking for specific details to bring the person's needs into sharper focus. For example, you can ask, "Could you describe for me what happened next," or "Tell me something about your reaction to (your concern or issue)," or "How do you feel about …?" Time should be allowed between questions for the person to respond fully. Health care providers often ask questions like this, but frequently do not provide enough time for the person to reflect on the question before thoughtfully responding. Remember that the use of silence can be a very effective communication technique.

Feelings are essential components of any health issue. People usually find it easier to talk about factual information related to an issue rather than to express their associated feelings and concerns. Feelings are typically more personal reflections. Nurses can help people connect important personal feelings with significant situations. For example, saying, "Can you tell me how you are feeling right now" or "It sounds as if you feel _____ because of _____" helps the person to express the relationship between what is occurring and its emotional impact. You can also ask directly, "What worries you the most about your health issue (or what we have talked about so far?)."

Understanding the person's perspective. Person-centred care requires understanding each person's illness experience with the broader framework of these factors:

- Life history, including unique personal and developmental issues
- Family history and level of social support
- Employment, school, and community background
- Cultural contexts and spiritual connections
- Quality of life, financial resources, and knowledge of support services (Scholl et al., 2014)

All involved health care providers have a legal and ethical responsibility to participate in helping people understand the nature of health issues as a basis for developing meaningful options in addressing them. Once the nurse and person develop a working definition of the health issue, the next step is to brainstorm the best ways to meet treatment goals. The brainstorming process occurs more easily when you as a nurse are open and willing to understand views that are different from your own. Brainstorming involves generating multiple ideas while suspending judgement until all possibilities are presented. However, having evidence-informed knowledge of potential treatment goals, the risk and benefits of different options are essential components of effective SDM.

The next step is to look realistically at options that could work, given the resources that the person has available right now and their preferences. Resistance to different options can be addressed with empathy and by listening to the person's concerns. Peplau (1997) suggests that a general rule of thumb in working with people is to "struggle with the health issue, not with the person" (p. 164).

The last component of the assessment process relates to determining the kind of support needed and who can best provide it. Careful consideration of the most appropriate sources of support is an important, but often overlooked, part of the assessment process needed in the planning phase.

Defining goals. Self-management goals should be based on the person's values, preferences, resources, and capabilities in relation to personalized goal achievement. Chosen health goals should have meaning to the person. For example, modifying the types of foods that follow normal adolescent eating habits, based on the input of an adolescent with diabetes, can facilitate acceptance of unwelcome dietary restrictions. The nurse conveys confidence in the person's capacity to solve their own health issues by encouraging the person to provide their own suggestions and to develop realistic goals. This strategy also helps ensure that the person's preferences and values are discussed and incorporated.

Working (Exploitation/Active Intervention) Phase

With relevant person-centred goals to guide nursing interventions and person actions, the conversation turns to active problem solving related to the identified health care needs. People are better able to discuss deeper, more difficult issues, and to experiment with new roles and actions in the working phase, when the nurse is viewed as a trustworthy guide. Corresponding to the implementation phase of the nursing process, the working phase focuses on self-directed actions related to personal health goals, the self-monitoring of changes, and the self-management of personal health care, to whatever extent is possible in promoting the person's health and well-being.

Supporting People's Self-Management Strategies

Helping people develop realistic self-management strategies is a key concept in caring for people experiencing chronic health conditions. Johnson et al. (2015) note, "Effective self-management requires autonomous action and active participation in health-related decision making and behaviors," (p. 666). Asking, "What is the most important outcome you hope to accomplish in managing your health issues?" is a good lead-in to this discussion. Through this discussion, the nurse can assist the person in identifying their priorities for self-management when they return home from hospital, and they can collaboratively identify ways the person's outcomes can be achieved.

Self-management includes the health care, physical, social, and lifestyle changes that the person carries out to live with their chronic health conditions. Self-management strategies identify the focus of action plans for health issues. Nurses should provide enough structure and guidelines for people to explore health issues and to develop realistic solutions. Lorig and Holman (2003) developed a seminal article on the history, meaning, tasks, and outcomes of self-management. Breaking a seemingly insoluble problem down into simpler pieces is a nursing strategy that makes doing difficult tasks more manageable. For example, a goal of eating three meals a day may seem overwhelming to a person suffering from nausea and loss of appetite associated with gastric health issues. A smaller goal of having small amounts of applesauce or chicken soup and a glass of milk three times a day may sound more achievable, particularly if the person can choose the times and the food. In difficult nursing situations, there are options, even if the choice is to die with dignity or to change one's attitude toward an illness or a family member. The nurse needs to accept the person's right to make decisions, provided they do not violate self or others, even when it runs contrary to the nurse's thinking. This action protects the person's right to autonomy.

Tuning in to the person's response patterns. Tuning in to the person's response patterns emphasizes shared information and joint actions that connect, collaborate, and create new possibilities for health and well-being. In the process of shared inquiry about the issues at hand, new possibilities can emerge, even in brief encounters. Nurses are in a position to be able to discuss and confirm the unique integration of biological and psychosocial processes that can influence a successful recovery process.

The art of nursing requires that nurses recognize differences in individual people's response patterns. Older people may need a slower pace. People in crisis usually respond better to a simple, structured level of support and may need repetition. It is not unusual for people and their families to completely forget what has been said in a stressful situation.

Throughout the working phase, nurses need to be attentive and assess whether a person is receptive or is no longer actively participating in the decision making. Looking at difficult issues and developing strategies to resolve those problems is not an easy process, especially when resolution requires significant behavioural changes. If the nurse is perceived as interfering rather than facilitative and supportive, communication breaks down.

Nurses have a responsibility to pace interactions in ways that offer support as well as challenge. Deciding whether to proceed or to pause to consider issues that may have arisen is a clinical judgement. This decision should be based on the person's verbal responses and overall body language. Warning signs that the pace may need adjustment include changes in facial expression, fidgeting, abrupt answers or changes in subject, and asking to be left alone.

Strong emotion should not necessarily be interpreted as reflecting a level of interaction stretching beyond the person's tolerance. Tears or an emotional outburst may reflect honestly felt emotion. A well-placed comment, such as, "I can see that this is difficult for you" acknowledges the feeling and may encourage further discussion.

Health issues can create distress and usually require adaptive changes in a person's life. In addition to providing direct care, nurses need to help people and families cope with unique emotional and reality challenges associated with the change in the person's health (see Chapter 17).

When unexpected responses occur as the person implements self-management strategies, they should be treated as temporary setbacks that provide new information about what needs to happen next. Helping people develop alternative strategies to successfully cope with unexpected responses can strengthen a person's problem-solving abilities. Alternative options (i.e., a Plan B) when an original plan does not bring about the desired results can be empowering.

Shared decision making (SDM). Barry and Edgman-Levitan (2012) identify SDM as the "pinnacle of person-centred care" (p. 780). Effective decision making represents both a cognitive and an interpersonal process. SDM is a shared process with the health care provider and person, with the goal of finding agreement on the best course of action (Land et al., 2017). Open communication is required because of the active involvement of people and their families considering the risks and benefits of treatment options. Decisions should reflect the person's priorities, preferences, and values, as well as the reality of the health situation. In addition to information about their health issue or injury, people need to have a clear understanding of treatment options and the potential outcomes and consequences, including what happens if no treatment is given.

Elwyn et al. (2012) outline three key steps in an effective SDM process model. They label these as follows:

- **Choice talk** consists of finding out what information the person has, how much information the person wants, and who should be involved in the decision-making process. Inquiry into person goals and concerns can help frame the option talk in the next step. Choice talk also requires assessing whether or not the information a person already has is the correct information.

- **Option talk** consists of providing sufficient and relevant, evidence-based information about potential treatment options, the risks involved, and the pros and cons of one option versus another. This discussion should consider what the health provider knows about the person's values, preferences, priorities, resources, and concerns. The extent of risk and the potential for outcome uncertainty should be included in the discussion. It is important to check in with people about their potential fears, expectations, and other ideas that they may have about different options.

Decision talk involves participatory active engagement, because this is when the person needs to make a decision. Whenever possible, people should not be forced to make a choice without being ready to make one. It is helpful to ask questions such as, "Are you ready to make a decision?" "Do you feel like you have enough information?" or "Do you need more time to think about it?" Some people need not only more time but also more information. They may want to consult with others who would be affected. It is critical that the decision be based on each person's informed choice. Having additional opportunities to revisit what led to the decision helps to confirm that the person is comfortable with the decision.

Defusing challenging behaviours. There is no unique way to approach a person and no single interpersonal strategy that works equally well with every person. Some people are more open and receptive to exploring self-management strategies and SDM while others are not. When trying to explore self-management strategies and SDM, some people may exhibit emotions such as anxiety, denial, fear, anger, hostility, disinterest, or a sense of powerlessness. Having to deal with health challenges can evoke all of these emotions. When a person seems unapproachable, it can be more difficult for you to maintain an empathetic response pattern. However, it is important to look beyond your own emotions to better understand why the person is responding in this way. Then, in a calm manner, remaining nonjudgemental and empathetic while actively listening, try to understand what the person is conveying in their behaviours. Once you have a better understanding of the reasons guiding the person's emotions and how you can assist in addressing them, you can then look at moving forward in supporting self-management strategies.

Case Example

I tried, but he just wasn't interested in talking to me. I asked him some questions, but he didn't really answer me. So I tried to ask him about what he liked to do. It didn't matter what I asked him; he just turned away. Finally, I gave up because it was obvious that he just didn't want to talk to me.

From the nurse's perspective in this case example, the behaviour of the person may represent a lack of desire for a relationship. However, in most cases, the rejection is not personal. Anxiety expressed as anger or unresponsiveness may be the only way a person can control fear in a difficult situation. Rarely does it have much to do with the interpersonal approach used by the nurse, unless the nurse is truly insensitive to the person's feelings or the needs of the situation. In this situation, the nurse might say, "It seems to me that you don't want to talk right now. Is there something that is bothering you?" If the person still doesn't respond, you can say, "I would like to help you, so I'll come back later and check in with you." Most of the time, people appreciate the nurse's willingness to stay involved.

For novice nurses, it is important to recognize that all nurses experience people at one time or another that demonstrate emotions expressing their distress through behaviours such as anger or withdrawal toward them. It is helpful to explore whether the timing was right, whether the person was in pain, or was feeling overwhelmed without being able to process the reasons why, and—potentially—what other circumstances might have contributed to the person's behaviours. Behaviours that initially seem negative may appear quite adaptive when the full circumstances of the person's situation are understood. A question you might want to consider is, "You seem upset right now. Can you tell me how you are feeling?" or "What has helped you deal with difficult situations or when you are feeling angry or anxious, in the past?

Giving constructive feedback. Preserving the person's personal dignity is a basic human right that nurses should always keep in mind, irrespective of the person's external behaviours, but depending on the situation, you may want to address the person's behaviours (Stievano et al., 2013). This can be challenging and anxiety provoking for the nurse. Before doing this, you should consider what possible outcomes may occur and what you would like to achieve from providing constructive feedback. In deciding what to say, reflect on how you want to convey the message and focus on the key points while still maintaining the therapeutic relationship. As you have the discussion, be self-aware of your feelings. If you start to feel negative as you speak to the person, try to relax, pause, and deep breathe, before responding. Visualize yourself responding in a caring and empathetic way. Self-talk can also help to remind yourself of your role of being therapeutic when someone is distressed (Balzer Riley, 2017). To be effective, constructive discussions are best attempted when the following criteria have been met:

- The nurse has established a firm, trusting relationship with the person.
- The timing and environmental circumstances are appropriate. For example, the person is not in pain, and privacy can be maintained.
- The discussion is delivered in a private setting, in a non-judgemental, calm, and empathetic manner.
- Describe the behaviours you want to discuss using "I" statements, describing the observed behaviour, the impact of the behaviour, and the follow-up discussion on how to move forward.
- Only those behaviours the person is capable of changing are up for discussion.
- The nurse supports the person's autonomy and right to self-determination as long as it does not interfere with the rights of others.

Case Example

Mary Kiernan is 5 feet 2 inches tall and weighs 118 kg (260 pounds). She has attended weekly weight management sessions for the past 6 weeks. Although she lost 4.5 kg (10 pounds) the first week, 1.8 kg (4 pounds) in week 2, and another 1.8 kg by week 5, her weight loss seems to have hit a plateau. Claudia Bernard, her primary nurse, notices that Mary seems to be able to stick to the diet until she gets to dessert, but then she cannot resist temptation. Mary is very discouraged about her lack of further progress. Consider the effect of each response on the person.

Response A

Nurse: You're supposed to be on a 1200-calorie-a-day diet, but instead, I see you eating desserts with your meals. If you eat dessert when you're on a diet, you won't lose the weight and be healthier.

Response B

Nurse: I can understand your discouragement, but you've done quite well in losing 7.3 kg (16 pounds). It seems as though you can follow your diet until you get to dessert. Do you think we need to talk more about what happens when you see the desserts? Do

you want to consider finding some alternatives that would help you get back on track?

The first statement is direct, valid, and concise, but the person is likely to disregard it or experience it as lacking caring and compassion. The person already knows the information the nurse has shared. In the second response, the nurse reframes a behavioural inconsistency as a temporary setback. By initially introducing an observed strength of the progress achieved so far, the nurse provides encouragement and reaffirms trust in the person's resourcefulness, while proposing that the issue might be resolved in a different way. Both responses require similar amounts of time and energy on the part of the nurse; however, the person is likely to accept the nurse's second comment as being more supportive if constructive criticism is paired with an acknowledgment of the person's achievements.

Caring for a person who is crying. There will be times in a therapeutic relationship or when supporting self-management strategies and SDM when the person may start to cry. Ryde and Hjelm (2016) describe how the nurse needs to respond to the person, keeping in mind that every person and situation is unique and requires individualized care. Crying is a natural way of expressing emotions such as sadness, grief, frustration, anger or joy. Crying can have positive outcomes as it is a way of communicating and understanding emotions (Ryde & Hjelm). Being present, actively listening, and staying close to the person as they cry conveys empathy, support, caring, and compassion. Even the simple act of finding the person some tissues to wipe their eyes conveys that you care about them. Try to ensure privacy, such as taking the person to a private room or even closing the curtain around their bed. The nurse should also assess, through the person's verbal, nonverbal, and cultural contexts, if physical contact such as holding someone's hand or touching them on the arm is appropriate. When a person begins to stop crying, the nurse can ask open questions in a soft tone about their feelings, for example, "Tell me what you're feeling that causes you to cry?" If the person doesn't want to talk about it, you can respond by saying, "I understand you don't want to talk about it right now, but I'm here for you, if you would like to talk about it later."

In situations where the person starts to cry, the nurse remains calm, caring, and empathetic while supporting them. There may be times when you become overwhelmed by emotion and find yourself crying with the person. People and their families are often very moved to find that the nurse cares enough about them and their circumstances to cry. When speaking to the person, you can say that you are "so moved by what is happening to them that you couldn't help yourself from becoming emotional." It is important that if you should cry with the person, it is appropriate and the person doesn't end up having to comfort you. As the nurse, you are there to support the person and family. If you become overemotional and not able to control your emotions to care for the person and family, then you should remove yourself from the situation and find someone immediately to be with the person.

Self-disclosure. *Self-disclosure* refers to an intentional (limited) sharing of relevant personal data used to enhance the nurse–person relationship and improve understanding between the nurse and person. When sharing personal information, the nurse must make sure that any information provided relates to the person's care (College & Association of Registered Nurses of Alberta, 2020). Feminist theories identify that self-disclosure enhances engagement between the health care provider and person, humanizing the experience, decreasing power differentials, normalizing experiences, a focusing of advocacy strategies, and a decrease in social inequities, through liberating activities (Steuber & Pollard, 2018).

The following are guidelines for keeping self-disclosure at a therapeutic level:

1. Keep your disclosure brief and relevant to the person's situation.
2. Do not imply that your lived experience is exactly the same as the person's experience.
3. Do not share intimate details of your life.

The nurse, not the person, is responsible for regulating the amount of disclosure needed to facilitate the relationship. If the person asks a polite, superficial question, the nurse may answer briefly with a minimum of information and return to focusing on the person. Simple questions such as, "Where did you go to nursing school?" and "Do you have any children?" may simply represent the person's effort to establish common ground for conversation.

Answering the person briefly but returning the focus to the person is a good guideline. You can make a simple statement such as, "This is your time, and I think I can help you best by hearing more about …" (Identify the person's health concern, question, or reason for seeking care.) Simulation Exercise 11.5 provides an opportunity to explore self-disclosure in the nurse–person relationship.

Termination Phase

Unlike social relationships, therapeutic relationships have a predetermined ending. They typically end when treatment outcomes have been achieved or the person has been discharged or transferred to another health care provider or setting. When possible, the ending of the relationship should be identified and prepared for with the person well before it actually occurs. In the termination phase, the nurse and person jointly evaluate the person's responses to care provided and explore the meaning of the relationship and what goals have been achieved. Discussing the person's achievements and person-centred plans for the future are activities with relevance for the termination phase.

Termination is a significant issue in long-term settings such as bone marrow transplant units, rehabilitation units, and self-management group activities. Meaningful long-term relationships can and do develop in these settings. As a student, you may have developed relationships caring for people during your clinical placements. If the relationship has been effective, real work has been accomplished. Nurses need to be sufficiently aware of their own feelings so that they may use them constructively without imposing them on the person. It is appropriate for nurses to share

---

SIMULATION EXERCISE 11.5   Self-Disclosure: Assessing Nurse Role Limitations in Self-Disclosure

Purpose
To help students differentiate between a therapeutic use of self-disclosure and spontaneous self-revelation

Procedure
1. Write **one** example for each category below that describes your own personality or make up examples for each category:
   A = I could share this with someone I provide nursing care to while maintaining a therapeutic relationship.
   B = If disclosed, this behaviour characteristic might affect my ability to function in a therapeutic manner.
2. Share your responses with the group.

Discussion and Reflective Analysis
1. What criteria did you use to determine the appropriateness of self-disclosure?
2. How much variation was there in what each student would feel comfortable sharing with others in a group or clinical setting, and why?
3. Were there any behaviours commonly agreed on that would never be shared with a person?
4. What interpersonal factors or behaviours of a person would facilitate or impede self-disclosure by the nurse in the clinical setting?
5. What did you learn from doing this exercise that could be used in future encounters with people in your care?

some of the meaning the relationship held for them, as long as such sharing fits the needs of the interpersonal situation and is not excessive or too emotionally intense.

Termination of a PCC relationship should be final. To provide the person with even a hint that the relationship will continue is unfair. Continuing to communicate with a person through social media can be an unintentional boundary violation. It keeps the person emotionally involved in a relationship that no longer has a health-related goal. All provincial and territorial nursing standards identify the importance of maintaining professional boundaries. This can be a difficult issue for nursing students, who often see no harm in telling the person they will continue to keep in contact. However, it is important to help the person move to the next step of their journey. When the person is unable to express feelings about endings, the nurse may recognize them in the person's nonverbal behaviour.

Case Example

A teenager who had spent many months on a bone marrow transplant unit had developed a real attachment to her primary nurse, who had stood by her during the frightening physical side effects and changes in her appearance caused by the treatment. The teenager was unable to verbally acknowledge the meaning of the relationship with the nurse directly, despite having been given many opportunities to do so by the nurse. She told the nurse she could not wait to leave this awful hospital and that she was glad she did not have to see the nurses anymore. Yet, this same teenager was found sobbing in her room the day she left. The relationship obviously had meaning for her, but she was unable to express it verbally.

Gift giving. People sometimes wish to give nurses gifts at the end of a therapeutic relationship because they value the care provided by the nurse. Accepting gifts from people requires careful reflection and professional judgement by the nurse. Nurses should consider two questions: What meaning does the gift have for the relationship? and In what ways might accepting the gift change the dynamics of the therapeutic relationship? Token gifts, such as chocolates or flowers, may be acceptable. In general, nurses should not accept money or gifts of significant material value. Should this become an issue, you might suggest making the gift to the health care agency or a charity. It is always appropriate to simply thank the person for their generosity and thoughtfulness. Your provincial or territorial nursing standards outline boundaries on gift giving. Examples from the College & Association of Registered Nurses of Alberta

(2020) outlining principles to consider prior to accepting gifts from clients include the following:

- Cash gifts are never appropriate.
- Gifts of gratitude may be acceptable, but the nurse should consider their professional standards and policies within the health care organization.
- Nurses should never imply the care of the person is dependent on receiving gifts or donations.
- Nurses should refuse a gift if they feel they are being manipulated or forced to accept the gift.
- Nurses should never be the recipient in a will of a person cared for.

Simulation Exercise 11.6 is designed to help you think about the implications of gift giving in the nurse–person relationship.

Evaluation. Objective evaluation of health outcomes achieved in the nurse–person relationship should focus on the following:

- Was the identification of the issues adequate and appropriate for the person?
- Were the interventions chosen adequate, consistent with person preferences, and appropriate to address the person's health issues?
- Were the interventions implemented effectively and efficiently to both the person's and the nurse's satisfaction, within the allotted time frame?
- Is the person progressing toward maximum health and well-being?
- Is the person satisfied with their progress and the care received?
- What type of follow-up care or self-monitoring is needed?
- If follow-up care is indicated, is the person satisfied with the recommendation and able to carry forward their treatment plan in the community?

Adaptation for Brief Relationships

In today's health care environment, you may have only a short amount of time with people addressing their health concerns. Here are some suggestions for relating to people in brief therapeutic relationships. Four essential qualities between the nurse and person are needed to establish relatedness in short-term relationships: a sense of belonging, reciprocity (a shared exchange and dependence on one another), mutuality (negotiation between the person and nurse) and synchrony (the time together) (Moser et al., 2010). Developing a brief relationship with people represents a working therapeutic relationship with active support. The same recommendations for self-awareness, empathy, therapeutic boundaries, active listening, competence, mutual respect, partnership, and level of involvement hold true as key elements of even the briefest therapeutic relationships.

SIMULATION EXERCISE 11.6   Gift-Giving Role Play

Purpose

To help students develop therapeutic responses to people who wish to give them gifts

Procedure

Review the following situations and answer the discussion questions.

Situation

Nurse Terrell, a hospice nurse, has taken care of Mr. Aitken for the 3 months prior to him passing away. Nurse Terrell has been very supportive of the family. Because of Nurse Terrell's nursing care, Mr. Aitken and his son were able to resolve a long standing and very bitter conflict before he died. The whole family, particularly Mr. Aiken's wife, is grateful to Nurse Terrell for his special attention to her husband and family.

Role-Play Directions for Mrs. Aitken

You are very grateful to Nurse Terrell for all his help over the past few months. Without his help, you do not know what you would have done. To show your appreciation,

you would like Nurse Terrell to have a $300 online gift certificate. It is very important to you that Nurse Terrell fully understand how meaningful his caring has been to you during this very difficult time.

Role-Play Directions for Nurse Terrell

You have provided the Aitken family high-quality nursing care and you feel very good about it, particularly the role you played in helping Mr. Aitken and his son reconcile before Mr. Aitken's death. Respond as you think you might in this situation, based on the data provided.

Discussion

1. Discuss the responses made in the role-playing situation.
2. Discuss the other possible responses and evaluate the possible consequences.
3. Would you react differently if Mrs. Aitken gave you a $100 gift certificate or a $20 coffee gift card? If so, why?
4. What do your professional nursing standards say about receiving gifts?

Orientation Phase

Following introductions and initial comments, the therapeutic relationship begins with a "here and now" focus on health issues identification and an emphasis on quickly understanding the context of the health concerns. Start with what is most important to the person. A question to elicit this information could be, "What is most important to you right now in relation to your health concerns?" Questions can then follow based on their response and may include asking about the person's symptoms and personal and emotional contexts in which they occur. Allowing the person to tell their personalized story of a health concern or injury with minimum interruptions conveys respect and interest (Nicholson et al., 2010).

Listen for what is left out and watch the person's nonverbal communication. Pay attention to what the person's story elicits in you. Acknowledge the person's feelings with a statement such as "Tell me more about …" (with a theme picked up from the person's choice of words, hesitancy, or nonverbal cues), which usually prompts further explanations.

Anderson (2001) echoes Rogers' belief that all people have potential for self-managing behaviours. As you interact with the person, there will be opportunities to observe the person's strengths and comment on them. Every person has healthy aspects of who they are and personal

strengths that can be drawn on to facilitate individual coping responses. Building on a person's strengths assists the person in addressing their health concerns. Simulation Exercise 11.7 provides an opportunity to explore the value of acknowledging personal strengths in people with a chronic health condition.

Even the briefest therapeutic encounter should be person-centred, with an emphasis on understanding the person's personalized experience of an illness and its social context (Bardes, 2012). A simple statement posed at the beginning of each shift, such as, "What is your most important need today?" or "What is the most important thing I can do for you today?" helps focus the relationship on immediate concerns that are important to the person (Cappabianca et al., 2009). This type of concern allows both of you to develop a shared understanding of what is uniquely important to the person in the present moment. Researchers consider PCC as being "defined by a focus on outcomes that people notice and care about including, not only survival, but also function, symptoms and modifiable aspects of quality of life" (Rodriguez et al., 2013, p. 1795).

Focusing on Essential Information

The nurse's goal as a health care provider is to gather accurate, reliable information. Because the time frame for a

---

SIMULATION EXERCISE 11.7 Identifying Person's Strengths

Purpose

To identify personal strengths in people with serious illness

Procedure

1. Think about a person you have cared for with a serious or prolonged chronic health condition.
2. What personal strengths does this person possess that could have a healing impact? For example, strengths can be courage, patience, positive outlook, family, and so on.

3. Write a one-page description of the person and the personal strengths observed, despite the person's medical or psychological condition.

Discussion and Reflective Analysis

1. If you didn't have to write the description, would you have been as aware of the person's strengths?
2. How could you help the person maximize their strengths to achieve good quality of life?
3. What did you learn from this exercise that you can use in your future clinical practice?

---

person-centred relationship may be only a few hours or days, nurses need to focus on what is absolutely essential rather than on everything that might be nice to know.

Finding out how much the person already knows and their experiences can save time. You can obtain this information by asking the person, "Tell me what you know about your health concern." It is also important to ask whether people have accessed the Internet, including social media sites, for information related to their health needs and which sites they were using. This is to assess whether the websites were reliable and the information they have is accurate. You can then follow up with the question, "What is your greatest concern at this moment?" You can also examine the person's needs from a broader contextual perspective, one that takes into consideration which concerns, if treated, would most increase their health and well-being. The information obtained through the assessment can also then guide nurses to advocate for people with family members where necessary, and with other health care providers and team members. The information additionally facilitates making plans for discharge when people have to manage their health condition in home environments with less support.

The more actively engaged the person is in the assessment and planning process as an equal partner, the more person-centred the plan will be. Choosing goals that are the most important to the person, realistic, and attainable should be the focus. Two basic questions are, What does this health issue mean to the person and what is their primary concern? Adapting your nursing care and support to a person's level of motivation, and encouraging small, achievable steps are actions that help maximize interest and the effectiveness of self-management strategies (Greene & Hibbard, 2012).

As nurses are an important member within the interprofessional team and often know the most about the person, they are responsible for clarifying, integrating, advocating,

and coordinating different aspects of the person's care as part of the team (see Chapter 24). An important component of this responsibility is ensuring that the person and the family understand and are able to advocate and negotiate treatment initiatives with health care team providers. The nurse is frequently the liaison resource between the team and the person and family for follow-up explanations.

Working Phase

Brief relationships should be solution-focused right from the start. Giving people your undivided attention and using concise active listening responses are essential to understanding the complexity of issues people are facing.

Adapting one's lifestyle to compensate for the demands of chronic health conditions can be difficult (Friesen-Storms et al., 2015). A central focus, agreed on by the nurse and person, promotes related activities and coping skills needed to meet the person's goals. People tend to work best with nurses who appear knowledgeable and empathetic. One way of helping them discover the solutions that fit them best is by engaging them in determining and implementing activities to meet therapeutic goals at every realistic opportunity. Conveying a realistic, hopeful attitude that the goals developed with the person are likely to be achieved is important.

Action plans should be as simple and specific as possible. Changes in the person's heath condition or other circumstances may require treatment modifications that should be expected in short-term relationships. Keeping people and their families informed, and working with them on alternative solutions, is essential to maintain trust in short-term relationships.

Termination Phase

The termination phase in short-term relationships can include discharge planning, community health referrals, obtaining prescriptions, and arranging follow-up appointments in the community for the person and family. Anticipatory guidance in the form of simple instructions and a review of important skills is appropriate. Coordination of post-discharge plans with other health care disciplines, families, and communities to support positive health changes should be the norm, not the exception. It is important to check with the person's support network, where appropriate, about the level of assistance they will be able to provide. Usually, the nurse has never seen the person's home and knows little about the person's home life. Prior to the person being discharged from acute care, the nurse should ensure that the person and family have everything they need, such as information about community referrals and supports, prescriptions, appointments, and information about which health care provider to contact with concerns and what is needed for self-managing at home.

The importance of the PCC relationship, no matter how brief, should not be underestimated. Simulation Exercise 11.8 stimulates reflection and discussion on what is PCC. Sudden illness or exacerbation (worsening) of chronic health conditions dramatically change a person's life—often in unexpected ways. Although the person may be one of several you need to take care of during a day, the relationship may represent the only interpersonal or professional contact available to a lonely and frightened person. Even if contact has been brief, you should stop by to say goodbye and check that everything is in order before you leave at the end of your work day. The dialogue in such cases can be simple and short—for example, "Ms. Zhao, I will be finishing my shift in a few minutes. I enjoyed working with you. Nurse Almasi will be taking care of you this evening. Is there anything I can do for you before I go?" Check to see if the person has the call button within reach. If the person has a whiteboard with caregiver names on it, you should put the names of the next nurse and support staff who will be caring for them. If you will not be returning at a later date, you should briefly share this information with the person.

SUMMARY

The nurse–person relationship represents a purposeful use of self in all professional relations with people and the health care providers involved in their care. Respect for the dignity of the person and self, person-centred communication, and authenticity in therapeutic relationships are process threads underlying all communication responses.

Therapeutic relationships have professional boundaries, purposes, and behaviours. Boundaries keep the relationship safe for the person. They spell out the parameters of the therapeutic relationship, and nurses are ethically responsible for maintaining them throughout the relationship. Effective relationships enhance the well-being of the person and the professional growth of the nurse. The professional relationship goes through a developmental process characterized by four overlapping yet distinct stages: pre-interaction, orientation, working phase, and termination phase. The pre-interaction phase is the only phase of the relationship the person is not part of. During the pre-interaction phase, the nurse develops the appropriate physical and interpersonal environment for an optimal relationship, in collaboration with other health care providers and significant others in the person's life.

The orientation phase of the relationship defines the purpose, roles, and guidelines of the process and provides a framework for assessing people's needs. The nurse builds a sense of trust through consistency of actions. Data collection forms the basis for identifying the person's health issues and needs. The orientation phase ends with a therapeutic contract mutually defined by the nurse and person.

The working phase is the problem-solving phase of the relationship, paralleling the planning and implementation phases of the nursing process. As the person begins to explore difficult problems and feelings, the nurse uses a variety of interpersonal strategies to help the person develop new insights and methods of coping.

The final phase of the nurse–person relationship occurs when the essential work of the intervention phase

---

SIMULATION EXERCISE 11.8   What Is Person-Centred Care?

Purpose

To stimulate a reflective discussion of the dimensions of person-centred care (PCC)

Procedure

1. Watch the World Health Organization video, "What is people-centred care?" (https://www.youtube.com/watch?v=pj-AvTOdk2Q). Short video, less than 3 minutes, available on YouTube.

2. How can you implement person-centred care specifically in your clinical setting?

3. What fundamental changes would you need to implement to advance the purposes of PCC in your nursing practice?

is complete. The ending should be thoroughly and compassionately defined early enough in the relationship so that the person can process it appropriately. Primary tasks associated with the termination phase of the relationship include summarization and evaluation of completed activities and referrals when indicated. Short-term relationships incorporate the same skills and competencies as traditional nurse–person relationships but with a sharper focus on the here and now. The action plan needs to be as simple and specific as possible.

👤 ETHICAL DILEMMA

What Would You Do?

During the COVID-19 virus outbreak that began in 2020, the difficult decision was made to create a "no visitors" policy in health care organizations. Mr. Montano, who has a diagnosis of end-stage cancer, is admitted to hospital just prior to the COVID-19 virus outbreak in palliative care. As a nurse on the palliative care unit, you have developed a therapeutic relationship with Mr. Montano and his family. Following the no visitor policy being instituted, his family is no longer able to visit. A few days later, Mr. Montano's passing is imminent. When you speak to the family, his wife bursts into tears and begs you to allow her to be with her husband as he is dying. What do you do?

QUESTIONS FOR REVIEW AND DISCUSSION

1. In what ways do organizational structure and expectations in your clinical setting enhance or hinder development of therapeutic relationships in nursing care?
2. What does the phrase "being present in health care relationships" mean?
3. How does a therapeutic relational partnership support an effective person and family decision-making processes?
4. What do you see as the most important attribute of person-centred care? What is the basis for your choice?

REFERENCES

Anderson, H. (2001). Postmodern collaborative and person-centered therapies: What would Carl Rogers say? *Journal of Family Therapy, 23*(4), 339–360.

Balzer Riley, J. (2017). *Communication in Nursing* (8th ed.). Elsevier.

Bandura, A. (2012). On the functional properties of perceived self-efficacy revisited. *Journal of Management, 38*, 9–44.

Bardes, C. (2012). Defining patient-centered medicine. *Journal of Nursing Education, 366*, 782–783.

Barr, V. J., Robinson, S., Marin-Link, B. et al. (2003). The expanded chronic care model: An integration of concepts and strategies from population health promotion and chronic care model. *Healthcare Quarterly, 7*(1), 73–82. https://doi.org/10.12927/hcq.2003.16763. https://www.longwoods.com/content/16763.

Barry, M., & Edgman-Levitan, S. (2012). Shared decision making—The pinnacle of patient-centered care. *Journal of Nursing Education, 366*(9), 780–781.

Batalden, P., Ogrinc, G., & Batalden, K. (2006). From one to many. *Journal of Interprofessional Care, 20*(5), 549–551.

Bodenheimer, T., Wagner, E., & Grumbach, K. (2002). Improving primary care for patients with chronic illness: The chronic care model. *The Journal of the American Medical Association, 288*, 1775–1779.

Bridges, J., Nicholson, C., Maben, J. et al. (2013). Capacity for care: Meta-ethnography of acute care nurses' experiences of the nurse-patient relationship. *Journal of Advanced Nursing, 69*(4), 760–772.

British Columbia Ministry of Health. (2011). *Self-management support: A health care intervention.* https://www.selfmanagementbc.ca/uploads/What%20is%20Self-Management/PDF/Self-Management%20Support%20A%20health%20care%20intervention%202011.pdf.

Bruner, B., & Yonge, O. (2006). Boundaries and adolescents in residential treatment centers: What clinicians need to know. *Journal of Psychosocial Nursing and Mental Health Services, 44*(9), 38–44.

Canadian Academy of Health Sciences. (2017). *Review of chronic care: Commissioned by Veterans Affairs Canada.* https://www.cahs-acss.ca/wp-content/uploads/2017/09/Review-of-Chronic-Care_Veterans-Affairs-Canada.pdf.

Canadian Interprofessional Health Collaborative. (2010). *A national interprofessional competency framework.* http://www.ipcontherun.ca/wp-content/uploads/2014/06/National-Framework.pdf.

Canadian Nurses Association. (2011). *Interprofessional collaboration: CNA position.* https://cna-aiic.ca/~/media/cna/page-content/pdf-en/Interproffessional-Collaboration_position-statement.pdf.

Canadian Nurses Association. (2012). *Effectiveness of registered nurses and nurse practitioners in supporting chronic disease self-management.* https://www.cna-aiic.ca/~/media/cna/page-content/pdf-en/effectiveness_of_rns_and_nps_in_self-care_managment_e.pdf?la=en.

Canadian Nurses Association. (2017). *Code of ethics for registered nurses.* https://www.cna-aiic.ca/html/en/Code-of-Ethics-2017-Edition/files/assets/basic-html/page-1.html#.

Canadian Patient Safety Institute. (2017). *Patient safety education program—Canadian curriculum Module 7a: Patients as partners engaging patients and families: Patient and family centered care.* https://www.patientsafetyinstitute.ca/en/education/PatientSafetyEducationProgram/PatientSafetyEducationCurriculum/Documents/Module%2007A%20-%20Patients%20as%20Partners%20-%20Patient%20and%20Family%20Centred%20Care.pdf.

Cappabianca, A., Julliard, K., Raso, R. et al. (2009). Strengthening the nurse-patient relationship: What is the most important thing I can do for you today? *Creative Nursing, 15*(3), 151–156.

Carmack, B. (1997). Balancing engagement and disengagement in caregiving. *Image (IN), 29*(2), 139–144.

Carter, M. (2009). Trust, power, and vulnerability: A discourse on helping in nursing. *Nursing Clinics of North America, 44,* 393–405.

College & Association of Registered Nurses of Alberta. (2020*). Professional boundaries: Guidelines for the nurse-client relationship*. https://www.nurses.ab.ca/docs/default-source/document-library/guidelines/rn_professional-boundaries.pdf?sfvrsn=cc43bb24_20.

College of Nurses of Ontario. (2006). *Therapeutic nurse-client relationship: Revised 2006.* https://www.cno.org/globalassets/docs/prac/41033_therapeutic.pdf.

Covington, H. (2003). Caring presence: Delineation of a concept for holistic nursing. *Journal of Holistic Nursing, 21*(3), 301–317.

Crowe, M. (2000). The nurse-patient relationship: A consideration of its discursive content. *Journal of Advanced Nursing, 31*(4), 962–967.

Dinc, L., & Gastmans, C. (2012). Trust and trustworthiness in nursing: An argument-based literature review. *Nursing Inquiry, 19*(3), 223–237.

Dolansky, M., & Moore, S. (2013). Quality and safety education for nurses (QSEN). The key is systems thinking. *Online Journal of Issues in Nursing, 18*(3), 1.

Egan, G. (2014). *The skilled helper: A problem-management and opportunity-development approach to helping* (10th ed.). Brooks Cole: Cengage Learning.

Elwyn, G., Frosch, D., Thompson, R. et al. (2012). Shared decision making: A model for clinical practice. *Journal of General Internal Medicine, 27,* 1361–1367.

Entwistle, V., Carter, S., Cribb, A. et al. (2010). Supporting patient autonomy: The importance of clinician-patient relationships. *Journal of General Internal Medicine, 25*(7), 741–745.

Epstein, R. M., & Peters, E. (2009). Beyond patients' preference. *Journal of the American Medical Association, 302*(2), 195–197.

Fahlberg, B., & Roush, T. (2016). Mindful presence: Being "with" in our nursing care. *Nursing, 46*(3), 14–15.

Ferguson, L., Ward, H., Card, S. et al. (2013). Putting the 'patient' back into patient-centered care: An education perspective. *Nurse Education in Practice, 13,* 283–287.

Friesen-Storms, J., Bours, G., Van der Weijdedn, T. et al. (2015). Shared decision making in chronic care in the context of evidence based practice in nursing. *International Journal of Nursing Studies, 52,* 393–402.

Gallant, M., Beaulieu, M., & Carnevale, F. (2002). Partnership: An analysis of the concept within the nurse-client relationship. *Journal of Advanced Nursing, 2,* 149–157.

Government of Canada. (2019). *Prevalence of chronic diseases among Canadian adults.* https://www.canada.ca/en/public-health/services/chronic-diseases/prevalence-canadian-adults-infographic-2019.html.

Government of Ontario. (2019). *A healthy Ontario: Building a sustainable health care system: 2nd report from the Premier's Council on Improving Healthcare and Ending Hallway Medicine.* https://files.ontario.ca/moh-healthy-ontario-building-sustainable-health-care-en-2019-06-25.pdf.

Greene, J., & Hibbard, J. (2012). Why does patient activation matter? An examination of the relationships between patient activation and health-related outcomes. *Journal of General Internal Medicine, 27,* 520–526.

Hawley, M. P., & Jensen, L. (2007). Making a difference in critical care nursing practice. *Qualitative Health Research, 17*(5), 663–674.

Hibbard, J. H. (2017). Patient activation and the use of information to support informed health decisions. *Patient Education and Counseling, 100*(1), 5–7. https://doi.org/10.1016/j.pec.2016.07.006.

Hook, M. (2006). Partnering with patients—A concept ready for action. *Journal of Advanced Nursing, 56*(2), 133–143.

International Council of Nurses. (n.d.) *Nursing definitions.* www.icn.ch/nursing-policy/nursing-definitions.

Jasovsky, D., Morrow, M., Clementi, P. et al. (2010). Theories in action and how nursing practice changed. *Nursing Science Quarterly, 23*(1), 29–38.

Johnson, K., McMorris, B., MapelLentz, S. et al. (2015). Improving self-management through patient-centered communication. *Journal of Adolescent Health, 57*(6), 666–672.

Kelly, L. (2020). Burnout, compassion fatigue and secondary trauma in nurses. *Critical Care Nursing Quarterly, 43*(1), 73–80. https://doi.org/10.1097/CNQ.0000000000000293.

Land, V., Parry, R., & Seymour, J. (2017). Communication practices that encourage and constrain shared decision making in health care encounters: Systematic review of conversation analytic research. *Health Expectations, 20*(6), 1228–1247. https://doi.org/10.1111/hex.12557.

Lazenby, M. (2013). On the humanities of nursing. *Nursing Outlook, 61*(1), e9–e14.

Lenzen, S. A., Daniels, R., van Bokhoven, M. A. et al. (2018). Development of a conversation approach for practice nurses aimed at making shared decisions on goals and action plans with primary care patients. *BMC Health Services Research, 18,* 891. https://doi.org/10.1186/s12913-018-3734-1.

Levigne, D., & Kautz, D. D. (2010). The evidence for listening and teaching may reside in our hearts. *Medsurg Nursing, 19,* 194–196.

Lhussier, M., Eaton, W., Forster, N. et al. (2015). Care planning for long term conditions—A concept mapping. *Health Expectations, 18,* 605–624.

Lorig, K., & Holman, H. (2003). Self-management education: History, definition, outcomes, and mechanisms. *Annals of Behavioral Medicine, 26*(1), 1–7.

Maslow, A. (1970). *Motivation and personality* (2nd ed.). Harper & Row.

Matthias, M., Salyers, M., & Frankel, R. (2013). Re-thinking shared decision-making: Context matters. *Patient Education and Counseling, 91,* 176–179.

McCance, T., McCormack, B., & Dewing, J. (2011). An exploration of person-centeredness in practice. *Online Journal of Issues in Nursing, 16*(2), 1.

McCarthy, C., & Aquino-Russell, C. (2009). A comparison of two nursing theories in practice: Peplau and Parse. *Nursing Science Quarterly, 22*(1), 34–40.

McCormack, B., & McCance, T. V. (2006). Development of a framework for person-centred nursing. *Journal of Advanced Nursing, 56*(5), 472–479.

McCormack, B., & McCance, T. (2010). *Person-centered nursing: Theory and practice.* Wiley Blackwell.

McDonough-Means, M., & Kreitzer, I. (2004). Bell: Fostering a healing presence and investigating its mediators. *Journal of Alternative and Complementary Medicine, 10*(Suppl. 1), S25–S41.

McGrath, D. (2005). Healthy conversations: Key to excellence in practice. *Holistic Nursing Practice, 19*(4), 191–193.

McLeod, S. A. (2020). Maslow's hierarchy of needs. *Simply Psychology.* https://www.simplypsychology.org/maslow.html.

McShane, S. L., Steen, S. L., & Tasa, K. (2015). *Canadian Organizational Behaviour* (9th ed.). McGraw-Hill Ryerson.

Mitchell, M., Chaboyer, W., Baumeister, E. et al. (2009). Positive effects of a nursing intervention on family-centered care in adult critical care. *American Journal of Critical Care, 18*(6), 543–552.

Monat, J. (2017). The emergence of humanity's self-awareness. *Futures, 86*, 27–35.

Morgan, S., & Yoder, L. H. (2012). A concept analysis of person-centered care. *Journal of Holistic Care, 30*(1), 6–15.

Moser, A., Houtepen, R., Spreeuwenberg, C. et al. (2010). Realizing autonomy in responsive relationships. *Medicine, Health Care, and Philosophy, 13*, 215–223.

Nicholson, C., Flatley, M., Wilkinson, C. et al. (2010). Everybody matters 2: Promoting dignity in acute care through effective communication. *Nursing Times, 106*(21), 12–14.

Palmer, K., Marengoni, A., Forjaz, M. J. et al. (2017). Multimorbidity care model: Recommendations from the consensus meeting of the joint action on chronic diseases and promoting healthy ageing across the life cycle. *Health Policy, 122*(1), 4–11.

Peplau, H. E. (1997). Peplau's theory of interpersonal relations. *Nursing Science Quarterly, 10*(4), 162–167.

Picker Institute. (2017). *Principles of person-centered care.* http://pickerinstitute.org/about/picker-principles/.

Porter, S., O'Halloran, P., & Morrow, E. (2011). Bringing values back into evidenced based nursing: Role of patients in resisting empiricism. *Nursing Science Quarterly, 34*(2), 106–118.

Province of Alberta, (2014). *Alberta health act: Statutes of Alberta, 2010 Chapter A-19.5.* Alberta Queen's Press. https://www.qp.alberta.ca/1266.cfm?page=A19P5.cfm&leg_type=Acts&isbncln=9780779778065.

Reeve, B., Thissen, D., Bann, C. et al. (2017). Psychometric evaluation and design of patient-centered communication measures for cancer care settings. *Patient Education and Counseling, 100*, 1322–1328.

Registered Nurses' Association of Ontario. (2015). *Clinical best practice guidelines: Person-and family-centered care.* https://rnao.ca/sites/rnao-ca/files/FINAL_Web_Version_0.pdf.

Reynolds, W. (1997). Peplau's theory in practice. *Nursing Science Quarterly, 10*(4), 168–170.

Rodriguez, A., Mayo, N., & Gagnon, B. (2013). Independent contributors to overall quality of life in people with advanced cancer. *British Journal of Cancer, 108*, 1790–1800.

Ryde, K., & Hjelm, K. (2016). How to support patients who are crying in palliative home care: An interview study from the nurses' perspective. *Primary Health Care Research & Development, 17*(5), 479–488. https://doi.org/10.1017/S1463423616000037.

Scheick, D. (2011). Developing self-aware mindfulness to manage countertransference in the nurse-client relationship: An evaluation and developmental study. *Journal of Professional Nursing, 27*(2), 114–123.

Scholl, I., Zill, J. M., Harter, M. et al. (2014). An integrative model of patient- centeredness—A systematic review and concept analysis. *PLoS One, 9*(9), e107828.

Steuber, P., & Pollard, C. (2018). Building a therapeutic relationship: How much is too much self-disclosure? *International Journal of Caring Science, 11*(2), 651–657.

Stievano, A., Rocco, G., Sabatino, L. et al. (2013). Dignity in professional nursing: Guaranteeing better patient care. *Journal of Radiology Nursing, 32*(3), 120–123.

Street, R. L., Makoul, G., Arora, N. K. et al. (2009). How does communication heal? Pathways linking clinician-patient communication to health outcomes. *Patient Education and Counseling, 74*, 295–301.

Truglio-Londrigan, M., & Slyer, J. T. (2018). Shared decision–making for nursing practice: An integrative review. *The Open Nursing Journal, 12*, 1–14. https://doi.org/10.2174/1874434601812010001.

Van den Heever, A., Poggenpoel, M., & Myburgh, C. P. H. (2015). Nurses' perceptions of facilitating genuineness in a nurse-patient relationship. *Health SA Gesundheit, 20*, 109–117.

Wagner, E. H., Austin, B. T., Davis, C. et al. (2001). Improving chronic illness care: Translating evidence into action. *Health Affairs, 20*(6), 64–78.

Western Health Sciences. (n.d.). *Interprofessional education and practice.* https://www.uwo.ca/fhs/education/ipe/index.html.

World Health Organization. (2010). *World health organization: Framework for action on interprofessional education and collaborative practice.* Geneva Switzerland.

World Health Organization. (2016). *Framework on integrated, people-centred health services: Report by the secretariat.* https://apps.who.int/gb/ebwha/pdf_files/WHA69/A69_39-en.pdf?ua=1.

SUGGESTED READING

Ashton, K. (2016). Teaching nursing students about terminating professional relationships, boundaries and social media. *Journal of Nursing Education, 37*, 170–172.

Bernabeo, E., & Holmboe, E. (2013). Patients, providers and systems need to acquire a specific set of competencies to achieve truly patient centered care. *Health Affairs, 32*(2), 250–258. https://doi.org/10.1377/hlthaff.2012.1120.

Brunero, S., Lamont, S., & Coates, M. (2010). A review of empathy education in nursing. *Nursing Inquiry, 17*(1), 65–74.

Castro, E., Regenmortel, T., Vanhaecht, K. et al. (2016). Patient empowerment, patient participation and patient-centeredness in hospital care: A concept analysis based on a literature review. *Education and Counseling, 99*, 1923–1939.

Clark, A. (2010). Empathy: An integral model in the counseling program. *Journal of Counseling and Development, 88*(3), 348–356.

De Boer, D., Delnoij, D., & Rademakers, J. (2013). The importance of patient-centered care for various patient groups. *Education and Counseling, 90*, 405–410.

Elwyn, G., Dehlendorf, C., Epstein, R. et al. (2014). Shared decision making and motivation: Achieving patient-centered care across the spectrum of health care problems. *Annals of Family Medicine, 12*(3), 270–275.

Erikson, A., & Davies, B. (2017). Maintaining integrity: How nurses navigate boundaries in pediatric palliative care. *Journal of Pediatric Nursing, 35*, 42–49.

Errasti-Ibarrondo, B., Pérez, M., Carrasco, J. M. et al. (2015). Essential elements of the relationship between the nurse and the person with advanced and terminal cancer: A meta-ethnography. *Nursing Outlook, 63*(3), 255–268.

Fasulo, A., Zinken, J., & Zinkin, K. (2016). Asking 'what about' questions in chronic self-management meetings. *Patient Education and Counseling, 99*, 917–923.

Fumagalli, L., Radaelli, G., Lettieri, E. et al. (2015). Patient empowerment and its neighbours: Clarifying the boundaries and their mutual relationships. *Health Policy, 119*, 384–394.

Halldorsdottir, S. (2008). The dynamics of the nurse-patient relationship: Introduction of a synthesized theory from the patient's perspective. *Scandinavian Journal of Caring Sciences, 22*(4), 643–652.

Kitson, A., Marshall, A., Bassett, K. et al. (2013). What are the core elements of patient centered care? A narrative review and synthesis of the literature from health policy, medicine and nursing. *Journal of Advanced Nursing, 69*(1), 4–15.

Krau, S. (2015). Patient centered care and lifelong learning. *Nursing Clinics of North America, 50*(4), xi–xii.

Légaré, F., & Witteman, H. O. (2013). Shared decision making: Examining key elements and barriers to adoption into routine clinical practice. *Health Affairs (Millwood), 32*(2), 276–284.

Mazor, K., Street, R. L., Sue, V. M. et al. (2016). Assessing patients' experiences with communication across the cancer center continuum. *Patient Education and Counseling, 99*, 1343–1348.

McCorkle, R., Ercolano, E., Lazenby, M. et al. (2011). Self-management: Enabling and empowering patients living with cancer as a chronic illness. *CA: A Cancer Journal for Clinicians, 61*, 50–62.

Oshima Lee, E., & Emanuel, E. J. (2013). Shared decision making to improve care and reduce costs. *Journal of Nursing Education, 368*(1), 6–8.

Pulvirenti, M., McMillan, J., & Lawn, S. (2014). Empowerment, patient centered care and self-management. *Health Expectations, 17*, 303–310.

Rogers, C. (1958). The characteristics of the helping relationship. *Personnel and Guidance Journal, 37*(1), 6–16.

Shively, M. J., Gardetto, N. J., Kodiath, M. F. et al. (2013). Effect of patient activation on self-management in patients with heart failure. *Journal of Cardiovascular Nursing, 28*, 20–34.

Small, D., & Small, R. (2011). Patients first! Engaging the hearts and minds of nurses with a patient-centered practice model. *Online Journal Issues in Nursing, 16*(2). Manuscript 2.

Sommerfeldt, S. (2013). Articulating nursing in an interprofessional world. *Nurse Education in Practice, 13*, 519–523.

Street, R. L. (2013). How clinician-patient communication contributes to health improvement: Modeling pathways from talk to outcome. *Patient Education and Counseling, 92*, 286–291.

Street, R. L. (2017). The many "disguises" of patient-centered communication: Problems of conceptualization and measurement. *Patient Education and Counseling, 100*(11), 2131–2134.

Windover, A., Boissy, A., Rice, T. et al. (2014). The REDE model of health care communication: Optimizing relationship as a therapeutic agent. *Journal of Patient Experience, 1*(1), 8–13.

World Health Organization. (n.d.). WHO: What is people-centred care? [Video.] https://www.youtube.com/watch?v=pj-AvTOdk2Q

12

Bridges and Barriers in Therapeutic Relationships

Claire Mallette

Originating US Chapter by *Kathleen Underman Boggs*

OBJECTIVES

At the end of the chapter, the reader will be able to:

1. Analyze which nursing actions can promote person-centred communication, using respect, caring, empowerment, trust, empathy, mutuality, truth and honesty, and confidentiality.
2. Describe personal and organizational barriers to the development of effective communication.
3. Analyze which nursing actions best reduce barriers to communication.
4. Identify research-supported relationships between communication outcomes, such as person empowerment and improvements in self-care.
5. Apply findings from research studies to foster communication in clinical practice.

Health communication is a multidimensional process. It includes aspects from the sender and the receiver of a message. This chapter focuses on the communication components of the nurse–person relationship acting as bridges to promote person's health and safety outcomes. Effective communication improves person satisfaction, facilitates decision-making, and promotes successful self-management of health issues. Types of nursing communications have been shown to affect the person's participation (Tobiano et al., 2016). As nurses, we apply the concepts of respect, caring, empowerment, trust, empathy, and mutuality, as well as confidentiality and truthfulness. We actively engage people's participation in health decisions, a right recognized by the World Health Organization (WHO, 2016).

Implementing actions that convey feelings of respect, caring, warmth, acceptance, and understanding to the person is an interpersonal skill that requires practice. Novice students and nurses may encounter interpersonal situations that leave them feeling helpless and inadequate. Feelings of sadness, helplessness, anger, or embarrassment, while overwhelming, are common. Through practice, discussion

of these feelings in peer groups, and experiential learning activities, you gain skills to deal with these feelings.

BASIC CONCEPTS

Bridges to the Relationship

Comprehensive nursing communication about the person's condition is critical to the competent provision of high-quality, safe, and compassionate care. It also improves person outcomes (Koo et al., 2016). Safety issues and related communication tools are discussed in Chapters 2 and 24. Communication also affects us as health providers in terms of our job satisfaction and stress levels. The following concepts describe methods to help you improve your communication skills in bridging and avoiding barriers (Fig. 12.1).

Respect

Conveying genuine respect for the person assists in building professional relationships. Because your mutual goal is to maximize the person's health status, you need to convey respect for their knowledge, values, opinions, and life

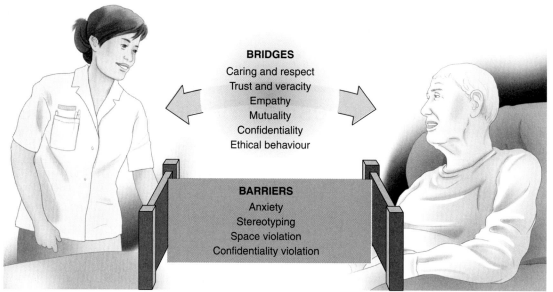

Fig. 12.1 Therapeutic relationships can move in a positive or negative direction, based on bridges and barriers to communication.

experiences. Asking them what they prefer to be called and always addressing them as such is a correct initial step. Using casual addresses such as "Honey," "Dear," or "Sweetie," or using the word "we" in the context of, "How are we feeling today?" needs to be avoided. It is important to remember that people who are hospitalized or have health care needs are defined by who they are, not by their disease or health issues. We should avoid these terms because they can contribute to people's sense of a loss of control in relation to interpersonal relationships with health care providers.

Lack of Respect

People report feeling devalued when they perceive that staff were avoiding talking with them or were unfriendly; they felt comforted when social conversations were included in communications. For example, if you see the person watching a sports show, you could ask them their thoughts on the team or game as you change their IV bag.

Collaborative Communication

In a true collaborative model, each team member conveys respect and assumes responsibility for initiating clear communication (Agency for Healthcare Research and Quality, 2017). Lack of respect among team members is associated with poor communication, leading to adverse health outcomes. In establishing person-centred care, we should treat every person as a respected member of the team, as suggested in Mr. Syds's case.

Case Example: Mr. Syds

Mr. Syds is recovering from pulmonary distress in an intensive care unit. This morning, as the team gathers at his bedside for rounds, he confides in his nurse about feeling a "sense of doom." Noting his anxious expression, falling oxygenation levels, and slightly elevated temperature, the nurse uses the C.U.S. TeamSTEPPS communication tool of three statements: "I'm concerned," "I'm uncomfortable," and "This is a safety issue" (Canadian Patient Safety Institute [CPSI], 2011), in saying "I am concerned about these changes." Mr. Syds's feedback, taken together with physiological data, prompts pattern recognition among team members. They explore the possibility that he may be developing pneumonia. In person-centred care, this type of person–nurse–team feedback loop might correlate with what Trainer et al. (2016) identify as flow of information crucial to person outcome.

Caring

Caring is an intentional human action characterized by commitment and a level of knowledge and skill to allow you to support basic integrity. You offer caring to the person and family by means of the therapeutic relationship. Nursing theorists such as Jean Watson describe the need to develop and sustain a helping, trusting, caring relationship with people and family. Watson's Human Caring Theory can guide human-to-human relationships and create a caring–healing environment to care for the person's body, mind, and spirit (Wei & Watson, 2019). The Canadian nursing theorist Sister Simone Roach (1992) describes the 6 C's of what nurses do when they are caring: compassion, competence, conscience, confidence, commitment, and comportment (professional presentation as a nurse). Everyone has an innate ability to care, based on their social environment, cultural and societal influences, and ongoing interaction with others (Kuper et al., 2007; Sokola, 2013). Your ability to care in your nursing practice develops from a natural response to help those in need, from respect for self and others, and from the knowledge that caring is a part of nursing ethics. As a caring nurse, you give person-centred care, recognizing and assisting people and families in their ability to achieve good health and well-being rather than simply doing things for them. They perceive care and empathy from your behaviours (Richardson, et al., 2015).

Providing a caring relationship that facilitates health and well-being is an expectation in all provincial and territorial nursing practice standards. For example, in the Standards of Practice for Licensed Practical Nurses (LPN) in Canada, it states, "LPNs are self-regulating and accountable for providing safe, competent, compassionate and ethical care within the legal and ethical framework of nursing regulation" (Canadian Council for Practical Nurse Regulators, 2013, p. 4). The Canadian Nurses Association [CNA] (2017) *Code of Ethics for Registered Nurses* also has principles related to providing a caring and compassionate relationship.

In the professional literature, the focus of the caring relationship is clearly placed on meeting the person's needs. You purposefully care for the person as an ethical responsibility. The behaviour of "caring" is not only an emotional feeling but also involves the following:

- Knowing: Nurses' knowledge and the person's needs
- Being: Verbal and nonverbal interactions that occur during the therapeutic relationship
- Doing: Nursing interventions that demonstrate caring while striving to achieve the best health outcomes (Swanson, 1991)

People want us to understand their unique health experiences. Health care providers tend to speak in a medical language that values facts and events. In contrast, people you care for tend to value associations and causes. To bridge this potential gap, you need to convey a sense that you truly care about the person's perspective. Families also need to experience a sense of caring from the nurse. Many families do not believe health care providers have a clear understanding of the issues they are encountering while caring for their family member. "Caring" interventions in the form of conferences where family members can express emotions and talk with experts, in conjunction with written materials, may help decrease anxiety. (Refer to Chapter 17, Table 17.2 for interventions to reduce family anxiety).

Lack of Caring

Although nursing has a long-standing commitment to person-focused care, sometimes you may observe a situation in which you feel a nurse is apathetic, trying to meet their own needs rather than the person's needs. Some nurses develop a detachment that interferes with expression of caring behaviours. At other times, nurses can be so rushed to meet multiple demands that they seem unable to focus on the person. Simulation Exercise 12.1 will help you focus on the concept of caring.

Empowerment

Empowerment is defined as assisting people to take charge of their lives. Chinn and Falk Raphael (2015) define *empowerment* as "growth of personal ability to enact one's will in the context of love and respect for others" (p. 65). Our nursing goal is to use communication skills that build bridges to form partnerships that foster the person and family's empowerment. We use the interpersonal process to provide information, tools, and resources that help people build knowledge and skills to reach their health goals. Empowerment is an important aim in every nurse–person relationship. Empowered people feel valued and are more likely to adopt successful coping and self-management strategies. Studies demonstrate that the more involved people are in their own care, the better the health outcomes.

Lack of Empowerment

People can experience disempowerment when they feel a "power over" them. This can occur based on their cultural

---

SIMULATION EXERCISE 12.1
Application of Caring

Purpose
To help you apply caring concepts in your nursing practice

Procedure
1. Based on the knowledge you have learned in this chapter, identify examples of "knowing, being, and doing" caring practices that can be applied to nursing practice. Work in a group to compile a list.

Discussion and Reflective Analysis
Discuss examples of how these caring practices could be implemented in a nurse–person situation.

contexts or through the use of power by others who enact rules, hierarchy, force, expediency (what is easy and readily available), or marginalization (Chinn & Falk Raphael, 2015). Some health providers exhibit a paternalistic attitude toward people, characterized by the attitude of "I know what's best for you or I can do it better." This attitude can occur when the health care provider tells the person what to do, rather than developing a person-centred care (PCC) relationship in exploring self-management health strategies through shared decision making, as discussed in Chapter 11. This disempowerment can lead to unsuccessful self-management activities and health outcomes. Empowerment should also extend to families. Lack of information about how to provide and support care, manage prescriptions, or recognize approaching crises can be major barriers to those who care for family members with health needs. Failure to assist people and their families in assuming self-management responsibility, or failure to provide appropriate resources and support, can inhibit empowerment.

Trust

Establishing **trust** is the foundation in all relationships. The development of a sense of interpersonal trust, a sense of feeling safe, is the keystone in the nurse–person relationship. Trust provides a nonthreatening, interpersonal environment in which people feel comfortable revealing their needs. The nurse is perceived as dependable, competent, and not causing harm. Establishment of this trust is critical toward enabling you to make an accurate assessment of health needs.

Trust is also the key to establishing effective health care team relationships. Lack of trust in the workplace has detrimental effects for the organization and for coworkers, undermining performance and commitment. According to Erikson (1963), trust is developed by experiencing consistency, sameness, and continuity during care by a familiar caregiver, while growing up. Trust develops based on past experiences. In the nurse–person relationship, maintaining an open exchange of information contributes to trust. For the person receiving care, trust implies a willingness to place oneself in a position of vulnerability, relying on health care providers to perform as expected. Truthfulness and honesty is a basic building block in establishing trust. Studies show that people and their families or substitute decision makers want "complete honesty," and most prefer complete disclosure. Box 12.1 lists interpersonal strategies that help promote a trusting relationship.

Mistrust

Mistrust has an effect not only on communication but on healing-process outcomes. Trust can be replaced with mistrust, as might occur if the nurse violates a person's confidentiality. Just as some managers treat employees as though they are not trustworthy, some nurses' behaviours lead to people not trusting them. An example might be a community health nurse who is inconsistent about keeping appointments or a pediatric nurse who indicates falsely that an injection will not hurt. Such behaviours create mistrust. It is hard to maintain trust in any situation when one person cannot depend on another. Having confidence in the nurse's knowledge, skills, commitment, and caring allows the person to feel confident in the person–nurse relationship, in focusing on the health situation requiring resolution. A person can also jeopardize the trust a nurse has in them; some people may not be truthful with the nurse when providing information. For example, the person may tell the nurse they are taking a prescribed medication, but they actually are not. While on an emotional level, the nurse may feel they can't trust the person, the nurse needs to explore the reasons why the person is not following the established health activities. Simulation Exercise 12.2 is designed to help students become more familiar with the concept of trust.

BOX 12.1 Techniques Designed to Promote Trust

- Convey respect.
- Consider the person's uniqueness.
- Show warmth and caring.
- Use the person's proper name.
- Use active listening.
- Give sufficient time to answer questions.
- Maintain confidentiality.
- Show congruence between verbal and nonverbal behaviours.
- Use a warm, friendly voice.
- Use appropriate eye contact.
- Smile.
- Be flexible.
- Provide for allowed preferences.
- Be honest and open.
- Give complete information.
- Provide consistency.
- Plan schedules.
- Follow through on commitments.
- Set limits.
- Control distractions.
- Use an attending posture: arms, legs, and body relaxed; leaning slightly forward.

Empathy

Empathy is the ability to experience what another person or family member is feeling and then communicate understanding. Empathy is the ability to put yourself into another's position. Characteristics associated with being empathetic include an individual's ability to understand and feel the person's experience, perspective, and feelings while remaining nonjudgemental; interpret nonverbal communication; and meet the person's needs through a therapeutic relationship (Dean et al., 2017; Kiosses, et al., 2016). Empathy and empathetic communication are crucial to developing a therapeutic relationship and nursing practice. The ability to effectively communicate empathy is associated with meeting the person's basic need to be understood and can lead to improved satisfaction and health outcomes.

An empathetic nurse perceives and understands the person's emotions accurately. Some nurses might term this as compassion, which has been identified as critical to the nurse–person relationship. In order to be compassionate, the nurse must have empathy (Durkin et al., 2018). Communication skills such as active listening are used to convey respect and empathy. Although expert nurses recognize the emotions a person feels, they hold on to their objectivity, maintaining their own separate identities. As a nurse, you try not to over-identify with or internalize the feelings of the person. If internalization occurs, objectivity is lost, together with the ability to help the person move through their feelings. It is important to recognize that these feelings belong to them, not to you.

Communicate your understanding of the meaning of a person's feelings by using both verbal and nonverbal communication behaviours: maintain direct eye contact, use attending open body language, and keep a calm tone of voice. Acknowledging the person's message about their feelings, difficulties, or pain helps create a positive connection (Williams et al., 2016). Remember to validate accuracy by restating what you understand the person is conveying, and have them confirm verbally that this is accurate. If you need more information about their feelings, ask them to expand on their message, perhaps asking, "Are there other things about your experience that are bothering you?" or "Is there anything else you think I should know?" Once you have all the information needed, you can identify, with the person, interventions to address their health needs.

Lack of Empathy

A failure to understand a person's needs may lead you to not provide required emotional support and educational support and meet the person's health needs. Major organizational barriers to empathy exist in the clinical environment, including a lack of time associated with heavy workloads. Several studies suggest that a lack of empathy affects the quality of care, results in less favourable health outcomes, and lowers satisfaction by the person and family. As providers, we can consciously choose to express empathy.

Mutuality

Mutuality is the recognition of reciprocity, in which we value and support the well-being of people (Berezin & Lamont, 2016). It means that the nurse and person agree on the person's health issues and the means for resolving them. Both parties are committed to enhancing the person's well-being. This is characterized by mutual respect for the autonomy and value system of the other. In developing mutuality, you maximize the person's involvement in all phases of the nursing process. Mutuality is collaboration in problem solving and guides the communication at the initial encounter. Evidence of mutuality is seen in the development of individualized goals and nursing actions that meet the person's identified, unique health needs. Simulation Exercise 12.3 provides practice in evaluating mutuality.

SIMULATION EXERCISE 12.3 **Evaluating Mutuality**

Purpose
To identify behaviours and feelings on the part of the nurse and the person that indicate mutuality

Procedure
Complete the following yes/no questions after terminating a relationship with a person you cared for; then bring them to class. Discuss the answers. How were you able to attain mutuality, or why were you unable to attain it?

1. Was I satisfied with the relationship?
2. Did the person express satisfaction with the relationship?
3. Did the person share feelings with me?
4. Did I make decisions for the person?
5. Did the person feel allowed to make their own decisions?
6. Did the person accomplish their goals?
7. Did I accomplish my goals?

Discussion and Reflective Analysis

1. In groups, analyze your responses for mutuality.
2. What practices did you do to support mutuality?
3. What could you have done differently?
4. How can you foster mutuality in your nursing practice?

As nurses, we respect interpersonal differences. We involve the person in the decision-making process as an equal partner. We accept their decisions even if we do not agree with them. Effective use of self-awareness and values clarification assists you to support people in decision making. Those who clearly identify their own personal values are better able to solve problems effectively. Decisions then have meaning to the person. There is a greater probability that they will work to achieve success. When a mutual relationship is terminated, both parties experience a sense of shared accomplishment and satisfaction.

Truthfulness and Honesty

Truthfulness and being honest in communication and actions is one of the most important aspects in upholding a high standard of ethical nursing. The CNA (2017) Code of Ethics for Registered Nurses states that "Nurses are honest and practise with integrity in all of their professional interactions" (p. 16). The Canadian Council for Practical Nurse Regulators (2013) Standards of Practice for Licensed Practical Nurses in Canada also states that

communication occurs in a "respectful, timely, open, and honest manner" (p. 9). Legal and ethical standards mandate specific nursing behaviours, such as confidentiality, beneficence, and respect for person autonomy. These behaviours are based on professional nursing values that stem from ethical principles. By adhering to these standards, nurses build their therapeutic relationships. When people know they can expect the truth, the development of trust is promoted and helps build the person–nurse relationship.

Barriers to Truthfulness and Honesty

Sometimes it is not as easy to maintain truthfulness as we would hope. For example, the physician may not have yet told the person what you already know, which is that the person has been diagnosed with Stage 3 cancer. Any deception (lies or omissions) erodes trust in care providers. There may be a need to balance truth-telling with following nursing practice standards, where communicating a diagnosis is not in the nurse's scope of practice. In situations like this, you can explore with the person what they are worried about and make every effort to have the physician speak with the person as soon as possible.

Person-Centred Communication

Within conversations between the person and nurse, the person should remain the focus. We should focus our attention on what the person is trying to tell us. We strive to use the "unconditional regard" advocated by Carl Rogers, in accepting and supporting the person regardless of what they say or do. For example, if the person informs you that they are misusing alcohol, you remain nonjudgemental and accept the person for who they are.

In social conversations, it is common to take turns and, when the other person speaks, you may not always give them your full focus. However, in professional person–nurse communication, you need to be actively listening, with 100% of your attention directed toward what the person is trying to tell you.

Acceptance

Everyone has conscious and unconscious biases. We need to make it a goal to be self-aware of our biases and recognize a person as a unique individual, both different from and similar to self. Acceptance of the other person needs to be total. Unconditional acceptance, as described by Rogers (1961), is essential in the therapeutic relationship. It does not imply agreement or approval; acceptance occurs without judgement. Mr. Rogers, the children's television show host, ended his programs by telling his audience, "I like you just the way you are." How wonderful if we, as nurses, could convey this type of acceptance through our words and actions. Simulation Exercise 12.4 examines ways of reducing nursing bias and stereotyping.

Stereotyping acts as a communication barrier. This is the process of attributing characteristics to a group of people as though all people in the identified group possess them. People may be stereotyped according to ethnicity culture, religion, social class, occupation, age, sexual orientation, and other factors. Even health issues can be the stimulus for stereotyping individuals. For example, alcohol addiction, mental health disorders, and sexually transmitted infections often have stereotypes, stigma, and biases attached to them. Stereotyping people in a group rather than looking at each person as an individual with unique characteristics leads to negative consequences in unconsciously influencing our judgement and responses to those we are stereotyping. Stereotypes develop through cultural contexts, communications, experiences with parents and peers, and behaviours portrayed in the media.

Stereotypes are never completely accurate. No attribute applies to every member of a group. All of us like to think that our way is the correct way, and that everyone else thinks about life experiences just as we do. The reality is that there are many perspectives and no one way of thinking is necessarily better than another. Emotions play a role in the value we place on negative stereotypes. Stereotypes based on strong emotions are called **prejudices** and racism, and these ways of thinking can result in discrimination.

Confidence

Having confidence as a nurse can lead to creating trusting relationships, empowerment, and resiliency, but it is important to recognize that having confidence does not substitute for or indicate competence (Owens & Keller, 2018). As a student or novice nurse, learning and growing in your knowledge and skills will assist you in feeling more confident in your role. By seeking out every learning opportunity possible, you will gain more competence, which will assist you in feeling more confident. You may feel nervous or anxious about seeking out new learning opportunities to develop your competence; a mild level of anxiety can foster learning

---

SIMULATION EXERCISE 12.4 Reducing Clinical Bias by Identifying Stereotypes

Purpose

To identify and reduce nursing biases and stereotyping. One component of identifying biases and maintaining high-quality, compassionate nursing care is to identify professional biases and stereotypes and how to then reduce them.

Procedure

Each of the following scenarios describes a stereotype. Identify the stereotype and explain how it might affect nursing care. As a nurse, what would you do to reduce the bias in the following situations?

Situation A

Mrs. Daniels is an obstetric nurse who believes in birth control. She comments about the person she is caring for, Mrs. Isaac, saying, "She's pregnant again. You know the one with six kids already! She can barely feed the children she already has. I don't know how she can continue to do this. Hasn't she ever heard of birth control?"

Situation B

Mr. Visser, a registered nurse on a medical unit, is upset with his 52-year-old patient. "If she rings that buzzer one more time, I'm going to disconnect it. Can't she understand that I have other people who need my attention more than she does? She just lies in bed all day long and doesn't do anything. It's no wonder she's overweight."

Situation C

Ms. Waters, a staff nurse in a nursing home, listens to the daughter of a 93-year-old resident, who says, "My mother, who is confused most of the time, receives very little attention from you nurses, while other people who are alert and clear-minded have more interaction with you. It's not fair! No wonder my mother is so confused. Nobody talks to her. Nobody ever comes in to say hello."

Situation D

To develop self-awareness, ask yourself whether there are any individuals or groups of people for whom you would not want to provide care (e.g., a woman with foul body odour experiencing homelessness; a person with high blood levels of alcohol; someone with a drug addiction; a person with a different skin colour or religion from your own)?

Discussion and Reflective Analysis

1. What stereotypes did you identify?
2. What other stereotypes and biases exist?
3. How do stereotypes and biases influence nursing care?
4. How can you begin to address your own and others' stereotyping behaviours in your nursing practice?

and decision making. For example, when you are feeling anxious that you need more experience caring for people who have pain, you can use this anxiety to push yourself out of your comfort zone and seek out these types of learning experiences. You can ask the nurse you are assigned to or your clinical instructor to assist you in finding new learning opportunities. When you are feeling nervous about doing a skill even though you have the knowledge and ability to perform it, you can try to convey confidence that you may not actually be feeling. Try doing self-talk to review what you know needs to be done and leverage your knowledge and experience to convey confidence. When you don't know what to do, ask for assistance. As a nurse, you have ethical and professional responsibilities to ask for assistance and not pretend you have the knowledge and ability to perform a skill. Asking for help is not a sign of incompetence. Instead, it is a sign of strength in knowing your competence and confidence in your own abilities.

Anxiety

Feeling anxious can become a personal barrier to communication in a person-centred relationship. Anxiety is a vague, persistent feeling of impending doom. It is a universal feeling; no one fully escapes it. The impact on the self is always uncomfortable. It occurs when one perceives a threat (real or imagined) to one's self-concept. Lower satisfaction with communication is associated with increased anxiety. Anxiety is usually observed through the physical and behavioural manifestations of the attempt to relieve the anxious feelings. Although individuals experiencing anxiety may not know they are anxious, specific behaviours provide clues that they are. Simulation Exercise 12.5 identifies behaviours associated with anxiety. Table 12.1 shows how an individual's sensory perceptions, cognitive abilities, coping skills, and behaviours relate to the intensity and level of anxiety experienced. Suggestions for reducing your anxiety or for destressing are listed in Box 12.2. Some of these suggestions can be adopted to address your own anxiety and taught to people you are caring for who are anxious.

Proxemics

Proxemics is the study of an individual's use of space and is the amount of personal space that a person feels comfortable setting between themselves and others. Invading a person's personal space potentially impacts negatively on person-centred communication. Personal space is an invisible boundary around an individual. The emotional personal space boundary provides a sense of comfort and protection. It is defined by past experiences, current circumstances, and our cultural contexts. Four

---

SIMULATION EXERCISE 12.5
Identifying Verbal and Nonverbal Behaviours Associated With Anxiety

Purpose

To broaden the learner's awareness of behavioural responses indicating anxiety

Procedure

List as many anxious behaviours as you can think of. Each column has a few examples to start. Discuss the lists in a group, and then add new behaviours to your list.

Verbal	Nonverbal
Quavering voice	Nail biting
Rapid speech	Foot tapping
Mumbling	Sweating
Defensive words	Pacing

Discussion and Reflective Analysis

1. What surprised you about the list of anxious behaviours?
2. What anxious behaviours from the list have you experienced or observed in others?
3. What nursing practices can you apply to help the person or yourself manage anxiety?

---

areas of personal space have been identified: the intimate zone (0–45 cm), personal zone (45cm–1 m), social zone (1m–4 m), and public zone (4 m and greater) (Jakubec & Astle, 2019).

Among the many factors that affect the individual's need for personal distance are cultural contexts. Some people will be comfortable with less space, while others will want more. Therapeutic touch, such as touching a person's arm or holding their hand, may be welcome by some and not by others. If a person is feeling anxious, they may want more space between you and them. Usually, people will tolerate someone standing close to them at their side more readily than directly in front of them. Direct eye contact can cause a need for more space. Placing oneself at the same level (e.g., sitting while the person is sitting or standing at eye level when they are standing) allows more access to the person's personal space because such a stance is perceived as less threatening. When considering a person's personal space, it is important to remember that every individual is unique. You will need to be assessing the person's verbal and nonverbal communication to determine whether you

TABLE 12.1 Levels of Anxiety With Degree of Sensory Perceptions, Cognitive and Coping Abilities, and Manifest Behaviours

Level of Anxiety	Sensory Perceptions	Cognitive and Coping Abilities	Behaviours
Mild	Heightened state of alertness; increased acuity of hearing, vision, smell, and touch	Enhanced learning, problem solving; increased ability to respond and adapt to changing stimuli; enhanced functioning*	Walking, singing, eating, drinking, mild restlessness, active listening, attending, questioning
Moderate	Decreased sensory perceptions; with guidance, able to expand sensory fields	Loss of concentration; decreased cognitive ability; cannot identify factors contributing to the anxiety-producing situation; with directions, can cope, reduce anxiety, and solve problems; inhibited functioning	Increased muscle tone, pulse, respirations; changes in voice tone and pitch, rapid speech, incomplete verbal responses; engrossed with detail
Severe	Greatly diminished perceptions; decreased sensitivity to pain	Limited thought processes; unable to solve problems even with guidance; cannot cope with stress without help; confused mental state; limited functioning	Purposeless, aimless behaviours; rapid pulse, respirations; high blood pressure; hyperventilation; inappropriate or incongruent verbal responses
Panic	No response to sensory perceptions	No cognitive or coping abilities; without intervention, death is imminent	Immobilization

*Functioning refers to the ability to perform activities of daily living for survival purposes.

BOX 12.2 Nursing Strategies to Reduce Anxiety

For the Person
- Use active listening to show acceptance.
- Be honest; answer all questions at the person's level of understanding.
- Explain procedures, surgery, and policies, and give appropriate reassurance based on data.
- Act in a calm, unhurried manner.
- Speak clearly, slowly, and firmly (but not loudly).
- Give information regarding laboratory tests, medications, treatments, and rationale for restrictions on activity.
- Set reasonable limits and provide structure.
- Encourage self-affirmation through positive statements such as "I will" and "I can."
- Use drawings or play therapy with dolls, puppets, and games with youth.
- Use touch where appropriate.
- Initiate recreational activities, such as physical exercise, music, card games, board games, crafts, and reading.

- Teach deep breathing and relaxation exercises.
- Use guided imagery.

For Nurses
- Ensure adequate amounts of sleep.
- Eat a healthy diet.
- Exercise.
- Practise mindfulness activities, such as meditating, daily (even if only for 5 minutes).
- Use guided imagery, positive attitude, and positive affirmations.
- Listen to music.
- Practise yoga.
- Do journalling.
- Do deep breathing exercises. Download the Breathe app, and have it remind you to do deep breathing periodically.
- Take your assigned breaks to do some of the above!

Modified from Gerrard, B., Boniface, W., & Love, B. (1980). *Interpersonal skills for health professionals.* Reston Publishing; TeamSTEPPS National Conference, June 2017.

may be invading their personal space. You can also ask the person if they feel comfortable with where you are communicating with them.

Violations of Personal Space

Hospitals are not home. Many nursing care procedures are a direct intrusion into the person's personal space. Commonly, procedures that require tubes (e.g., nasogastric intubation, administration of oxygen, catheterization, and intravenous initiation) restrict mobility, resulting in loss of control over personal territory. When more than one health provider is involved, the impact of the intrusion on the person may be even stronger. In many instances, personal space requirements are an integral part of a person's self-image. When people lose control over personal space, they may experience a loss of identity and self-esteem. A general recommendation is that you maintain a social physical body distance of approximately 1.2 meters (4 feet) when not actually giving care.

When people who are hospitalized are able to incorporate parts of their rooms into their personal space, it increases their self-esteem and helps them to maintain a sense of identity. This feeling of security is evidenced when a person asks, "Close my door, please." Freedom from worry about personal space allows the person to trust the nurse and fosters a therapeutic relationship. When invasions of personal space are necessary while performing a procedure, you can minimize the impact by explaining why a procedure is needed. Conversation at such times reinforces their feelings that they are human beings, worthy of respect, and not just objects being worked on. Advocating for the person's personal space needs is an aspect of the nursing role. This is done by communicating the person's preferences to other members of the health team and including those preferences in the care plan.

When caring for a person in their home, it is important to remember that you are the guest and you need to ask the person where it is best to provide care in their home.

Cultural Barriers

Cultural contexts and communication are discussed extensively in Chapter 7. Every interaction can encounter a basic challenge of communication when the culture of a person you're caring for differs from your own. Barriers include perceptions related to health needs that may differ from your own or health literacy needs. As Canada embraces multiculturalism, with multiple cultures coexisting while maintaining cultural differences, it is imperative that nurses acknowledge, respect, and support unique dynamic cultural identities of the people they care for.

Cultural safety communication is characterized by a willingness to try to understand and respond to the person's beliefs to safely meet their needs, expectations, and rights, given their own unique cultural contexts. Knowledge of your own and others' cultural contexts helps you acknowledge your own biases and stereotyping to provide culturally safe care.

Gender Differences

Gender is defined as the culture's attributions of masculine or feminine characteristics. The term *transgender* is used for people who express their gender in different ways from the established assigned gender at birth as being male or female (Baldwin et al., 2018; Merryfeather & Bruce, 2014). In Canada in 2019, 91% of the nursing population identified as female, yet from 2015 to 2019, the population of nurses who are male grew faster (an increase of 15.4% over nurses who are female 3.9%) (Canadian Nurses Association, 2020). Stereotyping and stigmas continue to exist related to the perception that nursing as a profession is only for women, that men in nursing are gay, or that men do not have the ability to care in the same way as nurses who are female. Learning environments often have cultural norms and educational practices that support the nursing profession as being firmly linked to feminine roles and identity, resulting in possible marginalization of students who are male or transgender (Sedgwick & Kellet, 2015). As educators, nurses, and students, we need to critically examine our own biases related to gender in nursing to create environments where being a nurse is gender neutral. One way to accomplish this, when communicating with others about the nursing role, is to highlight that caring as a nurse is gender neutral, and that it is based on professional knowledge and expertise, not the person's gender. There are times when a person may want a nurse of the same gender caring for them, for example based on religious beliefs. In these situations, where possible, a nurse of the same gender should be considered to provide nursing care. Where it is not possible, the nurse needs to be aware of the potential discomfort of the person and explore with them what would make them feel more comfortable while providing nursing care.

Organizational System Barriers

Communication barriers inherent in health care system agencies are commonly discussed in the professional literature. Frequent interruptions and lack of time are cited by Flick (2012), McGillis Hall et al. (2010), and many others. Often, such barriers to communication stem from cost-containment measures.

Heavy Workload

Heavy workload is often mentioned as a barrier to communication and developing therapeutic relationships. Lack of time is a result of the current demands of health care environments, with the emphasis on efficiency, cost containment, protocol-based care, and measurements of success and health outcomes. For nurses, this environment results in the expectation of nurses to complete multiple tasks with an increasing number of people to care for while completing an escalating number of administrative tasks. In our care for people with increasingly complex health problems and heavier workloads, we may think we lack the time to spend having meaningful communication. Nurses often believe that they can have only person-centred therapeutic communication when they sit down to speak with the person for a designated amount of time. While this is ideal and should try to be obtained, with increased workload expectations, nurses rarely have the time to do this. Instead of sitting down with the person, nurses can also try to incorporate these quality conversations while they are performing other care. For example, when doing a dressing change, the nurse could speak to the person about their concerns and the information they need to know. Reporting at the bedside and including the person as an active partner in the day's care goals can also identify their needs and incorporate them in care decisions. Simulation Exercise 12.6 assists you in fostering person-centred communication using awareness of bridges and barriers within limited amounts of time.

Time Allocation Expectations

The primary care literature describes demand for minimal appointment time with people in health care agencies. Primary care providers such as nurse practitioners are often constrained to focus just on the chief complaint to maximize the number of people seen, leading to "the 15-minute office visit." These system barriers limit the nurse's ability to develop substantial rapport with people. Adequate time is important in developing therapeutic communication to achieve effective care that is responsive to people's needs.

Inconsistent Caregivers

Along with workload barriers, another characteristic of organizations that creates communication barriers is lack of consistent nurse assignments and increased use of temporary staff, known as agency nurses, casual nurses, or float nurses. To overcome system barriers to communication, we need to work as a team to deliver consistent care. Working to develop open communications in our agencies leads to better communication and improved person safety (Agency for Healthcare Research and Quality, 2017).

 DEVELOPING AN EVIDENCE-INFORMED PRACTICE

Purpose

To explore the factors that affect nursing practices in person–nurse communication in intensive care units (ICUs) and increase awareness and understanding of Gottlieb's (2013) strengths-based strategies for person–nurse communication

Method

Qualitative study with semi-structured interviews asking 7 questions to 19 ICU nurses, in Montreal, Canada, to obtain data on nurse-to-patient communication in ICU's

Findings

Nurses believed person–nurse communication was inadequate. Factors affecting communication were related to the system, the team, the nurse, and the person and family.

Application to Clinical Practice

Reflective practices, promotion of empathetic and holistic communication with people and families, and sensitivity to the importance of team communication can assist in improved person–nurse communication.

Antonacci, R., Fong, A., Sumbly, P. et al. (2018). They can hear the silence: Nursing practices on communication with patients. *Canadian Journal of Critical Care Nursing, 29*(4), 36–39.

APPLICATIONS

Behaviours described in this chapter can be learned and are fundamental to your nursing role (Richardson et al., 2015). Many nursing actions recommended are mandated by the Canadian Council for Practical Nurse Regulators (CCPNR) Code of Ethics for Licensed Practical Nurses in Canada (2013), the CNA (2017) *Code of Ethics for Registered Nurses*, and provincial and territorial nursing standards. The actions specified include accountability, confidentiality, respect, dignity, autonomy, advocacy, beneficence, truthfulness, and justice. Mutuality characterized by mutual respect for the autonomy and value system of the other is also addressed in both Codes of Ethics (CNA, 2017; CCPNR, 2013) and within provincial and territorial nursing standards. Nurses with good communication skills have greater professional satisfaction and experience less job-related stress. Studies of person's perceptions generally show a correlation between good nurse communicators and good quality of care. Practice simulations and exercises provide you with opportunities to improve your skills. Part

SIMULATION EXERCISE 12.6 Building Communication Bridges Simulation

Purpose
To practise and evaluate current communication skills

Directions
1. In groups of three, role-play a person telling the nurse their story of some past unpleasant health experience while another student plays the nurse communicating with the person. The third person observes the interaction for bridges and barriers during the interaction. You have approximately 5–7 minutes for the interaction.

Discussion and Reflective Analysis
1. Both the person and nurse role-players reflect on how they felt during the interaction, including whether there was too little, too much, or just enough time for the interaction.
2. What parts of the interaction demonstrated empathy, respect, caring, mutuality, and so on?
3. Identify any barriers that occurred during the interaction.
4. What could have been done differently?
5. Observer should give the following types of feedback:
   a. Comment on positive verbal and nonverbal aspects observed.
   b. Offer constructive criticism.
   c. Identify any behaviours that served as barriers.
   d. Suggest alternative strategies the nurse could use.
   e. Think about times when you have used bridges and barriers in your own conversations.
6. How can you apply what you have learned from this exercise in your nursing practice?

of any simulation exercise to strengthen nursing communication is the offering of feedback and debriefing.

Steps in the Caring Process

The C.A.R.E approach focuses on person-centred communication with four steps to help you communicate C.A.R.E. with the person in your care:

C = First, *connect* with the person. Offer your attention. Here you introduce your purpose in developing a professional relationship (i.e., meeting their health needs). Use the person's formal name, and avoid terms of endearment such as "sweetie" or "honey." Show intent to care. Attentiveness is a part of communication skill

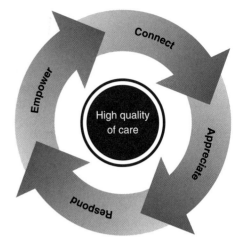

Fig. 12.2 C.A.R.E. Process

training even with time constraints, heavy workload, and so forth.

A = The second step is to *appreciate* the person's situation. Although the health care environment is familiar to you, it is a strange and perhaps frightening situation for the person. Acknowledge the person's point of view and express concern.

R = The third step is to *respond* to what the person needs. What are their priorities? What are their expectations for health care?

E = The fourth step is to *empower* the person to problem solve with you. The person gains strength and confidence from interactions with providers, enabling the person to move toward achievement of goals (Fig. 12.2).

The ability to become a caring professional is influenced by your previous experiences, social environment, cultural and societal influences, and ongoing interaction with others. A person who has received caring is more likely to be able to offer it to others. Self-awareness about feelings, attitudes, values, biases, and skills is essential for developing an effective, caring relationship. As a caring nurse, you give person-centred care, recognizing and assisting people in their ability to achieve good health and well-being.

Strategies for Empowerment

There is an increased focus on assisting people through person-centred care to actively participate as an equal partner in identifying and implementing self-management strategies to promote health and well-being. As nurses, we increasingly teach them new roles and skills to manage their health conditions. We may never fully understand the decisions some people make, but we support their right to make those decisions. Your method for empowering should include the following key strategies:

- Accept people as they are, by refraining from any negative judgements.
- Assess their level of understanding, exploring their perceptions and feelings about their health conditions and discussing issues that may interfere with self-care.
- Establish mutual goals for health care by forming a person-centred relationship, mutually deciding about their care.
- Find out how much information they need and want to know.
- Reinforce autonomy, for example, by allowing them to choose what self-management strategies they need information on and the best approach for the person to learn about them.
- Offer information in an environment that enables the person to use it.
- Ensure people actively participate in development and implementation of their care plans and self-management activities.
- Encourage networking with support groups and the use of applicable health apps (see Chapter 27).
- Support people in recognizing that they have ultimate decision-making power on health management activities for their health conditions.

Application of Empathy to Levels of Nursing Actions

Nursing actions that facilitate empathy can be classified into three major skills: (a) recognition and classification of requests, (b) attending behaviours, and (c) empathetic responses.

Recognition and classification of requests. There are two types of requests: for information and for action. Information requests do not involve interpersonal concerns and are easier to address. Action requests entail meeting the person's need for empathetic understanding.

Attending behaviours. Attending behaviours facilitate empathy and include an attentive, open posture; responding to verbal and nonverbal cues through appropriate gestures and facial expressions; maintaining appropriate personal space, using eye contact; and allowing the person's self-expression. Verbally acknowledging nonverbal cues shows you are attending, as does offering time and attention, showing interest in the person's issues, offering helpful information, and clarifying areas of concern. These responses encourage people to participate in their own healing.

Empathetic responses: You communicate empathy when you show people that you understand how they are feeling. This helps them identify emotions that are not readily observable and connect them with the current situation. For example, observing nonverbal cues such as a worried facial expression, and verbalizing this reaction with an empathetic comment, such as "I understand that this must be very difficult for you," validates what they are feeling and tells them you understand them. Using the actions listed in Table 12.2, the nurse applies attending behaviours and nursing actions to express empathy. Verbal

TABLE 12.2	Levels of Nursing Communication Behaviour	
Level	Category	Nursing Communication Behaviour
1. Process	Gathers data	Becomes aware of goals and person care plan
	Accepts	Uses person's correct name
		Maintains eye contact
		Adopts open posture
2. Act	Listens	Responds to cues
		Nods head
		Smiles
		Encourages responses
		Uses therapeutic silence
	Clarifies	Asks open-ended questions
		Restates the problem
		Validates perceptions
		Acknowledges confusion
	Informs	Provides honest, complete answers
		Assesses person's knowledge
		Confronts conflict
		Summarizes teaching points
3. Reflect	Analyzes	Identifies unknown emotions
		Interprets underlying meanings
		Evaluates outcomes
		Communicates with team to revise care plan

prompts such as "Hmm," "Uh-huh," "I see," "Tell me more," and "Go on," facilitate expression of feelings. The nurse uses open-ended questions to validate perceptions. Using informing behaviours listed in Table 12.2 provides new information to help the person better understand what is occurring and gives them feedback. Remember, demonstrating empathy as a communication behaviour has been shown to positively affect the outcome of your care.

Reduction of Barriers in Nurse–Person Relationships

Recognition of barriers is the first step in eliminating them, and thus enhancing the therapeutic process. Practice with exercises in this chapter should increase your recognition of possible barriers. Findings from many studies have emphasized the critical importance of honesty, cultural safety, and caring, especially in listening actively to suggestions and concerns from the person and family. Refer to Box 12.3 for a summary of strategies to reduce communication barriers in nurse–person relationships.

Respect for Personal Space

We need to assess a person's personal space needs. The minimum amount of space an individual needs is unique to each person. Assessment includes cultural and developmental factors that affect perceptions of space and reactions to intrusions. In some situations, if you need to increase the person's sense of personal space, you can decrease direct eye contact or position your body at an angle. This might occur when performing care that requires you to be quite close—for example, when bathing the person or changing their dressings. At the same time, it is important for you to talk gently during such procedures and to elicit feedback, if appropriate.

Actions to ensure private space and show respect in hospital settings where there is limited space for each person include the following:

- Closing the door slightly in private rooms or the curtains around the bed

---

- Providing privacy when disturbing matters are to be discussed
- Explaining procedures before implementation
- Entering another person's personal space with warning (e.g., knocking on the door or calling the person's name) and, preferably, waiting for permission to enter
- Providing an identified space for personal belongings and treating them with care
- Encouraging the inclusion of personal and familiar objects on the nightstand if the person is being hospitalized for a long period of time
- Minimizing bodily exposure during care
- Having only the necessary number of people present during any procedure
- Using touch appropriately

▐ SUMMARY

This chapter focuses on essential concepts that act as bridges in constructing a meaningful, effective nurse–person relationship, including caring, empowerment, trust, empathy, mutuality, and confidentiality. Respect for the person as a unique person is a basic component of each concept.

Caring is described as a commitment by the nurse that involves profound respect and concern for the unique humanity of every person and a willingness to confirm their personhood.

Empowerment is assisting people to assume responsibility of their own health.

Trust represents an individual's emotional reliance on the consistency and continuity of the health care experience. The person perceives the nurse as trustworthy—a safe person with whom to share difficult feelings about health-related needs.

Empathy is the ability to accurately perceive another person's feelings and to convey their meaning to the person. Nursing behaviours that facilitate the development of empathy are accepting, listening, clarifying and informing, and analyzing. Each of these behaviours implicitly recognizes the person as a unique individual, worthy of being listened to and respected.

Mutuality is characterized by reciprocity in setting goals and collaborating in methods to achieve the goals. To foster mutuality within the relationship, nurses need to remain aware of their own feelings, attitudes, and beliefs.

Barriers described include anxiety, stereotyping, overfamiliarity, and personal space violations, as well as organizational system demands such as a heavy workload and limited time for nurse–person communication. Solutions to overcome communication barriers include open

---

BOX 12.3   Tips to Reduce Relationship Barriers

- Establish trust.
- Demonstrate caring and empathy.
- Empower the person.
- Recognize and reduce anxiety.
- Maintain appropriate personal distance.
- Practise cultural safety.
- Use therapeutic, relationship-building activities such as active listening.
- Avoid medical terminology.

communication among all team members caring for the person, the person and family being active members of the health care team, and incorporating therapeutic communication while doing other activities.

👤 ETHICAL DILEMMA

What Would You Do?

There are limits to your professional responsibility to maintain confidentiality. Any information that, if withheld, might endanger the life or physical and emotional safety of the person or others needs to be communicated to the health team or appropriate people immediately.

Consider the teen who confides his plan to die by suicide. Can you breach confidentiality in this case? How about when you are caring for a woman in ER with a broken jaw who confides to you that her husband hit her but told you not to tell anyone as she is fearful he will cause her and her children harm.

QUESTIONS FOR REVIEW AND DISCUSSION

1. How could you apply the strategies for anxiety reduction and destressing provided in Box 12.2 to decrease your own anxiety and help develop resilience?
2. Reflect on which behaviours in Simulation Exercise 12.6 demonstrated empathy. Could you add the phrase, "That must have been difficult," to what the nurse role-player said? How do you think this would have changed the discussion?
3. Contrast stereotypes you have heard about in health care settings. Discuss them in a group. How can you begin to address stereotypes?
4. Analyze how proxemics changes in different situations. What is your own preferred space distance? To what do you attribute this preference? Under what circumstances do your needs for personal space change?

REFERENCES

Agency for Healthcare Research and Quality. (2017). *TeamSTEPPS, Webinar. (July, 2017). Introduction to the Fundamentals of TeamSTEPPS Concepts and Tools (Part 1 of 3)*. www.ahrq.gov/teamstepps/webinars/index.html.

Baldwin, A., Dodge, B., Schick, V. R. et al. (2018). Transgender and genderqueer individuals' experiences with health care providers: What's working, what's not, and where do we go from here?

Journal of Health Care for the Poor and Underserved, *29*(4), 1300–1318. https://muse.jhu.edu/article/708243.

Berezin, M., & Lamont, M. (2016). Mutuality, mobilization, and messaging for health promotion: Toward collective cultural change. *Social Science & Medicine*, *165*, 201–205.

Canadian Council for Practical Nurse Regulators. (2013). *Standards of practice for licensed practical nurses in Canada*. https://www.clpna.com/wp-content/uploads/2013/02/doc_CCPNR_CLPNA_Standards_of_Practice.pdf.

Canadian Nurses Association. (2017). *Code of ethics for registered nurses*. https://www.cna-aiic.ca/~/media/cna/page-content/pdf-en/code-of-ethics-2017-edition-secure-interactive.

Canadian Nurses Association. (2020). *Nursing statistics*. https://www.cna-aiic.ca/en/nursing-practice/the-practice-of-nursing/health-human-resources/nursing-statistics.

Canadian Patient Safety Institute. (2011). *Canadian framework for teamwork and communication: Literature review, needs assessment, evaluation of training tools and expert consultations*. https://www.patientsafetyinstitute.ca/en/toolsResources/teamworkCommunication/Pages/default.aspx.

Chinn, P. L., & Falk-Rafael, A. (2015). Peace and power: A theory of emancipatory group process. *Journal of Nursing Scholarship*, *47*(1), 62–69.

Dean, S., Williams, C., & Balnaves, M. (2017). Living dolls and nurses without empathy. *Journal of Advanced Nursing*, *73*(43), 757–759.

Durkin, M., Gurbutt, R., & Carson, J. (2018). Qualities, teaching, and measurement of compassion in nursing: A systematic review. *Nurse Education Today*, *63*, 50–58.

Erikson, E. (1963). *Childhood and society* (2nd ed.). Norton.

Flick, C. L. (2012). Communication: A dynamic between nurses and physicians. *MedSurg Nursing*, *21*(6), 385–387.

Gottlieb. L. (2013). *Strengths-based nursing care: Health and healing for person and family*. Springer.

Jakubec, S. L., & Astle, B. J. (2019). Communication and Relational Practice. In P. A. Potter, A. G. Perry, & J. C. Ross-Jerr et al. (Eds.), *Canadian Fundamentals of Nursing* (6th ed.). [E-reader edition]. Elsevier.

Kiosses, V. N., Karathanos, V. T., & Tatsioni, A. (2016). Empathy promoting interventions for health professionals: A systematic review of RCTs. *Journal of Compassionate Health Care*, *3*(7), 1–22.

Koo, L. W., Horowitz, A. M., Radice, S. D. et al. (2016). Nurse practitioners use of communication technologies: Results of a Maryland oral health literacy survey. *PLOS ONE*, 1–16.

Kuper, A., Reeves, S., Albert, M. et al. (2007). Assessments: Do we need to broaden our methodological horizons? *Medical Education*, *41*, 1121–1123.

McGillis Hall, L., Petersen, C., & Fairley, L. (2010). Losing the moment: Understanding interruptions of nurses' work. *Journal of Nursing Administration*, *40*(4), 169–176.

Merryfeather, L., & Bruce, A. (2014). The invisibility of gender diversity: Understanding transgender and transsexuality in nursing literature. *Nursing Forum*, *49*(2), 110–123.

Owens, K. M., & Keller, S. (2018). Exploring workforce confidence and patient experiences: A quantitative analysis. *Patient Experience Journal*, *5*(1), 97–105.

Richardson, C., Perry, M., & Hughes, J. (2015). Nursing therapeutics: Teaching student nurses care, compassion, & empathy. *Nurse Education Today, 35,* e1–e5.

Roach, S. M. (1992). *The Human Act of Caring.* Canadian Hospital Association Press.

Rogers, C. (1961). *On becoming a person.* Houghton-Mifflin.

Sedgwick, M. G., & Kellett, P. (2015). Exploring masculinity and marginalization of male undergraduate nursing students' experience of belonging during clinical experiences. *Journal of Nursing Education, 54*(3), 121–129.

Sokola. K. M. (2013). The relationship between caring ability and competency with caring behaviors of nursing students. *International Journal for Human Caring, 17*(1), 45–55.

Swanson, K. M. (1991). Empirical development of a mid-range theory of caring. *Nursing Research, 40*(3), 161–166.

Tobiano, G., Marshall, A., Bucknall, T. et al. (2016). Activities patients and nurses undertake to promote patient participation. *Journal of Nursing Scholarship, 48*(4), 362–370.

Trainer, R., Liske, L., & Nenadovic, V. (2016). Critical care nursing: Embedded complex systems. *The Canadian Journal of Critical Care, 27*(1), 11–16.

Wei, H., & Watson, J. (2019). Healthcare interprofessional team members' perspectives on human caring: A directed content analysis study. *International Journal of Nursing Sciences, 6,* 17–23. https://doi.org/10.1016/j.ijnss.2018.12.001.

Williams, B., Brown, T., McKenna, L. et al. (2016). Attachment and empathy in Australian undergraduate paramedic, nursing, and occupational therapy students: A cross-sectional study. *Collegian, 24*(6), 603–609. https://doi.org/10.1016/j.colegn.2016.11.004.

World Health Organization. (2016). *Framework on integrated, people-centred health services: Report by the secretariat.* https://apps.who.int/gb/ebwha/pdf_files/WHA69/A69_39-en.pdf?ua=1.

13

Communicating With Families

Olive Yonge

Originating US chapter by *Shari Kist, Elizabeth Arnold*

OBJECTIVES

At the end of the chapter, the reader will be able to:
1. Define *family* and identify its components.
2. Apply family-centred concepts to the care of the family in clinical settings, using standardized family-assessment tools.
3. Apply the nursing process to the care of families in clinical settings.
4. Identify nursing interventions for families in the intensive care unit (ICU).
5. Identify nursing interventions for families in the community.

The purpose of this chapter is to describe family-centred relationships and communication strategies that nurses can use to support family integrity in health care settings. This chapter identifies family theory frameworks and ways to maximize productive communication with family members. Practical assessment and intervention strategies address family issues that affect a person's recovery and support self-management of chronic health conditions or peaceful death in clinical practice.

BASIC CONCEPTS

Definition of Family

The term **family** has several definitions, particularly in today's society. The legal definition describes the family as individuals related through marriage, blood ties, adoption, or guardianship. As a biological unit, *family* describes the genetic connections among people. Two definitions of families exist, and they complement each other: census family (http://www12.statcan.gc.ca/census-recensement/2016/ref/dict/fam004-eng.cfm) and economic family (http://www12.statcan.gc.ca/censusrecensement/2016/ref/dict/fam011-eng.cfm). The term *census family* is the narrower concept, defined by couples living together, with or without children, and lone parents living with their children. The

term *economic family* is broader and refers to two or more persons living together who are related to each other by blood, marriage, common-law union, adoption, or a foster relationship. All people in a census family are part of one economic family. If there are additional relatives living with them, those people are also in the economic family. The additional relatives, if two or more, may also be in a census family among themselves, provided they are a couple with or without children or a lone parent with children.

A household may consist of a person living alone, or multiple unrelated individuals or families living together (Statistics Canada, 2016). However, as health care providers, it is more appropriate to use the Wright and Leahey (2013, p. 55) definition that "a family is who they say they are." Identified family members may or may not be blood related. Strong emotional ties and durability of membership characterize family relationships regardless of how uniquely they are defined. Even when family members are alienated or distanced geographically, they are still part of a family.

During times of crisis such as having a seriously ill family member, family members have a wide range of reactions to the situation and one another. Each family member responds in unique ways. Communication, even when reactive, is designed to maintain the integrity of the family.

Understanding the family as a system is relevant in today's health care environment as the family is an essential part of the health care team. Families have a profound influence on ill family members, as advisors, caretakers, supporters, and sometimes irritants. People who are very young or very old and those requiring assistance with self-management of chronic illnesses are particularly dependent on their families.

Support from the health care team during times of stress and crisis are necessary to provide information and empowerment to successfully adapt. Both resources and supports are essential for family empowerment (Trivette et al., 2010). Resources and supports include beliefs, past experiences, help-giving and -receiving practices, strengths, and capabilities; they are pieces of information that help explain person and family responses to health disruptions.

Conducting a family assessment is essential "to (1) assure that the needs of the family are met, (2) uncover any gaps in the family plan of action, (3) offer multiple supports and resources to the family" (Kaakinen et al., 2010, p. 104).

Family Composition

There is significant diversity in the composition of families, family beliefs and values, how they communicate with one another, ethnic heritage, life experiences, commitment to individual family members, and connections with the community. Families today are much more complex than in past generations. Box 13.1 identifies different types of family compositions. (Fig. 13.1).

Single-parent families must accomplish the same developmental tasks as two-parent families, but in many cases they do it without the support of the other partner or sufficient financial resources. Blended families have a different life experience from those in intact families because their family structure is often more complex. Children may be members of more than one family unit, linked biologically, physically, and emotionally to people who may or may not be a part of their daily lives. Parents, step- or half-brothers and sisters, two or more sets of grandparents, and multiple aunts and uncles may make up a blended family (Kaakinen et al., 2010, p. 135). The child may spend extended periods in separate households, each with a full set of family expectations that may or may not be similar. Initially, the parents in blended families may cohabitate, making for a sense of uncertainty for all involved (Jensen & Schafer, 2013). Blended families can offer a rich experience for everyone concerned, but they are more complex because of multiple connections. Table 13.1 displays some of the differences between biological and blended families. Issues for blended families include discipline, money, use of time, birth of an infant, death of a stepparent, inclusion at graduation, and marriage and health care decisions.

BOX 13.1   Types of Family Composition

- Nuclear family: a father and mother, with one or more children, living together as a single family unit
- Extended family: nuclear family unit's combination of second- and third-generation members, related by blood or marriage but not living together
- Three-generational family: any combination of first-, second-, and third-generation members living within a household
- Dyad family: husband and wife or other couple, living alone without children
- Single-parent family: divorced, never married, separated, or widowed adult and at least one child; most single-parent families are headed by women
- Stepfamily: family in which one or both spouses are divorced or widowed, with one or more children from a previous marriage who may not live with the newly reconstituted family
- Blended or reconstituted family: a combination of two families, with children from one or both families and sometimes children of the newly married couple
- Common law family: an unmarried couple living together, with or without children
- No kin: a group of at least two people sharing a nonsexual relationship and exchanging support, who have no legal, blood, or strong emotional ties to each other
- Polygamous family: one man (or woman) with several spouses
- Same-sex family: a same-sex couple living together, with or without children
- Commune: groups of individuals that may or may not be related, living together and sharing resources
- Group marriage: all individuals are "married" to one another and are considered parents of all the children

---

Theoretical Frameworks

Theoretical frameworks are used to provide a means for understanding certain processes and relationships between and among essential concepts. Numerous theoretical frameworks exist that can be used to understand family composition. Ludwig von Bertalanffy's (1968) general systems theory provides a conceptual foundation for family system models (Barker, 1998). Having a systems perspective allows one to examine the interdependence among all parts of the system to see how they support the system as a functional whole. Systems thinking maintains that the whole is greater than the sum of its parts, with each part reciprocally influencing its function. If one part of the system changes or fails, it affects the functioning of the whole. A clock is a useful metaphor. It displays time correctly,

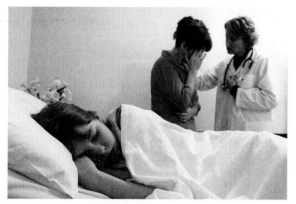

Fig. 13.1 Providing frequent updates and emotional support for family members is an important part of person-centred care. Copyright © Hemera Technologies/AbleStock.com/Thinkstock.

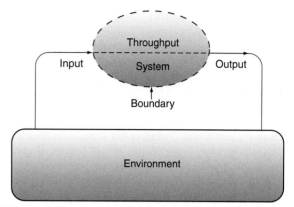

Fig. 13.2 Systems Model: Interaction With the Environment

the system of changes needed to achieve effective outputs. Fig. 13.2 identifies the relational components of a human system's interaction with the environment, using von Bertalanffy's model.

Systems theory can be applied to the human system. Individuals take in food, liquids, and oxygen to nourish the body (inputs). Within the body, a transformational process occurs through enzymes and metabolic processes (throughputs), so the body can use the inputs. This interactional process results in the human organism's growth, health, and capacity to interact with the external environment (outputs). Non-usable outputs excreted from the body include urine, feces, sweat, and carbon dioxide. A person's skin represents an important boundary between the environment and the human system.

Family systems have boundaries that regulate information coming into and leaving the family system. Family systems theory describes how families strive for harmony and balance (homeostasis), how the family is able to maintain its continuity despite challenges, (morphostasis), and how the family is able to change and grow over time in response to challenges (morphogenesis). Feedback loops describe the patterns of interaction that facilitate movement toward morphogenesis or morphostasis. These feedback loops impact goal setting in behavioural systems. The systems principle of equifinality describes how the same outcome or end state can be reached through different pathways. This principle helps explain why some individuals at high risk for poor outcomes do not develop maladaptive behaviours (Children's Services, Alberta Government, 2019).

Hierarchy is the term used to describe the complex layers of smaller systems that exist within a system. Communication can also be thought of as a complex system in which the message or output must be interpreted within an appropriate context.

TABLE 13.1 **Comparing Differences Between Biological and Blended Families**	
Biological Families	**Blended Families**
Family is created without loss.	Family is born of loss.
There are shared family traditions.	There are two sets of family traditions.
One set of family rules evolves.	Family rules are varied and complicated.
Children arrive one at a time.	Instant parenthood of children at different ages occurs.
Biological parents live together.	Biological parents live apart.

but only if all parts work together. If any part of the clock breaks down, the clock no longer tells accurate time.

A system interacts with other systems in the environment. An interactional process occurs when inputs are introduced into the system in the form of information, energy, and resources. Within each system, the information is processed internally as the system actively processes and interprets its meaning. The transformation process of raw data into desired outputs is referred to as *throughput*. The *output* refers to the result or product that leaves the system. Each system is separated from its environment by boundaries that control the exchange of information, energy, and resources into and out of the system. Evaluations of the output and feedback loops from the environment inform

Bowen's Systems Theory

Murray Bowen's (1978) family systems theory conceptualizes the family as an interactive emotional unit. He believed that family members assume reciprocal family roles, develop automatic communication patterns, and react to one another in predictable, connected ways, particularly when family anxiety is high. Once anxiety heightens within the system, an emotional process gets activated (Nichols & Schwartz, 2009), and dysfunctional communication patterns can emerge. For example, if one person is overly responsible, another family member may become less likely to assume normal responsibility. Until one family member is willing to challenge the dysfunction of an emotional system by refusing to play their reactive part, the negative emotional energy fueling a family's dysfunctional communication pattern persists.

Bowen developed eight interlocking concepts to explain his theoretical construct of the family system (Bowen Center for the Study of the Family, 2013).

- **Self-differentiation** refers to a person's capacity to define themselves within the family system as an individual having legitimate needs and wants. It requires making "I" statements based on rational thinking rather than emotional reactivity. Self-differentiation takes into consideration the views of others but is not dominated by them. Poorly differentiated people are so dependent on the approval of others that they discount their own needs (Hill et al., 2011). Individuals with a well-differentiated sense of self exhibit a balanced, realistic dependence on others and can accept conflict and criticism without an excessive emotional reaction. Self-differentiation serves as the fundamental means of reducing chronic anxiety within the family system and enhancing effective problem solving. Self-differentiation emphasizes thinking rather than feeling in communication.
- **Multigenerational transmission** refers to the emotional transmission of behavioural patterns, roles, and communication response styles from generation to generation. It explains why family patterns tend to repeat behaviours in marriages, child rearing, choice of occupation, and emotional responses across generations, without understanding why it happens.
- **Nuclear family emotional system** refers to the way family members relate to one another within their immediate family when stressed. Family anxiety shows up in one of four patterns: (1) dysfunction in one spouse, (2) marital conflict, (3) dysfunctional symptoms in one or more of the children, or (4) emotional distancing.
- **Triangles** refer to a defensive way of reducing, neutralizing, or defusing heightened anxiety between two family members by drawing a third person or object into the relationship (MacKay, 2012). If the original triangle fails to contain or stabilize the anxiety, it can expand into a series of "interlocking" triangles, for example, into school issues or an extramarital affair.
- **Family projection process** refers to an unconscious casting of unresolved anxiety in the family on a particular family member, usually a child. The projection can be positive or negative, and it can become a self-fulfilling prophecy as the child incorporates the anxiety of the parent as part of his or her self-identity.
- *Emotional cutoff* refers to a person's withdrawal from other family members as a means of avoiding family issues that create anxiety. Emotional cutoffs range from total avoidance to remaining in physical contact, but in a superficial manner. All people have unresolved emotional attachments, but the extent varies widely among individuals.
- **Societal emotional process** refers to parallels that Bowen found between the family system and the emotional system operating at the institutional level in society. As anxiety grows within a society, many of the same polarizations, lack of self-differentiation, and emotion-based thinking dominate behaviour and system outcomes.

Family Legacies

Family legacies have a powerful influence on family relationships and in shaping parenting practices (Fig. 13.3). Families of one generation tend to function in a similar manner to the previous generation. Knowledge of family relationships helps explain behaviours that would not be clear without having a family context. Helping families gain clarity about how their family heritage can be used as an asset in health care and what areas need work strengthens the potential for effective family-centred care.

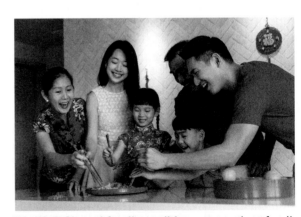

Fig. 13.3 Shared family traditions strengthen family bonds

Many theoretical frameworks exist that support understanding of family structure and function. Other family theories fall into three groupings related to structure, development, and resiliency theories. Table 13.2 identifies major characteristics of family theories. Other family-related theoretical frameworks based on the social sciences, family therapy, and nursing also exist (Kaakinen et al., 2010).

The challenge for health care providers is to be able to apply a theoretical understanding of family structure and function to an actual person-care situation (Wright & Leahey, 2013). In many settings, nurses tend to focus care on the individual. This is important, but the nurse must also understand that the family is impacted by even minor health deviations of a family member. Thus, understanding individuals as members of families from a theoretical perspective is necessary.

APPLICATIONS

Family-Centred Care

Family-centred care allows health care providers to have a uniform understanding of the person and family's knowledge, preferences, and values as the basis for shared decision making. This provides consistent information to all involved in the person's care and allows the family to identify any barriers that might arise with the care plan.

>> **DEVELOPING AN EVIDENCE-INFORMED PRACTICE**

This article describes the perceptions of cardiac health care providers (n = 368) concerning family presence (FP) during cardiopulmonary resuscitation (CPR).

A survey was conducted to explore the attitudes and beliefs of cardiac health care providers toward family presence during CPR, within five Edmonton and surrounding area hospitals. The response rate was 46%, with the greatest response from nurses and physicians. Of the respondents, 44.3% believed that family should have the option to be present during CPR, and 40.9% believed that family should be allowed at the bedside. Less than half of the respondents had experience with FP during CPR. The barriers identified toward FP were lack of support for families, belief that the experience would be too traumatic for families, belief that families would not understand the procedures, fear of families physically interfering with procedures, concern that FP would increase stress levels among staff, and tradition and politics that excludes FP. The researchers concluded that, despite that less than half of respondents supported FP, the majority endorsed development of policies and procedures to overcome barriers to FP during CPR (Jensen & Kosowan, 2011).

TABLE 13.2 Key Features of Other Family Theories

Theory	Key Elements	References
Structural family theory	Emphasizes how the family unit is structured (subsystems, hierarchies, and boundaries). Function is assessed in relation to instrumental functioning (completing tasks during times of health and illness) and expressive functioning (communication patterns, problem solving, and power structures). Families strive to maintain homeostasis.	Fivaz-Depeursinge et al., 2009; Minuchin, 1974
Developmental family theory	Eight specific developmental tasks are outlined, starting with a childless couple and ending with retirement. Traits that demonstrate successful family development are identified.	Antle et al., 2012; Duvall, 1958
Family stress theory	Family response to, and coping with, stressful events are explained. Factors associated with positive resolution include family system resources, flexibility, and problem-solving skills.	Frain et al., 2008; Lavee, 2013

Antle, B. F., Christensen, D. N., van Zyl, M. A. et al. (2012). The impact of the Solution Based Casework (SBC) practice model on federal outcomes in public child welfare. *Child Abuse & Neglect 36*(4), 342–353; Duvall, E. (1958). *Marriage and family development*. JB Lippincott; Fivaz-Depeursinge, E., Lopes, F., Python, M. et al. (2009). Coparenting and toddler's interactive styles in family coalitions. *Family Process 48*(4), 500–516; Frain, M., Berven, N., Chan, F. et al. (2008). Family resiliency, uncertainty, optimism, and the quality of life of individuals with HIV/AIDS. *Rehabilitation Counseling Bulletin, 52*(1), 16–27; Lavee, Y. (2013). Stress processes in families and couples. In G. W. Peterson, K. R. Bush (Eds). *Handbook of marriage and the family* (pp. 159–176). Springer; Minuchin, S. (1974). *Families and family therapy*. Harvard University Press.

Health events of one family member have the potential to affect the whole family. Trotter and Martin (2007) note, "Families share genetic susceptibilities, environments, and behaviors, all of which interact to cause different levels of health and disease" (p. 561). They are instrumental in helping persons appreciate the need for diagnosis and treatment and in encouraging the person to seek treatment. Family members are involved in a person's health care decisions, ranging from treatment options to critical decisions about end-of-life care. Families play a pivotal **advocacy** role in treatment by monitoring and insisting on quality care for a family member.

Nurses in family-centred care are to do the following:

- Understand the impact of a medical crisis on family functioning, dynamics, and health.
- Appreciate and respond empathetically to the emotional intensity of the experience for the family
- Determine the appropriate level of family involvement in holistic care of the person, based on an understanding of fundamental family system concepts.

Assessment

As defined at the beginning of this chapter, nurses should consider that "a family is who they say they are" (Wright & Leahey, 2013, p. 55). Regardless of how it occurs, any health disruption becomes a family event. For immediate health care purposes, *family* is defined as the significant people in the person's environment who are capable and willing to provide family-type support. However, even when the family is not directly involved in the family member's care, they will have feelings and opinions about the situation. Nonsupportive family responses have been associated with negative person outcomes, while supportive, positive family responses are associated with positive person outcomes (Rosland et al., 2012). Simulation Exercise 13.1 allows you to analyze positive and negative family responses. Box 13.2 provides examples of situations that could warrant family assessment and nursing intervention.

Assessment Tools

Initially, the nurse may not have the opportunity to complete a thorough family assessment. However, throughout the initial assessment and during ongoing nurse–person interactions, the nurse must be attentive to cues indicating potential family-related concerns. The nurse should take into consideration the anticipated health needs of the individual person upon discharge. For example, a 30-year-old person who had major reconstructive knee surgery and cannot bear weight on the affected leg for 4 weeks will require consistent personal assistance for a period of time. Family members are often called into action in such circumstances. However, if some type of family discord previously existed, the person may not feel comfortable requesting assistance from family members and may feel uncomfortable asking even close friends for assistance. In

---

BOX 13.2   Indicators for Family Assessment

- Initial diagnosis of a serious physical or psychiatric illness or injury in a family member
- Family involvement and understanding needed to support recovery of the person
- Deterioration in a family member's condition
- Illness in a child, adolescent, or adult who is cognitively impaired
- A child, adolescent, or adult child having an adverse response to a parent's illness
- Discharge from a health care facility to the home or an extended-care facility
- Death of a family member
- Health problem defined by family as a family issue
- Indication of threat to relationship (abuse), neglect, or anticipated loss of family member

---

SIMULATION EXERCISE 13.1   Positive and Negative Family Interactions

Purpose

To examine the effects of functional versus dysfunctional communication

Procedure

Answer the following questions in a brief essay:

1. Recall a situation in dealing with a person's family that you felt was a positive experience? What characteristics of that interaction made you feel this way?
2. Recall a situation in dealing with a person's family that you felt was a negative experience? What

characteristics of that interaction made you feel this way?

Discussion

Compare experiences, both positive and negative. What did you see as the most striking differences? In what ways were your responses similar to or dissimilar from those of your peers? What do you see as the implications of this exercise for enhancing family communication in your nursing practice?

this case, the nurse acts as intermediary to facilitate conversations among potential caregivers.

Other situations (see Box 13.2) require a more in-depth assessment of family structure and function. Wright and Leahey's (2013) 15-minute interview, consisting of the genogram, ecomap, therapeutic questions, and commendations provides a comprehensive look at family relationships. Assessment tools, such as the genogram, ecomap, and family time lines are used to track family patterns. The structured format of these tools focuses on getting relational data quickly and can sensitize clinicians to systemic family issues that affect patterns of health and illness.

Genograms

A **genogram** is defined as a diagram that uses a standardized set of connections to graphically record basic information about family members and their relationships over three generations. Genograms can be updated or revised as new information emerges. A genogram can be used to identify patterns of inheritable medical conditions, but when used as part of a family psychosocial assessment, it provides information about family relationships and the personal perspective of the individual providing the information (Chrzastowski, 2011). Such information may be used to guide in-depth family assessment and future interventions.

There are three parts to genogram construction: mapping the family structure, recording family information, and describing the nature of family relationships. Fig. 13.4 identifies the symbols used to map family structure, with different symbols representing pregnancies, miscarriages, marriages, deaths, and other family events. Male family members are noted with a square and females with a circle. The oldest sibling is placed on the left, with younger siblings following from left to right, in order of birth. In the case of multiple marriages, the earliest is placed on the left and the most recent on the right. Lines drawn between significant family members identify the strength of relational patterns that are overly close, close, distant, cut off, or conflicted. An example of a family genogram is presented in Fig. 13.5.

The genogram explores the basic dynamics of a multigenerational family. Its multigenerational format, which traces family structure and relationships through three generations, is based on the assumption that family relationship patterns are systemic, repetitive, and adaptive. Data about ages, birth and death dates, miscarriages, relevant illnesses, immigration, geographical location of current members, occupations and employment status, educational levels, patterns of family members entering or leaving the family unit, religious affiliation or change, and military service are written near the symbols for each person. The recorded information about family members allows families and health providers to simultaneously analyze complex family interaction patterns in a supportive environment. The impact of multiple generations on family relationships is more readily visible.

The genogram offers much more than a simple diagram of family relationship. Formal and informal learning about appropriate social behaviours and roles takes place within the family of origin. People learn role behaviours and responsibilities expected in different life stages experientially, by way of role modelling and through direct instruction. Simulation Exercise 13.2 provides practice with developing a family genogram.

Ecomaps

An ecomap visually illustrates relationships between family **members** and the external environment (Kaakinen et al., 2010). Beginning with an individual family unit or person, the diagram extends to include significant social and community-based systems with which they have a relationship. The diagram provides a quick visual of friends and community resource utilization. Adding the ecomap is an important dimension of family assessment, providing awareness of community supports that could be or are not being used to assist families. Ecomaps can point out resource deficiencies and conflicts in support services that can be corrected.

An ecomap starts with an inner circle representing the family unit, labelled with relevant family names. Smaller circles outside the family circle represent significant people, agencies, and social institutions with whom the family interacts on a regular basis. Examples include school, work, places of worship, neighbourhood friends, recreation activities, health care facilities or home care, and extended family. Lines are drawn from the inner family circle to outer circles indicating the strength of the contact and relationship. Straight lines indicate relationship, with additional lines used to indicate the strength of the relationship. Dotted lines suggest tenuous relationships. Stressful relationships are represented with slashes placed through the relationship line. Directional arrows indicate the flow of the relational energy. Fig. 13.6 shows an example of an ecomap. Simulation Exercise 13.3 provides an opportunity to construct an ecomap.

Family Time Lines

Time lines offer a visual diagram that captures significant family stressors, life events, health, and developmental patterns throughout the life cycle. Family history and patterns developed through multigenerational transmission are represented as vertical lines. Horizontal lines indicate the timing of life events occurring over the current life span. These include such milestones as marriages, graduations, and unexpected life events, such as disasters, war, illness, death of a person or pet, moves, births, and so forth (Fig. 13.7). Time lines are useful in

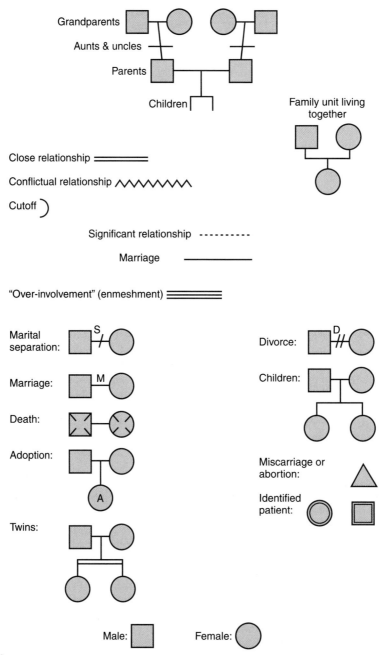

Fig. 13.4 Symbols for a genogram

looking at how the family history, developmental stage, and concurrent life events might interact with the current health concern. Fig. 13.6 is an Ecomap: A graphical representation that illustrates the shared relationships between family members and the external environment.

By completing a family assessment, the nurse is able to develop a personalized plan of care for both the person and the family. The findings of a family assessment should be documented for use by other members of the health care team and to avoid redundant collection of data.

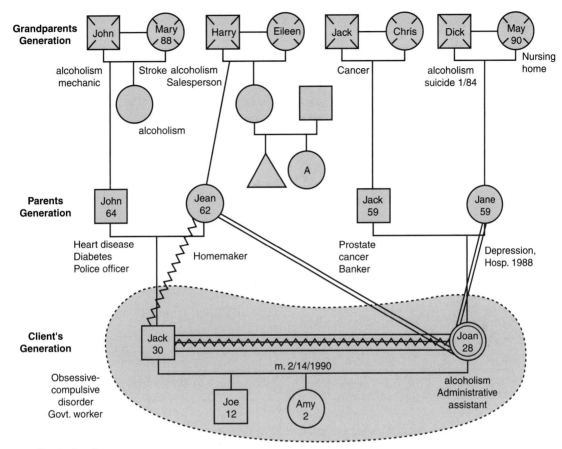

Fig. 13.5 Basic family genogram

SIMULATION EXERCISE 13.2 Family Genograms

Purpose
To practise creating a family genogram

Procedure
Students break into pairs and interview one another to gain information to develop a family genogram. The genogram should include demographic information, occurrence of illness or death, and relationship patterns for three generations. Use the symbols for diagramming in Fig. 13.2 to create a visual picture of the family information. Validate your genogram for accuracy with your informant.

Discussion
Each person displays the genogram they developed and discusses the process of obtaining information. Discuss strategies for obtaining information expediently yet sensitively and tactfully. Consider additional questions that could be used to gather additional information. Were you able to identify patterns that could be helpful in assisting individuals to cope with a health crisis? Discuss how genograms can be used by a nurse in a clinical setting.

Applying a Family-Centred Framework
Orienting the Family

The nurse–family relationship depends on reciprocal interactions between nurses and family members in which both are equal partners. Nurses should begin offering information to the family as soon as the person is admitted to the hospital or service agency. Orientation to the facility, location of the cafeteria and bathrooms, parking options, nearby lodging, and access to the hospitalist

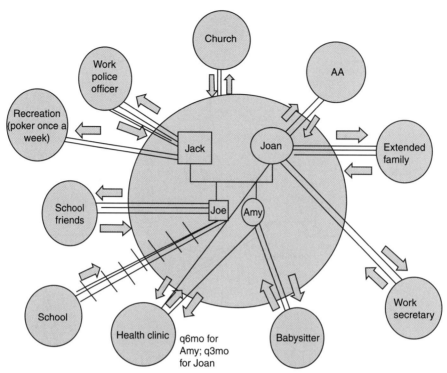

Fig. 13.6 Example of an ecomap. From Rempel, G. R., Neufeld, A., & Kushner, K. E. (2007). Interactive use of genograms and ecomaps in family caregiving research. *Journal of Family Nursing, 13*(4), 403–419.

SIMULATION EXERCISE 13.3   Family Ecomaps

Note: Simulation Exercises 13.3 and 13.4 can be carried out during the same interview.

Purpose
To practise creating a family ecomap

Procedure
Using the interview process, students break into pairs and interview one another to gain information to develop a family ecomap. The ecomap should include information about resources and stressors in the larger community system, such as school, religious institutions, health agencies, and interaction with extended family and friends, for each student's family.

Discussion
Each person displays their ecomap and discusses the process of obtaining information. Discuss strategies for obtaining information expediently yet sensitively and tactfully. Explain how additional information obtained from an ecomap improves understanding of a family. Analyze the ecomap for areas that could be problematic if the informant were faced with a serious health issue. Describe how ecomaps can be used by a nurse in a clinical setting.

---

or physician are important points to include in early family interactions.

The initial family encounter sets the tone for the relationship. How nurses interact with each family member may be as important as what they choose to say. Begin with formal introductions and explain the purpose of gathering assessment data. Even this early in the relationship,

you should listen carefully for family expectations and general **anxiety** or expressed concerns about the person, which may be revealed more through behaviour than through words.

When interacting with families, the nurse must ensure the person's right to privacy. With the implementation of the *Personal Information Protection and Electronic*

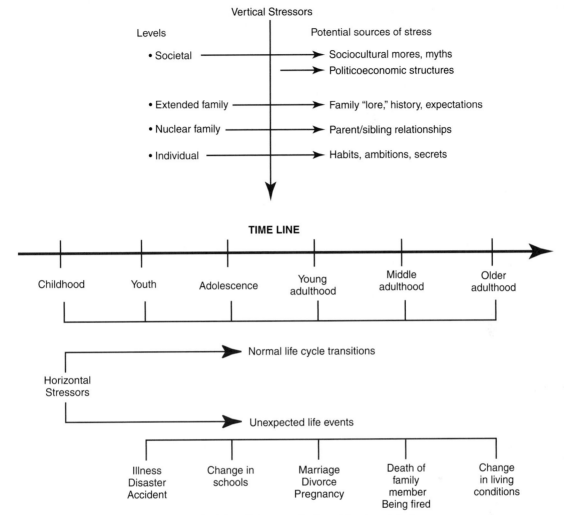

Fig. 13.7 Time line assessment example, identifying vertical and horizontal stressors

Documents Act (PIPEDA) (S.C. 2000, c.5), family members may receive information regarding person status only with the permission of either the person or their designee (Minister of Justice, 2019). This means that as a nurse, you cannot give out information regarding the health status of people in your care, either over the phone or in person, without the person's consent. Most facilities have developed strategies to ensure that staff members do not disclose unauthorized information. For example, some facilities have adopted the use of a "code word" that is established upon admission. The code word is shared with only those family members who the person wishes to receive information (McCullough & Schell-Chaple, 2013). If the person inquiring about the person does not know the code word, then the nurse should politely inform the individual that for privacy reasons information cannot be provided.

Gathering Assessment Data

Determining the association or relationship of the family member to the person is an initial step nurses can take in establishing a relationship. You might say, "I would like to hear what you think is the impact of your child's illness on the entire family." This statement guides your assessment but also reminds the family that each family member is of concern to the health care team (Health Council of Canada, 2009). Box 13.3 illustrates a framework for a family assessment with a person entering cardiac rehabilitation. Family participation in the assessment process enhances the

BOX 13.3   Family Assessment for Person Entering Cardiac Rehabilitation

Coping and Stress
- Who lives with you? _____
- How do you handle stress? _____
- Have you had any recent changes in your life (e.g., job change, move, change in marital status, loss)? _____
- On whom do you rely for emotional support? _____
- Who relies on you for emotional support? _____
- How does your illness affect your family members or significant others? _____
- Are there any health concerns about other family members? _____
- If so, how does this affect you? _____

Communication and Decision Making
- How would you describe the communication pattern in your family? _____
- How does your family address issues and concerns? _____
- Can you identify strengths and weaknesses within your family? _____
- Are family members supportive of each other? _____
- How are decisions made that affect the entire family? _____
- How are decisions implemented? _____

Role
- What is your role in the family? _____
- Can you describe the roles of other family members? _____

Value Beliefs
- What is your ethnic or cultural background? _____
- What is your religious background? _____
- Are there any particular cultural or religious healing practices in which you participate? _____

Leisure Activities
- Do you participate in any organized social activities? _____
- In what leisure activities do you participate? _____
- Do you anticipate any difficulty with continuing these activities? _____
- If so, how will you make the appropriate adjustments? _____
- Do you have a regular exercise regimen? _____

Environmental Characteristics
- Do you live in a rural, suburban, or urban area? _____
- What type of dwelling do you live in? _____
- Are there stairs in your home? _____
- Where is the bathroom? _____
- Are the facilities adequate to meet your needs? _____
- If not, what adjustments will be needed? _____
- How do you plan to make those adjustments? _____
- Are there any community services provided to you at home? (explain) _____
- Are there community resources available in your area? _____
- Do you have any other concerns at this time? _____
- Is there anything that we have omitted? _____
- Signature _____ (must be completed by R a health professional) Date/Time

Developed by Conrad, J., University of Maryland School of Nursing, 1993.

SIMULATION EXERCISE 13.4 Family Coping Strategies

Purpose

To broaden awareness of coping strategies among families

Procedure

Each student recalls a time when their family experienced a significant health crisis and how they coped. (Alternative strategy: Pick a health crisis you observed with a family in clinical practice.) Respond to the following questions:

1. Did the crisis cause a readjustment in roles?

2. Did the crisis create tension and conflict, or did it catalyze members into turning to one another for support? Look at the behaviour of individual members.

3. What would have helped your family in this crisis? Write a descriptive summary about this experience.

Discussion

Each student shares their experience. Discuss the differences in how families respond to crisis. Compile a list of coping strategies and helpful interventions on the board. Discuss the nurse's role in support of the family.

---

therapeutic relationship and completeness of the data. It is important to inquire about the family's cultural identity, rituals, values, level of family involvement, decision making, spiritual beliefs, and traditional behaviours as they relate to the health care of the person (Health Council of Canada, 2009).

Knowledge of a family's past medical experiences, concurrent family stressors, and family expectations for treatment are essential pieces of family assessment data. Suggested questions include the following:

- How does the family view the current health crisis?
- What is each family member's most immediate concern?
- Has anyone else in the family experienced a similar problem?
- Are there any other recent changes or sources of stress in the family that make the current situation worse (pileup of demands)?
- How has the family handled the problem to date?
- Can you tell me what you expect from the health care team?
- As you close the session, ask, "Is there anything else I should know about your family and this experience?"

Simulation Exercise 13.4 looks at assessment of family coping strengths.

Problem Identification

Based on assessment data (initial and ongoing), the nurse identifies whether problems related to family communication and functioning exist. Even if no problem is identified, the nurse must be alert for cues that indicate potential problems in family communication and function. Some problems related to family function may require referral to a social worker, family therapist, or other member of the health care team. In other instances, it may be appropriate for the nurse to provide assistance to the family. Health-related communication issues can involve unexpressed fears or anger management of uncertainty, or finding common ground for shared decision making.

Planning

The more the family can be involved in the planning process, the greater is the likelihood of successful adaptation (Kaakinen et al., 2010). The development of appropriate nursing actions should be based on mutually established goals. For the bedside nurse, these goals are often short term, focusing on improving awareness of areas to improve communication (see the following subsection regarding interventive questioning). Resources are available to help ensure family engagement.

Health care practitioners listen to and honour person and family perspectives and choices. Person and family knowledge, values and beliefs, and cultural backgrounds are incorporated into the planning and delivery of care. They do this in the following ways:

- Information sharing:

  Health care practitioners communicate and share complete and unbiased information with persons and families in ways that are affirming and useful. Persons and families receive timely, complete, and accurate information in order to effectively participate in care and decision making.

- Participation:

  Persons and families are encouraged and supported in participating in care and decision making at the level they choose.

- Collaboration:

  Persons, families, health care practitioners, and health care leaders collaborate in policy and program developments, implementation, and evaluation; in facility design; and in professional education, as well as in the delivery of care (Institute for Patient- and Family-Centered Care, n.d.).

The preceding resources provide overall guidelines for person- and family-centred care. As part of the overall plan of care, the nurse makes the most of communication skills to provide care to persons and families.

Interventive Questioning

Wright and Leahey (2009) identify questioning as a nursing intervention that nurses can use with families to identify family strengths; help family members sort out their personal fears, concerns, and challenges in health care situations; and provide a vehicle for exploring alternative options. Family-centred interventions relate to the following: "(1) providing direct care, (2) removing barriers to needed services, and (3) improving the capacity of the family to act on its own behalf and assume responsibility" (Kaakinen et al., 2010, p. 117).

Interventive questioning can be either linear or circular. Linear questions facilitate understanding of a situation by both the nurse and family members. **Circular questions** lead to introspection, greater depth of understanding, and behavioural change. They focus on family interrelationships and the effect that a serious health alteration has on individual family members and the equilibrium of the family system. Examples of therapeutic questions are found in Box 13.4. Both linear and circular questioning should be used as part of effective nursing care. The nurse uses information the family provides as the basis for additional questions.

The following case example demonstrates the use of circular questioning when the nurse asks a family, "What has been your biggest challenge in caring for your mother at home?"

In this example, each family member's concern is related but different. The therapeutic circular question opens a

---

BOX 13.4   Examples of Therapeutic Questions

- Who in the family is best at encouraging your family member to comply with her diet?
- What information do you still need to understand the prognosis of your disease? Who else would benefit from this information?
- Who is suffering the most?
- What do you feel when you see your family member in pain?
- If there was one question you could have answered now, what would it be?
- How can we best help you and your family?
- If your family member's treatment does not go well, who will be most affected?

Adapted from Wright, L. M., & Leahey, M. (2009). *Nurses and families: A guide to family assessment and intervention* (5th ed.). F. A. Davis.

---

discussion about each person's anxiety. As family members hear the concerns of other family members and as they hear themselves respond, their perspective broadens. The resulting conversation forms the basis for developing strategies that are mutually acceptable to all family members.

Case Example

Daughter: My biggest challenge has been finding a balance between caring for my mother and also caring for my children and husband. I've also had to learn a lot about the professional and support resources that are available in the community.

Son-in-law: For me, the biggest challenge has been convincing my wife that I can take over for a while so she can get some rest. I worry that she'll become exhausted.

Mother: I appreciate all the help they give me. My biggest challenge is to continue to do as much as possible for myself so I don't become too much of a burden on them. Sometimes I wonder about moving to a palliative care setting or a hospice (Leahey & Harper-Jaques, 1996).

Meaningful involvement in a person's care not only differs from family to family, it differs among individual family members (Health Council of Canada, 2009). Individual family members have different perspectives. Hearing each family member's perspective helps the family and nurse develop a unified understanding of significant treatment goals and implications for family involvement.

Although treatment plans should be tailored around personal goals for the person, acknowledging family needs, values, and priorities enhances compliance, especially if they are different from those of the person. Shared decision making and the development of realistic, achievable goals make it easier for everyone concerned to accomplish them with a sense of ownership and self-efficacy about the process. Taking small, achievable steps is preferred to attempting giant steps that misjudge what the family can realistically do. Simulation Exercise 13.5 provides practice with developing a family nursing care plan.

Implementation

Nurses can only offer interventions; it is up to the family to accept them (Wright & Leahey, 2013). Suggested nursing actions to promote positive change in family functioning include the following:

- Encouraging the telling of illness narratives
- Commending family and individual strengths
- Offering information and opinions
- Validating or normalizing emotional responses

SIMULATION EXERCISE 13.5 Developing a Family Nursing Care Plan

Purpose

To practise skills needed with difficult family patterns

Procedure

Read the case study, and think of how you could interact appropriately with this family.

Mr. Monroe, age 43 years, was chairing a meeting of his large, successful manufacturing corporation when he developed shortness of breath, dizziness, and a crushing, viselike pain in his chest. An ambulance was called, and he was taken to the hospital. Subsequently, he was admitted to the coronary care unit, with a diagnosis of an impending myocardial infarction (MI).

Mr. Monroe is married with three children: Steve, age 14; Sean, age 12; and Lisa, age 10. He is the president and majority stockholder of his company. He has no history of cardiovascular problems, although his father died at the age of 38 of a massive coronary occlusion. His oldest brother died at the age of 42 from the same condition, and his other brother, still living, had a severe disability after suffering two heart attacks, one at the age of 44 and the other at 47.

Mr. Monroe is tall, slim, suntanned, and very athletic. He swims daily; jogs every morning for 30 minutes; plays golf regularly; and is an avid sailor, having participated in every yacht regatta and usually winning. He is very health-conscious and has had annual physical checkups. He watches his diet and quit smoking to avoid possible damage to his heart. He has been determined to avoid dying young or becoming disabled like his brother.

When he was admitted to the coronary care unit, he was conscious. Although in a great deal of pain, he seemed determined to control his own fate. While in the unit, he acted in an exceedingly difficult way, a trial to the nursing staff and his physician. He constantly watched and listened to everything going on around him and demanded complete explanations about any procedure,

equipment, or medication he received. He would sleep in brief naps and only when he was totally exhausted. Despite his obvious tension and anxiety, his condition stabilized. The damage to his heart was considered minimal, and his prognosis was good. As the pain diminished, he began asking when he could go home and when he could go back to work. He insisted on being moved to a private room so that he could conduct some of his business by telephone.

When Mrs. Monroe visited, she approached the nursing staff with questions regarding Mr. Monroe's condition, usually asking the same question several times in different ways. She also asked why she was not being "told everything."

Interactions between Mr. Monroe and Mrs. Monroe were noted by the staff as Mr. Monroe telling Mrs. Monroe everything she needed to do. Little intimate contact was noted.

Mr. Monroe denied having any anxiety or concerns about his condition, although his behaviour contradicted his denial. Mrs. Monroe would agree with her husband's assessment when questioned in his company.

Discussion

1. What questions would you ask Mr. Monroe and his family to obtain data regarding their adaptation to crisis?
2. What family nursing diagnosis would apply with this case study?
3. What nursing interventions are appropriate to interact with Mr. Monroe and his family?
4. What other members of the health care team should be involved with this family situation?
5. How would you plan to transmit information to the family?
6. What outcomes and measures would you use to determine success or failure of the nursing care plan?

Developed by Conrad, J. (1993). University of Maryland School of Nursing, Baltimore, MD.

- Encouraging family support
- Supporting family members as caregivers
- Encouraging respite

Encouraging Family Narratives

Families need to tell their story about the experience of their loved one's illness or injury; this may be quite different from how the person is experiencing it. The differences can lead to a more complete understanding. Such sharing can help build mutual support and empathy (Novak et al.,

2020). Nurses play an important role in helping families understand, negotiate, and reconcile differences in perceptions without losing face.

Case Example

Frances has a diagnosis of breast cancer. When she sees her oncologist, Frances reports that she is feeling fine, eating, and able to function in much the same way as before receiving chemotherapy.

Her husband's perception differs. He reports that her appetite has declined such that she eats only a few spoonfuls of food and she spends much of the day in bed. What Frances is reporting is true. When she is up, she enjoys doing what she did previously, although at a slower pace, and she does eat at every meal. Frances is communicating her need to feel normal, which is important to support. What her husband adds is also true. Her husband's input allows Frances to receive the treatment she needs to stimulate her appetite and give her more energy.

Incorporating Family Strengths

Otto (1963) introduced the concept of *family strengths* as potential and actual resources that families can use to make their lives more satisfying and fulfilling when health care changes are required, and they usually are with persons suffering from serious illness or injury. Working through family strengths rather than focusing on deficits is useful. Viewing the family as having strengths to cope with a problem rather than being a problem is a healing strategy. The intent is not that the family comes away from a stressful event or period without blemish but instead that the existing skills and coping strategies are used in a healthy manner. While each family's experience with illness is unique, commonalities exist. The nurse should share strategies that families in similar situations have found effective.

Giving Commendations

Commendations are part of having positive and caring interactions between nurses and the people they care for (Porr, 2013). Commendations are particularly effective when the family seems dispirited or confused about an illness or accident. More than a simple compliment, commendations should reflect patterns of behaviour observed in the family unit over time. Wright and Leahey (2013) differentiate between a commendation ("Your family is showing much courage in living with your wife's cancer for 5 years.") and a compliment ("Your son is so gentle despite feeling so ill.") (p. 270). They suggest giving at least one commendation per interview. There may be situations that seem extremely dire, but by identifying even one positive factor, a family may feel empowered to push through the difficult situation. Simulation Exercise 13.6 provides practice with giving commendations.

Informational Support

Helping a family become aware of information from the environment and how to access it empowers families. By showing interest in the coping strategies that have and have not worked, the nurse can help the family recognize progress in their ability to cope with a difficult situation.

You can offer family members support related to talking with extended family, children, and others about the person's illness. You can help them prepare questions for meeting with physicians and other health providers. Encouraging family members to write down key points to be addressed with other family members and physicians can be helpful. Written instructions should also be provided upon discharge.

The statement that discharge planning begins at admission is very true when it comes to providing families with information. The nurse should anticipate assistance that will

---

SIMULATION EXERCISE 13.6 Offering Commendations

Purpose

To practise using commendation skills

Procedure

Students work in groups of three. Each student develops a commendation about the two other students in the group. The commendation should reflect a personal strength that the reflecting student has observed over a period of time. Examples might include kindness, integrity, commitment, persistence, goal-directedness, tolerance, or patience. Write a brief paragraph about the trait or behaviour that you observe in this person. If you can, give some examples of why you have associated this particular characteristic with the person. Each student, in turn, should read their reflections about the other two participants, starting the conversation with good eye contact, the name of the receiving student, and a simple orienting statement (e.g., "Kelly, this is what I have observed in knowing you …").

Discussion

Class discussion should focus on the thought process of the students in developing particular commendations, the values they focused on, and any consideration they gave to the impact of the commendation on the other students. Students can also discuss the effect of hearing the commendations about themselves and what it stimulated in them. Complete the discussion by considering how commendations can be used with families and how they can be used to counteract family resistance to working together.

be needed upon discharge that will require family involvement. Because family members are not always available consistently, the nurse should plan family teaching sessions prior to the time of discharge to create an environment more conducive to learning (Kornburger et al., 2013). The use of the "teach-back" method can be used with families and individual persons. Review Chapter 16 regarding health teaching.

If the person is seriously ill and is receptive, the nurse should see this as an opportunity to provide information regarding end-of-life decision making. Decisions regarding end-of-life care are best carried out when families are not in a crisis mode. Thus, you can engage with families in discussions about the cultural, ethical, and physical implications of using or discontinuing life-support systems. This is nursing's special niche, as these conversations are rarely one-time events, and nurses can provide informal opportunities for discussing them during care provision. Refer to Chapter 22 for additional information regarding advance directives and end-of-life care planning.

Case Example

Hilda Remple lives on the third floor of a long-term care facility in Winnipeg and she contracted COVID-19. Unfortunately, she cannot be isolated, but fortunately, at this point she is not seriously ill. She is to have no visitors. Her daughter Agatha travels from Brandon, Manitoba, on a monthly basis to visit her mother. When she is denied visitation, she becomes extremely upset. She insists the staff move her mother to the first floor so she can at least look at her through the window. The staff state there are no rooms available on the first floor. Agatha gets permission to have security cameras installed in her mother's room so she can at least see and monitor her mother.

Meeting the Needs of Families With Critically Ill Persons

The admission to an intensive care unit (ICU) is a stressful and traumatic experience for family members, causing a disruption in their life and requiring continuous adjustments on their part as the person's condition changes. As it frequently occurs without warning, the person's family is overwhelmed by the circumstances and needs to find new coping mechanisms to deal with the situation (Koukouli et al., 2018). See Box 13.5 for information for family of people who are critically ill.

Proximity to the Person Who Is Critically Ill

When someone is in the ICU, the need to remain near the person is a priority for many family members. Although

---

BOX 13.5   Caring for Family Needs in the Intensive Care Unit

Information for Families of Critically Ill Persons

- Seeing your family member in the ICU is very distressing because of the technology, level of illness and unknown outcome.
- If you have questions, please ask them. The staff are there to help you.
- Sometimes, your family member must be moved to another hospital because they need a different kind of specialty care.
- Your family member may not be able to communicate with you. If that happens, just sit by their bedside and touch them.
- Talk to them, even if they may not be able to talk back to you.
- Bring in some personal belongings, such as their favourite music.
- As your family member improves, you might want to assist with caregiving, like brushing their teeth.
- Choose one main contact from your family for communication with the hospital staff.
- Keep a diary of what is happening every day. It will help you see improvements and provide a record for the family member.
- Be careful to prevent infection by washing your hands before you enter the ICU.
- Your family member may act out of character, like being agitated. The staff will explain what is happening.
- Take care of yourself. You may feel very alone and exhausted. Ask for support from others.

---

the family may appear to hover too closely, it is usually an attempt to rally around the person in critical trouble (Shorofi et al., 2016). Viewed from this perspective, nurses can be more empathetic. As the family develops more confidence in the genuine interest and competence of the staff, the hovering tends to lessen.

Visitation policies may need to be adjusted based on the availability of family members and the person's needs (Hart et al., 2013). Staff need to be aware that family members may have obligations that prevent visits at expected times of day. When families visit loved ones in the ICU, the nurse should acknowledge them and provide any updated information that is available.

Families can be a primary support to persons, but they usually need encouragement and concrete suggestions for maximal effect and satisfaction. Family members feel helpless to reverse the course of the person's condition and appreciate opportunities to help their loved one. Suggested actions that family members can take at the bedside include doing range-of-motion exercises, holding the person's hand, positioning pillows, and providing mouth care or ice chips. Talking with and reading to the person, even if the person is unresponsive, can be meaningful for both the family and person.

Helping families balance the need to be present with the person's needs to conserve energy and have some alone time to rest or regroup is important. Family members also need time apart from their loved one for the same reasons. Tactfully explaining the need of critically ill persons to have family presence without feeling pressure to interact can be supportive. Encouraging families to take respite breaks is equally important. Providing information regarding dining and lodging can facilitate periods of rest for family members.

At the same time, nurses need to be sensitive to and respect a family member's apprehension or emotional state about their critically ill family member. Individual family members may need the nurse's support in talking about difficult feelings. Nurses can role model communication with persons, using simple caring words and touch. Families are quick to discern the difference between nurses who are able to connect with a critically ill person in this way and those who are not (Shorofi et al., 2016).

Breaking Bad News to Families

The physician is the provider who most often delivers life-threatening critical information to persons and families. It is often the nurse at the bedside who ensures that all have an adequate understanding of the information that has been provided. Additionally, nurses often notify the person and family members of significant changes in the person's status, such as poor wound healing, transfers, a need for further testing, and so forth (Edwards, 2010). Sometimes, this notification occurs over the telephone, which further complicates the communication process. In each instance, well-planned communication can facilitate positive coping and adaptation.

The situation, background, assessment, recommendation (SBAR) format (see Chapter 2) can be adapted to guide the communication of bad news to families. The nurse needs to plan for notifying persons and families of bad news in a similar manner to communicating with other health team members. Making notes of key points can assist the nurse to remember items that need to be addressed during a conversation. If the bad news is to be delivered in person, then the nurse needs to plan for a private, quiet setting (Pirie, 2012). If the news is to be delivered over the phone, the nurse should ask if it is a good time for a conversation. Present some background information

and alert the person that bad news is coming. The bad news needs to be presented in a factual, concise manner. Then the nurse should allow for a period of silence to show respect for the individual and to allow the person to process the information. In follow-up, the nurse should ask if the person understands the information that has been presented and ask for questions. The interaction needs to close with a summary of the treatment plan and when further communication can be expected (Pirie).

Providing Information

Families with family members in the ICU have a fundamental need for information, particularly if the person is unresponsive. Many families have stated, "Not knowing is the worst part." Providing updated information as a clinical situation changes is critical. This information is particularly critical when family members must act as decision makers for persons who cannot make them on their own (Shorofi et al., 2016). The use of a "family supportive care algorithm" that guides communication among family members and the health care team demonstrated families' improved sense of participation in decision making and perception of staff working as a team (Huffines et al., 2013).

Families of a person in the ICU need ongoing information on the person's progress, modifications in care requirements, and any changes in expected outcomes; opportunities to ask questions and clarify information empower families. Identifying one family member to act as the primary contact helps ensure continuity between staff and family. A short daily phone call when family members cannot be present maintains the family connection and reduces family stress (Shorofi et al., 2016).

Nurses in the ICU often serve as mediators between person, family, and other health providers to ensure that data streams remain open, coordinated, and relevant.

How health care providers deliver information is important. Even if the person's condition or prognosis leaves little room for optimism, the family needs to feel some hope and that the staff genuinely cares about what is happening with the person and family.

Caring for Families in the Pediatric Intensive Care Unit

Most parents of hospitalized children, particularly those in the pediatric intensive care unit (PICU), want to be with their children as much as possible (Kaakinen et al., 2010). Parents of children in the PICU need frequent reassurance from the nurse about why things are being done for their child and about treatment-related tubes and equipment. They want to actively participate in their child's care and have their questions answered honestly.

Families act as the child's advocate during hospitalization, either informally, by insisting on high-quality care, or formally, as the legal surrogate decision maker designated to make health care decisions on behalf of the child. The nurse is a primary health care provider agent in working with families facing these issues. A critical intervention for the family as a whole and its individual members is to help them recognize their limitations and hidden strengths and to maintain a balance of health for all members.

Family-Centred Relationships in the Community

"Major chronic diseases, including cardiovascular diseases (CVDs), cancer, chronic respiratory diseases (CRDs) and diabetes, are the cause of 65% of all deaths in Canada each year and are the leading causes of death globally" (Public Health Agency of Canada, 2017, p. 1).

Four modifiable risk factors (physical activity, obesity, smoking, and alcohol consumption) contribute substantially to the financial and emotional burden associated with chronic disease. Community-based nurses have many opportunities to educate and assist individuals to decrease risk factors and self-manage existing diseases. Many individuals are able to self-manage their disease, but an increasing number require family support with coping, self-management, and palliative care.

Nurses in nonacute care settings have multiple opportunities to provide screening and health teaching to newly insured families. A major portion of these interactions should focus on encouraging families to adopt a healthy lifestyle to decrease the incidence of disease and illness. Concurrently, the concept of person-centred care is becoming widely adopted throughout health care. For community-dwelling individuals, the concept of person-centred care focuses on empowering individuals to not only self-manage chronic diseases but also to make appropriate lifestyle modifications with the intent of either preventing disease or minimizing the effects of disease. Person-centred care should stimulate nurses to consider what constitutes effective communication when providing health education to families. Families need to feel empowered to take responsibility for their health state (Kaakinen et al., 2010). Family empowerment develops when well-designed interventions are appropriate to the needs and resources of the family unit. The concepts presented in Chapter 16 can be used within the context of family health teaching.

Family caregivers are common as more people live with chronic illness on a daily basis; the level of assistance required varies on a person-by-person basis. Healthy family members have concurrent demands on their time from their own nuclear families, work, religion, and community responsibilities.

A significant change in health status can exacerbate previously unresolved relationship issues, which may need advanced intervention, in addition to the specific health care issues. When individual family members are experiencing a transition—for example, ending or entering a relationship or a job change—they may not be as available to provide support and can experience unnecessary guilt. Nurses need to consider the broader family responsibilities people have as an important part of the context of health care in providing holistic care to a family.

Meeting Family Informational Needs

Providing information to family caregivers often starts when the person is discharged from an acute care facility. With the passage of time, the individual's needs for assistance may change, but the caregiver may lack the ability to adequately modify the care being provided. A sense of "preparedness" was identified as a factor in contributing to the hope and anxiety of caregivers (Henriksson & Arestedt, 2013). As a result, nurses in clinics and community-based centres should be responsive to cues from caregivers indicating deficient knowledge. Nurses can offer suggestions about how to respond to these changes and offer support to the family caregiver as they emerge. Helping family members access services, support groups, and natural support networks at each stage of their loved one's illness empowers family members because they feel they are helping in a tangible way.

Supporting the Caregiver

Discharge planning requires attention to caring for the caregiver as well as the person (Walton, 2011). Providing emotional support is crucial to helping families cope. Remaining aware of one's own values and staying calm and thoughtful can be very helpful to a family in crisis. Remember that your words can either strengthen or weaken a family's confidence in their ability to care for an ill family member. Focus initially on issues that are manageable within the context of home caregiving. This provides a sense of empowerment. The nurse can encourage the family to develop new ways of coping or can list alternatives and allow the family to choose coping styles that might be useful to them. Focus on what goes well, and ask the family to share their ideas about how to best care for the person. You can help normalize feelings of resentment and help family members set reasonable limits on overly dependent behaviour.

Many families will need information about additional home care services, community resources, and options needed to meet the practical, financial, and emotional demands of caring for a chronically ill family member. There are support groups available for family caregivers of persons with chronic illnesses. These are extremely helpful supports for family members. Not only can they provide practical ideas, but the support of being able to talk about your feelings, and finding that you are not alone, is healing for family members and indirectly beneficial for the person they are caring for.

Encouraging families to use natural helping systems increases the network of emotional and economic support available to the family in a time of crisis. The Canadian Association of Family Resource Programs (FRP Canada) is open to all families and provides numerous resources, from promoting wellness and celebrating diversity to focusing on the strengths that families bring to their situation (Prevnet, n.d.).

Validating and Normalizing Emotions

Families can experience many conflicting emotions when placed in the position of providing protracted care for a loved one. Compassion, protectiveness, and caring can be intermingled with feelings of helplessness and being trapped. Major role reversals can stimulate anger and resentment for both the person being cared for and the family caregiver.

Sibling or family position or geographic proximity may put pressure on certain family members to provide a greater share of the care. Criticism or advice from less-involved family members can be disconcerting, and conflicts about care decisions can create rifts in family relationships. Some caregivers find themselves mourning for their loved one, even though the person is still alive, wishing it could all end but feeling guilt about having such thoughts.

These emotions are normal responses to abnormal circumstances. Listening to the family caregiver's feelings and struggles without judgement can be the most healing intervention you can provide. Nurses can normalize negative feelings by offering insights about common feelings associated with chronic illness. Family members may need guidance as well as permission to get respite and recharge their commitment by attending to their own needs. Support groups can provide families with emotional and practical support and a critical expressive outlet.

Psychosocial concerns for parents with children who are chronically ill can cover many relationship issues—for example, how to respond to and discipline children with a chronic illness. Parents must balance caring for their chronically ill child along with parenting other children (Kaakinen et al., 2010). Healthy siblings may experience feelings of resentment, worry that they might contract a similar illness, or have unrealistic expectations of their part in the treatment process. Siblings need clear information about the sick child's diagnosis and care plan and the opportunity to experience their own childhood as fully as possible. Simulation Exercise 13.7 provides practice with using intervention skills with families.

Pitfalls to Avoid

While nurses strive to be effective in all communication, there are times that our communication efforts are less than

---

SIMULATION EXERCISE 13.7   Using Intervention Skills With Families

Purpose

To practise using intervention skills with families

Procedure

Describe a situation in which you have worked with a family. This may be from a clinical experience or other personal experience. Think about how you talked with the family regarding a specific problem.

Consider the following:

- Did you talk with the family about the problem and learn how they have dealt with the problem, their perception of the problem, and its impact on their family?
- What would be some approaches identified in the text to help them explore the problem in more depth and begin to develop viable options?
- Did you feel you were too intrusive or not assertive enough?

- Did you validate all members' perceptions and perspectives? Did you clarify information and feelings? Did you remain nonjudgemental and objective?
- Did you respect the family's values and beliefs without imposing your own? Did you assist the family in clarifying and understanding the problem in a way that could lead to resolution?

Discussion

In small groups, discuss your responses to the questions above. Be attentive to the experiences of others. Did they have similar experiences? Discuss strategies to facilitate goal-directed communication and problem resolution. How can nurses best provide support to families? How could families learn to use honest communication most of the time? How does one influence this in one's own family?

ideal. Wright and Leahey (2013) identified three common errors that occur in family nursing.

1. Failure to create context for change. In such instances, the nurse does not establish a therapeutic environment for open discussion of family concerns. Or a plan of care might be developed that would not be effective in light of the family situation (resources, distance, health state). To avoid this pitfall, the nurse should be respectful of each family member, obtain as much information about the family and its members as possible, and acknowledge the difficulty of the situation.

2. Taking sides. To minimize the risk of taking sides, the nurse should use questioning skills that help family members develop insight into the depth and scope of the problem. The use of circular questions, as discussed earlier, can be helpful.

3. Giving too much advice prematurely. Nurses inherently are in a position to provide persons and families with information and advice. However, it must be well timed and appropriate to the particular situation. To avoid this pitfall, obtain as much information from family members as possible before providing suggestions. Advice should be framed as a suggestion rather than a set of rules. Follow up with family members to get their reaction to your suggestion.

Using Technology to Enhance Family Communication

The use of the Internet and mobile technologies has progressed dramatically. Many community-dwelling individuals use electronic communication devices on a daily basis, whether via a cell phone or the Internet. The use of electronic communication with persons and families is less common but increasing rapidly. Federal regulations as outlined in the PIPEDA apply to all modes of communication and must be considered when communicating with family members in an electronic format.

Families today are often geographically separated. Encouraging and assisting persons to send email or call using a cell phone can decrease that distance. Simply hearing a person's voice can help to allay fear for distant relatives. Bridge2Health (http://www.bridge2health.ca) is an organization that offers free online resources for individuals undergoing serious health concerns. Online support groups are becoming more prevalent for those experiencing health issues and for family members and caregivers (van der Eijk et al., 2013). The nurse should assess family members' comfort level with the use of technology. Learning to use a smartphone, email, or other technology-based communication can add to the stress of an already anxious situation, and there are other educational modalities if the family member is not really interested. However, if there is interest, the searching the Web and watching certain YouTube videos can offer good information—seeing a skill presented on a video may be more useful than simple verbal instructions.

Evaluations

Evaluation should include both determining effectiveness of nursing interventions and self-reflection by the nurse regarding personal effectiveness. The nurse at the bedside may not see long-term benefits from family interactions due to the episodic nature of contemporary health care. It is important that the nurse provide closure to person interactions in any setting. You can accomplish this task by summarizing the interaction, asking the family if they have any questions, and providing information regarding follow-up. Bereaved families have reported that the support received from nurses played an important role in how they were able to cope (MacConnell et al., 2012). No matter how brief family and nurse interactions are, the impact may be substantial.

Referrals need to include a summary of the information gained to date and should be communicated by the health team member most knowledgeable about the person's condition. Persons and families should be provided with information related to referrals and next steps.

Self-evaluation and self-reflection by the nurse can be used to identify which communication strategies were successful in a given situation and which were not (Kaakinen et al., 2010). By identifying effective and ineffective family communication techniques, they can develop a repertoire of skills, thus enhancing the overall effectiveness of their communication and practice.

SUMMARY

This chapter provides an overview of family communication and the complex dynamics inherent in family relationships. Families have a structure, defined as the way in which members are organized. Family function refers to the roles people take in their families, and family process describes the communication that takes place within the family. Family-centred care is developed through a combination of strategies designed to gather information in a systematic, efficient manner, starting with the genogram, ecomap, and time line. Therapeutic questions and giving commendations are interventions nurses can use with families. Families with critically ill members need continuously updated information and the freedom to be with their family member as often as possible. Involving the family in the care of the person is important. Parents want to participate in the care of their acutely ill child. Nursing interventions are aimed at strengthening family functioning and supporting family coping during hospitalization and in the community.

👤 ETHICAL DILEMMA
What Would You Do?

Rosa is a 90-year-old woman living alone in a two-storey house. She has two daughters, Maria and Yolanda. Maria lives 200 kilometers away but works two jobs because her husband has been laid off for 9 months. Yolanda lives in another province. So far, Rosa has been able to live by herself, but within the past 2 weeks, she fell down a few stairs in her house and she has trouble hearing the telephone. Rosa has very poor vision, walks with a cane, and relies on her neighbours for assistance several times a week. Maria and her husband visit every 2 weeks to bring groceries. Both Maria and Yolanda worry about her and would like to see her in a nursing home. Rosa will not consider this option. As the nurse working with this family, how would you address your ethical responsibilities to Rosa, Maria, and Yolanda?

QUESTIONS FOR REVIEW AND DISCUSSION

1. Identify family communication situations (e.g., end of life, family discord) that you believe would be professionally challenging. Describe strategies that you, as a nurse, could use to be prepared to better manage those situations.
2. How would you personally feel as a nurse delivering bad news to a family?

REFERENCES

Barker, P. (1998). Different approaches to family therapy. *Nursing Times, 94*(14), 60–62.

Bowen, M. (1978). *Family therapy in clinical practice.* Jason Aronson.

Bowen Center for the Study of the Family. (2013). *Bowen theory: Societal emotional process.* http://www.thebowencenter.org/pages/conceptsep.html.

Children's Services, Alberta Government. (2019). *Well-being and resiliency: A framework for supporting safe and healthy children and families.* https://open.alberta.ca/publications/9781460141939.

Chrzastowski, S. K. (2011). A narrative perspective on genograms: Revisiting classical family therapy methods. *Clinical Child Psychology and Psychiatry, 16*(4), 635–644. https://doi.org/10.1177/1359104511400966.

Edwards, M. (2010). How to break bad news and avoid common difficulties. *Nursing & Residential Care, 12*(10), 495–497.

Hart, A., Hardin, S. R., Townsend, A. P., et al. (2013). Critical care visitation: Nurse and family preference. *Dimensions of Critical Care Nursing, 32*(6), 289–299. https://doi.org/10.1097/01.DCC.0000434515.58265.7d.

Health Council of Canada. (2009). *Teams in action: Primary health care teams for Canadians.* https://healthcouncilcanada.ca/files/2.42-teamsinaction_1.pdf.

Henriksson, A., & Arestedt, K. (2013). Exploring factors and caregiver outcomes associated with feelings of preparedness for caregiving in family caregivers in palliative care: A correlational, cross-sectional study. *Palliative Medicine, 27*(7), 639–646.

Hill, W. J., Hasty, C., & Moore, C. (2011). Differentiation of self and the process of forgiveness: A clinical perspective for couple and family therapy. *Australian and New Zealand Journal of Family Therapy, 32*(1), 43–57.

Huffines, M., Johnson, K. L., Smitz Naranjo, L. L., et al. (2013). Improving family satisfaction and participation in decision making in an intensive care unit. *Critical Care Nurse, 33*(5), 56–68.

Institute for Patient- and Family-Centered Care. (n.d.) *Patient- and family-centred care defined.* McLean. https://www.ipfcc.org/bestpractices/sustainable-partnerships/background/pfcc-defined.html.

Jensen, L., & Kosowan, S. (2011). Family presence during cardiopulmonary resuscitation: Cardiac health care professionals' perspectives. *Canadian Journal of Cardiovascular Nursing, 21*(3), 23–29.

Jensen, T., & Schafer, K. (2013). Stepfamily functioning and closeness: Children's views on second marriages and stepfather relationships. *Social Work, 58*(2), 127–136.

Kaakinen, J. R., Gedaly-Duff, V., Coehlo, D. P., et al. (2010). *Family health care nursing: Theory, practice and research.* F. A. Davis.

Kornburger, C., Gibson, C., Sadowski, S., et al. (2013). Using "teach-back" to promote a safe transition from hospital to home: An evidence-based approach to improving the discharge process. *Journal of Pediatric Nursing, 28*, 282–291.

Koukouli, S., Lambraki, M., Sigala, E., et al. (2018). The experience of Greek families of critically ill patients: Exploring their needs and coping strategies. *Intensive & Critical Care Nursing, 45*, 44–51. https://doi.org/10.1016/j.iccn.2017.12.001.

Leahey, M., & Harper-Jaques, S. (1996). Family-nurse relationships: Core assumptions and clinical implications. *Journal of Family Nursing, 2*(2), 133–152.

MacConnell, G., Aston, M., Randel, P., et al. (2012). Nurses' experiences providing bereavement follow-up: An exploratory study using feminist poststructuralism. *Journal of Clinical Nursing, 22*, 1094–1102.

MacKay, L. (2012). Trauma and Bowen family systems theory: Working with adults who were abused as children. *Australian and New Zealand Journal of Family Therapy, 33*(3), 232–241.

McCullough, J., & Schell-Chaple, H. (2013). Maintaining patients' privacy and confidentiality with family communications in the intensive care unit. *Critical Care Nurse, 33*(5), 77–79.

Minister of Justice, Government of Canada. (2019). Personal Information and Protection of Electronic Documents Act, S.C. 2000, c. 5. https://laws-lois.justice.gc.ca/ENG/ACTS/P-8.6/index.html.

Nichols, M., & Schwartz, R. (2009). *Family therapy: Concepts and methods* (9th ed.). Prentice Hall.

Novak, L., George, S., Wallston, K., et al. (2020). Patient stories can make a difference in patient-centered research design. *Journal of Patient Experience*, 1438–1444. https://doi.org/10.1177/2374373520958340.

Otto, H. (1963). Criteria for assessing family strength. *Family Process*, *2*, 329–338.

Pirie, A. (2012). Pediatric palliative care communication: Resources for the clinical nurse specialist. *Clinical Nurse Specialist*, *26*(4), 212–215.

Porr, C. J. (2013). Important interactional strategies for everyday public health nursing practice. *Public Health Nursing*, 1–7. https://doi.org/10.1111/phn.12097.

Prevnet. (n.d.) *Canadian Association of Family Resource Programs.* https://www.prevnet.ca/partners/organizations/canadian-association-of-family-resource-programs.

Public Health Agency of Canada. (2017). *How healthy are Canadians? A trend analysis of the health of Canadians from a healthy living and chronic disease perspective.* Ottawa: Ontario. https://www.canada.ca/en/public-health/services/publications/healthy-living/how-healthy-canadians.html.

Rosland, A., Heisler, M., & Piette, J. (2012). The impact of family behaviors and communication patterns on chronic illness outcomes: A systematic review. *Journal of Behavioral Medicine*, *35*(2), 221–239.

Shorofi, S. A., Jannati, Y., Moghaddam, H. R., et al. (2016). Psychosocial needs of families of intensive care patients: Perceptions of nurses and families. *Nigerian Medical Journal: Journal of the Nigeria Medical Association*, *57*(1), 10–18. https://doi.org/10.4103/0300-1652.180557.

Statistics Canada. (2016). *Household.* https://www23.statcan.gc.ca/imdb/p3Var.pl?Function=Unit&Id=96113.

Trivette, C. M., Dunst, C. J., & Hamby, D. W. (2010). Influences of family-systems intervention practices on patent-child interactions and child development. *Topics in Early Childhood Special Education*, *30*(1), 3–19.

Trotter, T., & Martin, H. M. (2007). Family history in pediatric primary care. *Pediatrics*, *120*(Suppl), S60–S65.

van der Eijk, M., Faber, M., Aarts, J., et al. (2013). Using online health communities to deliver patient-centered care to people with chronic conditions. *Journal of Medical Internet Research*, *15*(6), e115. https://doi.org/10.2196/jmir.2476.

von Bertalanffy. L. (1968). *General systems theory.* George Braziller.

Walton, M. (2011). Communicating with family caregivers. *American Journal of Nursing*, *111*(12), 47–53.

Wright, L. M., & Leahey, M. (2009). *Nurses and families: A guide to family assessment and intervention* (5th ed.). F. A. Davis.

Wright, L., & Leahey, M. (2013). *Nurses and families: A guide to family assessment and intervention* (6th ed.). FA Davis Company.

WEBSITE/RESOURCES LIST

Canadian Association of Family Resource Programs (FRP Canada) https://www.prevnet.ca/partners/organizations/canadian-association-of-family-resource-programs.

Canadian Critical Care Organization https://www.canadiancriticalcare.org/Patients-&-Families.

Canadian Patient Safety Institute https://www.patientsafetyinstitute.ca/en/Pages/default.aspx.

Families Canada https://familiescanada.ca/article/our-story/. https://www.canada.ca/en/employment-social-development/news/2018/09/support-for-families-with-critically-ill-loved-ones.html.

14

Resolving Conflicts Between Nurse and People Receiving Care

Olive Yonge
Originating US chapter by *Kathleen Underman Boggs*

OBJECTIVES

At the end of the chapter, the reader will be able to:

1. Define *conflict* and contrast the functional with the dysfunctional role of conflict in a therapeutic relationship.
2. Recognize personal styles of response to conflict situations and discriminate among passive, assertive, and aggressive responses to conflict situations.
3. Specify the characteristics of assertive communication strategies to promote conflict resolution in nurse–person relationships.
4. Practise strategies to de-escalate violence in the workplace.
5. Analyze findings from research studies and evidence-informed practice and discuss how they can be applied to communicating with people who hold differing values in your clinical practice.

Relational practice is a fundamental competency for nurses. It means intrapersonal, interpersonal, and contextual variables need to be considered if nurses are to have an impact on the people they care for, including individuals, families, and communities. Communication as a competency is the basis of collaboration and the ability to self monitor, use information technologies, articulate a nursing perspective, and contribute positively to the function of the health care team (Canadian Association of Schools of Nursing [CASN], 2015). It is through the application of these competencies that nurses have the ability to manage difficult communication situations.

Conflict is a natural part of human relationships. We all have times when we experience negative feelings about a situation or person, but in nursing, it can compromise the person's safety. When conflict occurs, direct communication is needed. This chapter emphasizes the dynamics of conflict and the problem-solving skills needed for successful resolution between you and the people in your care. Effective nurse–person communication is critical. According to nurses, open communication is a key factor in avoiding threatening situations (Avander et al., 2016). When conflict occurs, knowing how to respond calmly allows you to use feelings as a positive force. Some people approach their initial encounter with a nurse with verbal hostility or even physical aggression, as when we admit someone who is intoxicated to the emergency department. Maintaining safety for self and others in your care is paramount. To listen and respond creatively to intense emotion when your first impulse is to withdraw or retaliate demands a high level of skill, empathy, and self-control. Many of these skills can also be applied to the workplace conflicts discussed in Chapters 23 and 24.

BASIC CONCEPTS

Definition

Conflict is defined as disagreement arising from differences in attitudes, values, or needs, in which the actions of one party frustrate the ability of the other to achieve their expected goals. This disagreement results in stress or tension. Conflict serves as a warning that something in the relationship needs closer attention. **Dysfunctional conflict** occurs when information is withheld, feelings are expressed too strongly, the problem is obscured by a double message, or feelings are denied or projected onto others. Conflict is not necessarily a negative—it can become a positive force leading to growth in relationships. **Conflict resolution** is a learned process.

Nature of Conflict

All conflicts have certain things in common: (1) a concrete *content problem* issue and (2) relationship or *process* issues, which involves our emotional response to the situation. It is immaterial whether the issue makes realistic sense to you. It feels real to the other person and needs to be dealt with. Unresolved, such issues interfere with your and the person's success in meeting goals. Most people experience conflict as discomfort. Previous experiences with conflict situations, the importance of the issue, and possible consequences all play a role in the intensity of our reactions. For example, a person in your care may have great difficulty asking questions of the physician regarding treatment or prognosis but experience no problem asking similar questions of the nurse or family. The reasons for the discrepancy in comfort level may relate to previous experiences. Alternatively, it may have little to do with the actual people involved. Rather, the person may be responding to anticipated fears about the type of information the physician might give.

Causes of Conflict

Poor communication is the main cause of misunderstanding and conflict. Psychological causes of conflict include differences in values or personality as well as multiple demands causing high levels of stress. If your nursing care does not fit in with the cultural belief system of the people you care for, conflict can result. Recognize that our culture has moved toward greater incivility in mainstream society. This is reflected within the health care system.

Workplace Violence

A safe work environment is a prerequisite for providing good-quality care (Longo et al., 2016). Violence in the workplace is defined as an expression of anger by others, manifested as threats or attacks, either physical or psychological. Behaviours include negative dysfunctional aggression, expressed as verbal abuse, derogatory speech, harassment, bullying, pushing, hitting, or even attacks with weapons. Violence is classified as an occupational hazard.

Globally, nurses are at higher risk, owing to their direct contact with distressed people (International Council of Nurses [ICN], 2006; Nowrouzi & Huynh, 2016; Waschgler et al., 2013). At the same time, the incidence of violence is greatly under-reported (Campbell et al., 2016).

Conflict can escalate to violent threats or actions. Nurses need to be aware that the stressful nature of illness can aggravate factors that lead to violent behaviour on the part of people or their family members.

Incidence of Violence

Statistics show that violence against health care workers is increasing in every country and in every health care setting (Llor-Esteban et al., 2017; NICE Guideline #10, 2015; Wei et al., 2016; World Health Organization [WHO], 2012). Nurses and social workers are at three times greater risk for experiencing violence in the workplace than are other professionals. The highest risk exists in emergency departments, psychiatric settings, and nursing homes. From a Canada-wide survey conducted by the Canadian Federation of Nurses Unions, 61% of nurses reported abuse, harassment, and assault on the job during 2018 (Canadian Nurses Association & Canadian Federation of Nurses Unions, 2014; House of Commons Canada, 2019). A high percentage of nurses will experience violence, often physical violence, at some time during their careers (Brann & Hartley, 2016; Hahn et al., 2013; Llor-Estaban et al.).

Outcomes

Adverse outcomes for nurses include increased stress, job dissatisfaction, somatic illness, emotional trauma, increased absenteeism, post-traumatic stress disorder, self-medication abuse, and death (Avander et al., 2016). In addition to physical harm to the worker, the Canadian Centre for Occupational Health & Safety (2021) and other sources have identified problems for the health system, such as increased agency costs due to lost work days, job turnover, and occasionally, litigation.

Nurses educated in violence prevention and management are better prepared. Consider the case of Mr. Dixon.

Case Example: Mr. Dixon

Experienced staff RN Elaine Kaye works in a busy emergency department, where access to the treatment rooms is blocked by a locked security door. Staff do not wear necklaces or neck chains, nor do they carry implements, but Ms. Kaye does wear a medical alert bracelet. While Dr. Hughes is treating Donny, age 12, who appears to be suffering from convulsions related to overdosing on methylphenidate (Ritalin), Ms. Kaye notices that Mr. Dixon, who is in the waiting room, is becoming increasingly agitated.

Mr. D: "Why aren't you people doing more?"

Nurse (in a low tone of voice): "My name is Ms. Kaye and I am helping with your son. I'll be keeping you up to date with information as soon as we know anything. I know this is stressful ..."

Mr. D (interrupting in a louder voice): "I demand to know why you people won't tell me what is going on."

Nurse: "I see that you're really upset and feeling angry. Let's move over here to the conference area for privacy."

Mr. D: "You guys are no good."

Nurse: "I want to understand your point of view. You—"

Mr. D throws a chair.

Nurse: "This is an upsetting time for you, but violence is not acceptable. Please calm down and we will sit down. Let's both take a deep breath, and then you can explain to me what you need ..."

Strategies to prevent escalation of violent behaviour are discussed in the Applications section of this chapter. Suggestions for physical and organizational safeguards are available from The Centre for Occupational Health and Safety at https://www.ccohs.ca/.

Stage of Anger

- Mild Anger: Feels some tension, irritability. Acts argumentatively, sarcasticly, or is difficult to please
- Moderate Anger: Displays observably angry behaviours such as motor agitation and loud voice
- Severe Anger: Shows acting out behaviours, cursing, using violent gestures, but is not yet out of control
- Rage: Behaves in an out-of-control manner, being physically aggressive toward others or self

Goal: Work for Conflict Resolution

Unresolved nurse–person conflict impedes the quality and safety of the care you provide to people. It not only undermines your therapeutic relationship but can also result in your emotional exhaustion, leading to **burnout**. Energy is transferred to conflict issues instead of being used to build the relationship.

As nurses, our goal is to collaborate with people we care for to maximize their health. To accomplish this, we need to communicate clearly to prevent or reduce levels of conflict. We know that resolving a long-standing conflict is a gradual process in which we may have to revisit the issue several times to fully resolve it.

Conflict-Resolution Principles

It goes without saying that professionals must always demonstrate respect for the people they care for. Gender and

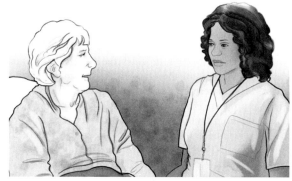

Fig. 14.1 Principles of conflict resolution: Identify the conflict issue

- Listen to the person's perspective
- Acknowledge you have heard by validating, using "I" sentences, avoiding "you"
- Stay focused on the current issue; know and control your own responses
- Use the "no blame" approach and discuss options, alternative solutions
- Negotiate and agree on a solution
- Summarize
- Follow through.

cultural factors that influence responses are described elsewhere. Fig. 14.1 lists some principles of conflict resolution. These principles may also be applied to conflicts with colleagues.

Understand Your Own Personal Responses to Conflict

Conflicts between nurses and the people they care for are not uncommon. First, gain a clear understanding of your own personal responses, since conflict creates anxiety that may prevent you from behaving in an effective, assertive manner. No one is equally effective in all situations. Completing Simulation Exercise 14.1 may help you identify your personal responses.

Recognize your own "triggers" or "hot buttons." What words or actions from others trigger an immediate emotional response in you? These could include having someone yelling at you or speaking to you in an angry tone of voice. Once you recognize the triggers, you can better control your own responses. It is imperative that you focus on the current issue. Put aside past experiences—listing prior problems will raise emotions and prevent resolution. Identify *available options*. Rather than immediately trying to solve the problem, look at the range of possible options. Create a list of these options and work with the other party to evaluate the feasibility of each option. By working

SIMULATION EXERCISE 14.1   Personal Responses to Conflict

Purpose

To increase awareness of how students respond in conflict situations and the elements in situations (e.g., people, status, age, previous experience, lack of experience, place) that contribute to their sense of discomfort

Anger	Competitiveness	Humiliation
Annoyance	Defensiveness	Inferiority
Antagonism	Devaluation	Intimidation
Anxiousness	Embarrassment	Manipulation
Bitterness	Frustration	Resentment

Procedure

Break the class up into pairs. You may do this as homework or create an online discussion. Think of a conflict situation that could be handled in different ways.

The following feelings are common correlates of interpersonal conflict situations that many people say they experienced in conflict situations that they have not handled well.

Although these feelings generally are not ones we are especially proud of, they are a part of the human experience. By acknowledging their existence within ourselves, we usually have more choice about how we handle them.

Reflective Analysis and Discussion

Construct different responses and then explain how the different responses might lead to different outcomes.

BOX 14.1   Nurse Behaviours That Can Create Anger in Others

- Violating someone's personal space
- Speaking in a threatening tone
- Providing unsolicited advice
- Judging, blaming, criticizing, or conveying ideas that try to create guilt
- Offering reassurances that are not realistic
- Communicating using "gloss it over" positive comments
- Speaking in a way that shows you do not understand the person's point of view
- Exerting too much pressure to make a person change their unhealthy behaviour
- Portraying self as an infallible "I know best" expert
- Using an authoritarian, sarcastic, or accusing tone
- Using "hot button" words that have heavy emotional connotations
- Failing to provide health information in a timely manner to stressed individuals

controls on the people they care for, who then often react by behaving in more difficult ways. Other behaviours of nurses that may lead to anger in people or their families are listed in Box 14.1. People who feel listened to and respected are generally receptive.

Situations that may cause nurses to become frustrated or angry include working with people who dismiss what they say or who ask for more personal information than nurses feel comfortable sharing, people who sexually harass or target them in a personal attack, or family members who make demands that nurses are unable to fulfill.

Develop an Effective Conflict Management Style

In the past, nurses were found to commonly use avoidance or accommodation when they were faced with a conflict situation (Sayer et al., 2012). Many felt that any conflict was destructive and needed to be suppressed. Current thinking holds that conflict can be healthy and can lead to growth when, with conflict-resolution training, we develop a collaborative problem-solving approach. Five distinct styles of response to conflict have been documented.

Avoidance is a common response to conflict. Nurses using avoidance distance themselves from the people they care for or provide them with less support. Sometimes, an experience makes you so uncomfortable that you want to avoid the situation or person at all costs, so you withdraw. This style is appropriate when the cost of addressing the conflict is higher than the benefit of resolution. Sometimes, you just have to "pick your battles," focusing your energy on the most important issues. However, the use of avoidance postpones the conflict, leads to future problems, and damages your relationship with the person, making it an "I lose, you lose" situation.

together, you shift expectations from adversarial conflict to an expectation of a win–win outcome. After discussing possible solutions, select the best one to resolve the conflict. Evaluate the outcome based on fair, objective criteria.

Know the Context

Second, understand the context or the circumstances in which the situation occurs. Most interpersonal conflicts involve some threat to one's sense of control or self-esteem. Nurses have been shown to respond to the stress of not having enough time to complete their work by imposing more

Accommodation is another common response. We surrender our own needs in a desire to smooth over the conflict. This response is cooperative but nonassertive. Sometimes, this approach involves a quick compromise or giving false reassurance. By giving in to others, we maintain peace but do not actually deal with the issue, so, often, it resurfaces in the future. It is appropriate only when the issue is more important to the other person. This is an "I lose, you win" situation. Harmony results. Goodwill may be earned that can be used in the future (McElhaney, 1996).

Competition is a response style characterized by domination. You exercise power to gain your own goals at the expense of the other person. It is characterized by aggression and lack of compromise. Authority may be used to suppress the conflict in a dictatorial manner. This leads to increased stress. It is an effective style only when there is a need for a quick decision, but it leads to problems in the long term, making it an "I win now but then lose and you lose" situation.

Compromise is a solution nurses still commonly use. By compromising, each party gives a little and gains a little. It is effective only when both parties hold equal power. Depending on the specific work environment and the issue in dispute, it can be a good solution, but since neither party is completely satisfied, it can eventually become an "I lose, you lose" situation.

Collaboration is a solution-oriented response in which we work together cooperatively to solve problems. To manage the conflict, we commit to finding a mutually agreeable solution. This approach involves directly confronting the issue, acknowledging our feelings, and using open communication. Steps for productive confrontation include identifying concerns of each party, clarifying assumptions, communicating honestly to identify the real issue, and working collaboratively to find a solution that satisfies everyone. Collaboration is considered to be the most effective style for genuine resolution. This is an "I win, you win" situation.

Structure Your Response

In mastering assertive responses, it may be helpful initially to use these steps:

1. Express empathy: "I understand that_____"; "I hear you saying _____." *Example:* "I understand that things are difficult at home."
2. Describe your feelings or the situation: "I feel that _____"; "This situation seems to me to _____." *Example:* "But your 8-year-old daughter has expressed a lot of anxiety, saying, 'I can't learn to give my own insulin shots.'"
3. State expectations: "I want_____"; "What is required by the situation is _____."

Example: "It is necessary for you to be here tomorrow when the diabetic teaching nurse comes so you can learn how to give injections and your daughter can, too, with your support."
4. List consequences: "If you do this, then _____ will happen" (state positive outcome); "If you don't do this, then _____ will happen" (state negative outcome). *Example:* "If you get here on time, we can be finished and get her discharged in time for her birthday on Friday." Focus on the present.
5. The focus should always be on the present. Focus only on the current issue. The past cannot be changed, so "stay in the moment."
6. Limit your discussion to one topic issue at a time to enhance the chance of success. Usually, it is impossible to resolve a multidimensional conflict with a single solution. By breaking the problem down into simple steps, you allow enough time for a clear understanding. You might paraphrase the person's words, reflecting the meaning back to them to validate its accuracy. Once the issues have been delineated clearly, the steps needed for resolution may appear quite simple.

Being assertive in the face of an emotionally charged situation demands thought, energy, and commitment. Assertiveness also requires the use of common sense, self-awareness, knowledge, tact, humour, respect, and a sense of perspective. Although there is no guarantee that the use of assertive behaviours will produce the desired interpersonal goals, the chances of a successful outcome are increased because the information flow is optimally honest, direct, and firm. Often, the use of assertiveness brings about changes in ways that could not have been anticipated. Changes occur because the nurse offers a new resource in the form of objective feedback, with no strings attached.

Use "I" Statements

Statements that begin with "You ..." sound accusatory and always represent an assumption because it is impossible to know exactly, without validation, why someone acts in a certain way. Because such statements point a finger and imply a judgement, most people respond defensively to them.

"We" statements should be used only when you actually mean to look at an issue collaboratively. Thus the statement, "Perhaps we both need to look at this issue a little more closely" may be appropriate in certain situations. However, the statement, "Perhaps we shouldn't get so angry when things don't work out the way we think they should" is a condescending statement, thinly disguised as a collaorative statement. What is actually being expressed in the second example is the expectation that both parties should handle the conflict in one way—the nurse's way.

The use of "I" statements is one of the most effective conflict management strategies. Assertive statements that begin with "I" suggest that the person speaking accepts full responsibility for their own feelings and position in relation to the conflict. "I" statements may seem a little clumsy at first and may take a little practice. The traditional format is as follows:

"I feel_____ (use a name to claim the emotion you feel)

when_____ (describe the behaviour non-judgementally)

because_____ (describe the tangible effects of the behaviour)."

Example: "I feel uncomfortable when someone's personal problems are discussed in the cafeteria because someone might overhear confidential information."

Make Clear Statements

Statements, rather than questions, set the stage for assertive responses to conflict. When questions are used, "how" questions are best because they are neutral in nature, they seek more information, and they imply a collaborative effort. Avoid "why" questions as they put people on the defensive, asking them to explain their behaviour. It is always important to state the situation clearly; describe events or expectations objectively; and maintain a strong, firm, yet tactful manner. Consider the case of Mr. Gow.

Case Example: Mr. Gow

Mr. Gow is a 35-year-old executive who has been hospitalized with a myocardial infarction. He has been acting seductively toward some of the young nurses but he seems to be giving Ms. O'Hara an especially hard time.

Mr. Gow: Come on in, honey, I've been waiting for you.

Nurse (using appropriate facial expression and eye contact, and replying in a firm, clear voice): Mr. Gow, I would rather you called me Ms. O'Hara.

Mr. G.: Aw, come on now, honey. I don't get to have much fun around here. What's the difference what I call you?

Nurse: I feel that it does make a difference, and I would like you to call me Ms. O'Hara.

Mr. G.: Oh, you're no fun at all. Why do you have to be so serious?

Nurse: Mr. Gow, you're right. I am serious about some things, and being called by my name and title is one of them. I would prefer that you call me Ms. O'Hara. I would like to work with you, however, and it might be important to explore the ways in which

---

this hospitalization is hampering your natural desire to have fun.

In this interaction the nurse's position is defined several times, using successively stronger statements before the shift is made to refocus on Mr. Gow's needs. Notice that the nurse labeled the behaviour, not the patient, as unacceptable. Persistence is essential when initial attempts at assertiveness appear too limited.

Use Moderate Pitch and Vocal Tone

The strength of a forceful, assertive statement depends on the nature of the conflict situation as well as the degree of confrontation needed to resolve the conflict successfully. Starting with the least amount of assertiveness required to meet the demands of the situation conserves energy and does not place you in a bind of overkill. It is not necessary to use all your resources at one time or to express your ideas too strongly. We sometimes lose effectiveness by becoming too long-winded. Long explanations detract from the spoken message. Get to the main point quickly, saying what is necessary in the simplest, most concrete way possible. This cuts down on the possibility of misinterpretation.

Pitch and tone of voice contribute to another person's interpretation of the meaning of your assertive message. A soft, hesitant, passive presentation can undermine an assertive message. The same is true if a harsh, hostile, aggressive tone is used. Try a firm but moderate presentation to effectively convey your message by doing Simulation Exercise 14.2.

Outcome: Positive Growth

Traditionally, conflict was viewed as a destructive force to be eliminated. Actually, conflicts that are successfully resolved lead to stronger relationships. The critical factor is the willingness to explore and resolve it mutually. Appropriately handled, conflict can provide an important opportunity for growth. Practice to develop conflict management skills is essential and effective.

Outcome: Dysfunction, Such as Unresolved Conflict

As mentioned, unresolved conflicts tend to resurface later, impeding your ability to give quality care. If the emotional aspect of the conflict is expressed too strongly, the nurse can feel attacked.

Nature of Assertive Behaviour

Assertive behaviour is defined as conveying confidence, including setting goals, acting on those goals in a clear, consistent manner, and taking responsibility for the consequences of those actions. Assertive communication is conveying this objective in a direct manner, without anger or frustration. The assertive nurse is able to stand up for their personal rights and the rights of others.

Components of assertive communication include the ability to (1) say no, (2) ask for what you want, (3) appropriately express both positive and negative thoughts and feelings, and (4) initiate, continue, and terminate the interaction. This honest expression of yourself does not violate the needs of others but does demonstrate self-respect rather than deference to the demands of others. Conflict creates anxiety, which may prevent you from behaving assertively. Assertive behaviours range from making a direct, honest statement about your beliefs to taking a very strong, confrontational stand about what will and will not be tolerated. Assertive responses contain "I" statements that take responsibility. This behaviour is in contrast with **aggressive behaviour**, which has a goal of dominating while suppressing the other person's rights. Aggressive responses often consist of "you" statements that fix blame on the other person. Box 14.2 lists characteristics of assertive behaviour. Remember that assertiveness is a learned behaviour and assertive responses need to be practised.

Nonassertive behaviour in a professional nurse is related to lower levels of autonomy. Continued patterns of nonassertive responses have a negative influence on you and on the standard of care you provide. Practise your own assertiveness in Simulation Exercise 14.3.

BOX 14.2   Characteristics Associated With the Development of Assertive Behaviour

- Express your own position, using "I" statements.
- Make clear statements.
- Speak in a firm tone, using moderate pitch.
- Assume responsibility for personal feelings and wants.
- Make sure verbal and nonverbal messages are congruent.
- Address only issues related to the present conflict.
- Structure responses so as to be tactful and show awareness of the person's frame of reference.
- Understand that undesired behaviours, not feelings, attitudes, and motivations, are the focus for change.

SIMULATION EXERCISE 14.2   Pitching the Assertive Message

Purpose
To increase awareness of how the meaning of a verbal message can be significantly altered by changing one's tone of voice

Procedure
Break class up into groups of five. Write on five slips of paper one of the following five vocal pitches: whisper, soft tone with hesitant delivery, moderate tone and firm delivery, loud tone with agitated delivery, and screaming.

In each group, have each person in turn pick one of five pieces of paper and demonstrate that tone, while the others in the group try to identify in which tone the assertive message is being delivered.

Reflective Analysis
Using information learned from the text to support your answer, justify how tone can affect perceptions of a message's content.

SIMULATION EXERCISE 14.3   Assertive Responses

Purpose
To increase awareness of assertiveness

Procedure
Role-play the following scenario:
 You are working full time, raising a family, and taking 12 credits of nursing classes. The teacher asks you to be a student representative on a faculty committee. You say the following:
1. "I don't think I'm the best one. Why don't you ask Karen? If she can't, I guess I can."

2. "Gee, I'd like to, but I don't know. I probably could if it doesn't take too much time."
3. "I do want students to have some input to this committee, but I am not sure I have enough time. Let me think about it and let you know in class tomorrow."

Reflective Analysis and Discussion
1. Critique the options, describing how they could be altered.
2. Select the most assertive response. Defend your choice using the text.

Safety

It is your responsibility to maintain your own safety and that of the people you care for. Mindfully, be aware. When you are confronted by an angry person or family member, use your skills to defuse the situation, addressing their concerns. If anger enters the rage stage (see above), leave and get help (College of Nurses of Ontario, 2018). Do not stay in a dangerous situation. It cannot be overemphasized that if you feel in danger, you must leave. Each agency should have a resource team to call for intervention assistance. Don't be a hero; CALL FOR HELP!

APPLICATIONS

It is essential to recognize the potential for conflict. TeamSTEPPS reminds us to use situation monitoring, continually scanning our environment to understand what is going on around us. Practising the following strategies can help you to improve your conflict-resolution skills. By doing so, we demonstrate that we are developing the competencies of relational practice (CASN, 2015).

Preventing Conflict

In addition to managing your own responses to provocations by others, model behaviour by adopting a professional, calm demeanor and low tone of voice. Use conflict-prevention strategies: signal your readiness to listen, with attending behaviours such as good body position, eye contact, and a receptive facial expression. Give your undivided attention to anyone you identify as potentially becoming aggressive. Multiple studies show that nurses' anti-communication attitudes act as a barrier. Increasing your positive appreciation of the person you are interacting with facilitates communication. As nurses, we hold the belief that all people have value as human beings. Try some of the strategies described in this chapter to help prevent or resolve conflict.

Assessing the Presence of Conflict in the Nurse–Person Relationship

To get resolution, you need to acknowledge the presence of conflict. Often, our awareness of our own feelings of discomfort is an initial clue. Evidence of the presence of conflict may be overt, that is, observable in the person's behaviour and

---

▶ DEVELOPING AN EVIDENCE-INFORMED PRACTICE

It is well documented that conflict in the workplace occurs more in health care than in other situations. Conflict management and de-escalation strategies are also documented. Ameliorating the effects of stress from workplace conflict was studied by Hersch and colleagues (2016), among others. They studied the effects of an online stress management program on 106 staff nurses and managers, from six hospitals, using a randomized pretest–post-test trial. Stress was measured using the "Nursing Stress Scale."

Results

Over a 3-month period, nurses in the experimental group, who accessed the web-based program, BREATHE: Stress Management for Nurses, reported significantly better handled (less) perceived stress. The BREATHE program was effective in moderating stress associated with conflict with doctors and other nurses, workload issues, inadequate preparation issues, and stress stemming from caring for people who are dying.

Application to Your Clinical Practice

An extensive literature review highlights the following effective strategies for coping with conflict:

- Paying attention to your own responses (emotional reactions may escalate conflict to aggression)
- Managing your own responses by staying calm; not overreacting; communicating nonverbal, nonthreatening messages; speaking softly, and using cognitive restructuring to replace negative ways of thinking
- Using relaxation and other coping strategies, including the online BREATHE program or downloading relaxation apps, and practising deep breathing immediately before responding
- Seeking to create a supportive work environment
- Identifying early risk factors in people, such as difficulty sleeping and concentrating, hostility or anger, and expression of threats
- Focusing on the person to discern the underlying problem
- Implementing de-escalation steps, confronting conflict immediately to prevent escalation to violence, and setting limits in a nonconfrontational way
- Showing respect to all, remaining empathetic and non-judgemental, and not dictating choices

Compiled from: Cheng, 2016; Crisis Prevention Institute (CPI; OSHA), (2017); Dwarswaard and van de Bovenkamp, 2015; Haugvaldstad and Husum, 2016; Hersch et al., 2016; Watkins et al., 2017.

expressed verbally–for example, someone you are looking after might criticize you. No one likes to be criticized, and a natural response might be anger, rationalization, or blaming others. But as a professional nurse, you recognize your response, recognize the conflict, and work toward resolution so that constructive changes can take place.

More often, conflict is covert and not so clear-cut. The conflict issues are hidden. The person talks about one issue, but talking does not seem to help and the issue does not get resolved; they continue to be angry or anxious. Subtle behavioural manifestations of covert conflict might include a reduced effort by the person to engage in self-care; frequent misinterpretation of your words; and behaviours that are out of character for the person, such as excessive anger. For example, the person you are caring for might become unusually demanding, have a seemingly insatiable need for your attention, or be unable to tolerate reasonable delays in having their needs met. Such problems may represent anxiety stemming from conflicting feelings. Behaviours are often negatively affected by feelings of pain, loss, helplessness, frustration, or fear. As nurses, we affect people's behaviour through our actions. This can lead to positive or negative outcomes. See Simulation Exercise 14.4 for practice in defining conflict issues.

Sometimes, the feelings themselves become the major issue, so that valid parts of the original conflict issue are hidden; consequently, conflict escalates. Consider how to respond to Mrs. Dentoni.

Case Example: Mrs. Dentoni

Mrs. Dentoni is scheduled for surgery at 8 a.m. tomorrow. As the student nurse assigned to care for her, you have been told that she was admitted to the hospital 3 hours ago and that she has been examined by the house resident. The anesthesia department has been notified of her arrival. Her blood work and urine have been sent to the laboratory. As you enter her room and introduce yourself, you notice that Mrs. Dentoni is sitting on the edge of the bed and appears tense and angry.

Mrs. D.: I wish people would just leave me alone. Nobody has come in and told me about my surgery tomorrow. I don't know what I'm supposed to do—just lie around here and rot, I guess.

At this point, you can probably sense Mrs. Dentoni's conflicting feelings, but it is unclear whether her emotions relate to anxiety about the surgery or anger about some real or imagined invasion of privacy because of the necessary laboratory tests and physical examination. She may also be annoyed by you or by a lack of information from the surgeon. She may

---

feel the need to know that hospital personnel see her as a person and care about her feelings. Before you can respond empathetically to Mrs. Dentoni's feelings, you will have to decode them.

Nurse (in a concerned tone of voice): You seem really upset. It's rough being in the hospital, isn't it?

Notice that the reply is nonjudgemental and tentative and does not suggest specific feelings beyond those the person has shared. There is an implicit request for her to validate your perception of her feelings and to link the feelings with a concrete issue. You process verbal as well as nonverbal cues. You express concern through your tone of voice and words. The content focus relates to the person's predominant feeling tone because this is the part of the conflict that is shared with you. It is important to maintain a non-anxious, relaxed presence.

Techniques for Conflict Resolution

Remember that your goal is to de-escalate the conflict. We need to model respect. Use the strategies for conflict resolution described in this section. Mastery takes practice. Although this may seem like a lot of information, an incident can occur in only a few minutes. Stay calm, and use the 3 Ps of **crisis de-escalation**:

- Position: face the person but remain closer to the exit, making eye contact only 60% of the time
- Posture: relax your stance, with uncrossed arms; rotate and relax your shoulders
- Proximity: stay 0.5 to 1 metre away

Reaching a common understanding of the problem in a direct, tactful manner is the first step in conflict resolution, moving you toward a goal of reaching a resolution that is acceptable to both parties (Fig. 14.2).

Prepare for the Encounter

Careful preparation often makes the difference between being successful or failing to assert yourself when necessary. Mentally visualize yourself responding assertively. Clearly identify the issue in conflict. For communication to be effective, it must be carefully thought out in terms of certain basic questions, such as the following:

- *Purpose.* What is the purpose or objective of this information? What is the central idea, the one most important statement to be made?
- *Organization.* What are the major points to be shared, and in what order?
- *Content.* Is the information to be shared complete? Does it convey who, what, where, when, why, and how?
- *Word choice.* Has careful consideration been given to the choice of words?

SIMULATION EXERCISE 14.4   Defining Conflict Issues: Case Analyses

Purpose

To help organize information and define the problem in interpersonal conflict situations

Procedure

In each conflict situation, look for specific behaviours (including words, tone, posture, and facial expression); feeling impressions (including words, tone, intensity, and facial expression); and need (expressed verbally or through actions).

Identify the behaviours, your impressions of the behaviours, and the underlying needs that the person is expressing in the following situations. Suggest an appropriate nursing action. Situation 1 is completed as a guide.

Situation 1

Mrs. Patel, a recent immigrant from India, does not speak much English. Her baby was just delivered by Cesarean section, and it is expected that Mrs. Patel will remain in the hospital for at least 4 days. Her husband tells the nurse that his wife wants to breastfeed, but she has decided to wait until she goes home to begin because she will be more comfortable there and she wants privacy. The nurse knows that breastfeeding will be more successful if it is initiated soon after birth.

Behaviours: Mrs. Patel's husband states that his wife wants to breastfeed but does not wish to start before going home. Mrs. Patel is not initiating breastfeeding in the hospital.

Your impressions of behaviours: Indirectly, she is expressing physical discomfort, possible insecurity, and awkwardness about breastfeeding. She may also be acting in accordance with cultural norms of her country or family.

Underlying needs: Safety and security. Mrs. Patel probably will not be motivated to attempt breastfeeding until she feels safe and secure in her home environment.

Suggested nursing action: Provide family support and guarantee total privacy for feeding.

Situation 2

Mrs. Moore is brought back to the unit from surgery after a radical mastectomy. The doctor's orders call for her to ambulate, cough, and deep breathe and to use her arm as much as possible in self-care activities. Mrs. Moore asks the nurse in a very annoyed tone, "Why do I have to do this? You can see that it is difficult for me. Why can't you help me?"

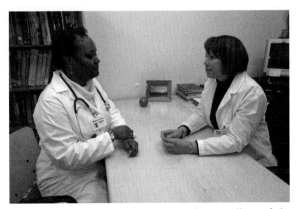

Fig. 14.2 Reaching a common understanding of the problem in a direct, tactful manner is the first step in conflict resolution.

Case Example: Mr. Pyle

Mr. Pyle is an 80-year-old bachelor who lives alone, in British Columbia. He has always been considered a proud and stately gentleman. He has a sister, 84 years old, who lives in Newfoundland. His only other living relatives, a nephew and his wife, also live in another province. Mr. Pyle recently changed his will so that it excludes his relatives, and he refuses to eat. When his neighbour brings in food, he eats it, but he won't fix anything for himself. He tells his neighbour that he wants to die and that he read in the paper about a man who was able to die in 60 days by not eating. As the visiting nurse assigned to his area, you have been asked to make a home visit and assess the situation.

If you wish to be successful, you must consider not only what is important to you in the discussion but what is important to the other person. Bear in mind the other person's viewpoint. The case featuring Mr. Pyle illustrates this idea.

The issue in this case example is not one of food intake alone. Any attempt to talk about why it is important for him to eat or expressing your point of view in this conflict immediately on arriving is not likely to be successful. Mr. Pyle's behaviour suggests that he feels that there is little to be gained by living any longer. His actions suggest further that he feels lonely and may be angry with his relatives. Once you correctly ascertain his needs and identify the specific issues, you may be able to help Mr. Pyle resolve his intrapersonal conflict. His wish to die may not be absolute or final because he eats when food is prepared by his neighbour, and he has not yet taken a deliberate, aggressive move to end his life. Each of these factors needs to be assessed and validated with him before an accurate nursing diagnosis can be made.

Organize Information

Plan your approach for a time and place conducive to collaborative discussion. Do not respond in the heat of the moment. Organizing your information and validating the appropriateness of your intervention with a knowledgeable person who is not directly involved is useful. Sometimes, it is wise to rehearse out loud what you are going to say. Remember to adhere to the principle of focusing on the conflict issue; avoid bringing up the past.

Manage Your Own Anxiety or Anger

Recognizing and controlling your own natural emotional response to upsetting behaviour may be one key factor in managing conflict. Refer to Chapter 12, Box 12.2, and use some immediate de-stressing behaviours, such as taking three deep breaths. Conflict produces anxiety and creates feelings of helplessness. You should see this discomfort as a signal that you need to deal with the situation. As mentioned earlier, part of an initial assessment of an interpersonal conflict includes recognition of the nurse's intrapersonal contribution to the conflict as well as that of the other person. It is not wrong to have ambivalent feelings about taking care of people with different lifestyles and values; however, you must acknowledge this to yourself. Remember that these feelings are about themselves, not about you.

Confronting the behaviour now should keep you from losing control later as the problem escalates. Most people experience some variation of a physical response when taking interpersonal risks. A useful strategy for managing your own anger is to vent to a friend, using "I" statements, as long as this does not become a complaining, whining session. Another strategy to manage your own anger is to take a break. A cooling-off period, doing something else for a few minutes or hours until your anger subsides, is acceptable. Take care that you re-engage, however, so that this does not become just an avoidance response style. Communicate with the correct person; do not take out your frustration on someone else. Focus on the one issue

involved. Try saying, "I would like to talk something over with you before the end of shift (or before I go)." Before you actually enter the person's room, do the following:

- Cool off. Wait until you can speak in a calm, friendly tone.
- Take a few deep breaths. Inhale deeply and count "1-2-3" to yourself. Hold your breath for a count of 2 and exhale, counting again to 3 slowly.
- Fortify yourself with positive statements (e.g., "I have a right to respect."). Anticipation is usually far worse than the reality.
- Defuse your own anxiety or anger before confronting the person.
- Focus discussion on one issue.

Time the Encounter

Timing is a determinant of success. Know specifically the behaviour you wish to have the person change. Make sure that they are capable, physically and emotionally, of changing the behaviour. Select a time when you both can discuss the matter privately, and use neutral ground, if possible. Select a time when the person is most likely to be receptive.

Timing is also important if an individual is very angry. The key to assertive behaviour is choice. Sometimes, it is better to allow someone to let off some "emotional steam" before engaging in conversation. In this case, the assertive thing to do is to choose silence accompanied by a calm, relaxed body posture. These nonverbal actions convey acceptance of feeling and a desire to understand. Validating the anger and reframing the conflict are useful steps. Comments such as, "I'm sorry you're feeling so upset" acknowledge the significance of the emotion being expressed without getting into the cause.

Put Situation Into Perspective

Do not play the blame game. Put the issue into perspective. How urgent is it to resolve this issue? How important is the issue? Will the issue be significant in a year? In 10 years? Will there be a significant situational change with resolution? This is another way of saying "pick your battles." Not every situation is worth expending your time and energy on. Remind yourself that anger may be caused by a problem in communicating; people you care for who are frustrated may become angry when they cannot make staff understand.

Use Therapeutic Communication Skills

Refer to the discussion on therapeutic communication in Chapter 11. Particularly useful is active listening. Really trying to understand what the person is upset about requires more skill than just listening to their words. Listening closely to what they are saying may help you understand their point of view. This understanding may decrease the stress. Repeat what the person said to make sure communication is crystal clear.

Nursing Communication Interventions: Following the CARE Steps

Riley (2017) adapted a CARE acronym to help nurses confront conflict situations. Refer to Box 14.3. Use the therapeutic nursing communication skills described in Chapter 11. Particularly useful in dealing with conflict situations is the use of active listening and paraphrasing.

C = Clarify

Choose direct, declarative sentences. Use objective words. Make sure verbal and nonverbal communication is congruent. Maintain an open stance and omit any gestures that might be interpreted as criticism, such as rolling your eyes or sighing heavily. Avoid mixed messages. One example of inappropriate communication might be found in the case of Larry, a staff nurse who works the 11 p.m. to 7 a.m. shift. Larry needs to get home to make sure his children get

on the bus to school. An older person routinely asks for a breathing treatment while Larry is reporting off. Instead of setting limits, Larry uses a soft voice and smiles as he tells her that he cannot be late in reporting off. Another example is Mr. Carl, the 29-year-old person who constantly makes sexual comments to a young student nurse. She laughs as she tells him to cut it out. Directly state the behaviour that is a problem.

A = Articulate why the behaviour is a problem

Acknowledge the feelings associated with the conflict, because it is emotions that escalate conflict.

R = Request a behaviour change

Avoid blaming. This would only make the person feel defensive or angry. Clearly request that they change the behaviour. Rather than just stating your position, try to use some objective criterion to examine the situation. Saying, "I understand your need to …, but the hospital has a policy intended to protect everyone we look after" might help you talk about the situation without escalating into anger. Psychiatric units have known rules against verbal abuse, violence such as throwing objects, violence against others,

---

BOX 14.3   Nursing Communication Interventions: Following the CARE Steps

| C | Clarify the behaviour that is a problem | Use communication skills, especially active listening skills, to identify issues of concern to the person.
• Use a calm tone and avoid conveying irritation.
• Paraphrase the person's message to be sure you understand.
• Ask for clarification if needed.
• Suggest simple interventions to decrease anxiety (deep breathing relaxation and guided imagery).
• Factually state the problem, focusing only on the current issue. |
| A | Articulate why the behaviour is a problem | Explain the institution's policies.
• Explain the limits of your role.
• Firmly sets limits. |

| R | Request a change in the problem behaviour | Work with the entire health team so all use the same approach to the person's demands.
• Develop a mutual health care plan: involve the person in care and setting goals.
• Review and re-evaluate whether you and the person have the same goals. |
| E | Evaluate progress | Provide education: explain all options, with outcomes.
• Verbalize incentives and withdrawal of privileges to modify unacceptable behaviour.
• Promote trust by providing immediate feedback. |

and so on. You can restate these "rules," together with their known violation outcomes (medication, seclusion, manual restraint), in a calm but firm voice.

There obviously will be situations in which such a thorough assessment is not possible, but each of these variables affects the success of the confrontation. For example, a person with dementia who makes a pass at a nurse might simply be expressing a need for affection in much the same way that a small child does; this behaviour needs a caring response rather than a reprimand. A 30-year-old person with all his cognitive faculties who makes a similar pass needs a more confrontational response.

Mutually generate some options for resolution. Focus on ways to resolve the problem by listing possible options. With the "fight-or-flight-or-freeze" response to stress, many people can respond to conflict only by either fighting or avoiding the problem. But brainstorming possible options and discussing pros and cons can turn the "fight" response into a more mutual "seeking a solution" mode of operations. Set mutual goals. Every member of the health care team needs to be "on the same page," presenting a similar approach to the person.

Readiness is vital. The behaviour might need to be confronted, but the manner in which the confrontation is approached and the amount of preparation or groundwork done beforehand may affect the outcome.

For longer-term behavioural problems, consider the use of a written contract, spelling out alternative behaviours, unacceptable ones, and their consequences.

E = Evaluate the conflict resolution

Encourage behaviour change by stating the outcomes, the positive consequences of changing, or the negative implications for failing to change. Evaluate the degree to which the interpersonal conflict has been resolved. Sometimes, a conflict cannot be resolved in a short time, but the willingness to persevere is a good indicator of a potentially successful outcome. Accepting small goals is useful when the attainment of a large goal is not possible. Your goal is open communication, with frequent feedback leading to successful problem solving.

For someone you are caring for, perhaps the strongest indicator of conflict resolution is the degree to which they are actively engaged in activities aimed at accomplishing tasks associated with the treatment goals. Here are some questions that you might want to address if modifications are necessary:

- What is the best way to establish an environment that is conducive to conflict resolution? What else needs to be considered?
- What self-care behaviours can be expected if these changes are made? These need to be stated in ways that are measurable.

Consider how to manage the case of Mr. Plotsky.

Case Example: Mr. Plotsky

Mr. Plotsky, age 29, has been employed for 6 years as a construction worker. About 4 weeks ago, while operating a forklift, he was struck by a train, leaving him with paraplegia. After 2 weeks in intensive care, he was transferred to a neurological unit. When staff members attempt to provide physical care, such as changing his position or getting him up in a chair, Mr. Plotsky throws things, curses angrily, and sometimes spits at the nurses. Staff members become very upset; several nurses have requested assignment changes. Some staff members try bribing him with food to encourage good behaviour; others threaten to apply restraints. The manager schedules a behavioural consultation meeting with a psychiatric nurse or clinical specialist in psychiatry. The immediate goal of this staff conference is to bring staff feelings out into the open and facilitate increased awareness of the staff's behavioural responses when confronted with Mr. Plotsky's behaviour. The outcome goal is to use a problem-solving approach to develop a behavioural care plan so all staff members respond to Mr. Plotsky in a consistent manner.

The Anger-Management Process: Nursing Behaviours to Avoid Violent Behaviour From Someone

Table 14.1 details nursing behaviours to avoid violence when you are dealing with an angry person or family member.

Maintain Self-Control

Once you identify that a person in a conflict situation may be so angry that they could be at risk for acting out or violent behaviour, your initial step is to maintain your self-control. Remember, you are modelling self-control. Early recognition is the key to preventing escalation. Illness generates feelings of powerlessness, where people you care for may feel they have little control. Anger is more powerful, so by focusing on their anger, they can feel more in control. This coping mechanism may work for them temporarily, but when you are the target, it can be difficult. Understanding this dynamic may help you to not take their behaviour personally.

To maintain the situation, you attempt to reduce strong emotion to a workable level by providing a neutral, accepting, interpersonal environment. Within this context, you can acknowledge their emotion as a necessary component of adaptation to life. You convey acceptance of the individual's legitimate right to have feelings. Say, "I'm not surprised that you are angry about ..." or simply stating, "I'm sorry you are hurting so much." Such statements acknowledge the person's uncomfortable emotions, convey an attitude of acceptance, and encourage them to express themselves. Once a feeling can be put into words, it becomes manageable because it has concrete boundaries. Remember, there is a continuum:

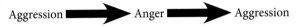

Aggression ➡️ Anger ➡️ Aggression

Talk About It

The second strategy in defusing a strong emotion is to talk the emotion through. For the other person, this someone is often the nurse. For the nurse, this might be a nursing supervisor or a trusted colleague. Unlike complaining, the purpose of talking the emotion through is to help the person bring the feeling up to a verbal level, which helps them to gain control. Verbalization helps the individual to connect with the personal feelings surrounding the incident.

Use Tension-Reducing Actions and Therapeutic Communication Skills

The third strategy is intervention. The specific needs expressed by the emotion suggest actions that might help the person deal with their emotion. Convey mutual respect and avoid any "put-down" type of comment. Sometimes, the most effective action is simply to listen. Active listening in a conflict situation involves concentrating on what the other person is upset about. Listening can be so powerful that it alone may reduce feelings of anxiety and frustration.

Physical activity can also reduce tension. For example, taking a walk can help control anxiety and defuse an emotionally tense situation. If the person is so upset that they constitute a danger, talk softly, in a calm tone; face the person but allow maximum space and an exit for yourself should it become necessary. Many hospitals and psychiatric units have a code word that is used to summon trained help.

TABLE 14.1	Five Steps for Nursing Behaviours with a Person Who Is Angry, to Avoid Violence	
Step	**Nurse**	**Person or Family Member Who Is Angry**
1. Control self	Appear calm, relax, and take two deep breaths. Remember to talk in low tone, monotone. Focus only on defusing anger or potential for violence. Remove any necklaces, cords around the neck (risk of being strangled). Do not respond to insults to self or team; do not become defensive. Avoid arguing, saying no, or hurrying.	Assess for unusually stressed individuals and potential for violence. Does the person appear out of control? If so, *leave!* Remember, showing your anxiety will increase the person's anxiety and anger. Reasoning with an individual who is enraged is impossible; focus on **de-escalation**. Devote only 3–5 minutes in attempting to de-escalate. (If it takes longer, it is not working.) Skip to the last step.
2. Nonthreatening body posture	Never touch a person who is angry; respect their personal space. Relax facial muscles; do not smile. Assume a neutral position, hands down by your sides, one foot in front of the other in a relaxed posture. Stay at same eye level; try to get the person to sit. If standing, do not position yourself face to face; be at an angle (so you can sidestep). Never turn your back. If standing, stay four times farther away than usual: do not crowd the person. Do not gesture; never point a finger. Always be closest to the door (so you can escape if necessary).	Allow the person to move around or pace (movement can help control stress). Allow the person to break eye contact; avoid a constant stare. Monitor the person's body position; watch for escalation in gestures.

(Continued)

TABLE 14.1 **Five Steps for Nursing Behaviours with a Person Who Is Angry, to Avoid Violence—cont'd.**

Step	Nurse	Person or Family Member Who Is Angry
3. Verbal de-escalation	Be nonconfrontational, nonjudgemental. Use the communication skills in Box 14.3 and therapeutic skills such as active listening and paraphrasing. Introduce yourself; call the person by name while making occasional eye contact. Communicate clearly and simply. Respond in a low, calm, gentle tone of voice; do not raise your voice. Be empathetic. Be neutral; avoid being defensive. Do not argue. Always be respectful. Do not dismiss any concern but always answer a request for information. Appeal to the person's cognitive rather than emotional self in trying to identify the underlying problem. Help the person verbalize their anger. Offer to work with the person to help them deal with the issue. Answer selectively, ignore generalized ranting comments, and focus on just giving the information requested. Set limits (empathize with the person's underlying feelings but not with their behaviour). State clearly that violence is *not* acceptable. Give the person options for alternative behaviour (e.g., "Let's take a break and have a [paper] cup of water"). If the person has a weapon, ask permission to move; do NOT be a hero.	Allow the person to ventilate some of their anger and discuss the problem. Help the person identify their own anger (e.g., "I notice you are clenching your fists and talking more loudly than usual. These are things people do when angry. Help me to understand."). Help the person identify the source of their anger. Have the person use a relaxation technique such as deep breathing. Give the person permission to feel angry, but set limits on acting out and violent behaviour (e.g., "It's okay to feel angry about … but not okay to act on it" or "It's natural to feel angry about … but throwing things isn't okay …"). Support the person's attempts to control their feelings. The person needs to know the consequences of their continued acting out behaviour.
4. Containment	Be aware of backup resources (orderlies, call to security, etc.). You can choose to leave. Use physical restraints if necessary. Place the person in seclusion or a locked isolation room if available. Use enforced chemical restraint (medication). Report all threats.	Implement agency violence code. Allow or ask the person to leave. Represent containment as a policy of the institution, not "I will restrain you." For some people with brain damage or a mental health disorder, it is appropriate to remove them from the source of their irritation to a calm environment, such as a locked room, to give them a time-out.
5. Debrief immediately: analyze and report	Reflect on the incident. What can be done to prevent a recurrence? Can you identify the trigger? Sometimes, too long a wait, too little information, or even an insensitive or hostile comment from staff can be a trigger.	After calming down, the person needs assistance to reflect on alternative ways of behaving and to plan for the future. Activate the person's support system.

Relaxation techniques may help the person regain control. Some can be taught quickly, such as deep breathing. Nurses frequently find the use of humour to be helpful. Humour can also be used as a means of reducing tension. To paraphrase a famous advice columnist, two of the most important words in a relationship are "I apologize." And this columnist recommended making amends immediately when you have made a mistake because "it is easier to eat crow while it's still warm." Is this advice easier to take (we will not say *swallow*) because it comes with a chuckle? Humour serves as an immediate tension reliever.

Containment

A priority is to maintain a safe environment for yourself and everyone receiving care at the agency. Isolation in a locked room is standard in many psychiatric facilities, as is the use of restraints and pharmaceutical tranquilizers. Sometimes, maintaining safety necessitates summoning agency resources, such as a critical incident response team, security, or the community police.

Evaluation: Immediate Debriefing

The final strategy is to do an evaluation of the effectiveness of responses. What was the trigger? Sometimes it was something simple, such as having had to wait too long to get information or hearing an insensitive or even hostile comment from a staff person. Your goal is to facilitate insight toward preventing future occurrences. It is not the responsibility of any nurse to help a person resolve all conflict—longstanding conflicts require more expertise to resolve; in such cases, refer them to the appropriate resource.

Each step in the process may need to be taken more than once and refined or revised as circumstances dictate.

Conflict Communication Skills

Be Assertive

Assertive communication means you convey objectives with directness but not with anger or frustration.

Demonstrate Respect

Responsible, assertive statements are made in ways that do not violate the rights of others or diminish their standing. They are conveyed by a relaxed, attentive posture and a calm, friendly tone of voice. Statements should be accompanied by the use of appropriate eye contact.

Clinical Encounters With People Who Are Being Demanding, Difficult

Every nurse encounters people who seem overly demanding of the nurse's limited time and resources. Although this may reflect a personality characteristic, most often, it is a sign of the person's anxiety. Box 14.1 describes behaviours that increase anger in others. Reflect on how to avoid these triggers. Conversely, ignoring inappropriate behaviour does not make it go away. For example in the case of Mr. Gow, discussed earlier, he is making inappropriate sexual suggestions. The nurse could have ineffectively responded by ignoring his verbal comments or by avoiding him. Instead, she responded assertively in a no-nonsense, professional manner. How would you handle such a situation? Try out some of the more therapeutic approaches outlined in Box 14.3 and Table 14.1. Usually, we tend to label people as "difficult to deal with" when our normal way of dealing with them has failed. Remember, we cannot change another's personality, but we can change the way we react to them.

Clinical Encounters With People Who Are Angry
Recognize Signs of Anger

You can expect to encounter people who express anger. This may take the form of refusal to comply with the treatment plan, withdrawal from any positive interaction with you, or display of hostile behaviours. Hostility may be verbalized, as when a person curses at you, or may even become physically violent. When you are dealing with a person who is behaving in a difficult manner, ask yourself what they are gaining from the violent behaviour. Some people have not learned how to communicate successfully, so they revert to behaviour that has gained them something in the past. For example, as children, they may have gotten needed attention only when they acted out in a negative way or when they pouted or sulked. Ask yourself whether a person who is behaving in a difficult way is being rewarded by becoming the focus of staff attention. Does such an individual only need to learn a more effective way of communicating? Remind yourself that usually a person's feelings centre on their disease or treatment and are not a reflection of their feelings about you. Do not take a person's frustration or anger personally.

Nonverbal clues to anger include grimacing, clenching of jaws or fists, turning away, and refusing to maintain eye contact. Verbal cues may, of course, include the use of an angry tone of voice, but they may also be disguised as witty sarcasm or as condescending or insulting remarks. To become comfortable in dealing with anger, the nurse must first become aware of their own reactions and learn not to feel threatened or respond in anger. Interventions include those listed in Table 14.1.

Help the Person Express Anger in an Acceptable Manner

Help people own their angry feelings by getting them to verbalize things that make them angry. Acknowledging their anger may prevent an expression of abusive ranting.

It is essential that you use empathetic statements or active listening to acknowledge their anger and maintain a non-threatening demeanor, *before* moving on to try to discuss an issue. Remember, your goal is to maintain safety while helping the person.

Defuse Hostility

Avoid responding to a person's anger by getting angry yourself. Verbal attacks follow certain rules; that is, the person behaving abusively expects you to react in specific ways. Usually, people respond by becoming aggressive and attacking back or by becoming defensive and intimidated. Keep your cool, using the strategies discussed earlier. Take a deep breath. Remember, if you lose control, you lose. If you become defensive, you lose. People acting abusively want to provoke confrontations as a means of controlling you.

- Use empathy in your communication. A person who is angry needs to have you acknowledge both the issue and their feelings about that issue. Only then can they begin to interact in a meaningful way. Deliberately begin to lower your voice and speak more slowly. When we get upset, we tend to speak quickly and use a higher tone of voice. If you do the opposite, the person may begin to mimic you and thus calm down.

Realistically Analyze the Current Situation That Is Disturbing the Person

- Be assertive in setting limits. If the behaviour persists, you need to assert limits, saying, for example, "Jim, I want to help you sort this out, but if you continue to curse at me and raise your voice, I'm going to have to leave. Which do you want?" Another response might be, "Yelling at me isn't going to get this worked out. I will not argue with you. Come back when you can talk calmly and I will try to help you."
- Help the person develop a plan to deal with the situation—for example, use techniques such as role-playing to help them express anger appropriately, using "I" statements such as, "I feel angry" rather than "You make me angry." Bringing behaviour up to a verbal level should help alleviate the need for acting out and other destructive behaviours.

Prevent Escalation of Conflict

In nurse–person confrontations, the recognition of "trigger" factors, which often lead to escalation, may help in prevention. Assess whether the person is intoxicated or disoriented, and whether there may be substance abuse. Using respectful, person-centred care approaches can help to prevent any escalation in interpersonal conflict. Hurt feelings or misunderstandings can quickly grow into a conflict. Keep the focus on the individual's *behaviour* rather than on

the person. If eye contact seems confrontational, then break eye contact. If the person is acting out by throwing or hitting, set limits: "No ___(e.g., hitting, spitting, cussing)___ behaviour is allowed here. Such behaviour is unacceptable." If you set limits, be sure to follow through. Ask the person to verbalize the anger (e.g., "Talk about how you feel instead of throwing things."). Use the strategies described in Table 14.1 for defusing conflict situations.

Strategies Useful in Clinical Encounters With People Who Are Violent

Your only goal is to lower the individual's level of rage and to protect them and yourself. Always leave yourself a clear exit.

- *Approach*. In an acute situation, you de-escalate and contain. If you are in danger of mortal harm, leave! Using "calming interventions" is recommended if there is no weapon.
- *Actions*. Table 14.1 lists some useful strategies for coping with individuals who are angry and potentially violent. Remember, your goal is to defuse the threat of violence if possible and to protect yourself and others from harm. Do not try for a rational discussion; just focus on calming interactions.
- *Reporting*. It has been estimated that a significant number of incidents go unreported; some say up to 80%. This is an international problem for nurses, and the ICN urges you to report all incidents of abuse or violence.
- *Analysis*. Post-incident analysis offers insight into how to prevent the next situation. Arbury et al. (2017) studied 12 workplace violence prevention training programs and found that most did not evaluate their effectiveness. They recommended collecting data, tracking incidents over time, and basing the evaluation on the behavioural theory used to set up the program. By doing this analysis, nurses can notify management of training gaps. Given health care workers experience physical and emotional consequences of violent incidents and people in your care also require physical and emotional safety, it is important to have the most effective, research-informed intervention possible.

Case Example: Sam

Sam, a man showing behaviours of extreme aggression, was admitted to a geriatric unit. Sam's behaviour ranged from bullying or pushing other people to noncompliance with his treatment. Staff tried setting clear limits and identifying specific negative outcomes, including restraints and medication, without success. They informed him that violence was not acceptable and at times had to move themselves from a potentially harmful situation. They knew the behaviour was not "evil" and was a result of his illness. They also were very aware that escalating conflict could be a threat to Sam and to themselves. They kept trying to be positive and eventually they were successful in their interventions, when they had a consistent response by all staff members and used a written contract for each of his unacceptable behaviours. Outcomes were specifically stated for both negative behaviours (restrictions) and positive, acceptable behaviours (rewards with his favourite activities) (Starcher, 1999).

An additional strategy for helping nurse–person problem interactions is the staff-focused consultation. Consider the following situation. Students are particularly prone to feeling rebuffed when they first encounter negative feedback from a person in their care. Support from staff, instructors, and peers, coupled with efforts to understand the underlying reasons for the person's feelings, can help you to resist the trap of avoiding the relationship. To develop these ideas further, you need to practise.

Defusing Potential Conflicts When You Are Providing Home Health Care

Recognizing potential situations that lend themselves to conflict is, of course, an important initial step. Caregivers have been shown to experience conflict through incompatible pressures suffered between caregiver demands and demands from their other roles, such as parenting their children or maintaining employment. In addition to this inter-role conflict, caregivers suffer pressures when a nurse comes into the home to participate in the care of a relative who is ill. A Canadian study of home health nurses and family caregivers of older relatives identified four evolving stages in the nurse–caregiver relationship. The initial stage is "worker–helper," with the nurse providing care to the ill person and the family helping. Next comes "worker-worker," when the nurse begins teaching the needed care skills to family members. Third is "nurse as manager; family as worker," as the family members learn needed care skills. The final stage, "nurse as nurse for family caregiver," occurs as the family member becomes exhausted (Butt, 2000). A source of conflict for nurses was the dual expectation of the family that the nurse would provide not only care for the identified person but also relief for the exhausted primary caregiver. When the nurse operated as manager and treated the caregiver as worker, the discrepancy in expectations and values resulted in increased tension in the relationship. Discussion of role expectations is essential. Solli and Hvalvik (2019), using qualitative research, asked nurses who worked with caregivers via telehealth in Norway how they managed tensions with at-home caregivers. The nurses admitted to the tension and provided strategies like teaching the caregivers to develop a sense of security by establishing mastery of their lives and using empathy. Because of the high cost of providing direct care to people with chronic conditions, home health nurses may be expected to quickly shift to teaching the necessary skills to family members. Although this shift in responsibility may result in a reduction of expensive professional time, it should not compromise commitment to the family.

SUMMARY

Conflict represents a struggle between opposing thoughts, feelings, or needs. It can be intrapersonal in nature—deriving from within a particular individual—or interpersonal, when it represents a clash between two or more people. This chapter focused on conflict between nurses and people in their care and their families.

All conflicts have certain features in common: a concrete content problem issue and relationship issues arising from the process of expressing the conflict. Generally, intrapersonal conflicts stimulate feelings of emotional discomfort. Strategies to defuse strong emotion were highlighted. Most interpersonal conflicts involve some threat, either to one's sense of power to control an interpersonal situation or to ways of thinking about the self. Giving up ineffective behaviour patterns in conflict situations is difficult because such patterns are generally perceived as safer because they are familiar.

Behavioural responses to conflict situations fall into five styles. In the past, nurses most commonly chose avoidance. However, this chapter describes other strategies (e.g., assertion) that have been more successfully used by nurses to manage person–nurse conflicts. Assertive behaviours range from making a simple statement, directly and honestly, about one's beliefs, to taking a very strong, confrontational stand about what will and will not be tolerated.

The principles of conflict management were described. To apply conflict management principles, you need to identify your own conflictive feelings or reactions. For internal conflict, feelings usually have to be put into words and related to the issue at hand before the meaning of the conflict becomes understandable. In conflict between the nurse and person in their care, you need to think through the possible causes of the conflict as well as your own feelings before making a response. To resolve these kinds of conflict, you need to use "I" statements and respond assertively. This chapter also discussed workplace violence and strategies to maintain or restore a safe environment.

ETHICAL DILEMMA

What Would You Do?

You are caring for Kim, born at the gestational age of 24 weeks in a rural hospital and transferred this morning to your neonatal intensive care unit. Today her father arrives on the unit. Seeing you taking a blood sample from one of the many intravenous lines attached to Kim, he yells at you to "Stop poking at her! What are you trying to prove by keeping her alive? Turn off those machines." This is both a communication problem and an ethics problem. How do you respond to his anger?

QUESTIONS FOR REVIEW AND DISCUSSION

1. Select a tone and pitch listed in Simulation Exercise 14.2. Describe how the tone and pitch affect a conflict situation.
2. Using the knowledge gained in this chapter and the behaviours listed in Box 14.1, design a response where you de-escalate a conflict.

REFERENCES

Arbury, S., Zankowski, D., Lipscomb, J. et al. (2017). Workplace violence training programs for health care workers: An analysis of program elements. *Workplace Health & Safety*, 65(6), 266–272. https://doi.org/10.1177/2165079916671534.

Avander, K., Heikki, A., Bjersa, K. et al. (2016). Trauma nurses' experience of workplace violence and threats: Short and long term consequences in a Swedish setting. *Journal of Trauma Nursing*, 23(2), 51–57.

Brann, M., & Hartley, D. (2016). Nursing student evaluation of NIOSH workplace violence prevention for nurses online course. *Journal of Safety Research*, 1–7. https://doi.org/10.1016/jsr2016.12.003.

Butt, G. (2000). Nurses and family caregivers of elderly relatives engaged in 4 evolving types of relationships. *Evidence-Based Nursing*, 3, 134.

Campbell, C. L., Burg, M. A., & Gammonley, D. (2015). Measures for incident reporting of patient violence and aggression towards healthcare providers: A systematic review. *Aggression and Violent Behavior*, 25, 314–322.

Canadian Association of Schools of Nursing. (2015). *National Nursing Education Framework: Final Report*. https://www.casn.ca/2016/09/national-nursing-education-framework/.

Canadian Centre for Occupational Health and Safety. (2021). Workplace Stress – General. OSH Answers Fact Sheet. https://www.ccohs.ca/oshanswers/psychosocial/stress.html.

Canadian Nurses Association & Canadian Federation of Nurses Unions. (2014). *Joint Position Statement: Workplace Violence and Bullying*. https://cna-aiic.ca/~/media/cna/page-content/pdf-en/Workplace-Violence-and-Bullying_joint-position-statement.pdf.

Cheng, F. K. (2016). Mediation skills for conflict resolution in nursing education. *Nurse Education in Practice*, 15, 310–313.

College of Nurses of Ontario. (2018). *Practice guideline conflict prevention and management*. https://www.cno.org/globalassets/docs/prac/47004_conflict_prev.pdf.

Crisis Prevention Institute. (2017). *Ten crisis prevention tips*. https://www.crisisprevention.com/en-CA/Blog/CPI-s-Top-10-De-Escalation-Tips-Revisited

Dwarswaard, J., & van de Bovenkamp, H. (2015). Self-management support: A qualitative study of ethical dilemmas experienced by nurses. *Patient Education and Counseling*, 98, 1131–1136.

Hahn, S., Muller, M., Hantikainen, V. et al. (2013). Risk factors associated with patient and visitor violence in general hospitals: Results of a multiple regression analysis. *International Journal of Nursing Studies*, 50, 374–385.

Haugvaldstad, M. J., & Husum, T. L. (2016). Influence of staff emotional reactions on the escalation of patient aggression in mental health care. *International Journal of Law and Psychiatry*, 49, 130–137.

Hersch, R. K., Cook, R. F., Deitz, D. K. et al. (2016). Reducing nurses' stress: A randomized controlled trial of a web-based stress management program for nurses. *Applied Nursing Research*, 32, 18–25.

House of Commons Canada. (2019). *Violence facing health care workers in Canada: A report of the Standing Committee on Health*. 42 Parliament, 1st Session. https://www.ourcommons.ca/Content/Committee/421/HESA/Reports/RP10589455/hesarp29/hesarp29-e.pdf.

International Council of Nurses (ICN). (2006). *Violence: A worldwide epidemic*. www.icn.ch/nursing-policy/position-statements.

Llor-Esteban, B., Sanchez-Munoz, M., Ruiz-Hernandes, J. A. et al. (2017). User violence towards nursing professionals in mental health services and emergency units. *The European Journal of Psychology Applied to Legal Context*, 9(1), 33–40. https://doi.org/10.1016/j.ejpal.2016.06.002.

Longo, J., Cassidy, L., & Sherman, R. (2016). Charge nurses' experience with horizontal violence: Implications for leadership development. *The Journal of Continuing Education in Nursing*, 47(11), 493–499.

McElhaney, R. (1996). Conflict management in nursing administration. *Nursing Management*, 27(3), 49–50.

NICE Guideline #10. (2015). *Violence and aggression*. British Psychological Society.

Nowrouzi, B., & Huynh, V. (2016). Citation analysis of workplace violence: A review of the top 50 annual and lifetime cited articles. *Aggression & Violent Behavior*, 28, 21–28.

Phillips, J. P. (2016). Workplace violence. *New England Journal of Medicine*, 374, 1661–1669.

Riley, J. B. (2017). *Communication in nursing* (8th ed.). Mosby/Elsevier Inc..

Sayer, M. M., McNeese-Smith, D., Leach, L. S. et al. (2012). An educational intervention to increase 'speaking-up' behaviors in nurses and improve patient safety. *Journal of Nursing Care Quality, 27*(2), 154–160. https://www.patientsafetyinstitute.ca/en/toolsResources/Creating-a-Safe-Space-Psychological-Safety-of-Healthcare-Workers/Documents/Manuscript%20Documents/1_Survey%20of%20Healthcare%20Providers%20Perceptions.pdf.

Solli, H., & Hvalvik, S. (2019). Nurses striving to provide caregiver with excellent support and care at a distance: A qualitative study. *BMC Health Serv Res, 19*, 893. https://doi.org/10.1186/s12913-019-4740-7.

Starcher, S. (1999). Sam was an emotional terrorist. *Nursing, 99*(2), 40–41.

Waschgler, K., Ruiz-Hernandez, J. A., Llor-Esteban, B. et al. (2013). Patients' aggressive behaviours towards nurses: Development and psychometric properties of the hospital aggressive behaviour scale-users. *Journal of Advanced Nursing, 69*(6), 1418–1427.

Watkins, L. E., Sippel, L. M., Pietrzak, R. H. et al. (2017). Co-occuring aggression and suicide attempt among veterans entering residential treatment for PTSD: The role of PTSD symptom clusters and alcohol misuse. *Journal of Psychiatric Research, 87*, 8–14.

Wei, C., Chiou, S., Chien, L. et al. (2016). Workplace violence against nurses: Prevalence and association with hospital organizational characteristics and health-promotion efforts: Cross-sectional study. *International Journal of Nursing Studies, 56*, 63–70.

World Health Organization. (2012). *Workplace violence.* Author. http://who.int/violence.injury.prevention/injury/work9/en/print.html.

15

Communication Strategies for Health Promotion and Disease Prevention

Olive Yonge
Originating US chapter by *Elizabeth C. Arnold*

OBJECTIVES

At the end of the chapter, the reader will be able to:
1. Define concepts related to health promotion and disease prevention.
2. Identify national agendas for health promotion and disease prevention.
3. Specify relevant conceptual frameworks for health promotion actions.
4. Apply health promotion and disease prevention strategies for individuals.
5. Apply health promotion and disease prevention strategies at the community level.
6. Explain the role of health literacy in health promotion and disease prevention strategies.

We are starting this chapter with a declaration that sets the tone for the chapter. In 2010, the Government of Canada made the following declaration:

"Creating a Healthier Canada: Making Prevention a Priority.

Through this Declaration on Prevention and Promotion, we [the Ministers of Health and of Health Promotion/ Healthy Living of Canada] express our view that the promotion of health and the prevention of disease, disability and injury are a priority and necessary to the sustainability of the health system" (Public Health Agency of Canada [PHAC], 2010).

This chapter focuses on the role of communication as a key nursing strategy in achieving specific health promotion and disease prevention goals. The chapter considers adverse psychosocial determinants of health as underlying challenges to achieving consistent, high-quality health promotion and disease prevention outcomes. Applications of communication strategies are designed to help individuals and targeted populations achieve a better health quality of life through education, and recommended lifestyle changes are presented.

BASIC CONCEPTS

Health care reform initiatives have created profound changes in how care is delivered, to whom it is delivered, and where it is delivered. The Declaration also addresses how governments must work together with private, nonprofit, municipal, academic, and community sectors, and with First Nations, Inuit, and Métis peoples, to improve health, reduce health disparities, and build and influence the physical, social, and economic conditions that will promote health and wellness and prevent illness so that Canadians can enjoy good health for years to come (PHAC, 2010).

Health promotion and disease prevention, with special attention to the underlying causes of a health problem, is increasingly recognized as a reimbursable, essential component of comprehensive health care. Evidence of the nation's commitment to health promotion and disease prevention includes new insurance reimbursement for preventive physicals and action plan generation for older people. Assisting people to practise positive health behaviours helps individuals prevent or delay chronic disease, functional decline, and related disability.

Definitions

Health is considered a fundamental human right, intimately tied to a nation's social and economic development (World Health Organization [WHO], 1997). **Health promotion** emphasizes "being able to function normally, experiencing well-being, and having a healthy lifestyle" (Fagerlind et al., 2010, p. 104). Factors such as genetics, environment, economics, and social circumstances influence health status. Some population groups are at higher risk for developing chronic health problems because of financial, personal, family, or environmental circumstances. Other factors include the availability of health services and new research findings—even opportunity and luck can enhance a person's ability to achieve optimal health status and well-being. Well-developed social skills, strong family bonds, consistent parenting skills, and active involvement in social institutions such as school, faith-based institutions, and the community provide more opportunities for health promotion and disease prevention strategies.

Health promotion is defined as "the process of enabling individuals to take control over their health" (WHO, 1986). Health-promoting activities can include the following:

- Health education
- Preventive health services
- Advocacy and development of public policies
- Safeguarding environmental health
- Community-based education in schools and workplaces
- Population-based targeted strategies for vulnerable populations
- Media outreach in the form of ads and blogs.

DISEASE PREVENTION

Disease prevention is the term used to describe actions designed to reduce or eliminate the onset, progression, complications, or recurrence of chronic disease. The goal of disease prevention is to help individuals "avoid the occurrence of a disease, disorder, or injury, to slow the progression of detectable disease and/or reduce its consequences" (WHO, 1997).

Relevant terminology includes risk and protective factors. *Risk and protective factors* are defined as personal and environmental characteristics that increase the probability of having a health problem *(risk factor)* or decrease the probability of its occurrence or progression *(protective factor)*. If a person is obese, eats too many carbohydrates, and leads a sedentary life, the combined risk factors can increase the probability of having a heart attack. Causal risk factors and social determinants of health play a major role in the onset and progression of emergent chronic disorders (PHAC, 2017; Canadian Nurses Association [CNA], 2018).

Some risk factors are modifiable. People with prediabetes can minimize progression to full symptoms through diet, regular exercise, and leading a balanced life. Smoking, overeating, and excessive alcohol consumption are associated with a range of chronic disorders, including cancer. It has been shown that aggressive reduction of potential threats to full health and well-being is effective. Regular health screenings can identify emerging treatable health problems such as osteoporosis, high blood pressure, and glaucoma. Individuals with a genetic predisposition to chronic diseases such as obesity, heart disease, arthritis, or diabetes can reduce the impact of inherited risk factors by actively embracing habits of healthy eating, adequate sleep, regular exercise, and an active lifestyle. The promotion of healthy behaviours involves more than just buzzwords. Many evidence-informed studies attest to the effectiveness of promoting health and well-being.

Protective factors are defined as circumstances, resources, and personal characteristics that delay the emergence of chronic disease or lessen its impact. Although protective factors do not guarantee a life free of serious illness or early death, they play a significant role in helping people improve their health and quality of life. Examples of protective factors include developing a healthy lifestyle, getting daily exercise, eating a healthy diet, having annual medical checkups, increasing the number of available support systems, obtaining health insurance, and so on. Health education, social marketing, and screening services help people to become aware of health risk factors.

Lifestyle

Lifestyle is defined as the typical way of life of an individual, group, or culture. The term was originally used by Austrian psychologist Alfred Adler. Components of a healthy lifestyle include eating healthy meals, staying active with adequate exercise, getting adequate sleep, managing stress, building supportive relationships, and nurturing one's spirit. Ideally, building a healthy lifestyle begins in childhood. As Frederick Douglass noted years ago, "It is easier to build strong children than to repair broken men" (Brainyquote.com, n.d.). Nurses serve as role models. You will have more credibility in advocating for healthy lifestyles if you practise what you preach.

Social Determinants of Health

The term **social determinants of health** defines a wide range of contextual factors influencing the health and well-being of individuals and communities. These social, economic, religious, and political factors are embedded at the level of the community as well as the larger society. They have a significant effect on health and well-being. *Social determinants of health* refer to a specific group of social and economic factors related to income, education, and employment. Experiences of discrimination, racism, and historical trauma are important social determinants of health for certain groups such as Indigenous peoples, LGBTQ2S+ and Black Canadians (Government of Canada, 2020a; PHAC, 2016; CNA, 2018).

Although each person enters the world with a distinct set of constitutional factors (size, gender, intellect, and personality), each grows up within social and community networks and, over time, incorporates the social values of those networks. One's environment interacts with personal factors to influence, enhance, or limit one's health behaviours. Larger social community systems create roles and expectations that further shape and modify the individual's health behaviours (Grey, 2017).

Health Inequity

The term *health inequities* describes fundamental differences in adverse health outcomes and lost opportunities to achieve optimal health and well-being as it relates to demographics, income, education, and access. (For further information on social determinants of health and health inequalities, visit www.canada.ca › Health Science, Research and Data › Determinants of Health › Social Determinants of Health and Health Inequalities.)

Social determinants associated with health disparities include lack of adequate health insurance, social isolation, cultural factors, access and availability of services, finances, lack of knowledge or education, food or job security, language barriers, health literacy, and poverty. Social determinants critically affect health, morbidity, and mortality. This means interventions for individuals or populations must be holistic. The Centers for Disease Control and Prevention (CDC, 2016) identify health disparities as a fundamental health concern requiring immediate, concentrated attention. The elimination of health disparities is a primary objective of our public health agenda (CDC, 2016).

Well-Being

Health promotion activities incorporate the WHO concept of a close connection between health and well-being. **Well-being** is defined as an individual's personal life satisfaction in terms of six dimensions: intellectual, physical, emotional, social, occupational, and spiritual (Government of Canada, 2019). People can experience well-being as being at peace with themselves. Being peaceful helps a person feel protected from stress and more resilient (Hanson, 2016). Fundamental changes in health habits and modifications in lifestyle typically improve health and well-being. Fig. 15.1 displays critical elements for maintaining health and well-being. A healthy lifestyle, a sense of purpose and supportive resources lead to health and well-being. Eighty-two point one percent of Canadian adults (18+ years) are satisfied with life every day or almost every day (Orpana et al., 2016).

GLOBAL AND NATIONAL HEALTH PROMOTION AGENDAS

Improving the quality of health promotion and disease prevention is a national and global health care reform

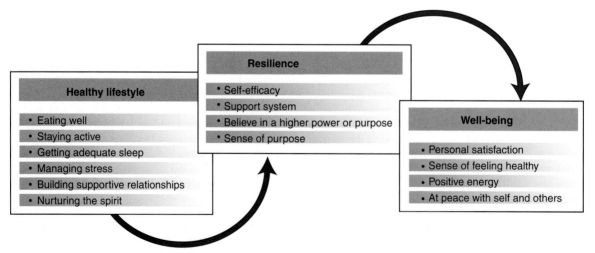

Fig. 15.1 Critical elements for maintaining health and well-being

initiative. As you read through this section, note the similar themes in virtually all national and global agenda goals. Strong recommendations appear about the need to explore the close interaction between personal, environmental, and social determinants of health and well-being and the provision of equal opportunity for high-quality health care.

Canada has a rich history in the field of health promotion. In 1974, the Lalonde Report, *A New Perspective on the Health of Canadians*, showed Canadians there were multiple influences on health (Lalonde, 1974). This was followed in 1986 by the WHO Ottawa Charter for Health Promotion and Epp's Achieving Health for All: A Framework for Health Promotion (Health and Welfare Canada, 1986). These reports established the principles of health promotion and proposed strategic frameworks for action. The WHO's *Ottawa Charter for Health Promotion* documented the essential prerequisites and resources needed for health promotion as "peace, shelter, education, food, income, a stable ecosystem, sustainable resources, social justice, and equity" (1986). The charter identified the prerequisites for improving health as follows:

1. Advocacy for health
2. Enabling equal opportunities and resources for people to achieve health
3. Mediation and coordinated action shared by community groups, health service agencies, and governments, targeted toward the pursuit of health

For Canada, our future lies in affirming and sharing the vision and values of health promotion:

- Affirming and sharing the vision and values of health promotion
- Emphasizing the creation of alliances across and between sectors
- Honing our knowledge, skills and capacity to improve health
- Emphasizing political commitment and the development of healthy public policies
- Strengthening our communities
- Ensuring that health systems reform promotes health both inside and outside the health care system (Canadian Public Health Association [CPHA], n.d.)

The Jakarta Declaration on Health Promotion is a global initiative that recommends the following to enhance health and well-being (WHO, 1997):

- Building healthy public policy
- Creating supportive environments for health
- Strengthening community action for health
- Developing personal skills
- Reorienting health services

Kushner and Sorensen (2013) suggest that "lifestyle medicine" may represent a new disciplinary approach for the management of chronic illness and disease prevention.

THEORY-BASED FRAMEWORKS

Theory frameworks for health promotion examine how people make choices and decisions about their health. Pender's Health Promotion Model, Prochaska's Transtheoretical Model, and Bandura's social learning theory are useful frameworks to guide health promotion strategies.

Pender's Health Promotion Model

A person's capacity to absorb and use health promotion information depends to a large degree on what people believe about their health, the seriousness of their health conditions, and the extent to which their personal actions can produce positive outcomes. Health promotion interventions target behavioural change. Nurses use Pender's revised health belief model to understand what motivates people to engage in personal health behaviours (Pender et al., 2011). The model expands on an earlier health belief model developed by Rosenstock and associates in the 1950s. This model (Fig. 15.2) proposes that a person's willingness to engage in health promotion behaviours is best understood by examining their personal beliefs about the nature and seriousness of a health condition and their capacity to influence its outcome.

Pender's model identifies perceived benefits, barriers, and ability to take action related to health and well-being as important components of people's health decision making. These dynamics act as internal or external "cues to action," which influence a person's decision to engage in health promoting activities. Cues to action include required school immunizations, interpersonal reminders, past experiences with the health care system, the mass media, and ethnic approval.

Case Example

Mary Nolan knows that walking will help diminish her risk for developing osteoporosis, but the threat of potentially having this problem in her 60s is not sufficient to motivate her to take action in her 40s. Mary does not feel any signs or symptoms of the disease, and it is easier to maintain a sedentary lifestyle. To create the most appropriate learning conditions and types of teaching strategies, the nurse will have to understand Mary's value system and other factors that influence Mary's readiness to learn. To remain healthy, Mary will have to effect positive change in her health habits.

Simulation Exercise 15.1 provides practice in applying Pender's model to common health problems.

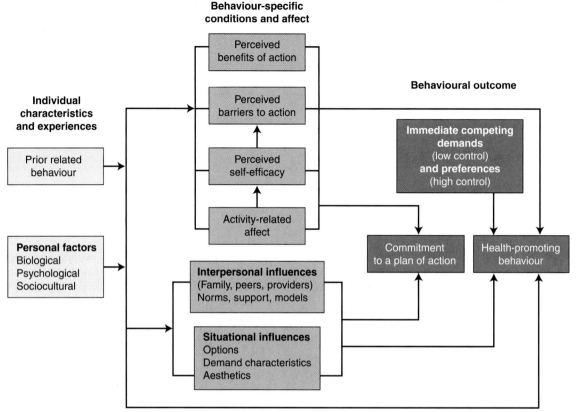

Fig. 15.2 Revised Health Promotion Model. From Pender, N., Murdaugh, C., & Parsons, M. (2011). Health promotion in nursing practice (6th ed., p. 45). Prentice Hall.

SIMULATION EXERCISE 15.1 Motivational Interviewing Using Pender's Model

Purpose

To help students understand the value of the health promotion model in assessing and promoting healthy lifestyles interview (CPHA, n.d.)

Procedure

1. Interview a person in the community about their perception of a common health problem (e.g., heart disease, high cholesterol, osteoporosis, breast or prostate cancer, obesity, or diabetes).
2. Record the person's answers in written diagram form, following Pender's model of health promotion. Identify the behaviour-specific thoughts and feelings that would best fit the person's situation.

3. Share your findings with your classmates, either in the general class or in a group of four to six students with a scribe to share common themes with the larger class.

Discussion

1. Were you surprised by anything the person said, their perception of the problem or interpretation of its meaning?
2. As you compare your findings with other classmates, do common themes emerge?
3. How could you use the information you obtained from this exercise in future health care situations?

Transtheoretical Model of Change

Prochaska's Transtheoretical Model is an evidence-informed model used to explore a person's motivational readiness to intentionally change their health habits (Prochaska & Norcross, 2013). The model identifies stages of readiness ranging from lack of acknowledgment of a problem to taking and maintaining constructive actions to correct unhealthy behaviours. Table 15.1 presents Prochaska's model with suggested approaches for each stage and corresponding sample statements.

In the *precontemplation* stage, a person either does not see a health problem (even though it may be obvious to others) or does not have any intention of modifying it in the foreseeable future. The *contemplation* stage is characterized by awareness of a problem. The person is thinking of change but is still ambivalent and lacks a strong commitment to take action. Prochaska and Norcross (2013) refer to contemplation as "knowing where you want to go but not being quite ready to go there" (p. 460). In this *preparation* stage, the person begins to take small tentative steps toward changing poor health habits but is not fully committed to consistent action. An important component in the preparation stage is the setting of goals and priorities. A strong commitment to change and taking consistent definitive actions to make behavioural changes a reality identify the *action* stage.

A *maintenance* stage, in which people stabilize and consolidate gains achieved during the action stage, follows. People can easily relapse and may need to recycle through previous stages several times before a new health behaviour is firmly established. Relapses are treated as temporary setbacks that provide information about triggers and high-risk situations people need to avoid.

TABLE 15.1 Prochaska's Stages of Change With Suggested Approaches and Sample Statements Applied to Alcoholism

Stage	Characteristic Behaviours	Suggested Approach	Sample Statement
Precontemplation	Person does not think there is a problem; is not considering the possibility of change	Raise doubt; give informational feedback to raise awareness of a problem and health risks	"Your lab tests show liver damage. These tests can be predictive of serious health problems and premature death."
Contemplation	Person thinks there may be a problem; is thinking about change; goes back and forth between concern and unconcern	Tip the balance; allow open discussion of pros and cons of changing behaviour; build motivation for change; help the person justify a positive commitment	"It sounds as though you think you may have a drinking problem but are not sure you are experiencing an alcohol problem. What would your life be like without alcohol?"
Preparation	Person decides there is a problem and is willing to make a change: "I guess I do need to stop drinking."	Help the person choose the best course of action for resolving the problem.	"What kinds of changes will you need to make to stop drinking? Most people find Alcoholics Anonymous (AA) helpful as a support. Have you heard of them?"
Action	Person engages in concrete actions to effect needed change	Help the person take active steps to resolve health problem; review progress; give feedback	"I am impressed that you went to two AA meetings this week and have not had a drink either. What has this been like for you?"
Maintenance	Person perseveres with positive behavioural change	Help the person identify and use strategies to sustain progress; point out positive changes; accept temporary setbacks and use steps from preparation phase if needed	"It's hard to let go of old habits, but you've been abstinent for 3 months now, and your liver tests are significantly improved."

SIMULATION EXERCISE 15.2   Assessing Readiness Using Prochaska's Model

Purpose

To identify elements in teaching that can promote readiness, using Prochaska's model

Procedure

Identify as many specific answers as possible to the following questions:

1. Patrick drinks four to six beers every evening. Last year, he lost his job. He has a troubled marriage and few friends. Patrick does not consider himself a person experiencing an alcohol problem and blames his chaotic marriage for his need to drink. There is a strong family history of alcoholism. What kinds of information might help Patrick want to learn more about his condition?

2. Lily has just learned she has breast cancer. Although there is a good chance that surgery and chemotherapy will help her, she is scared to commit to the process and has even expressed suicidal thoughts. What kinds of health teaching strategies and information might help Lily become ready to learn about her condition?

3. Shawn has just been diagnosed with epilepsy. He is ashamed to tell his friends and teachers about his condition. Shawn is considering breaking up with his girlfriend because of his newly diagnosed illness. How would you use health teaching to help Shawn cope more effectively with his illness?

Simulation Exercise 15.2 provides an opportunity to work with Prochaska's Transtheoretical Model.

Social Learning Theory

Bandura's (1997) contribution to the study of health promotion is the concept of self-efficacy. *Self-efficacy* is defined as a personal belief in one's ability to execute the actions required to achieve a goal. It represents a powerful mediator of behaviour and behavioural change.

Self-efficacy and motivation are reciprocal processes. Increased self-efficacy strengthens motivation, which in turn increases an individual's capacity to complete the learning task.

Bandura considers learning to be a social process. He identifies three sets of motivating factors that promote the learning necessary to achieve a predetermined goal: physical motivators, social incentives, and cognitive motivators. Physical motivators can be internal, such as memory of previous discomfort or a symptom that the person cannot ignore. Social incentives, such as praise and encouragement, increase self-esteem and give the person reason to continue learning. Bandura refers to a third set of motivators as cognitive motivators, describing them as thought processes associated with change.

In the following case example, the nurse combines the concept of a physical motivator with a social incentive related to something the person values (his grandson) and relates the process to the desired outcome. The intervention is designed to help Francis recognize how changes in his health behaviour can not only improve his health and well-being but also give him a social outlet that could be important to him.

Case Example

Nurse: "I'm worried that you are continuing to smoke because it affects your breathing. There is nothing you can do about the damage to your lungs that's already there, but if you stop smoking it can help preserve the healthy tissue you still have (physical motivator) and you won't have as much trouble breathing. I bet your grandson would appreciate it if you could breathe better and be able to play with him (social incentive)." Francis gives up smoking and notices that he is coughing less; this new perceptual knowledge will act as an internal cognitive motivator for him to remain abstinent.

DISEASE PREVENTION

Disease prevention frameworks are concerned with identifying modifiable risk and protective factors associated with specific diseases and mental disorders. Nurses use case-finding strategies to identify risk factors in individuals, families, and communities. The goal of prevention is to promote healthy living so all can be more productive and independent (PHAC, 2015). Three tiers of prevention—primary, secondary, and tertiary—represent a continuum of disease prevention focus.

- *Primary prevention* strategies target modifiable risk factors, with suggestions for health promoting activities to facilitate a healthy lifestyle—for example, promoting exercise and a healthy diet in order to prevent obesity and diabetes. Other examples include immunizations;

low-cost flu shots; safe-sex counselling; smoking cessation; the use of car seats, seat belts, and motorcycle helmets; and bans on texting while driving. Advocacy for these health protections is easily incorporated into ordinary nursing care.

- *Secondary prevention* strategies focus on early disease detection through regular health screenings for conditions such as prostate cancer, osteoporosis, and diabetes; regular mammograms and pap smears for women; periodic colonoscopies; and blood pressure screenings. Individuals with known risk factors such as family history, high cholesterol, elevated blood sugar, high blood pressure, and advanced age should be screened

periodically. With early case finding, the emergence or course of a chronic disease can be modified to allow a better quality of life. Screening for mental health problems during the course of primary care visits can help detect undiagnosed depression, anxiety, and substance abuse.

- *Tertiary prevention* strategies focus on minimizing the damaging effects of a disease or injury once it has occurred. The goal is to help people achieve a good quality of life regardless of their health circumstances.

Simulation Exercise 15.3 provides an opportunity to look at the role of potential risk factors in your personal health profile.

SIMULATION EXERCISE 15.3   Developing a Health Profile

Purpose

To help students understand the relationship between lifestyle health assessment factors and related health goals, from a personal perspective

Procedure

Out-of-class assignment: Develop a personal health profile in which you do the following:

1. Assess your own personal risk factors related to each of the following:
   a. Family history risk factors (diabetes, cardiovascular disease, cancer, osteoporosis)
   b. Diet and nutrition
   c. Exercise habits
   d. Weight
   e. Alcohol and drug use
   f. Safer sex practices

g. Perceived level of stress
h. Health screening tests: cholesterol, blood pressure, blood sugar

2. Identify unhealthy behaviours or risk factors
3. Develop a personalized action plan to identify strategies to address areas that need strengthening
4. Identify any barriers that might prevent you from achieving your personal goals

Discussion

1. In small groups, discuss findings that you feel comfortable sharing with others.
2. Get input from others about ways to achieve health-related goals.
3. In the larger group, discuss how doing this exercise can inform your practice related to teaching about lifestyle changes and health promotion.

⟫ DEVELOPING AN EVIDENCE-INFORMED PRACTICE

Background

It is very expensive for employers to have employees absent from work. One strategy to promote health among employees is to offer them workplace health promotion and wellness programs. At this time, it is not known how effective these programs are. The main purpose of this study was to use an intervention mapping approach to develop a workplace health promotion and wellness program.

Methods

The research was conducted at a large, international financial services company. Data were collected via a qualitative synthesis based on an intervention mapping

methodology. The researchers used systematic reviews of theoretical models for changing behaviour and stakeholder experience. This was then systematically operationalized into a program using discussion groups and consensus among experts and stakeholders.

Results

The top health problem impacting the workplace was mental health disorders. Depression and stress were the first and second highest cause of productivity loss, respectively. A multipronged program with detailed action steps was developed and directed at key stakeholders and health conditions. For mental health disorders, regular sharing focus groups, social networking, monthly

DEVELOPING AN EVIDENCE-INFORMED PRACTICE—cont'd.

personal stories from leadership using webinars and multimedia communications, expert-led workshops, lunch-and-learn sessions, and manager and employee training were part of a comprehensive program. Comprehensive, specific, and multipronged strategies were developed and aimed at encouraging healthy behaviours that impact presenteeism—for example, regular exercise, proper nutrition, adequate sleep, smoking cessation, socialization, and work-life balance.

Limitations

Limitations of the intervention mapping process included high resource and time requirements, the lack of external input and viewpoints skewed towards middle and upper management, and using secondary workplace data of unknown validity and reliability. The greatest issue will be for the employer to maintain this level of programming.

Conclusions

In general, intervention mapping was a useful method to develop a workplace health promotion and wellness program. The methodology provided a step-by-step process to unravel a complex problem. The process compelled participants to think critically, collaboratively, and in non-traditional ways.

Application to Your Clinical Practice

Nurses are very good at designing these kinds of programs for nonprofit agencies. They have many transferable skills that could be used in private industry. These programs are labour intensive and require coaching, teamwork, and a strong belief in the Health Promotion Model.

Modified from Ammendolia, C., Côté, P., Cancelliere, C. et al. (2106). Healthy and productive workers: Using intervention mapping to design a workplace health promotion and wellness program to improve presenteeism. *BMC Public Health*, 6, 1190. https://doi.org/10.1186/s12889-016-3843-x.

APPLICATIONS

The Canadian Association of Schools of Nursing (CASN, 2014), through an intensive consultation process funded by the PHAC, struck a task force that produced the Public Health Nursing Competencies in Undergraduate Nursing Education. The results of this work were the formalization of the following competencies outlined in five domains that every undergraduate baccalaureate student must achieve in their program: 1. public health sciences in nursing practice, 2. population and community health assessment and analysis, 3. population health planning, implementation, and rvaluation, 4. partnerships, collaboration and advocacy, and 5. communication in public health nursing.

Health promotion strategies should be a part of everyday nursing care. Education and coaching can be introduced informally as you provide care. Community-based interventions can be formally presented through education, screening programs, and social media.

Nurses need to be public advocates of health promotion actions as well as care agents. They are perceived as trustworthy informants about health matters because of their extensive knowledge base and close caregiving associations with people and their families.

Nurses can be influential in helping communities to create supportive health environments. For example, nurses can serve on health-related community advisory committees and provide relevant discussions regarding care and funding (Kemppainen et al., 2013). The provision of health fairs for area schools or community groups is another avenue nurses can use to support health promotion and disease prevention at the community level.

Health Education for Health Promotion

Health education is an essential component of effective health promotion and disease prevention strategies (Hoving et al., 2010). Clinical approaches to promote healthy behaviours with individuals include motivational interviewing, empowerment, social support, and self-management coaching.

Mol and colleagues (2010) note that good care involves "persistent tinkering in a world full of complex ambivalence and shifting tensions" (p. 14). People requiring the same educational information can demonstrate a wide range of learning, cognitive, experiential, and communication diversity. They differ in intellectual curiosity, learning preferences, motivation for learning, learning styles, and rate of learning, each of which will require adaptations to maximize learning. This is where the art of nursing comes in. It is important to select strategies that hold meaning for people.

Common examples of general health promotion include developing a healthy lifestyle, good nutrition, regular physical activity, adequate sleep patterns, and stress reduction. But in addition to these desired outcomes, engaging in meaningful health promotion activities supports the development of autonomy, personal competence, and social relatedness.

Choosing disease prevention topics of potential interest to higher-risk populations offers the best return on investment. For Indigenous peoples, a nurse would be interested in learning more about the following: human immunodeficiency virus (HIV), mumps, diabetes, chickenpox and HPV (Government of Canada, 2020b), as there is a higher risk for these conditions in this demographic.

Formal and informal instruction can focus on condition-specific topics. A wide variety of topics lend themselves to a health promotion focus, including the following:

- Alcohol, nicotine, and other types of drug abuse prevention
- Anger management
- Prevention, screening, and early detection of common chronic diseases, such as HIV, diabetes, cancer, heart disease, osteoporosis, and associated disorders
- Fall prevention strategies
- Stress reduction for informal caregivers and organizational work sites
- Healthy dietary practices
- Regular exercise habits
- Effective support systems

Health promotion interventions must be responsive to each individual's personal situation, as universal applications may not be appropriately sensitive to the social or economic factors associated with individuals or a target populations. For example, attempts to help people modify food choices or engage in physical activity may mean different things to various cultural and socioeconomic groups.

Motivational Interviewing

Treatment for many chronic diseases such as cancer, heart disease, asthma, diabetes, and arthritis often require significant ongoing lifestyle changes. People are charged with taking a much more active role in designing and implementing the sometimes significant lifestyle changes that are required to live a purpose-filled life, while coping with chronic illness. Motivational interviewing is a useful strategy in dealing with people who are ambivalent but must make significant lifestyle changes (Brobeck et al., 2011).

Motivational interviewing is an evidence-informed clinical framework designed to help people incorporate the functional abilities and skills they will need to fully engage in health promotion and disease prevention activities. An overarching goal of individuals who need to improve their health is to develop a better health-related quality of life. To achieve this goal, people must want to change behaviours that compromise their health.

The incorporation of people's preferences and cultural understandings is an essential component of an effective health promotion strategy. Miller and Rollnick (2013) assert that "When you understand what people value, you have a key to what motivates them" (p. 75). People put energy into actions that they believe are essential to their well-being. If they do not understand the link between their actions and their well-being, they are unlikely to sustain their efforts.

Motivational interviewing is "theoretically congruent" with the Transtheoretical Model of behaviour change (Arkowitz et al., 2015). A motivational intervention encompasses a person's values, beliefs, and preferences incorporated into relevant functional abilities and learned skills. Motivation is seen as a state of readiness rather than a personality trait (Dart, 2011). The motivational interview fits well with concepts of person-centred care (Howard & Williams, 2016) and is used with a growing range of chronic health conditions, such as diabetes or obesity exacerbated by unhealthy lifestyle behaviours (Lukaschek et al., 2019).

Since making positive changes in health behaviours is basically the person's responsibility, it requires a strong commitment of self to engage in such behaviours. Motivational interviewing emphasizes an individual's capacity to take charge of their personal health and control lifestyle factors that interfere with optimal health and well-being. Although, initially, a motivational interview approach takes longer, it is likely to be more effective because the person chooses actions that have personal meaning and will be more committed to them.

The underlying premise of motivational learning is that learning takes root from within a person. It occurs when the learner is ready and *wants* to learn because they believe that it will make a positive difference. The person must also believe that success is achievable with their personal efforts and resources. The decision to change, the choice of goals, and the commitment to developing new behaviours is always under the person's control.

Readiness to change can be influenced. Nurses can better understand and influence a person's deeper perception of a problem through Socratic questioning. This type of questioning allows nurses to point to discrepancies between a person's goals or values and their current behaviours without argument or direct confrontation. Motivational interviewing help people address resistance and ambivalence about making health-related lifestyle changes in a nonjudgemental environment (Hall et al., 2012). Therapeutic strategies centre on resolving problem behaviours, increasing committed collaboration, and using joint decision making (Miller & Rollnick, 2013).

Case Example

Person: "I'm ready to go home now. I know once I get home, I'll be able to get along without help. I've lived there all my life and I know my way around."

Nurse: "I know that you think you can manage by yourself at home. But most people need some rehabilitation after a stroke to help them regain their strength. If you go home now without rehabilitation, you may be shortchanging yourself by not taking the time to develop the skills you need to be independent at home. Is that something that's important to you?"

Motivational interviewing is an intervention in which the nurse uses empathetic exploration to help someone become aware of discrepancies in their behaviour that are hurting their health and well-being. This exploration is coupled with teaching them new skills to achieve healthy life goals (Baumann, 2012).

1. What does the person need to know?

Negotiating behaviour change is conceptualized as a shared endeavor in which both the person and the provider examine the person's potential and willingness to change destructive health behaviours (Arkowitz et al., 2015). When motivational strategies match an individual's readiness to change, this match increases the likelihood of positive, intentional behavioural lifestyle changes.

Miller and Rollnick (2013) describe two phases of motivational interviewing. The first phase focuses on mutually exploring and resolving ambivalence to change as a collaborative endeavor. This is accomplished through weighing the pros and cons of the current situation and the actions one would have to take to make change possible. With the person in charge of determining change activities, the second phase emphasizes strengthening and supporting the person's commitment to change based on the person's choice and capacity for change.

A good starting point is a simple introductory question, such as, "I wonder if you could tell me what you do to keep yourself healthy? This type of question helps you to see what the person values or even if they think about taking a personal role in achieving and maintaining healthy behaviours. It also provides an opportunity to assess for possible issues that actually may be counterproductive.

Case Example

Anju is a 77-year-old woman with osteoporosis. She is health conscious and walks regularly to build bone strength. She wears a weighted vest to increase her workout strength and recently upped this weight to 15 pounds without consulting her physician. This change caused pain, and Anju was advised to decrease the weight. In this case, the concept of bone strengthening was appropriate, but its application had become inappropriate.

When someone begins to tell you about their personal health habits, you can reflect on the relevant details and ask for clarification. The purpose of the dialogue is to deepen the person's understanding. Use empathy in your responses. For example, "It sounds like you have been having a tough time and not getting a lot of support."

Open-ended questions allow people the greatest freedom to respond. Asking someone if he regularly exercises may yield a one-sentence answer. Inviting the same person to describe his activity and exercise during a typical day and what makes it easier or harder for him to exercise can provide stronger data. Potential concerns and inconsistency with values, preferences, or goals are more readily identified.

Person and family perspectives on disease and treatment are not necessarily the same as those of their health care providers. For example, you may think that a woman who is emaciated or obese would be worried about her weight and would want to modify it because she values the way she looks. On the other hand, her culture or family values and traditions may be in conflict with making significant behavioural changes. Until the person can understand a health-related value for making a change, she will not put serious effort into doing so. This level of data allows nurses to tailor interventions based on the person's readiness to change and the availability of a support system.

As people progress to the contemplative stage, nurses provide coaching guidance, information, and practical support to help them consider different choices and potential solutions. The pros and cons of each possible choice are explored. Empathy for the challenges faced by the person and affirming the person's reflection process encourages them to consider alternative options and choose the most viable among them (Arkowitz et al., 2015). A critical component of motivational interviewing is acceptance of the person's right to make the final decision and the need for the nurse to honor the person's right to do so.

In the preparation stage, your role is to help people establish realistic goals and develop a plan for achieving them. Goals should be realistic, person-centred, and achievable. For example, the goal of losing 10 pounds in 3 months sounds more doable than a goal to simply lose weight (too vague) or to lose 75 pounds (potentially overwhelming). Incremental goals build a sense of confidence as the person sequentially meets them.

Personalizing goals and treatment plans for people in your care is critical. Each person has a unique life situation, support system, and way of coping with problems. Unhealthy habits are cumulative and hard to break. Work with people to monitor their progress, offering suggestions, revising goals or plans when needed, and reminding them of progress made. It is useful to help people proactively identify potential obstacles and to anticipate the next steps. You can offer additional suggestions, empathize or commend people's efforts, and revisit actions from the preparation stage if goals need revision. For example, you could say, "You have really worked hard to master your exercises" or "I'm really impressed that you were able to avoid eating sweets this week." Availability to help people solve problems or rethink plans, if needed, is also key.

Empowerment Strategies

Werbrouck and colleagues (2018) distinguish between empowerment as a *goal* in having control over the determinants of one's quality of life and as a *process* in which one has control over problem formulation, decision making, and the actions one takes to achieve relevant health goals. Empowerment takes place through clinician-initiated person-centred care approaches and through actions people take on their own initiative (Holmstrom & Roing, 2010).

As a process strategy, empowering people to take the initiative with their own health and well-being supports a person's ability to maintain their role as a functioning adult and facilitates the self-management of chronic disorders (Sachdeva, 2019).

Case Example

"When Mrs. Hixon [who'd had a stroke] was relearning how to dress herself, it initially took her an hour. With much practice, and with guidance from the occupational therapist, this time finally dropped to 25 minutes. Even so, I confess I practically had to sit on my hands as I watched her struggle… It would have been so much faster to do it for her, but she had to learn and I had to let her" (Collier, 1974, p. 80).

Other enabling strategies include a focus on knowledge and skills, tailored education and training, previous successes in solving problems, social support the person can lean on, and reviewing the existing supportive assets. It is empowering to learn as much as possible about healthy lifestyles and how they support the self-management of chronic conditions (Goele et al., 2019).

Using the Internet as a Resource

The Internet is a powerful resource for knowledge. People you care for and their families can find specific information on the web, regardless of the stage of their illness. Helping people use technology to find information and access related health resources is a form of enabling people to take charge of their health. Online support groups, chat rooms, and sharing blog experiences provide additional support for people who live in areas that are not geographically convenient to person-to-person contact. People can connect with others coping with issues such as weight control and exercise and can share practical strategies online.

Nurses can help people and their families select and critically evaluate relevant web data. Not all data are completely accurate or relevant to a particular situation. If the person or family does not use technology, then flyers, fact sheets, and direct dialogue with opportunity for questions and follow-up can be used to reinforce information.

A participatory learning format that encourages different ways of thinking and opportunities to try out new behaviours is more effective than giving simple instructions to a person or family or than offering people a demonstration without enabling feedback (Durkin et al., 2018). When time is short, focus on topics that address the most pressing lifestyle changes. Literacy involves more than a person's capacity to read (Alberta Education, n.d.). People need to be able to turn information into meaningful actions to meet life and health goals. Teaching strategies presented in Chapter 16 can be used or modified for health promotion teaching.

Empowerment Through Social Support

Amdam (2011) suggests that "Empowerment implies a gathering of power, in a dynamic way, over a period of time" (p. 50). Social support from friends and family is an important empowerment resource in health promotion activities. **Social support** describes a person's "integration within a social network," and "the perceived availability of support" when it is needed (MacGeorge et al., 2011, p. 320). The interested support of significant others can strengthen a person's resolve, provide input for innovative solutions, and nurture the development of self-efficacy.

Health-related support groups in the community are available for a wide variety of diagnoses, providing relevant information, direct assistance, referral to appropriate resources, and the opportunity to simply interact with others experiencing similar challenges. For example, Alzheimer societies (Alzheimer.ca) hold regularly scheduled support groups in most major locations to assist family members. Community-based cancer support groups provide valuable information and support for many common cancer diagnoses. Educational and referral supports enable people and their families to learn the skills they need to effectively manage chronic conditions and live healthy lives.

Health Promotion as a Population Concept

Community is defined as a group of people who share something in common, like physical, work, social, or spiritual arenas, but who may have different priorities, needs, cultures, and expectations. They share attributes by the strength of the connections among them. There are multiple groups that can be described by place or venue or that have common goals. (Goodman et al., 2014). The community offers a natural social system with special significance for facilitating health promotion activities, particularly for people who are economically or socially disadvantaged. It is difficult to change attitudes and lifestyles to promote health when a person's social or economic environment does not support prevention efforts.

Successful community-based health promotion activities start with a community analysis of health issues identified by the community. Consciousness raising is critical, as engagement and buy-in of the community in which the activity is to take place is essential. The WHO notes that health promotion activities should be "carried out by and with people, not on or to people" (WHO, 1997). The active participation of individuals, communities, and systems means a stronger and more authentic commitment to the establishment of the realistic regulatory, organizational, and sociopolitical supports that will be needed to achieve targeted health outcomes (CPHA, n.d.). Simulation Exercise 15.4 provides an opportunity to analyze community health problems when using health promotion interventions.

Health Inequities and Empowerment

Major advances in health promotion and prevention have not benefited all segments of the nation's population equally (CPHA, n.d.). Health inequities are differences in health between specific population groups that are systematic, avoidable, unfair, and unjust (Kirst et al., 2017). People with the greatest health burdens often have inadequate financial resources and the least access to information, communication technologies, health care, and supporting social services. Individuals living in extreme poverty do not have access to preventive care, adequate nutrition, or the opportunity to live in a healthy environment. When they are living at the survival level, most people are not in a position to think about health promotion techniques to acquire a better quality of life. Being mindful of the person's environment helps nurses proactively tailor interventions to engage and meet their health promotion and disease prevention needs.

Equity and empowerment related to health care are the expected outcome of health promotion activities at the community level. Equity corresponds to the WHO directive that all people should have an equal opportunity to enjoy good health and well-being. Key health issues in economically disadvantaged communities are often those with social roots, such as violence or abuse, substance abuse, teen pregnancies, and acquired immunodeficiency syndrome (AIDS) (Donaldson & Rutter, 2017).

Empowerment is a process endowing individuals or communities to create change while having autonomy and

---

SIMULATION EXERCISE 15.4   Analyzing Community Health Problems for Health Promotion Interventions

Purpose

To develop an appreciation for the multidimensional elements of a community health problem

Procedure

In groups of three to five students, brainstorm about health problems you believe exist in your community and develop a consensus about one public health problem that your group would prioritize as being most important.

Use the following questions to direct your thinking about developing health promotion activities for a health-related problem in your community.

- What are the most pressing health problems in your community?
- What are the underlying causes or contributing factors to this problem?
- In what ways does the selected problem affect the health and well-being of the larger community?

- What is the population of interest you would target for intervention?
- What additional information would you need to have to propose a solution?
- Who are the stakeholders, and how should they be involved?
- What step would you recommend as an initial response to this health problem?
- What is one step the nurse would take to increase awareness of this problem as a health promotion issue?

Discussion

How hard was it for your group to arrive at a consensus about the most pressing problem? Were you surprised with any of the discussion that took place about this health problem? How could you use what you learned in doing this exercise in your nursing practice?

control. This means they have the power to make decisions and to mobilize resources (Painter et al., 2011).

This type of empowerment is fueled by both public policy and targeted education. Successful health promotion programs require individuals, groups, and organizations to act as active agents in shaping health practices and policies that have meaning to a target population. Specific interventions are designed to engage those people who are most involved as active participants in a common environmental concern related to health. Proactive social and political action to enhance health services can augment educational efforts to ensure program viability.

Health promotion activists recognize the community as their principal voice in promoting health and well-being. Health promotion represents a multidisciplinary approach, also inclusive of health education, public health, and environmental health (Corcoran, 2013). Health promotion strategies are relevant in clinics, schools, communities, and faith-based communities; they can be introduced during many aspects of routine care in hospitals.

Health Promotion Models for Community Empowerment

Community empowerment strategies are used to help identify and address environmental and social issues needed to improve the overall health of the community. This strategy is sometimes referred to as "capacity building." Community-focused empowerment strategies build on the personal strengths, community resources, and problem-solving capabilities already existing among individuals and within communities that can be used to address potential and actual health problems. Capacity building requires the inclusion of informal and formal community leaders as valued stakeholders. Networking, partnering, and creating joint ventures with Indigenous and local religious organizations is a powerful consensus-building strategy that communities can use for effective health education planning and implementation. Box 15.1 outlines a process for engaging the community in health promotion activities.

Health Literacy in Health Promotion and Disease Prevention

The Institute of Medicine has specified that health literacy must be incorporated as an essential component in undergraduate nursing curricula (Mosley & Taylor, 2017). Health literacy differs from overall literacy and IQ. People with inadequate health literacy may be highly intelligent but functionally unable to fully grasp medical terminology due to lack of education or language differences. Many of the words and meanings associated with medical terminology are complex and not easily understood by the lay public.

BOX 15.1 Guiding Principles for Community Engagement

Five interconnected practices that lead to community change:
1. Collective impact: How can you mobilize collaboration across sectors for systems change?
2. Community engagement: How can you engage the community to create and realize bold visions for the future?
3. Collaborative leadership: How can you bring the right people together in constructive ways?
4. Community innovation: How can you create, test, and scale new approaches?
5. Evaluating impact: How can you identify and amplify what works?

https://www.tamarackcommunity.ca/communityengagement

Health Literacy Is Central to Achieving Good Health and Well-Being

"**Health literacy** skills are cognitive and social skills which determine the motivation and ability of individuals to gain access to, understand, and use information in ways which promote and maintain good health" (Rowlands, 2014, p. 2130). A lack of health literacy has disastrous implications for self-management, as indicated in the following case example.

Case Example

Jonathan is a 14-year-old adolescent who was recently discharged from a mental health unit. This was his fourth admission over an 18-month period. His mother assumed responsibility for making sure that he took his medications as directed. She knew the names of his medications and faithfully monitored him taking them. But Jonathan's behaviour began to deteriorate again. At one of Jonathan's follow-up visits, the nurse asked him to show her the medications he was on, and how he was taking them. It turned out that Jonathan's mother could not read, got the medications mixed up, and was administering the daily medication three times a day and the thrice daily medication once daily.

Responsibility for health literacy is a collaborative initiative that lies with both providers and people receiving care. Special attention needs to be given to people disadvantaged by social determinants that limit their understanding of health-related materials. A more proactive approach needs to be extended to lower socioeconomic groups and minority populations, as health illiteracy disproportionately affects these population groups. People need to be encouraged to ask questions about anything they do not understand. You can reinforce the expectation that people should ask questions for complete understanding, by saying something like, "Many people find it difficult to fully understand what is going on with their health. They ask a lot of questions and I'm hoping you will too." "Teach-back" (see Chapter 16), in addition to written instructions, also helps people grasp complex clinical instructions. See Simulation Exercise 15.5, Developing Relevant Teaching Aids, to assist you in learning about teaching aids.

Literacy is not just about reading and writing. It is also about speaking, listening for understanding, asking questions for clarification, and checking in with people to see that the messages sent are the same as those received. Simply providing information to people with low literacy using "plain language" is *not* sufficient to encourage behavioural changes. Even when people seem to understand information at the time, they may have trouble keeping complex information straight, afterward. It can be difficult to comprehend and retain new and complex information.

Health literacy can be compromised by background noise, individual visual or auditory impairment, diminished mental alertness, fatigue, and acute illness. For example, a person who is deaf or hard of hearing may not hear the words correctly and assign meanings that are incorrect. A person with poor vision can misread a medication label or misinterpret individual words on a consent form. It is important to ask relevant questions or to use teach-back strategies (see Chapter 16) to ensure understanding.

Functional health literacy is defined as an individual's capacity to obtain, process, and understand basic health information and services.

Health illiteracy can include inability to understand the complexity and implications of medical treatments or essential system navigation skills (Kobayashi et al., 2016). A few well-placed questions can reveal this problem. People with inadequate health literacy skills often do not know what to do about their health or how to manage a chronic condition. They may not understand why their medical management is important, especially if they have not previously been exposed to medical settings. Even when people can comprehend the words, their level of understanding may be too limited to weigh possible alternative meanings or to know what questions to ask for a better interpretation or to effectively make appropriate choices. Table 15.2 presents examples of the core constructs of health literacy.

A less common but related literacy skill is numeracy. Alberta Education defines *numeracy* as the ability, confidence, and willingness to engage with quantitative and spatial information to make informed decisions in all aspects of daily living (Alberta Government, n.d.). Lack of numeracy skills can affect a person's ability to understand expiration dates and timing related to medications as well as to comprehend the dosing of oral medications, the importance of time intervals between medications, and so forth. Inadequate numeracy is particularly relevant for people who rely on prescribed medications given at different times, and as-needed medications, to cope with their illness. People with decreased numeracy skills who have cancer may have a diminished ability to accurately assess and personalize health risks (Donelle et al., 2008).

Partial understanding or a lack of full, step-by-step instructions can result in unintentional noncompliance. Some people try to hide the fact that they have trouble understanding the meaning of complex words or making sense of numbers. They may fake an ability to understand by appearing to agree with the nurse by saying they will read the instructions later, or by not asking questions. Here

---

SIMULATION EXERCISE 15.5 Developing Relevant Teaching Aids

Purpose
To develop skill in adapting learning materials for people with limited literacy.

Procedure
1. Develop a one-paragraph case study, preferably from the experience of someone you provided care for.
2. Choose a related health promotion topic such as exercise, diet, stress reduction, or medication adherence.
3. Use the topic to develop a simple poster or teaching aid for someone with limited literacy skills.
4. Use clear plain language consistent with a Grade 6 to 8 reading level to develop your project.

5. Check your content for accuracy.
6. Use your teaching aid with a person you are caring for and ask for feedback about the person's understanding of your message and reaction to the teaching aid.

Discussion
How difficult was it to develop the teaching aid? What factors did you have to take into consideration to make it interesting and informative for the person you are caring for? Were you surprised at any of the feedback you received from the person? Would you do anything differently as a result of the feedback?

TABLE 15.2 Core Constructs of Health Literacy With Application Examples

Core Construct	Application Examples
Basic literacy or comprehension	Reading various texts, such as appointment cards
	Interpreting medical tests, dosages and instructions, side effects, contraindications
	Understanding what is read, including brochures, medication labels, informed consent, insurance documents
Interactive and participatory literacy (able to engage in two-way interactions)	Provision of appropriate and usable information
	Comprehension and ability to act on information
	Mutual decision making
	Remembering and acting on information
Critical literacy	Ability to weigh critical scientific facts; capacity to assess competing treatment options

Adapted from Marks, R. (2009). Ethics and patient education: Health literacy and cultural dilemmas. *Health Promotion Practice*, *10*(3), 328–332.

are some issues people and their significant caregivers present, related to poor health literacy:

- Inability to adequately describe symptoms or health problems
- Taking instructions too literally
- Having a limited ability to generalize information to new situations
- Decoding one word at a time rather than reading a passage as a whole
- Skipping over uncommon or hard words
- Thinking in individual rather than categorical terms

Case Example

A 2-year-old is diagnosed with an inner ear infection and prescribed an antibiotic. Her mother understands that her daughter should take the prescribed medication twice a day. After carefully studying the label on the bottle and deciding that it does not tell how to take the medicine, she fills a teaspoon and pours the antibiotic into her daughter's painful ear. (Parker et al., 2003, p. 150)

People who are educationally disadvantaged or functionally health illiterate are interested in learning, but nurses need to adapt teaching situations to accommodate literacy learning differences. Use a shame- and blame-free approach. Have materials written at a Grade 6 to Grade 8 reading level and provide lists of key instructions for use after visits. Using symbols and images with which the person is familiar makes the material easier to comprehend. Taking the time to understand a person's use of words and phrases provides the nurse with concrete words and ideas that may be more familiar to the person and their family. If

you have any concerns about a person's ability to interpret or understand health-related instructions, it is important to check with the person or caregiver about the availability of additional supports needed for self-management strategies. Do not assume that the person understands the implications of a clinical recommendation without some form of dialogue. Use a combination of multimedia teaching strategies based on sound educational theories (RNAO, 2012).

It is important to check with the person or their family about any circumstances that might get in the way of understanding any other special directions. Health literacy is both content and context specific (RNAO, 2012).

Case Example #1

Annika is a nurse practitioner in an inner-city pediatric clinic. After examining a child with strep throat, she prescribed an antibiotic for him. She instructed the mother to give her child the medication two times a day and to store it in the refrigerator between doses. She asked the mother if she had any questions or concerns. The mother indicated that she did not have any. But as the mother and child were leaving the exam room, the mother turned to the nurse practitioner and said, "We don't have a refrigerator. Will anything happen if I don't refrigerate the medication?"

If you were the nurse in this situation, how would you respond to this person?

Case Example #2

Jose is filling out a routine clinical information form that asks questions about his health, use of medications, past surgeries, and family history of illnesses.

Jose fills out his personal identifying information because he understands this section. There is a lot of reading involved in filling out the rest of form, and he is puzzled by some of the other medical history questions. He leaves these questions blank because he is not sure what they mean. He signs his name and returns the form. Working on filling out a clinical form as a joint exercise between nurse and person may make the difference between understanding and unintentional noncompliance.

The following are guidelines for improving communication with people and their caregivers who may have a low level of health literacy:

1. Use common, concrete words rather than abstractions or medical terminology—for example, "Call the doctor on Monday if you still have pain or swelling in your knee."

2. Use the same words to describe the same thing. Name the medication or procedure and use the same words to describe it each time. Otherwise, there can be slippage as a person struggles to understand whether the different words mean the same thing. The same instructions, written exactly as they were spoken, act as a reminder once the person leaves the actual teaching situation.

3. Sequence the content logically, beginning with the most important core concept.

4. Remember that someone with low health literacy may not be able to read or interpret the label instructions on the bottle. Go over the instructions verbally, with them holding the bottle.

5. Medications for children often have dosing charts, which identify age and weight recommendations for dose requirements. This can be confusing when the correct age or weight on the medication bottle does not match the reality of the child's presentation.

6. *Guide the person to think about the following sequence when taking a new medication*:
   What do I take?
   How much do I take?
   When do I take it?
   What will it do for me?
   What do I do if I experience a problem or a side effect?

7. If there are multiple oral medications, describe each medication's appearance and let the person actually see the medication.

8. *Apply common, simple, concrete words*, such as "You should take your medicine when you're not having a meal" instead of "Take this medication on an empty stomach." Sophisticated terminology, while accurate, may not be understood.

9. Whenever possible, *link new information and tasks with what the person already knows*. This strategy builds on previous knowledge and reinforces self-efficacy in mastering new concepts.

10. Keep sentences short and precise (no more than 15–20 words).

11. The use of active verbs helps people better understand what you are teaching. It is easier to understand "Take this medication three times a day" than "This medication is taken by the patient three times a day." When technical words are necessary for people to communicate about their condition with health providers, people may need additional instruction or coaching about the appropriate words to use.

12. When it is the concept rather than the words that is complex, you may need to guide the person through the explanation. For example, you may have to explain the meaning and clinical implications of certain lab tests, offer help with filling out insurance forms, and so on.

Developmental Level

Developmental level affects both teaching strategies and the delivery of content. You will work with people at all levels of the learning spectrum in regard to their social, emotional, and cognitive development.

Developmental learning capability is not necessarily age-related; it is easily influenced by culture and stress. Social and emotional development does not always parallel cognitive maturity or literacy. Mirroring the person's communication style and framing messages to reflect cultural characteristics helps improve comprehension and understanding. Parents and other family members can provide information about their child's immediate life experiences and suggest commonly used words to be incorporated into the nurse's health teaching.

Avoid information overload and giving vague or conflicting health information to older people, particularly if there is any evidence of cognitive processing difficulties (Baur, 2011). For example, it is better to say, "This plastic box has 31 little bins. Each bin holds all the pills you should take in the morning. It is coloured yellow, so think of the sunrise. This other plastic box also has 31 little bins. Each bin holds all the pills you need to take in the evening. It is coloured dark blue, so think of the night sky." To reinforce messages, use written instructions along with verbal ones. Another issue for older people is that they often have multiple medications, some of which may look alike.

Incorporating Cultural Understandings

Cultural understandings add to the complexity of health promotion strategies in health care (Lie et al., 2012). Values, norms, and beliefs are an integral part of each person; they influence individual and community lifestyles and health perceptions (see Chapter 7).

Respecting a person's cultural values increases their trust of individual care providers. Eliciting and integrating explanatory information regarding health and illness into health teaching promotes better understanding *and* greater acceptance of health promotion and disease prevention recommendations. Cultural sensitivity includes knowledge of the preferred communication styles of different cultural groups. For example, Indigenous people are known for learning through stories. The tradition of oral storytelling is a primary means of teaching that nurses can use for health promotion purposes. You can also promote motivation and participation through the use of Indigenous teachers and counsellors. If health literacy is related to language, qualified interpreters should be used for the translation and preparation of written materials.

Nurses participate routinely in community health promotion and disease prevention activities. They have an ethical and legal responsibility to maintain the expertise and interpersonal sensitivity required to promote effective learning.

SUMMARY

This chapter focuses on communication strategies nurses can use, to help people increase understanding of personal health care across clinical settings. National and global agendas reinforce the importance of developing public health policies to create supportive health environments. Specific attention to reducing health disparities and negative social determinants through strengthened community action for health, along with increased access for all, are advocated. Optimal health and well-being are considered the desired outcomes of health promotion activities.

Three individual health promotion frameworks are presented. Pender's Health Promotion Model identifies perceptions of benefits, barriers, and ability to take action related to health and well-being as components of the individual's willingness to engage in health promotion activities.

Prochaska's Transtheoretical Model is used to explore a person's readiness to intentionally change their health habits. This theory serves as the foundation for motivational interviewing, developed by Miller and Rollnick (2013).

Bandura's social learning theory explores the role of self-efficacy in empowering people to use health promotion and disease prevention recommendations to take better care of their health.

Community-based interventions are critical in addressing broader causal influences on health, referred to as social determinants. This chapter also describes the important

role of health literacy. Culture, developmental status, and lack of health literacy are described as factors that can compromise a person's ability to fully engage in healthy lifestyle behaviours.

🔲 ETHICAL DILEMMA
What Would You Do?

Jack Marks is a 16-year-old adolescent who comes to the clinic complaining of symptoms of a sexually transmitted infection (STI). He receives antibiotics and you give him information about safer sex and preventing STIs. Two months later, he returns to the clinic with similar symptoms. It is clear that Jack has not followed instructions and has no intention of doing so. He tells you he's a regular jock and just can't get used to the idea of condoms. He says he cannot tell you the names of his partners—there are just too many of them. As his nurse, what are your ethical responsibilities in caring for Jack? What are the implications of your potential decisions?

QUESTIONS FOR REVIEW AND DISCUSSION

1. In what ways are the concepts of health literacy and functional health literacy different and alike, and why is this important?
2. Why are health promotion and disease prevention strategies receiving so much emphasis in contemporary health care?
3. How would you implement Pender's model to enhance personal responsibility for health promotion and disease prevention practices?
4. Discuss how you could use motivational interviewing as a tool for helping people learn self-management strategies.

REFERENCES

Alberta Education. (n.d.). *What is literacy?* https://education. alberta.ca/literacy-and-numeracy/literacy/everyone/what-is-literacy/.

Alberta Government. (n.d.) *Fact Sheet: Numeracy.* https://education. alberta.ca/media/3402195/num-fact-sheet.pdf.

Amdam, R. (2011). *Planning in health promotion work: An Empowerment Model.* Routledge.

Arkowitz, H., Miller, W. & Rollnick, S. (2015). *Motivational interviewing in the treatment of psychological problems* (2nd ed.). The Guildford Press.

Bandura, A. (1997). *Self-Efficacy: The exercise of control.* W. H. Freeman.

Baumann, S. (2012). Motivational interviewing for emergency nurses. *Journal of Emergency Nursing, 38*, 254–257.

Baur, C. (2011). Calling the nation to act: Implementing the national action plan to improve health literacy. *Nursing Outlook, 59*, 63–69.

Brainyquote.com. (n.d.) *Frederick Douglass.* http://www.brainyquote.com/quotes/quotes/f/frederickd201574.html.

Brobeck, E., Bergh, H., Odencrants, S. et al. (2011). Primary health care nurses' experiences with motivational interviewing in health promotion practice. *Journal of Clinical Nursing, 20*, 33322–33330.

Canadian Association of Schools of Nursing. (2014). Entry-to-Practice public health nursing competencies for undergraduate nursing education. https://casn.ca/wp-content/uploads/2014/12/FINALpublichealthcompeENforweb.pdf.

Canadian Nurses Association. (2018). *Position statement: Social determinants of health.* https://www.cna-aiic.ca/-/media/cna/page-content/pdf-en/social-determinants-of-health-position-statement_2018_e.pdf?la=en&hash=AE82392EB4843FBB1D43FAB26B8F85012D7AC636.

Canadian Public Health Association. (n.d.). Action statement for health promotion in Canada. https://www.cpha.ca/action-statement-health-promotion-canada.

Centers for Disease Control and Prevention. (2016). *Health equity: Strategies for reducing health disparities 2016.* https://www.cdc.gov/minorityhealth/strategies2016/index.html.

Collier, S. (1974). Mrs. Hixon was more than the "CVA in 251". *Nursing, 4*(11), 78–80.

Corcoran, N. (2013). *Communicating health: Strategies for health promotion* (2nd ed.). Sage Publications.

Dart, M. (2011). *Motivational interviewing in nursing practice.* Jones & Bartlett.

Donaldson, L., & Rutter, P. (2017). *Healthier, fairer, safer: The global health journey, 2007–2017.* World Health Organization.

Donelle, L., Arocha, J. F., & Hoffman-Goetz, L. (2008). Health literacy and numeracy: Key factors in cancer risk comprehension. *Chronic Diseases in Canada, 29*(1). (https://www.canada.ca/content/dam/phac-aspc/migration/phac-aspc/publicat/hpcdp-pspmc/29-1/pdf/cdic29-1-1eng.pdf).

Durkin, M., Gurbutt, R., & Carson, J. (2018). Qualities, teaching, and measurement of compassion in nursing: A systematic review. *Nurse Education Today, 63*, 50–58. https://doi.org/10.1016/j.nedt.2018.01.025.

Fagerlind, H., Ring, L., Feltelius, N. et al. (2010). Patients' understanding of the concepts of health and quality of life. *Patient Education and Counseling, 78*(1), 104–110.

Goele, J., Lenzen, S., Van Pottelbergh, G. et al. (2019). Self-management among community-dwelling people with chronic conditions: Adapting evidence-based group programs using intervention mapping. *Patient Education and Counseling, 103*(3), 589–596. https://doi.org/10.1016/j.pec.2019.10.001.

Goodman, R. A., Bunnell, R., & Posner, S. F. (2014). What is "community health"? Examining the meaning of an evolving field in public health. *Preventive medicine, 67 Suppl 1*(Suppl 1), S58–S61. https://doi.org/10.1016/j.ypmed.2014.07.028.

Government of Canada. (2019). *Well-being framework.* https://www.canada.ca/en/department-national-defence/corporate/reports-publications/transition-guide/well-being-framework.html.

Government of Canada. (2020a). *Social determinants of health and health inequity.* https://www.canada.ca/en/public-health/services/health-promotion/population-health/what-determines-health.html.

Government of Canada. (2020b). *Diseases that may affect First Nations communities.* https://www.sac-isc.gc.ca/eng/1569867927914/1569867958318.

Grey, M. (2017). Lifestyle determinants of health. Isn't it all about genetics and environment? *Nursing Outlook, 65*(5), 501–505.

Hall, K., Gibbie, T., & Lubman, D. (2012). Motivational interviewing techniques: Facilitating behavior change in the general practice setting. *Australian Family Physician, 42*, 660–667.

Hanson, R. (2016, Nov 9). What is your sense of peace? [Blog] https://www.psychologytoday.com/us/blog/your-wise-brain/201611/what-is-your-sense-peace.

Health and Welfare Canada. (1986). *Achieving health for all: A framework for health promotion.* http://www.hc-sc.gc.ca/hcs-sss/pubs/system-regime/1986-frame-plan-promotion/index-eng.php.

Holmstrom, I., & Roing, M. (2010). The relation between patient-centeredness and patient empowerment: A discussion on concepts. *Patient Education and Counseling, 72*(2), 167–172.

Hoving, C., Visser, A., Mullen, P. D. et al. (2010). A history of patient education by health professionals in Europe and North America. *Patient Education and Counseling, 78*(3), 275–281.

Howard, L., & Williams, B. (2016). A focused ethnography of baccalaureate nursing students who are using motivational interviewing. *Journal of Nursing Scholarship, 48*(5), 472–481. https://doi.org/10.1111/jnu.12224.

Kemppainen, V., Tossavainen, K., & Turunen, H. (2013). Nurses' roles in health promotion practice: An integrative review. *Health Promotion International, 28*(4), 490–501. https://doi.org/10.1093/heapro/das034.

Kirst, M., Shankardass, K., Singhal, S. et al. (2017). Addressing health inequities in Ontario, Canada: What solutions do the public support? *BMC Public Health, 17*(1), 7. https://doi.org/10.1186/s12889-016-3932-x.

Kobayashi, L., Wardle, J., Wolf, M. et al. (2016). Aging and functional health literacy: A systematic review and meta-analysis. *The Journals of Gerontology: Series B, 71*(3), 445–457. https://doi.org/10.1093/geronb/gbu161.

Kushner, R. F., & Sorensen, K. W. (2013). Lifestyle medicine: The future of chronic disease management. *Current Opinion in Endocrinology, Diabetes and Obesity, 20*(5), 389–395.

Lalonde, M. (1974). *A new perspective on the health of Canadians.* Minister of Supply and Services Canada. http://www.phac-aspc.gc.ca/ph-sp/pdf/perspect-eng.pdf.

Lie, D., Carter-Pokras, O., Braun, B. et al. (2012). What do health literacy and cultural competence have in common? Calling for a collaborative health professional pedagogy. *Journal of Health Communication, 17*(Suppl. 3), 13–22.

Lukaschek, K., Schneider, N., Schelle, M. et al. (2019). Applicability of motivational interviewing for chronic disease management in primary care following a web-based E-learning course: Cross-Sectional Study. *JMIR Ment Health, 6*(4), e12540. https://doi.org/10.2196/12540.

MacGeorge, E., Feng, B., & Burleson, B. (2011). Chapter 10: Supportive communication. In M. Knapp, & J. Daly (Eds.), *The Sage handbook of interpersonal communication.* (pp. 317–354). Sage.

Miller, W., & Rollnick, S. (2013). *Motivational interviewing: Helping people change* (3rd ed.). Guildford Press.

Mol, A., Moser, I., & Pols, J. (Eds.). (2010). *Care in practice: On tinkering in clinics, homes and farms.* www.transcript-verlag.de/ts1447/ts1447.php.

Mosley, C., & Taylor, B. (2017). Integration of health literacy content into nursing curriculum utilizing the health literacy expanded model. *Teaching and Learning in Nursing, 12*(2), 109–116.

Orpana, H., Vachon, J., Dykxhoorn, J. et al. (2016). Monitoring positive mental health and its determinants in Canada: The development of the Positive Mental Health Surveillance Indicator Framework. *Health Promotion and Chronic Disease Prevention in Canada, 31,* 1–12. https://doi.org/10.24095/hpcdp.36.1.01.

Painter, J., Dominelli, L., Macleod, G. et al. (2011). *Connected communities: Connecting localism and community empowerment.* https://ccednet-rcdec.ca/sites/ccednet-rcdec.ca/files/2011-connectinglocalismandcommunityempowerment-discussionpaperpainter.pdf.

Parker, R., Ratzan, S., Lurie, N. et al. (2003). A policy challenge for advancing high-quality health care. *Health Affairs (Millwood), 22*(4), 147–153.

Pender, N., Murdaugh, C., & Parsons, M. (2011). *Health promotion in nursing practice* (6th ed.). Prentice Hall.

Prochaska, J., & Norcross, J. (2013). *The transtheoretical model in systems of psychotherapy: A transtheoretical analysis* (8th ed.). Cengage Learning.

Public Health Agency of Canada. (2010). Creating a healthier Canada: Making prevention a priority. https://www.canada.ca/en/public-health/services/health-promotion/healthy-living/creating-a-healthier-canada-making-prevention-a-priority.html#v.

Public Health Agency of Canada. (2015). *Improving health outcomes: A paradigm shift. Centre for Chronic Disease Prevention Strategic Plan 2016–2019.* https://www.phac-aspc.gc.ca/cd-mc/assets/pdf/ccdp-strategic-plan-2016-2019-plan-strategique-cpmc-eng.pdf.

Public Health Agency of Canada. (2016). *Social determinants of health. Canadian best practices portal.* https://cbpp-pcpe.phac-aspc.gc.ca/public-health-topics/social-determinants-of-health/

Public Health Agency of Canada. (2017). *How healthy are Canadians? A trend analysis of the health of Canadians from a healthy living and chronic disease perspective.* https://www.canada.ca/en/public-health/services/publications/healthy-living/how-healthy-canadians.html.

Registered Nurses' Association of Ontario. (2012). Facilitating client centred learning. https://rnao.ca/sites/rnao-ca/files/BPG_CCL_2012_FA.pdf.

Rowlands, G. (2014). Health literacy. *Human vaccines & immunotherapeutics, 10*(7), 2130–2135. https://doi.org/10.4161/hv.29603.

Sachdeva, J. (2019). Stages of behavioral change and their effects. In A. Abd-Elsayed (Ed.), *Pain.* Springer. https://doi.org/10.1007/978-3-319-99124-5_83.

Werbrouck, A., Swinnen, E., Kerckhofs, E. et al. (2018). How to empower patients? A systematic review and meta-analysis. *Translational Behavioral Medicine, 8*(5), 660–674. https://doi.org/10.1093/tbm/iby064.

World Health Organization. (1986). *Ottawa charter for health promotion: First international conference on health promotion.* Ottawa. http://www.who.int/healthpromotion/conferences/previous/ottawa/en/.

World Health Organization. (1997). *Jakarta declaration on leading health promotion into the 21st century.* www.who.int/hpr/NPH/docs/jakarta_declaration_en.pdf.

SUGGESTED READING

Dennison-Himmelfarb, C. R., & Hughes, S. (2011). Are you assessing the communication "vital sign"? *Journal of Cardiovascular Nursing, 26,* 177–179.

Dudas, K. (2011). *Patient centered care: Assessment of health literacy.* http://qsen.org/patient-centered-care-assessment-of-health-Literacy.

Elliot, D. L., Goldberg, L., MacKinnon, D. P. et al. (2010). Patients' understanding of the concepts of health and quality of life. *Patient Education and Counseling, 78,* 104–110.

Heinrich, C. (2012). Health literacy: The sixth vital sign. *Journal of the American Association of Nurse Practitioners, 24*(4), 218–223.

Institute of Medicine (IOM). (2011). *Health literacy implications for health care reform.* National Academies Press.

Institute of Medicine (IOM). (2012). *Primary care and public health: Exploring integration to improve population health.* National Academies Press.

Jager, A. J., & Wynia, M. K. (2012). Who gets a teach-back? Patient-reported incidence experiencing a teach-back. *Journal of Health Communication, 17*(Suppl. 3), 294–302.

Lorig, K., & Halsted, R. H. (2017). Self-management education, outcomes and mechanisms. *Annals of Behavioral Medicine, 26*(1), 1–7.

Miller, W. R., & Rollnick, S. (2014). The effectiveness and ineffectiveness of complex behavioral interventions: Impact of treatment fidelity. *Contemporary Clinical Trials, 37,* 234–241.

Saint Onge, J. M., & Krueger, P. M. (2017). Health lifestyle behaviors among US adults. *Society for Social Medicine & Population Health, 3,* 89–98.

Sheridan, S. L., Halpern, D. J., Viera, A. J. et al. (2011). Interventions for individuals with low health literacy: A systematic review. *Journal of Health Communication, 16*(Suppl. 3), 30–54.

Sørensen, K., Van den Broucke, S., Fullam, J. et al. (2012). Health literacy and public health: A systematic review and integration of definitions and models. *BioMed Central Public Health, 12* Article 80.

Yip, M. (2012). A health literacy model for limited English speaking populations: Sources, context, process, and outcomes. *Contemporary Nurse, 40*(2), 160–168.

WEBSITE/RESOURCES LIST

https://alzheimer.ca/en/Home

https://www.canada.ca/en/public-health/services/publications/healthy-living/how-healthy-canadians.html.

https://www.canada.ca/en/public-health/services/health-promotion/healthy-living/creating-a-healthier-canada-making-prevention-a-priority.html#v.

https://www.canada.ca/en/public-health/services/health-promotion/population-health/what-determines-health.html.

https://casn.ca/wp-content/uploads/2014/12/FINALpublichealthcompeENforweb.pdf.

https://cbpp-pcpe.phac-aspc.gc.ca/public-health-topics/social-determinants-of-health/.

https://www.ccsa.ca/sites/default/files/2019-04/CCSA-Motivational-Interviewing-Summary-2017-en.pdf.

https://www.cdc.gov/minorityhealth/strategies2016/index.html

https://www.cpha.ca/.

https://www.cpha.ca/action-statement-health-promotion-canada.

https://www.definitions.net/definition/lifestyle.

https://education.alberta.ca/literacy-and-numeracy/literacy/everyone/what-is-literacy/.

https://education.alberta.ca/media/3402195/num-fact-sheet.pdf.

http://www.health.gov/healthliteracyonline/.

http://healthliteracy.worlded.org/.

www.hsph.harvard.edu/healthliteracy.

www.jointcommission.org/NR/rdonlyres/D5248B2E-E7E6-4121-8874-99C7B4888301/0/improving_health_literacy.pdf.

http://www.nifl.gov/mailman/listinfo/Healthliteracy.

https://www.phac-aspc.gc.ca/cd-mc/assets/pdf/ccdp-strategic-plan-2016-2019-plan-strategique-cpmc-eng.pdf.

https://www.sac-isc.gc.ca/eng/1569867927914/1569867958318

16

Communication in Health Teaching and Coaching

Olive Yonge

Originating US chapter by *Elizabeth C. Arnold*

OBJECTIVES

At the end of the chapter, the reader will be able to:
1. Describe person-centred health education.
2. Identify the domains of learning.
3. Discuss theoretical frameworks used in person-centred health teaching.
4. Discuss health teaching applications in different settings.
5. Describe coaching strategies for the self-management of chronic conditions.
6. Apply the teach-back strategy.

This chapter examines evidence-informed patient education communication strategies in health care. Health teaching is a defined professional standard for professional nurses. Nurses are legally and ethically charged with providing relevant, health-related education to people they provide care for, their families, caregivers, and the community across clinical settings (Baur, 2011). This chapter identifies selected theories of teaching and learning as an evidence-informed foundation for effective **health teaching** and coaching needed for people to self-manage their chronic illness and work effectively with community resources to maximize their health and well-being (Deek et al., 2016).

BASIC CONCEPTS

Patient education represents a focused form of instructional communication. Its purpose and design are to provide people in your care and their families with the specific knowledge, life skills, and practical and emotional support needed to do the following:
- Cope with diagnosed health disruptions
- Self-manage and minimize the effects of chronic disorders
- Make effective health-related decisions
- Slow or prevent disease progression
- Promote attainment of a high quality of life

The Complexity of Patient Education

Chronic illness usually requires long-term consistent self-management. Patient education is complex, particularly for the long-term treatment of people with chronic illnesses. The overarching goals of patient education are to assist people and caregivers to do the following:
- Understand the nature of their chronic conditions
- Develop personally relevant lifestyle changes to cope with chronic health problems and to maximize health and well-being

The "learner" can be someone in your care, a family member or caregiver, a school group, or a community group. Regardless of a person's medical diagnosis, each learning experience is uniquely human and creates different realities for people with different cultural beliefs, life experiences, personal perception of impact, and financial or social resources. Learning characteristics of people and their families from different socioeconomic, educational, cultural, and life experience backgrounds vary across the spectrum and are further complicated by degrees of interest. The goals of patient education are presented in Fig. 16.1.

Health teaching related to chronic conditions extends beyond simple medical and clinical data. Each teaching situation requires an individualized teaching approach and "learner buy-in" to ensure successful outcomes. Assessment of a person's readiness to learn and learning style are important details in developing tailored nursing approaches with

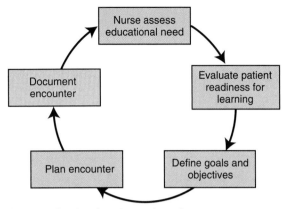

Fig. 16.1 Goals of patient education

people and their families. Self-management skills require people and their families to do the following:

- Develop personalized problem-solving strategies related to their particular health care and related needs
- Identify, access, and use resources across clinical settings
- Demonstrate mastery of skill, reflecting an understanding of underlying skill dynamics (Registered Nurses' Association of Ontario [RNAO], 2012). There has been a shift away from nurses teaching and telling people what to do and toward one of partnership between people and nurses. Promoting health is a key competency for nurses, and this is best facilitated by being person-centred and drawing on educational theory (RNAO).

Documentation of patient-specific education provided to people about treatment options in a language they can fully understand is required for informed consent. Although the informed consent document is the physician's responsibility, nurses play an important role in providing appropriate preparatory and follow-up health teaching, particularly with people who have limited mental or literacy capacity and with surrogate decision makers (Menendez, 2013).

BASIC CONCEPTS

Theoretical Frameworks

Carl Rogers

Carl Rogers' (1983) learner-centred approach engages learners as active partners in all aspects of the learning process. In health care, nurses act as health guides for people, their families, and ancillary personnel. Rogers advises that the "teacher" must start where the learner is. For example, some people initially are disinterested and others have a natural desire to learn. Relationship conditions of

unconditional positive regard, empathy, and authenticity in interpersonal relationships are conceptual threads in health teaching environments.

Participatory strategies build on personal strengths. They support a person's effectiveness in learning new behaviours because they incorporate skills that a person is already practising. When information is provided in a meaningful context, it has greater impact (Benner et al., 2010; Su, Herron, & Osisek, 2011). The learner is in charge of processing and acting on personally relevant information, in partnership with health care providers. In health teaching situations, nurses should offer sufficient background information, specific instructions, coaching, and emotional support about the topic under discussion but no more than is required to reinforce forward movement. Each person should be encouraged to take responsibility for personal self-management. Health teaching related to self-management strategies must be a participatory sport—it has to be a shared endeavour, with both the person and the nurse working together to achieve specific goals. Without this alliance, optimal outcomes may be compromised.

Science of Teaching

Andragogy refers to the "art and science of helping adults learn" (Knowles et al., 2011). Adult learners tend to be self-directed, action-oriented, and practical; they want to see the usefulness of what they are learning. Generally, adults favour a problem-focused approach to learning. They want to be directly engaged in developing the skills needed to master immediate life problems. The adult learner expects the nurse to inquire about previous life experience and to incorporate this knowledge into a jointly agreed-upon teaching plan. Fig. 16.2 presents Knowles's model of adult learning principles.

Pedagogy describes the processes used to help people learn, including children. Children need direct health education, but they come to the learning experience with far less life experience that can be tapped as resources for learning. They pass through cognitive and psychosocial stages, which dictate different teaching formats for successful participation (see Chapter 19).

A key difference between pedagogy and andragogy is the need to provide the child learner with additional direct guidance and structure in learning content. Parent participation is critical to successful education with school-aged children. It provides both oversight management guidance and essential emotional support (Kelo et al., 2013).

Bastable (2017) describes learning approaches in older adulthood as *geragogy*. In normal aging, a person's knowledge changes, and asking about the particular life experiences of older people is essential for successful health teaching. It can be much harder for some older people to

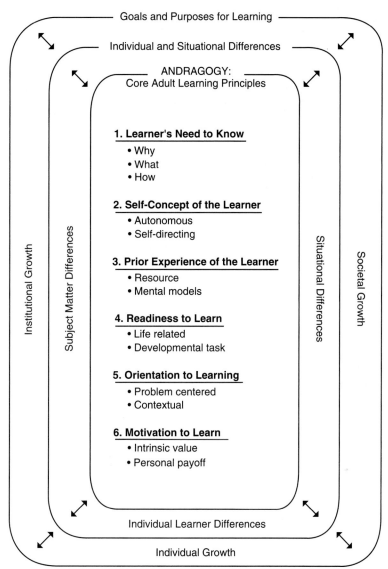

Fig. 16.2 Andragogy Model: A core set of adult learning principles. From Knowles, M., Holton. E., Swanson. R. (1998). *The adult learner: The definitive classic on adult education and training.* Butterworth-Heinemann, p. 182.

adapt to new ways of managing their health. Others may have significant mobility or sensory deficits that interfere with ease in learning formats. These impairments can make performing self-management skills challenging.

Older people may need a slower pace, as many are likely to be cautious about trying new self-management strategies. Simple accommodations such as cueing, brighter lighting, and enlarged print can facilitate learning. Encouragement and positive reinforcement also improve motivation, self-efficacy, and performance. More communities are making community-based efforts to provide free or low-cost exercise and stress-management programs for older people. Specific targeted classes on fall prevention and bone strengthening are available in many communities.

Bandura's Social Cognitive Model

Bandura's social cognitive model links successful behavioural changes to a person's perception that they have the capability to carry out the actions (self-efficacy) required to meet identified goals (outcome expectancy) within their unique social context. If people think they have the skills or can easily learn them, they tend to be more confident and are more likely to succeed.

Health teaching is a dynamic, interactive process. A person's knowledge about the reasons for using the skill and the steps involved provides a stronger foundation in the cognitive domain. For example, health teaching for a person with a recent diagnosis of diabetes might include knowledge of the disease; the roles of diet, exercise, and insulin in diabetic control; and guidance about how to identify trouble signs requiring immediate attention. Concrete information—provided through verbal discussions, images and line drawings, written instructions, and web data—can help to explain the steps needed to achieve negotiated health goals. Paying attention to the emotional impact of a diabetes diagnosis allows people to work through emotional issues that could potentially compromise compliance with essential treatment. Emotions are a powerful backdrop for self-efficacy and motivation.

Bloom's Taxonomy: Classifying Behavioural Objectives

Objectives are essentially guides to action related to achieving goals. Nurses use Bloom's taxonomy as a guide to writing behavioural objectives in health care. The utility of the taxonomy, originally described by Bloom and associates, is that it provides "a common language about learning goals to facilitate communication across persons and subject matter" (Krau, 2011, p. 305).

Bloom's taxonomy identifies a hierarchy of learning objectives ranging from simple to the most complex. Fig. 16.3 shows levelled objectives using this model.

These objectives were revised in the twenty-first century to represent verbs rather than nouns (Krau, 2011).

The revised Bloom's taxonomy consists of the following:

- **Remembering**: recognizing, recalling information and facts
- **Understanding**: interpreting, explaining, or constructing meaning
- **Applying**: carrying out or executing a procedure, using information in a new way
- **Analyzing**: considering individual components of the whole and how they relate to each other and the whole
- **Evaluating**: making judgements, critiquing, prioritizing, selecting, verifying
- **Creating**: putting material together into a coherent whole, reorganizing material into a new pattern, creating something new (Kadiyala et al., 2017; Krau, 2011).

Behavioural objectives begin with the phrase "The person will," followed by step-by-step achievable, measurable behaviours toward treatment goals. Ideally, there should be an objective for each significant component of the teaching session. An example of levelled objectives applied to teaching people about diabetes is presented in Fig. 16.3.

Simulation Exercise 16.1 provides practice with developing behavioural objectives.

DOMAINS OF LEARNING

There are three domains of learning: cognitive, affective, and psychomotor. The cognitive domain consists of the knowledge base for the self-management skill and an understanding of the nature and dimensions of the

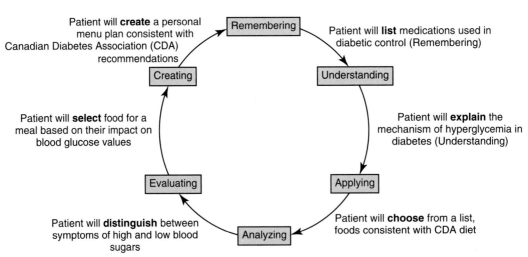

Fig. 16.3 Levelled objectives using Bloom's revised taxonomy. Text adapted from Krau, S. (2011). Creating educational objectives for patient education using the new Bloom's taxonomy. *Nurs Clin North Am 46*(3), 302.

SIMULATION EXERCISE 16.1 **Developing Behavioural Goals**

Purpose

To provide practical experience with developing teaching goals

Procedure

Establish a nursing diagnosis related to health teaching and a teaching goal that supports the diagnosis in each of the following situations:

1. Jimmy is a 15-year-old adolescent who has been admitted to a mental health unit with disorders associated with impulse control and conduct. He wants to lie on his bed and read Stephen King novels; he refuses to attend unit therapy activities.
2. Maria, a 19-year-old single woman, is in the clinic for the first time because of cramping. She is 7 months pregnant and has had no prenatal care.

3. Jennifer is overweight and desperately wants to lose weight. However, she cannot walk past the refrigerator without stopping, and she finds it difficult to resist the snack machines at work. She wants a plan to help her lose weight and resist her impulses to eat.

Discussion

1. What factors did you have to consider in developing the most appropriate diagnosis and teaching goals for each person?
2. In considering the diagnosis and teaching goals for each situation, what common themes did you find?
3. What differences in each situation contributed to variations in diagnosis and teaching goals? What contributed to these differences?
4. In what ways can you use the information in this exercise in your future nursing practice?

---

underlying medical and psychological issues associated with the person's diagnosis.

Learning in the **affective domain** focuses on emotional attitudes related to acceptance, compliance, valuing, and taking personal responsibility. It is more complex because of its association with values and beliefs. Objectives focusing on affective understanding are useful when people demonstrate compliance issues or seem stalled in moving forward. Learning in the affective domain helps to keep the person on track when challenges arise and to maintain the emotional commitment needed to achieve success.

The **psychomotor domain** focuses on hands-on practice (performance learning). Performance learning promotes greater understanding than reading or hearing about a skill. Think of the first time you rode a bike. Chances are it was not until you made the bike move through your personal efforts that you really "owned" the skill of bike riding. Coaching a person through a psychomotor skill step by step is a helpful strategy to achieving competence. Encouragement and teach-back in which the person verbally goes through the steps can reinforce psychomotor task performance. Developing proficiency in performing the required psychomotor skill also involves building personal confidence and the coping skills needed to adjust when challenged with unexpected circumstances.

Case Example

Jack "knows" that following his diabetic diet is essential to control his diabetes. He can tell you everything there is to know about the relationship of diet to diabetic control. Although he follows his diet at home, he eats snack foods at work and insists on extra helpings at dinner, especially when he is stressed. He says he does not mind taking extra insulin and that it is his choice to do so. Jack's problem with compliance lies in the affective domain; he resents having a lifelong condition that limits his food selections. Motivational interviewing might be useful in working with Jack to look at his health picture from a broader perspective. This strategy would allow him to explore his ambivalence and frustration at dietary restrictions imposed by his health condition. Without such a discussion, his behaviour is unlikely to change.

CORE DIMENSIONS OF CONTEMPORARY PATIENT EDUCATION

Contemporary health education embraces a broad spectrum of related activities (Farin et al., 2013). Taking personal actions to achieve health goals helps people connect the dots related to physical, social, and lifestyle modifications needed for self-managed health promotion and treatment compliance, as presented in the following paragraphs.

Person's Perspective

In 2012, the RNAO developed the L.E.A.R.N.S. Model (Listen, Establish, Adopt, Reinforce, Name, and Strengthen), illustrated in Fig. 16.4 (RNAO, 2012). The whole concept of person-centred teaching is represented in the model. The

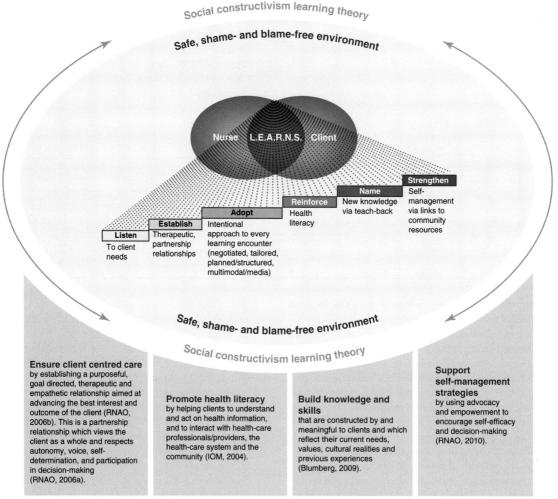

Fig. 16.4 The L.E.A.R.N.S. Model. Source: Registered Nurses' Association of Ontario (2012). *Facilitating Client Centred Learning.* Toronto, Canada: Registered Nurses' Association of Ontario.

key concepts are: person-centred learning, self-efficacy, and decision making. Both the person and the nurse are in a shame-free environment, allowing them to work together as partners. It is a partnership that facilitates and respects the person's autonomy, voice, and self-determination. People are therefore able to require new knowledge, apply new skills, see how they could apply the skills to their own environments, and gain mastery, which results in self-efficacy and self-management. This process is ongoing throughout one's life.

Self-Management

Self-management strategies are designed to optimize chronic disease management for people and their families, in the home and community. The focus is on skill enhancement, with full engagement of people in clinical decision making and consistent self-management activities.

New models related to self-management skill development are competency-based. Teaching strategies include coaching, shared decision making, and personal self-management of the individual's health condition(s). Strategies start with obtaining an active nurse–person collaborative commitment to setting realistic, achievable health goals.

The next step is to mutually identify specific learning outcomes with the person and incorporate the support of essential others in the coaching process. This step is followed by developing specific action plans to meet learning outcomes and evaluating their effectiveness (Su et al., 2011). What is taught and how it is taught are critical elements of competency-based health teaching. Applications are grounded in evidence-informed and nursing practice guidelines tailored to each person's presenting needs, preferences, and available resources. The linkage between assessment needs and tailored actions should be transparent to everyone involved with the person's care.

Tailoring interventions begins with listening for hidden emotional cues. Accommodating individual differences into teaching plans whenever possible shows respect for the person's preferences. For example, a person with normal cognitive functioning might respond well to a suggestion to shower, while a person with a mental health disorder or mild dementia might respond poorly. Accommodations for some flexibility in timing, built into the teaching process, can make a major difference. When self-management health-related tactics fit within a person's daily routine, they are more likely to be followed with cooperation. Scheduled times for exercising and taking medications also help new habits assume a regular place in the person's life.

People are expected to be active participants and to take responsibility for their health care with collaborative support from their health care team. Contemporary patient education involves multilevel interventions linked to a common purpose of maximizing a person's health and well-being. Nurses use evidence-informed knowledge and guidelines to facilitate and support individualized person and family decision making (Inott & Kennedy, 2011). Meaningful person-centred teaching does more than supply a basis for action; this process can improve the person's self-esteem and reduce health anxiety (Ortiz, 2018).

Opportunities for Health Teaching

Person-centred education is evidenced as a continuous thread, extending across health care settings and community systems. Opportunities for health teaching occur in the community, school, parish, home, hospital, and clinic (Dreeben, 2010). Teaching formats range from informal, one-to-one health sessions to formal, structured group sessions, family conferences, and scheduled presentations in the care setting or community. Health teaching can occur spontaneously during home visits as the nurse observes people having specific difficulties with aspects of health care. Referred to as *guided care*, this type of on-the-spot health teaching is targeted to respond to specific health issues as they appear. The media provides health-related information related to primary prevention (e.g., safer sex and drug use prevention commercials) to targeted community groups. Health fairs for children and preventive screenings for adults provide natural health teaching spot opportunities in the community.

Using Plain Language

Plain language is defined as a major instructional strategy for making written and oral information easier to understand, especially for individuals with lower literacy capabilities, those who speak English as a second language, and older people. Key elements of plain language include the following:

- Organizing information so that the most important points come first
- Breaking complex information into easily understandable chunks
- Using simple language and defining technical terms
- Using the active voice
- Writing at a reading level of Grades 6 to 8
- Using less than 15 words in each sentence
- Using phrasing that is easy to understand

Technology Integration

Technological advances have expanded the depth and breadth of health information available to the health consumer. In addition to basic tailored health information, decision support systems can assist people in making better health care decisions (Urmimala & Lipika, 2020). The Internet provides instant health information, with a wide range of learning resources to accommodate different levels of knowledge and learning styles. For example, MedlinePlus, from the U.S. National Library of Medicine, provides accurate, current information about the most common health conditions, palliative care, and drug information (Smith, 2013). People can type in a layperson's description of a problem and quickly receive links to tutorials and appropriate websites. Information on reliable sites on the Internet is searchable, up to date, inexpensive to obtain, and accessible at any time of day. Search engines allow people to type in a few key words that grant immediate access to websites related to their diagnosis (Gordon, 2011)—for example, for information on diabetes, they can go to https://www.diabetes.ca. These and other websites offer specific ideas for self-management, with a wide range of information and learning tools.

Although it is a powerful learning resource, the Internet has human and resource limitations. People have free access to computers in public libraries and selected community centres (Bastable, 2017). But many people do not have easy access to computers or know how to use them. Also, not all health information is equally relevant or directly applicable. Nurses can educate people on how to begin searches and how to access information as well as evaluate its quality (Gordon, 2011). People receiving care and their families find it helpful to share online with others coping with similar health conditions.

Holt and colleagues (2011) describe using cell phone technology as a health teaching aid. They created an app consisting of personalized, step-by-step photos, beginning with essential equipment and accompanied by voice memo directions for complicated self-management of wound care.

DEVELOPING AN EVIDENCE-INFORMED PRACTICE

Purpose:
The goal of this scoping review study was to provide a comprehensive review of the different beneficial and challenging aspects of participation in self-management education programs for people living and coping with chronic illness.

This scoping review of the literature searched eight evidence-informed literature databases. The Arksey and O'Malley framework was used to guide the review process, and thematic analysis was used to synthesize the extracted data.

Results:
Forty-seven articles met the criteria for inclusion in this literature review. Positive benefits of participation in the education programs included less symptom distress, improved execution of self-management strategies, peer support, increased hope, and better learning.

Application to Your Clinical Practice:
The results of this review study can assist health care providers in developing and carrying out effective education programs related to self-management strategies.

Stenberg, U., Haaland-Overby, M., Fredriksen, K. et al. (2016). A scoping review of the literature on benefits and challenges of participating in patient education programs aimed at promoting self-management for people living with chronic illness. *Patient Education and Counseling, 99*(11), 1759–1771.

APPLICATIONS

Professional, Legal, and Ethical Mandates for Patient Education

Within the last decade, the International Joint Commission established standards requiring health care agencies to provide systematic health education and training for people and their families. These include the following:

- Information sufficient for people to make informed decisions and to take responsibility for self-management activities related to their needs
- Information provided to people and their families in a manner understandable to them and designed to accommodate various learning styles
- Information including documentation that people and their families have received appropriate health information and their response to this medical information

(2015). Note: There are a number of Joint Commissions between Canada and the United States because we share a common border, water, and air. Both countries develop standards in many areas, resolve disputes, and work jointly on projects.

DEVELOPING AND IMPLEMENTING INDIVIDUALIZED TEACHING PLANS

Preparation

Health Teaching Responsibilities

Individualized teaching plans follow the nursing process, beginning with an assessment of people's learning needs, strengths, and limitations and ending with an evaluation of clinical outcomes. Common categories of health teaching responsibilities are featured in Fig. 16.5.

Health teaching is a complex nursing intervention consisting of many interlocking parts. Research demonstrates that structured, individualized teaching is more effective than generalized approaches (Friedman et al., 2011). As a health provider, you are responsible for the quality of health teaching, even though only the person you provide care for can assure the outcome. Prior to beginning the teaching process, you should review evidence-informed care guidelines for the person's condition. Taking time to look over key concepts and verifiable, bottom-line information needed to achieve designated health goals for the person facilitates later content discussion. Effective teaching plans provide people and their families with new or reorganized knowledge, skills, and attitudes, based on scientific evidence and personally tailored to people's needs, resources, preferences, and values.

Case Example

Dakota returned to his hospital room from abdominal surgery with a nasogastric tube. It was attached to a suction pump. Hour after hour, he watched the drainage bottle fill, being too shy to ask the nurse if this was normal. A student nurse was assigned to him on the evening shift and asked him if he had any questions about his surgery or the suction pump. He simply nodded and said he did not know what was going on. The student explained that the nasogastric tube was used to alleviate nausea, vomiting, and gastric distention. She then checked to ensure that the tube was securely attached to Dakota's nose and pinned to his gown. She looked at the head of the bed to ensure it was elevated and instructed Dakota never to lie flat to avoid the risk of aspiration. She finished her care

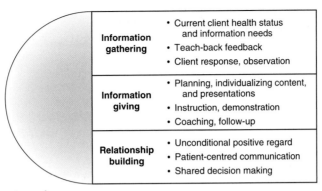

Fig. 16.5 Health teaching categories

by giving Dakota mouth care, explaining that since the tube obstructed one nostril, many people preferred mouth breathing. As she left, Dakota thanked her for the explanations because he believed he was dying, watching all the green fluid leave his body.

Coaching

As people assume stronger collaborative responsibility for the self-management of their conditions, coaching becomes a major nursing strategy in health education. The nurse acts not only as an information provider but also as a guide, resource, and knowledgeable emotional support. As guides, nurses coach people on actions they can take to improve their health. They offer suggestions on modifications as their condition changes. As information providers, they help people become more aware of why, what, and how they can learn to take better care of themselves. As resource supports, nurses help people connect with appropriate community social and health supports to promote health and well-being while preventing the emergence of chronic disorders and disability.

Nurses act as a knowledge source and emotional support, encouraging positive learning efforts by helping people minimize the impact of temporary setbacks and never giving up on them. For example, helping people anticipate actual and potential effects of a medication or treatment reduces anxiety and the incidence of errors.

Self-Awareness

It is easier to remain engaged with self-directed, motivated learners. It takes energy and imagination to stimulate interest in learning when a person sees little reason to participate in making essential lifestyle changes.

Health teaching is a two-way process. This means rising above personal stereotypes to fully understand and appreciate each person's unique world view. Incorporating a discovery approach to health teaching means encouraging questions and using the person's life experiences whenever possible to help them apply new knowledge. Try to imagine yourself in the person's or their family members' health situation. Empathy and understanding of motivational commitment broaden health-teaching perspectives and convey respect for the person and family.

Assessment Data for Health Teaching and Coaching

Each learning situation has a past and a present reality. Patient education and coaching begins with a comprehensive assessment of each person's needs, issues, strengths, and concerns. Start with what people already know about their health condition and treatment. When what a person "already knows" is inaccurate, a different set of evidence-informed data should be shared with them. Sometimes, such data has meaning for people. If not, new data can be presented as another source of information.

Past experience and beliefs about illness, medications and treatments, cultural values, and the reactions of others produce assumptions that directly affect motivation and the acceptance of health teaching. Finding out what the person feels is their primary health concern is important, as this may differ from the reason that the person is seeking treatment.

Apart from a person's symptom history, contextual factors such as impact on work or social relationships are often of considerable concern to people. Asking open-ended questions can help nurses understand people's unique learning needs and those of their families in a practical way. Box 16.1 provides examples of questions nurses can use to assess people's learning needs—for example, "What has this illness been like for you so far?"

Assessing Personal Learning Characteristics

Personal learning characteristics have a significant influence on achieving positive clinical outcomes. Preferred

---

BOX 16.1   Questions to Assess Learning Needs

- What does the person already know about their condition and treatment?
- In what ways is the person affected by it?
- In what ways are those people intimately involved with the person also affected by the person's condition or treatment?
- What does the person identify as their most important learning need?
- To what extent is the person willing to take personal responsibility for seeking solutions?
- What goals would the person like to achieve?
- What will the person need to do to achieve those goals?
- What resources are available to the person and their family that might affect the learning process?
- What barriers to learning exist?

BOX 16.2   Characteristics of Different Learning Styles

Visual
Learns best by seeing
- Likes to watch demonstrations
- Organizes thoughts by writing them down
- Needs detail
- Looks around; examines situation

Auditory
Learns best with verbal instructions
- Likes to talk things through
- Detail is not as important
- Talks about situation and pros and cons

Kinetic
Learns best by doing
- Hands-on involvement
- Needs action and likes to touch, feel
- Loses interest with detailed instructions
- Tries things out

---

learning style, developmental stage, learning readiness and motivation, and low health literacy affect successful learning (Bastable, 2017).

Preferred Learning Style

There are three major types of learning styles: visual, auditory, and kinesthetic. A visual learner learns best by reading or viewing web-based material and graphic images rather than listening to explanations. Auditory learners need to hear the information and appreciate discussion rather than strictly depending on visual material. Kinesthetic learners learn best with demonstration and hands-on practice. Beagley (2011) notes that although most people can learn using any of these learning styles, each person has a preference and responds best when their preference is incorporated into the teaching plan. Box 16.2 presents the characteristics of different learning styles.

Learning Readiness

Learning readiness refers to a person's mindset and openness to engaging in a learning or counselling process for the purpose of adopting new behaviours. Motivational interviewing is a widely used strategy designed to assess and enhance the potential for learning readiness when internal motivation seems to be lacking. Nurses use empathy, acceptance, and respect for the person's autonomy to help people choose and commit to positive health behaviour changes. Rather than challenging a person's resistance directly, nurses should guide them from wherever they are on the continuum of assuming responsibility for health promotion. Four stages

of change applicable to current behaviours and the person's investment in making positive behavioural change (precontemplation, contemplation, action, and maintenance) direct the teaching–learning process (Prochaska & Velicer, 1997).

Emotional issues can increase learning readiness as well as interfere with it. Crisis anxiety (if it is not extreme) can create an immediate need to learn (Mezirow, 1990). If people experience professional support as a helpful relationship, they may be more receptive to less crisis-oriented teaching interventions related to chronic conditions.

Ability to Learn

Some people are ready to learn but are unable to do so using traditional learning formats. Assessing the person's ability to learn and adapting the learning format to the learner's unique characteristics makes a difference. For example, a person's physical condition or emotional state can temporarily preclude teaching. When people are in pain, they can focus on little else. Nausea or weakness makes it difficult for people to sustain attention. Medications, or a temporary period of disorientation after a diagnostic test or surgical procedure, can inhibit concentration.

Accurately assessing and managing a person's level of anxiety before health teaching is essential, as is choosing a time when the person's level of energy makes it most likely they will be receptive (RNAO, 2012). The shock of a difficult diagnosis may require teaching in small segments or postponement of serious teaching sessions until the person has understood the diagnosis. People with significant thought disorders have difficulty processing information. They may need simple, concrete instructions and frequent prompts to perform adequately. Comorbid health problems, if not recognized, can interfere with the goals of patient education. For example, an exercise program might be useful for a person who is overweight, but if the person also has asthma or another activity-limiting issue, the intervention might require modification. Elevated stress and anxiety affect a person's ability to focus attention and process material.

Health Literacy

Health literacy is critical so people can be informed and make good decisions. During the pandemic beginning in 2020, it became apparent that vast amounts of data had to be quickly analyzed and synthesized, but this was not easy to do because there was often conflicting information from virologists, epidemiologists, doctors, nurses, different levels of government, and the media (Sentell et al., 2020). People in your care can sense this confusion if they cannot understand what is being taught, and learning does not take place. When people are in crisis mode, they do not always ask questions. Anxiety limits cognitive skills even in the best of us, and medical vocabulary can be daunting.

"Health literacy skills are cognitive and social skills which determine the motivation and ability of individuals to gain access to, understand, and use information in ways which promote and maintain good health" (Rowlands, 2014, p. 2130). This broader definition heightens awareness of the social aspects of health literacy, which are sometimes overlooked in immediate, hectic teaching situations. Low literacy is related to but not the same as low health literacy; medical vocabulary can be daunting for many people (Kobayashi et al., 2016). People now first search for descriptions of their illness on the Internet before seeing their doctor. This behaviour is to be applauded since people are trying to manage their self care, but there are also issues with the quality of the information, depending on the trustworthiness of the websites they use. Online information needs to used as a complement to information from health care providers (Tonsaker et al., 2014).

Case Example

Mr. Dion was to be discharged and needed health teaching on how to change the bandage on his thigh. He had burned himself when a pot of hot water had slipped from his hand and splashed onto his right thigh. His nurse, Mr. King, was unsure how much English Mr. Dion knew, given he conversed mainly with French-speaking health care staff. Mr. King decided that he had to use visuals, so he wrote French phrases on a poster and broke down the process into simple steps for Mr. Dion. He demonstrated for Mr. Dion and then asked for a return demonstration. It was done correctly. However, to reinforce the learning, he asked Mr. Dion to verbally repeat how and why he changed the bandage to keep the burned skin as clean as possible.

In addition to being able to read and understand words and numbers, literacy includes being able to "orally express oneself, understand and recall spoken instructions, make inferences, utilize technology, critically weigh options and make decisions, and sustain often complex behaviors" (Wolf et al., 2012, p. 1302). Since nurses are identified as key providers of patient education across clinical settings, it is especially important for us to incorporate health literacy strategies in all aspects of care. Baker et al. (2011) suggest using a limited set of essential learning goals related to the following:

- Explaining the outcome behaviour
- Essential background information to understand the recommended behaviour
- Explanation of how the behaviour change will help the person feel better
- The barriers that exist and how they can be overcome to produce the desired result (p. 11)

People with limited literacy struggle harder to understand and usually need more time to process information. They tend to decode messages one word at a time and may not grasp the whole message. Ensure resource materials are at an appropriate reading level. To facilitate understanding, use fewer rather than more words to explain a concept and allow extra time to practise psychomotor skills with ongoing feedback. Learning goals should be simple and stated in words that are familiar to the learner. Provide only essential, basic information, in a sequential format, and avoid information overload. Using open-ended questions and other listening responses can help you clarify the information for the person. Question them to determine if reading material in their preferred language would be helpful.

Some people have adequate literacy skills but a limited background or lack of interest in medical matters. This makes it difficult for them to understand medical terminology and complex medical explanations. The advice to keep information simple and straightforward applies to all health education situations (Kobayashi et al., 2016).

Developmental Factors

The person's developmental learning factors significantly influence their ability to learn (Bastable, 2017).

TABLE 16.1 Recommended Teaching Strategies at Different Developmental Levels	
Developmental Level	**Recommended Teaching Strategies**
Preschool	Allow child to touch and play with safe equipment. Relate teaching to child's immediate experience. Use child's vocabulary whenever possible. Involve parents in teaching.
School age	Give factual information in simple, concrete terms. Focus teaching on developing competency. Use simple drawings and models to emphasize points. Answer questions honestly and factually.
Adolescent	Use metaphors and analogies in teaching. Give choices and multiple perspectives. Incorporate the person's norm group values and personal identity issues in teaching strategies.
Adult	Involve the person as an active partner in the learning process. Encourage self-directed learning. Keep content and strategies relevant and practical. Incorporate previous life experience into teaching.
Older person	Explain why the information should be important to the person. Incorporate previous life experience into teaching. Accommodate for sensory and dexterity deficits. Use short, frequent learning sessions (<30 minutes).

Children at different levels of cognitive development need health teaching that is specifically tailored to their developmental level. For example, children who cannot think abstractly will not understand a conceptual explanation of what is happening to them. Instead, they need simple, concrete explanations and examples. Recommended teaching strategies for learners at different developmental levels are presented in Table 16.1.

Social Determinants

Socioenvironmental factors can undermine the effectiveness of health teaching and even produce dangerous outcomes. Commonly overlooked potential barriers include transportation difficulties, lack of follow-up facilities, lack of access to grocery stores and health facilities, cultural considerations, and choice of priorities. People may not have enough money for medication. Health illiteracy can be a product of poverty as well as culture (Lowenstein et al., 2009). Nurses need to explore the level and types of situational support available to people and their families as part of any teaching plan.

Planning

Family Involvement

Health teaching similar to what is provided to the person should also be given to anyone actively involved in the

person's care as a primary caregiver or reliable supportive influence. Information and anticipatory guidance about what to expect when the person goes home, and early warning signs of complications or potential problems, should also be given to family members. It is critical for them to know when to seek professional assistance and resource support. Examples of appropriate goals for family teaching relate to empowerment of family members in using equipment, understanding what is happening to their family member, and promoting direct involvement in therapeutic care.

Note changes in the level of support from primary caregivers, as this circumstance can affect a person's willingness or ability to learn. When these supports are no longer available through death, incapacity, or for other reasons, the person may lack not only motivation but also the skills to cope with complex health problems.

Case Example

Edward Flanigan, an 82-year-old, recently widowed man, has severe diabetes. There is no evidence of memory problems, but there are significant emotional components to his current health care needs. All his life, his wife pampered him and did everything for him, from meal preparation to monitoring his diabetes. Since her death, Edward has taken no interest in controlling his diabetes. He does not follow his pre-scribed diabetic diet and is not consistent in taking his medication. Predictably, his diabetes has become increasingly unstable. His family worries about him, but he is unwilling to consider leaving his home of 42 years. To enhance Edward's learning readiness, how could his teaching plan related to diabetic self-care management skills be individualized?

Considering Special Learning Needs
Cultural Diversity

People interpret health care messages within the context of their culturally bound traditions, beliefs, and values. Tailoring teaching interventions to meet people's specific cultural needs and resources is key to improving outcomes through patient education (Peek et al., 2012). Explanatory models for why symptoms develop, and personalized cultural attitudes toward common treatment protocols, are important to know, primarily because they may be wrong or harmful. Inquire about home remedies and applicable spiritual influences. It is critically important to know about the use of Indigenous traditional medicine and recommendations from Indigenous health informants and providers. Differences should be treated with the utmost respect. When you are working with people who are culturally different from you, it is important to provide health resources in a way that fits with their culture, if at all possible. Doing so can be a collaborative venture in which you ask the person to tell you how the health problem would be treated in their culture and negotiate for an acceptable treatment option. Culturally unique perspectives and preferences for treatment can be incorporated in many situations if they are not harmful. When this is not the case, negotiating an acceptable compromise respects a person's cultural values and, most important, the person exhibiting them.

There are several reasons for including cultural values. People whose culture is different from yours may be more likely to trust traditional health care solutions than modern medical approaches. They may prefer a teaching plan that integrates cultural practices with mainstream biomedical approaches because the traditional sounds familiar. They may be more likely to follow suggestions that correspond with their preferences and to use the provider relationship as a valued resource.

Focusing on accurate information without destroying the credibility of influential cultural health advisors is part of the art of health teaching. Nothing is gained by injuring the reputation of someone who gave the person information, and only those findings with potentially adverse health consequences should be addressed. To stimulate further discussion, you could say, "There have been some new findings that I think you might be interested in…" or "Current thinking suggests that (and give a relevant example) works well in situations like this." With this type of statement, you can expand the person's thinking without challenging the status of someone they consider as expert. (See Chapters 7 and 15 for more ideas tailoring communication and teaching strategies to use in teaching people whose culture is different from yours.)

Sometimes, there is a tendency for people to speak louder when instructing someone from a different culture. Instead, speak more *slowly*, in a normal conversational tone. When teaching a person for whom English is a second language, keep in mind that words from one language do not necessarily translate with the same meaning in another. Certain concepts may not exist or the phrases used for expressing and describing them may differ significantly. It is best to use simple, concrete words and images in explaining options and to ask frequently for validation of understanding. When preparing teaching materials for translation, the following ideas are important:

- Use nouns rather than pronouns and simple unambiguous language.
- Use short, simple sentences of less than 16 words each.
- Avoid the use of metaphors and informal language or slang.
- Avoid verb forms that have more than one meaning or include *would* or *could* (p. 181).

If someone still is unable to understand important concepts with accommodations, enlisting the services of a trained medical interpreter becomes an essential intervention.

Adaptations for Cognitive Processing Deficits

Learners with memory deficits, lack of insight, poor judgement, or limited problem-solving abilities require accommodations. Learners with special needs respond best when the content is presented in a consistent, concrete, and patient manner, with clear and frequent cues to action. Patience and repetition of key ideas are essential. Illustrated materials can result in greater comprehension and recall, but they should be simple, without distracting details (Friedman et al., 2011). If the deficit is more than minimal, it may be helpful to include significant others in the teaching session, as this may increase the chance that the person will follow the instructions.

Creating and Implementing a Successful Teaching Plan

Teaching plans provide a guide for choosing and sequencing content and for identifying the best approach. Box 16.3

provides a sample format for developing a relevant teaching plan.

- What essential information does the person need to have for self-management of their disease process?
- What attitudes does the person hold that could enable or hinder the learning process?
- What specific skills does the person need for self-management?
- What does the person want from this health experience to improve their quality of life?
- What cultural or socioenvironmental factors could facilitate or sabotage the learning process?

Periodically asking the person and primary caregivers, "Do you have any questions for me?" gives nurses a sense of what is most important to the person or what may not be fully understood. Suggest that if the person has questions about anything later, they should ask for further clarification. Often, hours or days after health teaching takes place, people have questions or concerns about the information they have received. You can offer additional opportunities for discussion after the person has had time to absorb the initial information, and ask questions to determine comprehension.

Health Teaching Goals

Setting realistic, collaborative goals with people, with periodic reviews, not only helps motivate people but also serves as a benchmark for evaluating changes. Establish goals *with* the person rather than *for* the person. Clear, step-by-step learning goals that the person agrees to are more likely to be met.

Identify outcome goals with a general statement of what the person needs to achieve as a result of the teaching (e.g., "After health teaching, the person will maintain dietary control of her diabetes"; an interim goal might be, "After health teaching, the person will develop an appropriate diet plan for 1 week"). Setting realistic goals prevents disappointment.

Developing Measurable Objectives

Objectives help organize content and identify logical action steps. Box 16.4 provides guidelines for developing effective health teaching goals and objectives.

Collaboratively developed objectives should describe an immediate action step-by-step plan for goal achievement, based on the person's most pressing clinical issues (Edwards, 2013). Each action step should build on the previous one for maximum effectiveness. Objectives should be achievable within the allotted time frame. To determine whether an objective is achievable, consider the person's level of experience, educational level, resources, skills, and motivation. This information helps ensure that the objectives are defined in specific, measurable behavioural terms. Objectives also should directly relate to medical and nursing diagnoses and support the overall health outcome.

Timing

Health teaching is an essential nursing intervention; it is not an add-on. Teaching interventions should never be eliminated because the nurse lacks time. Even in the most limited situation, schedule a block of time for health teaching. Because time is a precious commodity in health care, choosing the most effective and efficient ways to achieve identified clinical goals is vital (RNAO, 2012). You need to consider how much time is required to learn a particular skill or body of knowledge and build this into the learning situation. Complicated skill development may require blocks of time for repeated practice with feedback. Pick times for teaching when energy levels are high, there are no distractions, it is not visiting time, and the person is alert and not in pain. Careful observation of the person helps determine the most appropriate times for health teaching.

Even under the best of circumstances, people can absorb only so many details and fine points at a time. Keep the teaching session short, interesting, and to the point. Ideally, teaching sessions should last no longer than about 20 minutes, including time for questions. Otherwise the person may tire or lose interest. By scheduling shorter sessions with time in between to process information, you can help to prevent information overload and reinforce teaching points.

Nurses also have opportunities for informal teaching during the course of providing care. Simple, spontaneous health teaching takes minutes but can have significant effects. Teaching can be enhanced by asking people questions such as, "How are you feeling right now?" before the nurse does health teaching. If the person is in pain, this will be a barrier to their learning. Ask the person directly what they know already or would like to learn. Ask them how they like to learn or what help they need to learn (RNAO, 2012).

Implementation

Each teaching session should be a collaborative process, with a reciprocal exchange of information, feedback, and opportunities to ask questions.

Building a Logical Information Teaching Flow

No one teaching strategy can meet everyone's needs (Su et al., 2011). Introductory content should build on the person's experiences, abilities, interests, motivation, and skills. Most people learn best when there is a logical flow and a building of information from simple to complex. Begin by presenting a simple overview of what will be taught and why the information is important to learn. Include only essential information in your overview; for example, give a brief explanation of the health care problem, risk factors, treatment, and self-care skills the person will need to manage at home. Incorporate or ask about previous related experience.

Concrete application of knowledge in a meaningful context increases learning (Benner et al., 2010). Ideally, you should solicit input frequently and offer opportunities for the person to provide feedback and questioning. Complex information can be delivered in smaller, stepwise learning segments. For example, diabetic teaching could include the following segments:

- Introduction, including what the person already knows
- Basic pathophysiology of diabetes (keep description simple and short)
- Diet and exercise
- Demonstration of insulin injection with return demonstration
- Recognizing signs and symptoms of hyperglycemia and hypoglycemia
- Care of skin and feet
- How to talk to the doctor

A strong closing statement summarizing major points reinforces the learning process. Simulation Exercise 16.2 provides practice with developing a mini teaching plan.

Using Clear Concrete Language

Use simple, familiar words and limit the number of ideas in each learning segment. General or vague language leaves the learner wondering what the nurse actually meant. For example, "Call the doctor if you have any problems" has more than one meaning. "Problems" can refer to side effects of the medication, a return of symptoms, problems with family acceptance, changed relationships, and even alterations in self-concept. You could say, "If you should develop a headache or feel dizzy in the next 24 hours, call

---

SIMULATION EXERCISE 16.2 Developing Teaching Plans

Purpose
To provide practice with developing teaching plans

Procedure
1. Using the teaching plan format, develop a mini teaching plan for someone you are providing care for. Alternative: Develop a mini teaching plan for one of the following situations:
   a. Jim Dolan feels stressed about returning to work after his accident. He is requesting health teaching on stress management and relaxation techniques.
   b. Adrienne Parker is newly diagnosed with diabetes. Her grandfather had diabetes.
   c. Marion Hill just gave birth to her first child. She wants to breastfeed her infant but she is afraid that she does not have enough milk.
   d. Barbara Scott weighs 210 pounds and wants to lose weight.
2. Include the following data: a brief statement of the person's learning needs and a list of related nursing diagnoses in order of priority.
3. For one nursing diagnosis, develop a mini teaching plan outlining objectives, topical content, planned teaching strategies, time frame for planned activities, and evaluation criteria.

the emergency department (or doctor) right away." Provide the phone number (and physician's name, if appropriate).

Checking with people to confirm a common understanding of words and concepts is critical to knowledge transfer in health teaching. It is helpful to seek feedback from the person to determine if they understood the content. To do this, ask them questions, watch their nonverbal behaviour, and have them explain to you what they have learned (see Table 16.1). Concrete examples help people understand abstract material. You also can ask the person for relevant examples to make a point.

Written directions should demonstrate similar language clarity. From a study of input from people about written care instructions, Buckley et al. (2013) suggest highlighting key words—for example, "After cleaning, you can apply antibiotic ointment, Neosporin or bacitracin, to the wound and then put on a clean bandage" (p. 556).

Incorporating Visual Aids

Line drawings and simple diagrams of body parts or physiology related to a procedure help to increase comprehension. Simple images and plain language work better than complicated visual aids and technical terms. For example, an illustrated chart showing how the heart pumps blood might help a person understand the anatomy and physiology of a cardiac problem better than words. Various media formats are useful in teaching people with limited reading skills. They have the advantage of allowing people to watch them again at their convenience. Related discussions help to correct misinterpretations and emphasize pertinent points.

Preparing Written Handouts

Written materials reinforce learning. Attention to the person's reading level and health literacy helps ensure that the pamphlets will be read (Centers for Disease Control and Prevention [CDC], 2009). Most reading materials should be geared to a Grades 6 to 8 reading level. Even people with adequate health literacy comprehend written information better when the language is simple and clear, using layperson's language. Large-print pamphlets and online videos are helpful learning aids for those with sight problems and for those who are auditory learners.

Guidelines for preparing effective written materials include the following:

- Present the most important information first.
- Use clear illustrations and diagrams designed to enhance clarity and appeal.
- Make sure that the content is current, accurate, objective, *and* consistent with information provided by other team members.
- Use simple language at a literacy level that the reader can understand easily.

- Use at least a 12-point font size and avoid using all capital letters, for reading ease.
- Define technical terms in lay language (plain language); avoid medical jargon.
- Make important points in bold.
- Check for spelling errors and avoid complicated sentences.
- Include resources with contact information that the person can refer to for further information or for help.

Advance Organizers

Advance organizers are methods of presenting introductory materials ahead of time, to help people remember and understand difficult concepts; they may consist of cue words, phrases, or letters related to more complex data. One type, mnemonics, give the person a useful tool for remembering related concepts—for example, each letter in the word *diabetes* can represent an action for diabetes control. In the case of diabetes, the following mnemonic can be useful:

D = diet
I = infections
A = administering medications
B = basic pathophysiology
E = eating schedules
T = treatment for hyperglycemia or hypoglycemia
E = exercise
S = symptom recognition

Evaluation and Documentation
Teach-Three and Teach-Back

Teach-back is a simple, effective means of checking the person's comprehension of care concepts and how to execute self-management skills post-discharge. People are initially taught up to three key actions, knowledge concepts, and care skills related to self-management of a condition. This information should be delivered in small chunks of data or skill demonstrations, using terminology that the person can easily understand (see Fig. 16.6).

The first step in the process is to determine what the person knows about their medical condition. Listen to questions, explain the person's condition in terms they can understand, and use teach-back or "show me" as a participatory evaluation method. This method allows you to confirm the person's understanding of or ability to execute self-management skills, through demonstration or explanation of major points. The person explains relevant information and treatment instructions in their own words. Teach-back offers nurses valuable data about areas of skill learning needing additional attention (Paterick et al., 2017).

Start with a statement such as, "I just want to be sure that I have explained everything you need to know. Can you tell me, in your own words, how you will determine that your blood sugar is low, and what you will do if it is?" Encourage the person to ask questions. If the content is complex, consider using teach-back after each segment, before moving on to the next concept. Repeat instructions if needed. Document your use of teach-back and the person's response (Simulation Exercise 16.3).

Documenting Health Teaching

The International Joint Commission (2015) requires written documentation of all health teaching. Notes about the initial assessment should be succinct but comprehensive and objective. Teaching content should be linked to assessment data, including the person's preferences, previous knowledge, and values. Included in the documentation are the teaching actions, the person's response, and any clinical issues or barriers to compliance. If family members are involved, you should identify their role, content provided, and teaching outcomes in your documentation. Accurate documentation promotes continuity of care and prevents duplication of teaching efforts.

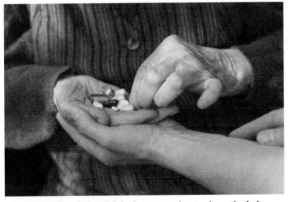

Fig. 16.6 "Teach-back" helps people anchor their knowledge about important aspects of self-management. Copyright © Ocskaymark/iStock.com

The record informs other health care providers of completed teaching and what areas need further work.

Self-Management Strategies

People are living much longer than in years past, and the contemporary focus on helping people and their families develop self-management strategies in contemporary health care reflects the expanded extent of chronic illness reform. Examples of chronic illnesses requiring self-management include cancer, diseases that cause dementia, asthma, osteoporosis, diabetes, multiple sclerosis, arthritis, hypertension, macular degeneration, cardiovascular disorders, chronic obstructive pulmonary disease, stroke, and chronic mental health disorders. Cystic fibrosis, developmental delays and abnormalities, type I diabetes, sickle cell anemia, and childhood cancer are significant chronic disorders seen particularly in younger people. Participatory self-management related to chronic disorders represents a logical way of reducing health costs while still providing quality care (Peeters et al., 2013).

Skill support for people and their families requires more than basic informative education about a person's medical information and treatment (The International Joint Commission, 2015).

COMPONENTS OF SELF-MANAGEMENT PATIENT EDUCATION

The British Columbia Ministry of Health (2011) identifies essential self-management skills such as the following:
- "Has knowledge of his/her condition and/or its management
- Adopts a self-management care plan agreed and negotiated in partnership with health professionals
- Actively shares in decision making with health professionals

---

SIMULATION EXERCISE 16.3 Teach-Back

Purpose
To help students understand the teach-back process

Procedure
Review what you learned in class about the teach-back method. Break into groups of three students: the nurse, person, and observer. Each student takes a turn being the nurse, the person, and the observer. Using one medication that the person is on for the first time, role-play the teach-back process. Rotate roles so each student has the opportunity to role-play the part of the nurse.

Discussion
After *each* teach-back role-play, discuss the following:
1. The nurse reflects on what they did well or would have changed.
2. The observer provides feedback on what the nurse did well and what they could have done better.
3. The person receiving the teaching aids should add their perspective and anything that was not addressed by the other two participants.

- Monitors and manages signs and symptoms of his/her condition
- Manages the impact of the condition on physical, emotional, occupational and social functioning
- Adopts lifestyles that address risk factors and promotes health by focusing on prevention and early intervention
- Has access to and confidence in the ability to use support services" since this is a direct quote, the page number is 8.

Simple, direct pieces of information help people and their families understand and effectively support their management of chronic disorders. You can reinforce relevant information with a guidebook or checklist. Collaborative development of a self-management plan helps people feel more committed to a self-management plan in line with their values, health and life needs, and resources.

Learning self-management strategies takes time and social support. Approaches must be tailored to each person's unique life situation, values, opportunities, and skills. Care plans and self-management plans can be useful in facilitating people's discussion of self-care actions and lifestyle management. Organizational factors affect opportunities for professionals to support people's self-care management. These include time, resources, the opportunity for open access to appointments, and early referral to other professional groups.

SELF-MANAGEMENT SKILL DEVELOPMENT

Mickley et al. (2013) define self-management as "the skills and activities necessary to control symptoms of a chronic condition" (p. 323). Development of self-management skills requires a problem-based teaching approach. In addition to acquiring specific knowledge and skills, people and their families need to learn how to cope effectively with a chronic illness. This usually involves special attention to the social consequences and lifestyle changes occurring as a result of the chronic condition.

A multistrategy approach is useful, including the activation of essential resources such as accessing social services, joining support groups, choosing different activities, and so forth (British Columbia Ministry of Health, 2011). Children usually require consistent parental support and encouragement to follow through with care tasks and reinforcement for small successes. Because of their developmental needs, children may require special adaptations to lead normal, healthy lives. It is critically important to be aware of the school and community supports available for children with chronic disabilities.

Active participation of the person with the support of the person's family is essential in the daily management of chronic medical conditions (Udlis, 2011). Participatory decision making is a vital component of meaningful action planning, and tailoring of teaching strategies for people and their families is a critical dimension. Repetition is important, as is careful inquiry with open-ended questions about new issues. People must understand why an action is important, what can be expected with a medication or treatment protocol, what the risks and benefits of treatment options are, and what the warning signs of adverse reactions are. A specific plan about what to do when something goes wrong is essential content. Unforeseen factors affecting the self-management process, such as changes in the environmental context, interactions with health providers, and changes imposed by the chronic illness make this information essential content. Incomplete patient education, resulting in people not knowing how to self-monitor symptoms and recognize side effects, is not only unsafe but also ethically indefensible (Redman, 2011). People need support as they take the first steps toward autonomously assuming responsibility for self-care and whenever a health situation changes. Living with chronic illness produces unexpected transitions in care requirements associated with exacerbations. Self-monitoring should focus on changes in symptoms and achieving treatment goals. Input from the person and family, combined with professional contributions, is essential for the development of personalized self-care applications. They help to incorporate specific self-management actions into a person's daily routine.

COACHING

Coaching involves the use of evidence-informed skillful conversation to engage others in health behaviour change (Huffman, 2016). The aim of coaching is to support people to set and achieve healthy living goals using a peer-led self-management approach. There is evidence that people benefit from being coached by their peers as this can offer more authentic support in a relationship that is equality-based. This approach also helps people reconnect with their community. People are more likely to listen and change their behaviour when working with a peer who is similar to themselves (British Columbia Ministry of Health, 2011, p. 49).

For example, you can help people and their families choose the most appropriate questions to ask their provider. A coaching intervention can be as simple as helping people seek information from several sources rather than calling only one and waiting for a response (Huffman, 2016).

Coaching "builds on the patient's strengths rather than attempting to fix weaknesses" (Dossey & Hess, 2013, p. 10). A coaching process emphasizes the person's autonomy in acquiring self-management skills because the person is always in charge of the pace and direction of the learning.

Coaching involves a number of skills presented in Fig. 16.7. Start an assessment with an examination of a person's current health issue, followed by an exploration of its meaning in the person's life. This dual dialogue provides a basis for looking at current options through the lens of personal values and beliefs. The next step is to encourage people to think critically about the elements of a situation. Only then is it possible to consider multiple options and new perspectives. The final step is to evaluate the appropriateness of choosing one option over another and to choose a course of action.

The coaching process involves taking the person step by step through a procedure or activities, with the person taking the lead in choice of actions. The secret of successful coaching is to provide enough information and support to help the person take the next step without taking over for them (Fig. 16.7).

Coaching strategies can include supervised skill practice and role-playing. For example, role-playing a potentially difficult conversation can inform the person about timing of actions and potential outcomes. The exercise highlights areas that need special attention, and related issues

that might not otherwise emerge in a teaching situation. Simulation Exercise 16.4 provides practice with coaching as a teaching strategy.

Providing Transitional Cues

People sometimes have difficulty learning essential information because they do not see how it fits together when applied to their particular circumstances. Transitional cues should do the following:

- Link purpose with action—for example, follow the purpose of taking a medication or doing an exercise with the actions you want the person to take. This dual approach helps fix the process in the person's mind and makes it easier for them to remember related instructions.
- Specify what is important, and why. When you tell someone that a medication should be taken with meals, be specific about what this means and why it is important.
- Ask the person (teach-back) how they will implement essential health management skills such as using an inhaler or adhering to a therapeutic diet. Ask the person if they have any issues or concerns that you have not addressed. Visual cues such as a sticky note to

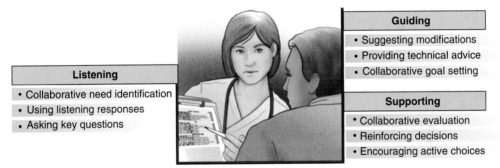

Listening
- Collaborative need identification
- Using listening responses
- Asking key questions

Guiding
- Suggesting modifications
- Providing technical advice
- Collaborative goal setting

Supporting
- Collaborative evaluation
- Reinforcing decisions
- Encouraging active choices

Fig. 16.7 The nurse's role in coaching people

SIMULATION EXERCISE 16.4   Coaching

Purpose
To help students understand the process of coaching

Procedure
Identify the steps you would use to coach someone currently in your care or a person with one of the chronic health conditions listed below. Use Fig. 16.1 as a guide to develop your plan.
1. A person returning from hip replacement surgery
2. A person recovering from a myocardial infarction
3. A person with newly diagnosed type II diabetes

4. A child with partially controlled asthma
Share your suggestions with your classmates.

Discussion
1. What were the different coaching strategies you used with the person?
2. In what ways were your coaching strategies similar to or unlike those of your classmates?
3. How could you use the information you gained from this exercise to improve the quality of your coaching?

remember to take medication or to keep an appointment are helpful too. Ask people to keep a self-report log and share it with you as needed.

Giving Feedback

Feedback is of central importance in successful health coaching. Giving immediate feedback is important with learning psychomotor tasks. To appreciate its significance in learning new skills, consider the effect on your performance if you never received feedback from your instructor. For maximum effectiveness, give feedback as soon as possible after the learning event or observation. Consider the impact on the person. Encourage the person's reflection by asking open-ended questions such as, "How did you feel about doing your treatment by yourself?" "Is there anything you would do differently next time?"

Indirect feedback—provided through nodding, smiling, and sharing information about the process and experiences of others—also reinforces learning. When providing feedback, keep it participatory and simple. Focus only on behaviours that can be changed. Include strengths as well as areas needing improvement. Simulation Exercise 16.5 provides practice with giving feedback.

BEHAVIOURAL APPROACHES

Behavioural approaches are based on the work of B. F. Skinner (1971). Behaviourists believe that **reinforcement** strengthens learner responses. Reward must have meaning to the learner in order to be effective. This is critical because what is reinforcing to one person may not be so for another. Positive reinforcement of an individual's behaviours tends to lead those behaviours to increase. Reward withdrawal and ignoring behaviours tend to diminish their occurrence. Different types of reinforcement and punishment, with examples, are found in Table 16.2. Reinforcement schedules describe the timing of rewards. Schedules start with

---

SIMULATION EXERCISE 16.5   Usable Feedback

Purpose

To give students perspective and experience in giving usable feedback

Procedure

1. Divide into working groups of three or four students.
2. Present a 3-minute sketch of some aspect of your current learning situation that you find difficult (e.g., writing a paper, speaking in class, coordinating study schedules, or studying certain material).
3. Each person, in turn, offers one piece of usable informative feedback to the presenter. In making suggestions, use the guidelines on feedback given in this chapter.
4. Place feedback suggestions on a flip chart or chalkboard.

Discussion

1. What were your thoughts and feelings about the feedback you heard in relation to resolving the problem you presented to the group?
2. What were your thoughts and feelings in giving feedback to each presenter?
3. Was it harder to give feedback in some cases than in others? In what ways?
4. What common themes emerged in your group?
5. In what ways can you use the self-exploration about feedback in this exercise in teaching conversations with people?

TABLE 16.2   Types of Reinforcement

Concept	Purpose	Example
Positive reinforcer	Increases probability of behaviour through reward	Stars on a board, smiling, verbal praise, candy, tokens to "purchase" items
Negative reinforcer	Increases probability of behaviour by removing aversive consequence	Restoring privileges when the person performs desired behaviour
Punishment	Decreases behaviour by presenting a negative consequence or removing a positive one	Negative punishment: losing privileges Positive punishment: Time-outs, denial of privileges
Ignoring	Decreases behaviour by not reinforcing it	Not paying attention to whining, tantrums, or provocative behaviours

continuous reinforcement for each completed attempt. Once a new behaviour is in place, interval schedules in which reinforcement is given after a certain number of successful attempts (fixed interval) or amount of time (fixed interval), or after a random number of responses (variable ratio) or amount of time (variable interval) are introduced. Tangible rewards are gradually replaced with social reinforcement such as praise. Over time, improved health outcomes become a source of reinforcement to people. For example, significant weight loss and the way it makes a person feel about their personal appearance is a strong motivator to continue with a healthy diet.

A behavioural approach starts with a careful description of a concrete behaviour requiring change. Describe each action as a single behavioural unit (e.g., failing to take medication, cheating on a diet, or not participating in unit activities). It is important to start small so that the person will experience success.

A behavioural approach requires the cooperation of the person and a shared understanding of the problem. Count the number of times the person engages in a behaviour as a baseline before implementing the behavioural approach. This allows the nurse and the person to monitor progress as the process progresses.

Behavioural objectives should be action oriented. They reframe the problem in a solution statement (e.g., "The person will lose 2 pounds"). Begin with the simplest and most likely behaviour to stimulate interest in the person. Identify the tasks in sequential order; define specific consequences, positive and negative, for behavioural responses; and solicit the person's cooperation.

Behavioural Strategies

Modelling describes learning a behaviour by observing another person who is performing it. Nurses model behaviours in their normal conduct of nursing activities and teaching situations. Bathing an infant, feeding an older person, and talking to a scared child in front of significant caregivers provides informal modelling.

Shaping refers to the reinforcement of successive approximations of the target behaviour. The long-term goal is broken down into smaller steps. The person is reinforced for any behaviour (successive approximations) that gets them closer to accomplishing the desired behaviour.

Learning Contracts

A learning contract with the person serves as a formal commitment to a behavioural learning process. Contracts spell out the responsibilities of each party, expected behaviours, and reinforcements. Contracts are especially useful as part of learning self-management strategies for school-aged children. The contract should include the following:

- Behavioural changes that are to occur
- Conditions under which they are to occur
- A reinforcement schedule
- A time frame punctuation

Initially, each instance of the expected behaviour should be rewarded. If the person is noncompliant or needs to pay more attention to a particular aspect of behaviour, the nurse can say, "This (name the behaviour or skill) needs a little more work." One advantage of a behavioural approach is that it never considers the person as bad or unworthy.

Group Presentations

Group presentations offer the advantage of teaching a number of people at one time. Group formats allow people to hear other people's questions and learn from their experiences and approaches (Tucker, 2013). Health teaching topics that lend themselves to a group format include care of a newborn, diabetes, oncology, and prenatal and postnatal care (Belton, 2017).

Formal group teaching should occur in a space large enough to accommodate all participants. The learner should be able to hear and see the instructor and visual aids without strain. Technical equipment (if used) should be available and in working order. Should the equipment not work, it is better to eliminate the planned teaching aid completely than to spend a portion of the teaching session trying to fix it. Preparation and practice can ensure that your presentation is clear, concise, and well spoken.

Establish rapport with your audience. Extension of eye contact to all participants communicates acceptance and inclusion. Make eye contact immediately and continue to do so throughout the presentation. An initial quote capturing the meaning of the presentation or a humorous opening grabs the audience's attention. Logical organization of the material is essential. Strengthen content statements with careful use of specific examples. Citing a specific problem and the ways another person dealt with it offers a broader perspective. Repeating key points and summarizing them again at the conclusion of the session helps reinforce learning.

Use of electronic presentation formats identify key points and help the presenter stay on track and move through the agenda. The font should be large enough to be seen from a distance (32 point is recommended). Use presentation slides and include no more than four or five items per slide. Face the audience, not the presentation. Practise your presentation to ensure that you keep within the time frame and allot time for short discussion points. It is up to the presenter to set the pace. No matter how interesting the presentation and the dialogue that it stimulates, running out of time is frustrating for the audience.

Anticipate questions and be on the alert for blank looks. No matter how good a nurse educator you are, from time to time, you will experience the blank look. When this occurs, it is appropriate to ask, "Do you have any questions about anything I have said so far?" Give reinforcement for comments, such as, "I'm so glad you brought that up," or "That's a really interesting question (or comment)." Smiling and nodding are nonverbal reinforcers. If a participant has a question that you cannot answer, do not bluff. Instead, say, "That's a good question. I don't have an answer at this moment, but I will get back to you with it." This should not be the end point. Sometimes, another person will have the required information and will share it. Handouts provide reinforcement. Make sure the information is accurate, complete, easy to understand, logical, and—very important—that you have enough for all participants. Simulation Exercise 16.6 provides an opportunity to practise health teaching in a group setting.

Health Teaching in the Home

Health teaching in the home includes assessment of the home environment, family support, and resources, as well as the needs of the person and their family. In many ways, the home offers a teaching laboratory unparalleled in the hospital. The nurse can "see" improvisations in equipment and technique that are possible in the home environment. Family members may have ideas that the nurse would not have thought of, and the nurse can see the obstacles the family faces. Nurses should review the basic pathophysiology and course of the person's health condition with the person and family. Everyone needs to understand the nature of chronic illness and the potential for exacerbation episodes. Teach-back evaluation helps reinforce learning.

The nurse is a guest in the person's home. Always call before going to the person's home. This is common courtesy; it also protects the nurse's time if the person is going to be out. Teaching in home care settings is rewarding. Often, the nurse is the person's only visitor. Family members often display a curiosity and willingness to be a part of the learning group, particularly if the nurse actively uses knowledge of the home environment to make suggestions about needed modifications.

Teaching in home settings should centre on self-management essentials. Encourage people or caregivers to write down their questions between visits, so critical issues can be addressed during the home visit. Start each session with an open-ended question as to how things are going. Ask if there are any new or unresolved concerns.

You need to review medications with the person or caregiver on every visit. Tips for teaching people and their caregivers about medications are presented in Box 16.5. Other content reflects specific information the person and their family need to support self-care management.

Expert nurses know that people often can be a source of information about resources the nurse may not know about.

Constructing the Teaching Plan

Health teaching consists of three interrelated components: information gathering, information sharing, and relationship building, as shown in Fig. 16.5.

Essential content in all teaching plans includes information about the health care problem, risk factors, and self-care skills needed to manage at home. The person's learning needs help define relevant teaching strategies. Assessment

---

SIMULATION EXERCISE 16.6   Group Health Teaching

Purpose

To provide practice with presenting a health topic in a group setting

Procedure

1. Plan a 15- to 20-minute health presentation on a health topic of interest to you, including teaching aids and methods for evaluation. Suggested topics:

Nutrition	Weight control
Drinking and driving	Mammograms
High blood pressure	Safer sex

2. Present your topic to your class group.

BOX 16.5   Medication Teaching Tips

- Provide people with written drug information, particularly for metered-dose inhalers and high-alert medications such as insulin.
- Include family or caregivers in the teaching sessions for people who need extra support or reminders.
- Do not wait until discharge to begin education about complex drug regimens.
- Clearly explain directions for using each medication.
- Always require repeat demonstrations or explanations about medications to be taken at home, particularly for those requiring special drug administration techniques.
- Use the time you already spend with people during assessments and daily care to evaluate their level of understanding about their medications.
- Keep medication administration schedule as simple and easy to follow as possible.

Modified from Institute for Safe Medication Practices. (2006). *Patient medication teaching tips.*

for purposes of constructing a teaching plan centres on three areas: What does the person already know? What is important for the person to know? What is the person ready to learn?

SUMMARY

This chapter describes the nurse's role in health teaching. Theoretical frameworks, person-centred teaching, as well as developmental and behavioural approaches guide the nurse in implementing health teaching. Teaching is designed to access one or more of the three domains of learning: cognitive, affective, and psychomotor. Box 16.1 provides characteristics associated with each of these domains.

Several teaching strategies, such as coaching, use of mnemonics, and visual aids, are described. Repetition of key concepts and frequent feedback make the difference between simple instruction and teaching that informs. Nurses use teach-back methods to confirm understanding. They are also responsible for documenting their patient education activities, thereby informing other health care workers what has been taught and what areas need to be addressed in future teaching sessions (International Joint Commission, 2015).

ETHICAL DILEMMA:

What Would You Do?

Louisa, who has a low level of literacy, is at the mental health clinic and wants a refill of her medication. She states that she has reduced her medication to every other day rather than every day because she thinks it "works better for her." She does not want to lower her dose. She also tells the nurse that she gave several of her extra pills to her brother because he ran out of his pills. Although she listens politely to the nurse's concerns, Louisa tells her that she thinks her current regimen is appropriate for her. She sees nothing wrong with sharing her medications with her brother as he is on the same medication. If you were the nurse, how would you respond to Louisa?

QUESTIONS FOR REVIEW AND DISCUSSION

1. How can you best integrate chronic disease–related personal self-management skills with lifestyle and other aspects of the person's life?

2. Discuss what is meant by the following statement: "Patient education is essential to safe, ethical, clinical practice."

3. What *specific* strategies would you use to help people with low literacy learn essential health information?

REFERENCES

Baker, D., DeWalt, D., Schillinger, D., et al. (2011). Teach to goal: Theory and design principles of an intervention to improve heart failure self-management skills of patients with low literacy. *Journal of Health Communication, 16*(Suppl. 3), 3–88. 7.

Bastable, S. (2017). *Nurse as educator: Principles of teaching and learning for nursing practice* (5th ed.). Jones & Bartlett.

Baur, C. (2011). Calling the nation to act: Implementing the national action. *Nursing Outlook, 59*(2), 63–69. https://www.bccnp.ca/Standards/all_nurses/harmonized/Pages/Default.aspx.

Beagley, L. (2011). Educating patients: Understanding barriers, learning styles, and teaching techniques. *Journal of Perianesthesia Nursing, 26*(5), 331–337.

Belton, A. (2017). *The how to of patient education.* https://books.google.ca/books?id=ehMxswEACAAJ.

Benner, P., Sutphen, M., Leonard, V., et al. (2010). *Educating nurses: A call for radical transformation.* Jossey-Bass.

British Columbia Ministry of Health. (2011). *Self management support: A health care intervention,* 6. https://www.selfmanagementbc.ca/uploads/What%20is%20Self-Management/PDF/Self-Management%20Support%20A%20health%20care%20intervention%202011.pdf.

Buckley, B. A., McCarthy, D. M., Forth, V. E., et al. (2013). Patient input into the development and enhancement of ED discharge instructions: A focus group study. *Journal of Emergency Nursing, 39*(6), 553–561. https://doi.org/10.1016/j.jen.2011.12.018.

Centers for Disease Control and Prevention. (2009). *Simply put: A guide to creating easy-to-understand materials.* https://www.cdc.gov/healthliteracy/pdf/Simply_Put.pdf.

Deek, H., Hamilton, S., Brown, N., et al. (2016). Family-centered approaches to healthcare interventions in chronic diseases in adults: A quantitative systematic review. *Journal of Advanced Nursing, 72*, 968–979.

Dossey, B., & Hess, D. (2013). Professional nurse coaching: Advances in global healthcare transformation. *Global Advances in Health and Medicine, 40*(2), 10–16.

Dreeben, O. (2010). *Patient education in rehabilitation.* Jones & Bartlett Publishers.

Edwards, A. (2013). Asthma action plans and self-management: Beyond the traffic light. *Nursing Clinics of North America, 48*, 47–51.

Farin, E., Gramm, L., & Schmidt, E. (2013). Predictors of communication preferences in patients with chronic low back pain. *Patient Prefer Adherence, 7*, 1117–1127.

Friedman, A. J., Cosby, R., Boyko, S., et al. (2011). Effective teaching strategies and methods of delivering for patient education: A systematic review and practice guideline recommendations. *Journal of Cancer Education, 26*, 12–21.

Gordon, J. (2011). Educating the patient: Challenges and opportunities with current technology. *Nursing Clinics of North America, 46,* 341–350.

Holt, J. E., Flint, E. P., & Bowers, M. T. (2011). Got the picture? Using mobile phone technology to reinforce discharge instructions. *American Journal of Nursing, 111*(8), 47–51.

Huffman, M. (2016). Advancing the practice of health coaching: Differentiation from wellness coaching. *Workplace Health Safety, 64*(9), 400–403. https://doi.org/10.1177/21650799 16645351.

Inott, T., & Kennedy, B. (2011). Assessing learning styles: Practical tips for patient education. *Nursing Clinics of North America, 46*(3), 313–320.

Kadiyala, S., Gavini, S., Kumar, D. S., et al. (2017). Applying Bloom's taxonomy in framing MCQs: An innovative method for formative assessment in medical students. *Journal of Dr. NTR University of Health Sciences, 6*(2), 86–91. https://doi.org/10.4103/2277-8632.208010.

Kelo, M., Eriksson, E., & Eriksson, I. (2013). Pilot educational program to enhance empowering patient education of school-age children with diabetes. *Journal of Diabetes & Metabolic Disorders, 12,* 18.

Knowles, M., Holton, E., & Swanson, R. (2011). *The adult learner: The definitive classic on adult education and training* (7th ed.). Elsevier.

Kobayashi, L., Wardle, J., Wolf, M., et al. (2016). Aging and functional health literacy: A systematic review and meta-analysis. *The Journals of Gerontology: Series B, 71*(3), 445–457. https://doi.org/10.1093/geronb/gbu161.

Krau, S. (2011). Creating educational objectives for patient education using the new Bloom's taxonomy. *Nursing Clinics of North America, 46,* 299–321.

Lowenstein, A. A., Foord-May, L. L., & Romano, J. J. (2009). *Teaching strategies for health education and health promotion.* Jones & Bartlett.

Menendez, J. (2013). Informed consent: Essential legal and ethical principles for nurses. *JONAS Healthcare Law, Ethics, and Regulation, 15*(4), 140–144.

Mezirow, J. (1990). *Fostering critical reflection in adulthood: A guide to transformative and emancipatory learning.* Jossey-Bass.

Mickley, K., Burkhart, P., & Sigler, A. (2013). Promoting normal development and self-efficacy in school age children managing chronic conditions. *Nursing Clinics of North America, 48*(2), 319–328.

Ortiz, M. R. (2018). Patient-centered care: Nursing knowledge and policy. *Nursing Science Quarterly, 31*(3), 291–295. https://doi.org/10.1177/0894318418774906.

Paterick, T. E., Patel, N., Tajik, A. J., et al. (2017). Improving health outcomes through patient education and partnerships with patients. *Proceedings (Baylor University. Medical Center), 30*(1), 112–113. https://doi.org/10.1080/08998280.2017.11929552.

Peek, M., Harmon, S., Scott, J., et al. (2012). Culturally tailoring patient education and communication skills training to empower African Americans with diabetes. *Translational Behavioral Medicine, 2*(3), 296–308.

Peeters, J., Wiegers, T., & Friele, R. (2013). How technology in care at home affects patient self-care and self-management: A scoping review. *International Journal of Environmental Research and Public Health, 10*(11), 5541–5564.

Prochaska, J. O., & Velicer, W. F. (1997). The transtheoretical model of health behavior change. *American Journal of Health Promotion: AJHP, 12*(1), 38–48. https://doi.org/10.4278/0890-1171-12.1.38.

RNAO (Registered Nurses' Association of Ontario. (2012). *Facilitating client centred learning.* https://rnao.ca/sites/rnao-ca/files/BPG_CCL_2012_FA.pdf.

Redman, B. K. (2011). Ethics of patient education and how do we make it everyone's ethics. *Nursing Clinics of North America, 46,* 283–289.

Rogers, C. (1983). *Freedom to learn for the '80s.* Merrill.

Rowlands, G. (2014). Health literacy. *Human Vaccines & Immunotherapies, 10*(7), 2130–2135. https://doi.org/10.4161/hv.29603.

Sentell, T., Vamos, S., & Okan, O. (2020). Interdisciplinary perspectives on health literacy research around the world: More important than ever in a time of COVID-19. *International Journal of Environmental Research and Public Health, 17*(9), 3010.

Skinner, B. F. (1971). *Beyond freedom and dignity.* Knopf.

Smith, L. (2013). Help your patients access government health information. *Nursing, 2013,* 32–34.

Su, W. M., Herron, B., & Osisek, P. (2011). Using a competency-based approach to patient education: Achieving congruence among learning, teaching and evaluation. *Nursing Clinics of North America, 46*(3), 291–298.

The International Joint Commission. (2015). Sentinel Event. [webpage]. www.jointcommission.org/sentinel_event.aspx.

Tonsaker, T., Bartlett, G., & Trpkov, C. (2014). Health information on the Internet: Gold mine or minefield? *Canadian family physician Medecin de famille canadien, 60*(5), 407–408.

Tucker, M. (2013). *Older diabetes patients benefit from group education.* Medscape.

Udlis, K. (2011). Self-management in chronic illness: Concept and dimensional analysis. *Journal of Nursing and Health Care in Chronic Illness, 3*(2), 130–139.

Urmimala, S., & Lipika, S. (2020). How effective are clinical decision support systems? *British Medical Journal, 370,* m3499.

Wolf, M., Curtis, L., & Baker, D. (2012). Literacy, cognitive function, and health: Results of the LigCog study. *Journal of General Internal Medicine, 27*(100), 1300–1307.

SUGGESTED READING

Bennett, H., Coleman, E., Parry, C., et al. (2010). Health coaching for patients with chronic illness. *Family Practice Management, 17*(5), 24–29.

de Boer, D., Delnoij, D., & Rademakers, J. (2013). The importance of patient-centered care for various patient groups. *Patient Education and Counseling, 90*(3), 405–410.

Durham, B. (2015). The nurse's role in medication safety. *Nursing, 45*(4), 1–4.

Dykes, P., & Collins, S. (2013). *Building linkages between nursing care and improved patient outcomes: The role of health information technology.* http://www.nursingworld.org/Main MenuCategories/ANAMarketplace/ANAPeriodical.

Hudon, C., Tribble, D., Bravo, G., et al. (2013). Family physician enabling attitudes: A study of patient perceptions. *BMC Family Practice, 14*, 8–16.

Koh, H., Brach, C., Harris, M., et al. (2013). A proposed 'Health Literate Care Model' would constitute a systems approach to improving patients' engagement in care. *Health Affairs, 32*(2), 357–367.

Masters, K. (2017). *Role development in professional nursing.* Jones & Bartlett.

Speros, C. L. (2011). Promoting health literacy: A nursing imperative. *Nursing Clinics of North America, 46*(3), 321–333.

Ward, B. W. (2014). Multiple chronic conditions among US adults: A 2012 update. *Preventing Chronic Disease, 11*, E62.

WEBSITE/RESOURCES LIST

www.cdc.gov/healthliteracy/pdf/Simply_Put.pdf.

https://www.diabetes.ca.

www.nlm.nih.gov/medlineplus/healthtopics.html.

https://www.swselfmanagement.ca/uploads/ResourceTools/ Webinar-%20Teach%20Back%20-March%2018,%202014.pdf.

17

Communication in Stressful Situations

Olive Yonge
Originating US Chapter by *Elizabeth C. Arnold*

OBJECTIVES

At the end of the chapter, the reader will be able to:
1. Define stress and associated concepts.
2. Describe biological and psychosocial models of stress.
3. Identify concepts related to coping with stress.
4. Discuss stress assessment strategies.
5. Describe stress reduction strategies nurses can use in stressful situations.
6. Identify stress management therapies.
7. Address burnout in nurses.

Stress is both a cause and a consequence of illness and injury; it stems from functional disruptions and unrealistic self-expectations. Stress has been linked to the six leading causes of death, including heart disease, cancer, lung ailments, accidents, cirrhosis of the liver, and suicide (Government of Canada, 2008; Canadian Mental Health Association [CMHA], 2016).

When a person is admitted to the hospital, they enter a new and usually unfamiliar world. This circumstance in itself represents a stressful situation. This chapter focuses on understanding the role of stress, and helping people develop coping strategies to reduce the impact of stress reactions in health care relationships. Included in this chapter are descriptions of biological and psychosocial models of stress reactions and the types of coping mechanisms used to deal with stress. Nurses and other primary providers of care, especially those working in highly acute nursing situations, are especially vulnerable to stress and burnout. This chapter identifies communication strategies nurses can use to help people and their families reduce stress levels in health care situations.

BASIC CONCEPTS

Definition

Hans Selye (1950) defined **stress** as a nonspecific response of the body to any demand made upon it, regardless of whether it is caused by a pleasant or unpleasant situation. McEwen (2012) describes *stress* as a state of mind "involving both brain and body as well as their interactions" (p. 17180). A stress response is a common reaction to serious illness that affects quality of life for all family members as well as the person's ability to function (Haugland et al., 2013).

Stress represents a natural physiological, psychological, and spiritual response to the presence of a stressor. A stress reaction differs from a crisis situation. Unlike crises, stress responses usually are less dramatic and may not lessen over time. Strengthening a person's capacity to cope effectively with stress has important implications for clinical outcomes as well as the person's **motivation** and capacity to perform self-management (Jaser et al., 2012). A stress assessment should be incorporated as part of the complex data needed to support a person's ability to adapt to chronic illness.

A **stressor** is defined as any demand, situation, internal stimulus, or circumstance that threatens an individual's personal security or integrity. Internal stressors such as pregnancy, fever, menopause, or emotions originate within the body. External stressors—such as social or work stressors, accidents, debt, and exams—start outside the self. **Crisis** (detailed in Chapter 21) represents an extreme acute stressor situation for which coping mechanisms fail and the person is unable to function normally. By definition, a crisis situation resolves within 6 weeks.

Sources of Stress

Stress is a common part of life. For each individual, stress represents a personal experience. What is stressful for one person may not be for another. Stress can develop over time or can strike without warning. Stressors can affect many people at the same time—for example, due to war, hurricane, earthquake or severe flood damage, community mass murders in a school, or 9/11. They can be cumulative, continuous, or just minor hassles. Personal stress can be related to a major life change (marriage, divorce, death, moving to a new area, becoming a parent, graduating from college, starting a new job) or an illness or injury. A new diagnosis, loss of social ties, premature death, and potential damage from adjuvant therapy are common health-related stressors (Antoni, 2013). Some of the more common personal sources of stress are identified in Box 17.1.

In health care situations, sources of emotional stress include watching a loved one steadily decline physically or mentally, concern about finances, uncertainty about the future, balancing other family responsibilities with a person's care, and coping with personal frustration. Stressors likely to stimulate an intense stress response are those where a person has limited control over the situation, the situation is ambiguous, or aspects of the current situation resemble past unresolved stressful events.

The intensity and duration of stress varies according to the circumstances, level of social support, and the person's emotional state. Significant or prolonged stress can increase the impact of a current stressful situation (Meyers, 2011). People with mental health disorders have a double set of chronic stressors as some stems from their disorder, which lowers a person's threshold for stress and diminishes a person's capacity to act effectively to reduce the stress (Lavoie, 2013). Daily hassles (traffic jam, child misbehaviour, too many competing tasks, computer crashes) are mild stressors that can turn into chronic stress, especially when they are cumulative. The stress response is commonly present in most health care situations.

Levels of Stress

Selye used the term **eustress** to describe a mild level of stress, which is a positive response with protective and adaptive functions. Mild stress heightens awareness and can motivate people to master challenges and develop new skills. Coping skills learned in mastering a stressful situation help people cope better with other life circumstances as well (Centre for Studies on Human Stress [CSHS], 2019).

Distress, defined as a negative stress level, creates a level of anxiety exceeding a person's normal coping abilities. Distress diminishes performance and quality of life. High stress levels interfere with a person's ability to function. Severe, chronic stress weakens the immune system, thereby contributing to the development of stress-related illnesses (CSHS, 2019).

Chronic stress is implicated in the development and exacerbation of cardiac conditions, migraine, and digestive disorders. Stress and coping are said to account for up to 50% of the variation in psychological symptoms (CSHS, 2019).

Acute stress requires immediate attention. It creates a very intense form of anxiety, which is disabling for the person experiencing it. Once the situation is resolved, homeostasis is re-established. Untreated, severe mental stress reactions associated with traumatic events can develop into post-traumatic stress disorder, a clinical syndrome requiring psychiatric intervention.

Variation in Stress Responses

Although stress is a universal occurrence, it is a subjective, personal experience. People have different tolerance levels for stress. Some people are extremely sensitive to any stressor. Others are laid back and appear less disturbed by unexpected stressful circumstances.

Stress that is more than mild reduces the efficiency of cognitive functions and clouds perceptual acuity. Secondary stressors, such as insomnia caused by worry and financial issues, can heighten the impact of primary stressors on a person's personal life and routines (Wittenberg-Lyles, 2012). The level of social and resource support that a person receives when stressed can reduce the impact of a stressor.

BOX 17.1 Personal Sources of Stress

Physical Stressors
- Acute or chronic illness
- Trauma or injury
- Pain
- Insomnia

Psychological Stressors
- Mental health disorder
- Loss of job or job security
- Loss of a significant person or pet
- Significant change in residence, relationship, work
- Personal finances
- Work relationships
- High-stress work environment
- Caretaking (older people, children)
- Significant change or loss of role

Spiritual Stressors
- Loss of purpose
- Loss of hope
- Questioning of values or meaning

Current research suggests that men and women respond to stress differently. Men respond with patterns of "fight or flight," whereas women use a "tend and befriend" approach (CSHS, 2019). Women use nurturing activities to reduce stress and promote safety for self and others as priority interventions. They seek social support from others, particularly from other women. Children express stress through behaviour, usually corresponding with their developmental stage and family patterns. Acting-out behaviours and psychosomatic illness can mask a child's distress.

STRESS MODELS

Systemic Physiological Response

Cannon (1932) described stress as a systemic physiological response to a perceived threat. It occurs in a similar way regardless of the stressor. Cannon believed that when people feel physically well, emotionally centred, and personally secure, they are in a state of **homeostasis (also dynamic equilibrium)**. Stress disturbs homeostasis. Physiologically, the sympathetic nervous system sets in motion an immediate hormonal cascade designed to mobilize the body's energy resources to cope with the acute stress.

Cannon proposed that people attempt to adapt to stress using either a "fight or flight" response. The "fight" response refers to a person's inclination to act against a threat. This response is used if the threat appears to be resolvable. People use a "flight" response if they perceive that the threat cannot be overcome through personal effort. Today, the fight or flight response to threats has been updated to "freeze, flight or fight," with "freeze" describing the response of feeling immobilized in the face of a threat.

General Adaptation Syndrome

Hans Selye (1950) described stress as a physiological whole-body response to stress, evidenced primarily through the endocrine and autonomic nervous systems. Referred to as **adaptation**, this set of symptoms "was so general that it was like a single burglar alarm that sounds, no matter what intrudes" (Meyers, 2011, p. 275). The same physiological response occurs regardless of whether a stressor is psychological or physical.

Selye described a three-stage progressive pattern of nonspecific physiological responses: alarm, resistance, and exhaustion. The *"alarm stage"* is similar to Cannon's acute stress response. If the stressor is not resolved in the initial alarm stage, a second-level adaptive phase, the *"resistance stage,"* occurs as the body tries to accommodate for the stressor. In the resistance stage, overt alarm symptoms subside as the immune system helps the body to adapt to the demands of the stressor. If the body fails to adapt or is unable to resist the continued stress, it leads to the *"exhaustion stage."* At this point, the person becomes a higher risk for a stress-related illness or mental health disorder. The longer the physiological stress response remains elevated, the greater is the negative impact on the person.

Allostasis

Allostasis is a short-term adaptation to stress, and when the stress becomes malapative or toxic, it is called *allostatic load*. It is the person's brain that interprets whether the person is threatened and in turn stressed—the greater the severity of the threat, the more the person will be stressed (McEwen and Gianaros, 2011).

Allostatic accommodation is the physiological process through which the brain tries to find a new homeostasis, using a range of adaptive functioning (Simandan, 2010). The interaction between stressors and physical responses is ongoing, such that individuals become more or less susceptible to the negative consequences of stress over time. Inclusion of genetic risk factors, early life events, and adaptive lifestyle behaviours offers a way to understand the interaction between stressful events and physiological adaptation processes (McEwen, 2012). Fig. 17.1 identifies the relationships in the model.

Stress hormones protect the body against short-term acute stress (through allostasis). Stress mediators, such as social support, can provide protective effects. When slight or moderate levels of stressor exposure are encountered and social support is available, coping with stress can actually work to strengthen well-being and quality of life.

Complex or prolonged stress levels are more problematic. Early life experiences with stress can have implications for later life (Simandan, 2010). If a stressor presents continued challenges, or coping responses are ineffective, there is "wear and tear" on the body, which can have a damaging effect. The term *allostatic load* was coined by McEwan & Stellar (1993) to describe this phenomenon. The allostatic load can be negligible, severe, or protracted enough to result in significant illness or death if untreated.

Psychosocial Frameworks
Critical Life Events

Holmes and Rahe (1967) consider stressful life events—such as marriage, divorce, death, and losing a job—as stimuli sufficient to disrupt homeostasis and thus create stress. In the Holmes and Rahe scale, each life event has a weighted numeric score reflecting its potential impact. Stressors requiring a significant change in the person's lifestyle have greater impact, as do the number of cumulative stresses on the scale. A higher score reflects a person's potential for the later development of physical illness (Sheldon et al., 2019).

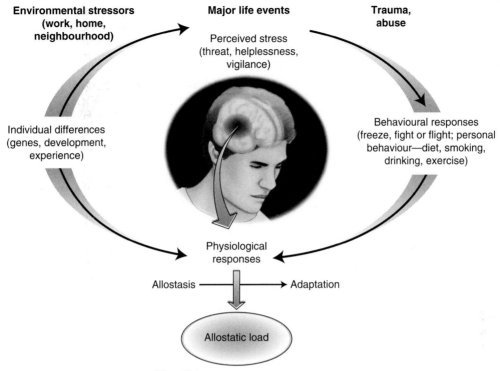

Fig. 17.1 Allostasis Model of Stress

Transactional Model of Stress

Lazarus and Folkman's 1984/1991 transactional appraisal model of stress is widely used in health care (1991). Basically, this is a psychological model; it considers stress as a two-way interactive process involving both the stressor and the individual's interpretive response to the stressor. According to the transactional model of stress and coping, when stress occurs, the stressor creates a significant adaptive demand, requiring a response from the individual. It does not matter if the stressor is a hassle or a major life event (Fig. 17.2).

The transactional model helps explain individual differences in personal responses to stressors that objectively could be thought of as having the same stress value. There are two forms of appraisal. A primary appraisal examines the strength of a person's belief about the potential harm that a stressor holds. The stronger the perceived threat to self-integrity, the greater the stress response. The secondary appraisal considers a person's perception of personal coping skills and availability of appropriate social environmental resources to reduce a stressor's impact. Both appraisals are required to determine whether a stressor will be considered a harmful threat or challenge. People experience stress if they appraise the stressor to be threatening

or feel incapable of meeting the stressor's demands with available resources.

COPING

Coping is "defined as the constantly changing cognitive and behavioural efforts to manage specific external or internal demands that are appraised as taxing or exceeding the resources of the person (Bayuo & Agbenorku, 2018, p. 47). In a classic work, Pearlin and Schooler (1978) define coping as "any response to external life strains that serves to prevent, avoid, or control emotional distress" (p. 2). They identify three purposes of coping strategies:

- To change the stressful situation (problem focused)
- To change the meaning of the stressor (meaning focused)
- To help the person relax enough to take the stress in stride (emotion focused)

In general, using problem-focused coping strategies to actively reduce the impact of a stressful situation and make it less stressful is more effective in controllable situations (Thoits, 2010). By contrast, emotion or meaning-focused strategies have a stronger impact when less controllable situations are causing the stress. Meaning-focused strategies are designed to diminish the importance of the stressor.

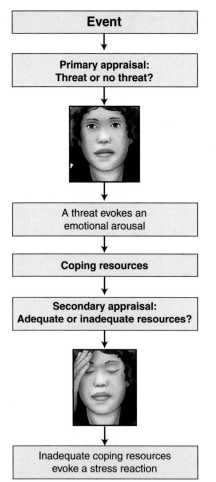

Fig. 17.2 Primary and secondary appraisal in stress reactions

They work best when work or financial issues are not easily reducible through active efforts.

COPING STRATEGIES

Culture plays a role in determining a person's stress and coping behaviours in these ways:
1. By shaping the types of stressors a person is likely to experience
2. By influencing the person's appraisal of stress
3. By affecting the choice of coping strategies
4. By providing different resources and institutional mechanism as coping options (Aldwin, 2010, p. 564)

A fundamental problem in defining coping is that it is a comprehensive term that includes many behaviours. For example, in certain collective cultures like China, Korea, and Japan, *distress* is commonly expressed through somatic symptoms (Grover, S., & Ghosh, 2014). In addition to cultural differences, previous stressful experiences, financial assets, and social and self-management support influence a person's and family's ability to solve problems and cope effectively with their health conditions.

People learn coping strategies from their parents, peers, and life experiences. Those with varied life opportunities and supportive people in their lives have an advantage over those who lack opportunity or support systems (or both). People who have been overprotected or were repeatedly exposed to danger without support generally lack adequate coping skills. Simulation Exercise 17.1 is intended to help identify common personal coping strategies.

Types of Coping

Appraisal theory describes *coping* as "a process by which a person makes cognitive and behavioural efforts to manage

---

SIMULATION EXERCISE 17.1   Examining Personal Coping Strategies

Purpose
To help students identify the wide range of adaptive and maladaptive coping strategies

Procedure
1. Identify all of the ways in which you handle stressful situations.
2. List three personal strategies that you have used successfully in coping with stress.
3. List one personal coping strategy that did not work and identify why you think it was inadequate or insufficient to reduce your stress level.

4. On a whiteboard or flip chart, list the different coping strategies identified by students.

Discussion
1. What common themes did you find in the ways people handle stress?
2. Were you surprised at the number and variety of ways in which people handle stress?
3. What new coping strategy might you use to reduce your stress level?
4. Are there any circumstances that increase or decrease your automatic reactions to stress?

psychological stress" (Bippus & Young, 2012, p. 177). The two most common coping strategies are an approach, problem-focused style and an avoidant, emotion-focused style (Wagland et al., 2015). **Problem-focused coping** strategies are purposeful, active, task-oriented methods to reduce stress. Examples include confronting a problem directly, negotiating for a different solution, seeking social support, constructive problem solving, and taking action. In general, problem-focused coping strategies have been found to be the most effective in reducing stress. For example, Jaser et al. (2012) found that adolescents who used problem-solving strategies to control their diabetes demonstrated better diabetic control and experienced a higher quality of life than those who did not.

People who use **emotion-focused coping** strategies act in a different way to minimize the influence of stress in their mind. These strategies can be effective when the stressor is perceived as an overwhelming, irreversible situation or the person needs respite from overthinking about a stressful situation. Emotion-focused coping strategies—such as meditation, yoga, or spirituality—are constructive when a person deliberately chooses to let go of negative feelings associated with an unmanageable stressor and employs other strategies.

Most people use both types of coping strategies, with the choice of strategy dependent on the nature of the stressor and a person's typical coping style. Awareness of personal and external resources adds options. Individuals who believe they have options are generally better able to cope with stress. Common personal coping assets, referred to as *resource options*, include health, energy, problem-solving skills, the amount and availability of social supports, and other material resources to cope effectively with the stressor.

Meaning-focused coping strategies help to reframe the meaning or significance of the stressor so that it loses its power as an overwhelming challenge and becomes a challenge in need of a change in focus level. The stressor may still exist, but the greater calmness inherent in the focused coping strategies provides a realignment of its impact. Simulation Exercise 17.1 provides an opportunity to examine your personal use of coping strategies.

Defensive Coping Strategies

Although some forms of coping yield positive results to reduce stress, others are negative influences. Rumination, denial, anger, excessive anxiety, and use of drugs or alcohol can increase the effects of stressors and further add to distress. **Ego defence mechanisms** are defined as a coping style that people use to protect the self from full awareness of challenging conflict situations. They are designed to protect the ego from anxiety and loss of self-esteem by denying, avoiding, or projecting responsibility for a challenging conflict to an external source.

Ego defence mechanisms can be temporarily adaptive by minimizing the threat of a potentially overwhelming stressor (Cherry, 2021; Shpancer, 2018). Persistent use of the ego defence mechanisms presented in Table 17.1 is considered pathological. As a primary stress reducer, defence mechanisms are ineffective because avoidant behaviour typically delays action and compromises trust in relationships. Some defence mechanisms—humour, anticipation, affiliation (asking for help), and sublimation—can be adaptive if not used exclusively as coping strategies (Reich et al., 2010).

Case Example

Lynn was diagnosed as having high cholesterol and was advised to lose weight. She sees no purpose in going on a diet because "it's all in the genes." Both her parents had high cholesterol and died of heart problems. Lynn claims that there is nothing she can do about it, even though her physician advised her differently. Her defensive interpretation prevents her from taking actions needed to reduce her risk for cardiovascular disease. Motivational interviewing (see Chapter 15) offers guidelines for gently casting doubt, providing new information, and introducing problem solving to people who are resistant. Her nurse enquires about Lynn's personal health goals and provides her with information about the link between diet, exercise, and heart disease. Linking information to Lynn's stated life goals provides her with a different frame of reference.

Resilience

Resilience is a concept linked to well-being and burnout prevention (Arrogante & Aparicio-Zaldivar, 2017). It is defined as the ability of individuals who are exposed to highly disruptive stressors to remain relatively stable and functional despite the stress (Garcia-Dia et al., 2013). Resilience explains why some people seem to weather stress and adversity more easily than others and are able to grow from the experience. Through development of a strong internal sense of control and a positive attitude, people can develop the skills needed to override their stress and move forward despite stressful life events (Marsiglia et al., 2011).

Characteristics of resilience include empowerment and creativity (Lin et al., 2013). Resilient people develop coping mechanisms that allow them to see a situation as it is, focus on what can be changed, and accept what cannot be altered. Helping people develop clear goals, shape relevant problem-solving skills, and take baby steps toward

TABLE 17.1 Ego Defence Mechanisms

Ego Defence Mechanism	Clinical Example
Regression: returning to an earlier, more primitive form of behaviour in the face of a threat to self-esteem	Julie was completely toilet trained by 2 years of age. When her younger brother was born, she began wetting her pants and wanting a pacifier at night.
Repression: unconscious forgetting of parts or all of an experience	Elizabeth has just lost her job. Her friends would not know from her behaviour that she has any anxiety about it. She continues to spend money as if she were still getting a paycheque.
Denial: unconscious refusal to allow painful facts, feelings, or perceptions into awareness	Bill has had a massive heart attack. His physician advises him to exercise in moderation, with caution. Bill continues to jog 6 miles a day.
Rationalization: offering a plausible excuse or explanation for unacceptable behaviour	Ann Marie tells her friends she does not misuse alcohol, even though she has blackouts, because she drinks only on weekends and when she is not working.
Projection: attributing unacceptable feelings, facts, behaviours, or attitudes to others; usually expressed as blame	Ruby just received a critical performance evaluation from her supervisor. She tells her friends that her supervisor does not like her.
Displacement: redirecting feelings onto an object or person considered less of a threat than the original object or person	Mrs. Jones took Mary to the doctor for bronchitis. She is not satisfied with the doctor's explanation and feels he was condescending, but she says nothing. When she gets to the receptionist's desk to make the next appointment, she yells at her for not having the prescription ready and taking too much time to set the appointment.
Intellectualization: unconscious focusing on only the intellectual and not the emotional aspects of a situation or circumstance	Johnnie has been badly hurt in a car accident. There is reason to believe he will not survive surgery. His father, waiting for his son to return to the ICU, asks the nurse many questions about the equipment and philosophizes about the meaning of life and death.
Reaction formation: unconscious assumption of traits that are the opposite of undesirable behaviours	John has a strong family history on both sides of misusing alcohol. He abstains from drinking alcohol, both at home and in social gatherings.
Sublimation: redirecting socially unacceptable unconscious thoughts and feelings into socially approved outlets	Bob has a lot of aggressive tendencies. He decided to become a butcher and thoroughly enjoys his work.
Undoing: verbal expression or actions representing one feeling, followed by expression of the direct opposite	Barbara criticizes her subordinate, Carol, before a large group of people. Later, she sees Carol on the street and tells her how important she is to the organization.

identified goals is a means of improving personal resilience. A person develops resiliency through practice, social support, and learning self-efficacy strategies (CMHA Fort Francis, n.d.). Examples of relevant strategies include developing an organized way of coping with challenges and cultivating a meaningful support system. A strong faith and sense of purpose are other factors associated with resilience (Rahmati et al., 2017).

Hardiness

Hardiness is considered a protective factor that can minimize the effects of stress. The concept of *hardiness* consists of three basic elements:
- *Challenge:* looking at stressors and characterizing the need for change as an opportunity for personal growth
- *Commitment:* developing a sense of purpose and a strong involvement in directing one's life

- *Taking control:* believing that one can help to influence one's life's outcomes (Stein & Bartone, 2020).

Resilience and hardiness act as protective factors that influence a person's ability to view global stress events as ultimately being manageable.

APPLICATIONS

Stress Assessment

Stress is an unwelcome part of most illnesses and injury; it is rarely a personal choice. People experience and cope with stress in different and sometimes unexpected ways. Nurses can be instrumental in helping people cope with stress effectively so that their anxiety does not dominate their health experience and they are able to function effectively. Factors that influence the impact of stress are identified in Box 17.2.

Addressing stress issues and teaching people related coping strategies enhances clinical outcomes and recovery potential. An initial assessment should include the following from the person:

- Perception of current stressors

- Perception of the stressor causing the greatest stress
- Insights about the value or meaning attached to the stressor
- Identification of usual coping strategies used to manage stressful situations
- Assessment of linked issues such as developmental stage, culture, family ways of coping, and level of support
- Religious and spiritual beliefs and activities

Understanding how a stressful event relates to other life issues, including stressors from the past and current financial or family concerns, is helpful. Ask open-ended questions about changes in daily routines and new roles and responsibilities. Explore the person's and family's current understanding of diagnosis and treatment options. Pay close attention to cultural values. What is a small stressor in one culture can be huge in another, and normal coping strategies can be quite different.

Sources of Stress in Health Care

All health disruptions create a sense of vulnerability. Health-related stressors for people and their families include fear of death, uncertainty about diagnosis, clinical outcomes, changes in roles, disruption of family life, and financial

---

►► DEVELOPING AN EVIDENCE-INFORMED PRACTICE

The purpose of this qualitative exploratory study was to describe occupational stressors and ways they could be reduced from the nurse's perspective. Thirty-eight registered nurses (RNs) participated in six focus groups to discuss sources of occupational stress and possible ways to reduce the stress.

Results

This same group of nurses identified high workloads, shift work, unsupportive management, unavailability of physicians, poor parking facilities and other human resource issues, and issues regarding people and their relatives as sources of stress. Suggestions for modification included workload and shift hour changes, organizational development, better work conditions, and acknowledgment from management.

Application to Your Clinical Practice

All nurses have a responsibility to participate in making health care environments better and less stressful. Nurse managers should make opportunities available to discuss occupational stressors and encourage nurses to engage in stress reduction activities.

From Happell, B., Dwyer, T., Reid-Searl, K. et al. (2013). Nurses and stress: Recognizing causes and seeking solutions. *Journal of Nursing Management, 21*(4), 638–647.

BOX 17.2   Factors That Influence the Impact of Stress

- Magnitude and demands of the stressor on self and others
- Multiple stressors occurring at the same time
- Suddenness or unpredictability of a stressful situation
- Accumulation of stressors and duration of the stress demand
- Level of social support available to the person and family
- Previous trauma, which can activate unresolved fears
- Presence of an associated mental health disorder
- Developmental level of the person
- Normal attitude and outlook
- Knowledge, expectations, and perceptions

concerns. Hospital-related sources of stress include physical discomfort, strange noises and lights, unfamiliar people asking personal questions, and strange equipment. People and their families experience stress when someone is transferred to the intensive care unit (ICU), again when the person is transferred to a step-down or regular unit, and still again when people are transitioning to home (Lee et al., 2017). Providing immediate practical and emotional support during such transitions helps reduce excessive stress.

A person-centred approach pays attention to the *type* of stress a person is experiencing. When stress presents as anxiety, the nurse might suggest problem-solving techniques. However, if the stress is related to a significant loss, the nurse would want to focus on the loss and work with the person from a grief perspective. Box 17.3, developed by a nursing student, provides an assessment and intervention tool that you can use to organize assessment data and plan interventions.

Behavioural Observations

Stress behaviours are sometimes hard to understand or accept. Distress often presents through behaviour rather than through words. For example, anxiety can present in the form of heart palpations, shortness of breath, sweating,

and muscle tension (Heart and Stroke Foundation & CMHA, 2013). Other physical and mental symptoms of stress include the following:

- Significant changes in eating or sleeping habits
- Headaches, gastric problems, muscular tension, aches and pains, tightness in the throat
- Restlessness and irritability
- Inability to cope with normal, everyday concerns and obligations
- Inability to concentrate

Anger and Hostility

Anger and hostility are common stress responses associated with feeling helpless or psychologically threatened. People and their families become hostile when they feel threatened about what is happening or feel they have little control in a situation. Anxiety usually exists as the underpinning of anger people or families who have hostile behaviours need understanding, comfort, and human caring.

Blame is a frequent form of hostility. Family members blame each other for undesired outcomes, or the physician for operating (or not operating) on a loved one. They criticize the nurse for not responding quickly enough.

BOX 17.3   Assessment and Intervention Tool

Assessment

1. Perception of stressors
1. Major stress area or health concern
2. Present circumstances related to usual pattern
3. Experienced similar problem in the past? How was it handled?
4. Anticipation of future consequences
5. Expectations of self
6. Expectations of caregivers

2. Intrapersonal factors
1. Physical (mobility, body function)
2. Psychosociocultural (attitudes, values, coping patterns)
3. Developmental (age, factors related to present situation)
4. Spiritual belief system (hope and sustaining factors)

3. Interpersonal factors
1. Resources and relationship of family or significant others as they relate to or influence interpersonal factors

4. Environmental factors
1. Resources and relationships of community as they relate to or influence interpersonal factors

Prevention as Intervention

1. Primary
1. Classify stressor
2. Provide information to maintain or strengthen strengths
3. Support positive coping mechanisms
4. Educate person and family

2. Secondary
1. Mobilize resources
2. Motivate, educate, involve person in health care goals
3. Facilitate appropriate interventions; refer to external resources as needed
4. Provide information on primary prevention or intervention as needed

3. Tertiary
1. Attain/maintain wellness
2. Educate or re-educate as needed
3. Coordinate resources
4. Provide information about primary and secondary interventions

Developed by Conrad, J. (1993). *Assessment and Intervention Tool*. University of Maryland School of Nursing.

Recognizing hostility as a cry for help in coping with escalating stress makes it easier to respond empathetically. Nurses can help a person stabilize an out-of-control situation by providing a calming, supportive presence and working with the person to find a viable resolution to personal anxiety.

Carefully listening to a person's concerns goes a long way toward neutralizing anger and hostility. The person feels heard, even if the issues cannot be fully resolved to the person's satisfaction. In the course of the conversation, both the nurse and the person can sort out how the person experiences a stressor. This data can serve as a basis for choosing productive solutions. Set limits if necessary, but do so with a calm attitude and empathetic, matter of fact manner. If the person's or family member's expectations are unrealistic, or cannot be met in the current situation, you can introduce alternative explanations and suggestions. Simulation Exercise 17.2 is designed to address the relationship between anger and anxiety.

Social Withdrawal

Stress does not always look like a "stressor response" to observers. Some people internalize stress. Culture and circumstance play a role. People may withdraw or seem disengaged from an obvious stressor when they are feeling stressed. Unexpressed emotions of anxiety and anger are toxic and debilitating. Nurses can help people externalize their stress. Putting their observations into words helps people link emotional states to specific stress reactions using words rather than behaviour to express them. Words put limits on the stress experience and make it more manageable. For example, you might say, "This (name stressor) must be very upsetting," or "It seems like you are pretty anxious about . . ." Offering your presence, together with a simple statement such as "When people put their stress into words, they usually experience less anxiety," can help to normalize the feelings.

Assessment of Coping Skills

Assessment of a person's coping behaviours and social support network is critical to understanding stress from a holistic perspective. Ask about coping strategies a person has used in the past and what they are currently doing to resolve stress. Relevant issues include culturally sanctioned coping approaches and typical family coping strategies. The questions might include the following:

- What do you do to relieve your stress?
- Who can you rely on when you are feeling stressed?

Discussing stress can be difficult in part because it is so uncomfortable. People feel more comfortable when their nurse presents an open, nonthreatening stance and a calm attitude. Use an informal conversational format. Being

---

SIMULATION EXERCISE 17.2   Relationships Between Anger and Anxiety

Purpose
To help students appreciate the links between anger and anxiety and understand how anger is triggered

Procedure
1. Think of a time when you were really angry. It need not be a significant event, or one that would necessarily make anyone else angry.
2. Identify your thoughts, feelings, and behaviour in separate columns of a table you construct. For example, what were the thoughts that went through your head when you were feeling this anger? What were your physical and emotional responses to this experience? Write down words or phrases to express what you were feeling at the time. How did you respond when you were angry?
3. Identify what was going on with you before experiencing the anger. Sometimes it is not the event itself but your feelings before the incident that make the event the straw that breaks the camel's back.
4. Identify underlying threats to your self-concept in the situation (e.g., you were not treated with respect, your

opinion was discounted, you lost status, you were rejected, you feared the unknown).

Reflective Analysis Discussion
1. In what ways were your answers similar to and different from those of your classmates?
2. What role did anxiety and threat to your self-concept play in the development of the anger response? What percentage of your anger related to the actual event and to your self-concept?
3. In what ways did you see anger as a multidetermined behavioural response to threats to your self-concept?
4. Did this exercise change any of your ideas about how you might handle your feelings and behaviour in a similar situation in future?
5. What are the common threads in the events that made people in your group angry?
6. In what ways could experiential knowledge of the close association between anger and anxiety be helpful in your nursing practice?

patient and willing to listen is important. The person's reactions will serve as a guide for how much and how quickly the information can be gathered.

Social Support

Social support is an essential buffer against stress. Families can be a major support for people in managing health-related distress (Antoni, 2013). To be sure that everyone is on the same page, nurses should inquire about the following as part of the initial assessment:

- What are the family's expectations of care?
- In what ways, if any, are family, person, and provider expectations different?
- What does the family or person need from you as the nurse? From each other?
- Is there a family spokesperson?
- What are the family's cultural, religious, and other values concerning the meaning of the stressor?
- What do family members identify as sources of strength and hope? Are these sources similar or different from sources on the person's list?

Community resources include support groups, social services, and other public health agencies that provide practical support, as well as social contacts. Nurses need to be aware of community support services. Simulation Exercise 17.3 is designed to help you become better acquainted with resources in your community.

Belief in a personal god or higher power provides interested people with an personal resource. Multiple studies reveal that spiritual interventions can help prevent and improve physical illnesses and have helped people cope with chronic pain and death (Moeini et al., 2014). Some people rely on faith to facilitate their acceptance of a reality that cannot be changed. Assessing and providing spiritual comfort to people is an important consideration in caring for people experiencing stress. For example, the Plains Cree tend to use spirituality and religious activities as preferred coping strategies (Graham & Martin, 2016).

Assessing Impact on Family Relationships

Stress Issues for Children

Health disruptions create special stress for children; they lack the words and life experience to sort out the meaning of illness, either their own or that of a significant family member. Children express their stress through behaviour (HealthLinkBC, 2019). Signs of distress, such as academic decline, gastric distress, and headaches, can alert the nurse to unvoiced stress. In the hospital, children withdraw, demonstrate clinging behaviours, or have frequent meltdowns. Uncertainty creates stress for both parents and children (Abela et al., 2020). A new professional that has joined the health care team is the child life professional. They are educated in how children and adolescents grow and develop, how to manage fears and anxiety, and more, and they make a significant contribution to a more positive hospitalization experience for the family and their child.

Parents may need help with communicating information about serious illness to children, with anticipating their child's reactions, or with setting realistic limits with a child who is ill.

Children need to have their questions answered simply and honestly, consistent with their developmental stage. Hearing information from someone they trust is important in modifying the uncertainty of a serious illness. Small children can be encouraged to express their stress feelings through drawings and manipulating puppets.

SIMULATION EXERCISE 17.3 Identifying Community Resources for Stress Management

Purpose

To help students become aware of the community resources available for stress management

Procedure

1. Contact a community agency, social services group, or support group in your community that you believe can help people cope with a particularly stressful situation. Look in the newspaper, community flyers, or online for ideas.
2. Find out how a person might access the resource, what kinds of cases are treated, what types of support are offered, the costs involved, and what you as a nurse can do to help people learn about and take advantage of the resource.

Reflective Analysis Discussion

1. How did you decide which community agency to choose?
2. How difficult or easy was it to access the information about the agency?
3. What information about the community resource did you find that surprised or perplexed you?
4. In what ways could you use this exercise in planning care for people in your care?

STRESS ISSUES FOR OLDER PEOPLE

Stress issues for older people often relate to multiple health challenges and an increased potential for loss of important interpersonal supports during this phase of life. Worry about finances and fears of not being able to live independently are common. Older people living alone often feel vulnerable about their safety or ability to reach help, should they experience a fall or sudden physical change. The loss of significant supportive people, isolation, and loneliness can complicate treatment issues.

Stress management strategies for older people from a health promotion perspective include maintaining an active social life and a healthy lifestyle to keep mind and body actively engaged with life. Developing leisure or volunteer interests helps older people build a well-balanced lifestyle that not only reduces stress but also improves quality of life. Sometimes all it takes are simple suggestions and well-timed questions about recreational activities or hobbies that the older person has not considered. Many communities have low-impact exercise programs, seniors centres, continuing education, and social programs for older people. Activities provide a venue for socialization that may not be available otherwise. Caregivers of people with dementia can benefit from some of the suggestions in Chapter 20 to reduce stress as they care for a family member with dementia.

STRESS REDUCTION STRATEGIES

In stressful situations, normal feelings are overlaid by anxiety. The initial goal is to help people and families feel secure. A calm, empathetic approach helps establish a safe holding environment. It creates the space people need to express fears, anger, and negative feelings. Slowing the pace is essential to allow feelings to emerge. Name the feelings—for example, "You seem to be really struggling right now." This can be followed by a simple question, such as, "How can I best help you?"

Providing Information

Information is an essential stress reducer. Relevant information can range from providing basic data about visiting hours, the timing of tests and procedures, plans for discharge, or contact phone numbers, to complex facts about the person's condition or treatment. Information sharing should begin with orienting people and their families to the health care situation or unit. Types of information people and families find helpful during a hospital stay include the following:

- What will happen during tests or surgery?
- Who is likely to interview the person, and why?
- How can the person best collaborate in their treatment process?

In stressful situations, the perceptual field narrows. Information and directions given in the first 48 hours of an admission should be repeated, usually more than once, because this is a time of high stress. The same is true when there is a change in treatment plans or prognosis. A calm approach and repetition help people in stressful situations relax enough to hear new information. Providing simple written instructions, particularly about medications, that can be discussed at the time and then left with the person or family, enhances understanding. Allow time to answer questions and provide the person's family with the health provider's contact numbers to call if other issues arise.

Processing Strong Feelings

When strong stress feelings get bottled up, constructive problem solving ceases. Often, nurses can tell that people are stressed from their body language, even when they deny strong feelings. Helpful statements include, "This must be very difficult for you to absorb" or "Can you tell me what you are experiencing?" Your immediate goal is to help people step back and take a second look at their situation from a broader perspective.

A calm, accepting presence and willingness to listen to the person's story allows nurses and the people they care for to develop a shared understanding of a stressful event. You can help someone normalize stressful feelings when people say things like, "I think I'm losing my mind," with probes such as, "What you are feeling is not unusual; although it feels that way, you're having a normal response to a sudden, overwhelming situation. Can you tell me what worries you the most?" Notice that in both probes, the nurse acknowledges the legitimacy of feelings as a normal response to an abnormal situation. Once the person begins to calm down, it becomes possible to look at the situation more realistically.

Simulation Exercise 17.4 provides practice with helping people handle stressful situations.

Reappraisal of either the stress event itself (primary appraisal) or of coping and personal resources (secondary appraisal) can help a person change the meaning of a stress event from a failure to a challenge or opportunity for personal growth. Jamieson and colleagues (2011) propose that when people believe they have the resources to cope with stressors, they begin to perceive a stressful situation as a challenge rather than a threat. Pointing out personal or community resources the person has not considered can reduce the impact of the stressor and may strengthen coping efforts. Group formats provide social support and practical education. It is important to help people choose supports that are convenient and compatible with their stage

---

SIMULATION EXERCISE 17.4 Role-Play: Handling Stressful Situations

Purpose
To give students experience in responding to stressful situations

Procedure
Use the following case study as the basis for this exercise.
  Dave is a 66-year-old man with colon cancer. In the past, he had a colostomy. Recently, he was readmitted to your unit and had an exploratory laparotomy for small-bowel obstruction. Very little can be done for him because the cancer has spread. He is in pain, and he has to have a feeding tube. His family has many questions for the nurse: "Why is he vomiting?" "How come the pain medication isn't working?" "Why isn't he feeling any better than he did before the surgery?" You have just entered the person's room; his family is sitting near him, and they want answers now.

1. Have different members of your group role-play the person, the nurse, the son, the daughter-in-law, and the wife. One person should act as observer.
2. Identify the factors that will need to be clarified in this situation to help the nurse provide the most appropriate intervention.
3. Using the strategies suggested in this chapter, intervene to help the person and family reduce their anxiety.
4. Role-play the situation for 10 to 15 minutes.

Reflective Analysis Discussion
1. Have each player identify the interventions that were most helpful.
2. From the nurse's perspective, which parts of the person's and family's stress were hardest to handle?
3. How could you use what you learned from doing this exercise in your clinical practice?

---

of life, other commitments, and health issues (Köpsén & Sjöström, 2020). Concrete assistance with negotiating appropriate referral resources may be needed.

Developing Realistic Goals

Without command over controllable parts of life, most people feel helpless and stressed. Relevant goals for stress reduction should relate to assessment data—for example, self-identified needs, strengths, resources, barriers, and goal achievement priorities. Treatment goals and objectives should build on past successful coping efforts and preferences. Choosing personal responses to stress is empowering and has a ripple effect on the person's self-efficacy around other health issues.

Coping mechanisms such as negotiation, specific actions, seeking advice, and rearranging priorities can significantly diminish stress through direct action. Once stressors are named, nurses can use health teaching formats and coaching that help people to do the following:

- Develop a realistic plan to offset stress
- Deal directly with obstacles as they emerge
- Evaluate action steps
- Make needed modifications in the plan and make essential lifestyle adjustments

---

Case Example

Dong-hyun received a diagnosis of prostate cancer after a routine physical examination. His way of coping (problem focused) included obtaining as much information on the disease as possible. He researched treatment options and sought advice from physician friends as to which surgeons had the most experience with this type of surgery. As he shared his diagnosis with friends and colleagues, he found several men who had successfully survived without a cancer recurrence. Dong-hyun used the time between diagnosis and surgery to finish projects and delegate work responsibilities. He attended a support group with his wife and was able to obtain valuable advice on handling his emotional responses to what would happen. When the time came for his surgery, Dong-hyun experienced less stress because of his actions before surgery.

Priority Setting

People do not always know where to start when faced with a stressful situation. Priority setting helps reduce hesitation and offers a stepwise framework for resolving stress. You can help people determine which task elements are critical and achievable and which can be addressed later. Break objective tasks into smaller, manageable, progressive segments. The most important tasks should be scheduled during times when the person or family has the most energy and freedom from interruption.

The next step is to help people identify the concrete tasks needed to achieve treatment goals, including the people involved, necessary contacts, amount of time each task will take, and specific hours or days for each task.

Some tasks are more important than others in reducing stressful situations, and not everything can be handled at once. A helpful suggestion might be, "Let's see what you need to do right now and what can wait a little while." Tasks that someone else can do and those that are not essential to the achievement of goals should be delegated or ignored for the moment.

Anticipatory Guidance

Fear of the unknown intensifies the impact of a stressor. **Anticipatory guidance** is a nursing intervention characterised by psychological preparation to help relieve the fear and anxiety of an event or future concerns and expectations that are anticipated to be stressful. It is also used to prepare someone for the next stage of a process (Ramos et al., 2017).

In framing a response, you might reflect on the following:

- What type of information would be most helpful to this person at this particular time, given what the person has told me?
- How would I feel if I was in this person's position?
- What would I want to know that might bring me comfort in this situation?

Providing anticipatory guidance can put needless worry to rest. You can prepare people for a procedure, beginning with a simple statement like, "You've never had this procedure before. Let me explain how it works." When you are providing anticipatory guidance, do not offer more than what the situation dictates. Encourage the person to expand on suggestions rather than outlining a full plan. The growth in the person's ability to set priorities, develop a plan with personal meaning, and establish benchmarks to measure progress stimulates self-confidence and decreases stress.

Anticipatory guidance should relate only to behaviours that can be changed. Stress-related questions about uncertainties do not qualify—for example, "If I take this chemotherapy, will I be cured, or am I going to die anyway?" The reality is that there may be no single answer. It helps to ask the person what prompted the question and to have a good idea of the person's level of knowledge before answering. Honest communication is essential, but sensitivity to the person's experience also is critical.

Social Support

Social support is the physical and emotional comfort given to us by our family, friends, co-workers and others. It's knowing that we are part of a community of people who love and care for us and value and think well of us. The concept functions in helping people reduce stress levels by enhancing close, supportive relationships, providing opportunities for support in conjunction with other health services, and reducing isolation by improving social support (CMHA Fort Francis, n.d.). A person's social networks are drawn from family, friends, faith-based institutions, work, social groups, or school. Being able to contact family and friends when you need an emergency babysitter or an extra set of hands in a stressful situation immediately lessens stress. Not only does sharing with others reduce stress by "externalizing" negative emotions, but family, friends, and support groups can provide a sounding board, practical assistance, and tangible encouragement. Seeking help can empower both seeker and provider of emotional support. Sharing a laugh, eating a meal with others, and being in good company helps people feel more relaxed, which in turn reduces stress levels.

Social support does not have the same meaning for all cultures in terms of self-disclosure. Some cultures may be more comfortable with an implicit form of social support that does not require the sharing of thoughts. Examples of implicit social support include showing kindness, caring, acceptance, and positive regard for a person (Ishii et al., 2017).

Helping Families Reduce Health-Related Stress

Contemporary health care environments with advanced technology, shorter stays, and multiple caregivers are complex and anxiety producing. It is important to have the voices of families heard and for health care providers to work in collaboration with them. Families want to have regular communication, and providing updated information about a family member's condition is a key component of stress reduction. Listen carefully to the family. Statements such as "Most people would feel anxious in this situation," or "It would be hard for anyone to have all the answers in a situation like this" can normalize difficult situations (Wolf et al., 2017).

Ongoing direct family contact can sometimes provide additional information about the person's preferences, health care needs, and resources. This strategy is particularly helpful when the person is unable to provide information. It also helps family members feel more connected (CMHA Fort Francis, n.d.).

Nurses play an important role in helping families reduce their stress to a workable level in health care. They can explore the presence of stress by linking the immediate health situation with expected feelings, with statements like, "Seeing your husband like this must be a terrible shock. I suspect you might be wondering how you're going to cope with his care at home." This type of statement normalizes feelings and introduces subjects that are difficult but necessary to talk about. Nurses can help families process complex information and address specific concerns. Topics should focus on what will happen next, how to explain the illness to others, or what the person or family is experiencing related to the stressor. Table 17.2 identifies interventions to decrease family stress.

TABLE 17.2	**Nursing Interventions to Decrease Family Anxiety**
Recommendation	**Specific Actions**
Identify a family spokesperson and support people involved in decision making	Choose a person the family and person trusts; establish mechanisms for contact.
Identify a primary nursing contact for the family	If possible, choose the nurse most in contact with the person. Meet with the family within 24 hours of admission to explain roles of each health care team member. Provide a contact number to the family spokesperson.
Discuss family access to the person	Arrange for visitation based on unit protocols, the person's condition and needs, and family preferences. Educate the family about visiting hours, how to reach the physician/hospitalist, when rounds occur. Involve the family in the person's care whenever possible and desired.
Call the family about any changes in the person's condition or treatment	Inform the family of changes as they occur. Provide frequent status reports. Allow time for questions.
Provide complete data in easily understandable terms	Ask questions about what the person and family understand about the person's condition, how they are coping, and what they fear. Check for misunderstandings and incomplete information. Provide information based on family needs. Respect cultural and personal desire for the level of information disclosure.
Actively involve the person and family in all clinical decisions	Hold formal care conferences for important care decisions. Take into account and respect person preferences as well as spiritual and cultural attitudes. Allow time for questions. Strive for consensus in decisions.
Connect family with support services	Provide information about support groups and hospital-based social, spiritual, American, hospice, home care, and other care services as needed.
Ensure collaborative rapport and support among health care team members	Maintain clear communication among health care team members. Avoid conflicting messages to the family. Provide opportunities for staff to decompress and discuss difficult situations and feelings.

Shafipour, V., Moosazadeh, M., Jannati, Y. et al. (2017). The effect of education on the anxiety of a family with a person in critical care unit: A systematic review and meta-analysis. *Electronic Physician*, *9*(3), 3918–3924. https://doi.org/10.19082/3918; Scott, P., Thomson, T., & Shepherd, A. (2019). Families of people in ICU: A scoping review of their needs and satisfaction with care. *NursingOpen*, *6*(3), 698–712. https://doi.org/10.1002/nop2.287; Ontario Hospital Association. (2011). *Leading Practices in Emergency Department Patient Experience*. Health Quality Ontario. http://www.hqontario.ca/Portals/0/modals/qi/en/processmap_pdfs/resources_links/leading%20practices%20in%20emergency%20department%20patient%20experience%20from%20oha.pdf.

In critical care situations, families have a strong need to remain physically close to the person; there is a strong correlation between proximity to the person and satisfaction with care. It is important to support the presence of key family members in "every area of the hospital, including the emergency department and the intensive care unit" (Alsharari, 2019).

Family members often want to provide support and comfort to people who are critically ill. They want to be full "partners in care." Being able to "do something" for the person helps them feel less helpless and defuses stress. Allowing family members to provide comfort measures and participate in the person's care—to whatever extent is possible for the person and comfortable for the family—can be a meaningful experience for both.

Even the most dedicated family members, however, need respite periods. A helpful strategy is suggesting that family members take short breaks. Family members may need "permission" to go to a movie or eat in a restaurant outside the hospital. Sometimes, they will do so with an assurance that they will be called should there be any change in the person's condition.

Promoting a Healthy Lifestyle

Encouraging a healthy lifestyle is an essential but sometimes overlooked component of stress-management strategies. Good health habits improve stress resistance. Eating a healthy diet and avoiding emotional eating gives people a sense of control and well-being. Too much caffeine and alcohol can exacerbate stress. Laughter dissolves it and reduces stress levels.

Quality sleep is restorative. Healthy nighttime habits, such as establishing a scheduled bedtime and having a small snack before bedtime, encourage sleep. Regular exercise helps the body release tension as well as contributes to fitness. Exercise can be accomplished in a social setting, for example, hiking or biking. Certain exercise programs such as yoga or tai chi meditation, deep breathing, and muscle stretching are well known stress reducers. Stress can be reduced by organizing time and deliberately choosing activities that energize rather than stress, balancing work with leisure activities, and eliminating unnecessary obligations.

Therapeutic Approaches for Chronic Stress Management

Cognitive Behavioural Approaches

Cognitive-behavioural approaches have proven useful in addressing stressful, negative attributions about oneself and modifying negative core beliefs. The cognitive behavioural therapy (CBT) model (Beck & Beck, 2011) uses a person-centred approach aimed at helping individuals troubled by faulty thinking reframe the meaning of difficult situations. According to Beck, the relationship between a person's thoughts and feelings influences the person's behaviours. Optimistic or neutral thoughts can lead to positive emotions and tend to create cooperative, constructive actions. Negative thinking does the opposite. Faulty thinking causes a person to interpret neutral situations in unrealistic, exaggerated, or negative ways. Helping people become aware of and modify negative or dysfunctional thoughts, beliefs, and perceptions (cognitive distortions) makes it possible for them to change behaviour patterns. Awareness can result in a more constructive approach to a problem situation.

Stress symptoms look similar on the surface, but the cognitive beliefs supporting the stress reaction can be quite different. **Cognitive restructuring** is a strategy that "involves teaching clients to question the automatic beliefs, assumptions, and predictions that often lead to negative emotions and to replace negative thinking with more realistic and positive beliefs" (Schacter et al., 2010, p. 599). The focus of CBT is not on the behaviour itself but on the inner perceptions and thoughts that create and perpetuate negative self-evaluations and self-defeating behaviours.

Automatic negative thoughts are classified as **cognitive distortions**. Examples include magnifying or minimizing the impact of a single behaviour as a commentary on the person. Failing a test is experienced as, "I am stupid," instead of "I messed up on a test—what can I do so this doesn't happen again?"

Mind reading or having rigid rules about what a person "should" do is another example of a cognitive distortion. Over time, a person develops a set of related, automatic distortions referred to as a *schema*. The person uses core schemas to filter incoming information and determine its meaning related to self, others, and the world. Schemas become a template for understanding the meaning of incoming information and appraising its value to the self. They are pervasive and hard to dislodge. Although distortions seem to be legitimate assessments, they are not valid.

Nurses can help people challenge distortions through Socratic questioning. By gathering and weighing evidence to support a different position, people are able to distinguish between a distorted perception and a realistic appraisal of its validity. Ridding oneself of unrealistic expectations and negative self-thoughts allows cognitive space for thinking about possible options and broader choices. Once a problem is appropriately categorized, solutions become more apparent. You can help people understand that they have choices and that no matter what feeling they have, it is not permanent. Initially, people have to force themselves to challenge negative thoughts and replace them with more balanced thoughts. As time passes, this becomes easier.

Nurses can use open-ended questions such as the following:

- What is the worst thing that can happen?
- If (worst thing) did happen, what could you do?

Mind–Body Therapies

There are numerous interventions to assist people, families, and health care providers to cope with stress (Tran et al., 2020)—for example, meditation, relaxation, guided imagery, yoga, and cognitive restructuring.

Meditation is a stress-reduction strategy that people use to develop a sense of inner peace and tranquillity.

Meditation clears the mind of disturbing thoughts and neutralizes toxic feelings. This activity helps to reduce the concentration of stress hormones attached to stressful thinking. A guide to meditation is provided in Box 17.4.

Mindfulness meditation uses a non-judgemental, personal, conscious awareness related to the present moment and what is happening in the here and now. Mindfulness is a stress management tool that can be used at any point. It can be as simple as focusing on deep breathing. Paying full attention to breathing, music, or what is happening in the current moment forces a person to at least momentarily let go of stressful thoughts. It is an easy way of quieting the mind and decreasing the intensity of stressful feelings.

Progressive Relaxation

Progressive relaxation is a technique that focuses the person's attention on conscious control of voluntary skeletal muscles. Originally developed by Edmund Jacobson (1938), the technique consists of alternately tensing and relaxing muscle groups. Anxiety Canada (n.d.) has published guidelines explaining techniques for progressive muscle relaxation.

A variant of progressive relaxation is deep breathing. This can be accomplished anywhere and at any time a person experiences stress. Try doing it, as follows:

- Deeply inhale to the count of 10 and hold your breath.
- Exhale slowly, again to the count of 10.
- As you do this exercise, concentrate only on your breathing.
- Feel the tension leave your body.

BOX 17.4   Meditation Techniques

1. Choose a quiet, calm environment with as few distractions as possible.
2. Get in a comfortable position, preferably a sitting position.
3. To shift the mind from logical, externally oriented thought, use a constant stimulus: a sound, word, phrase, or object. Close your eyes if you use a repetitive sound or word.
4. Pay attention to the rhythm of your breathing.
5. When distracting thoughts occur, discard the thought(s) and redirect your attention to repeating the word or gazing at the object. Distracting thoughts will occur and do not mean you are performing the techniques incorrectly. Do not worry about how you are doing. Redirect your focus to the constant stimulus and assume a passive attitude.

Modified from Benson, H. (1975). *The relaxation response.* Morrow.

Focusing your mind on the continuous rhythm of inhaling and exhaling turns the mind away from thinking about specific stressors. To experience the progressive relaxation technique, use Simulation Exercise 17.5.

Yoga and Tai Chi

Yoga is a mind–body exercise practice rooted in ancient India. The practice of yoga has proven useful as a treatment for depression and for promotion of physical and mental health (Rao et al., 2013). Yoga emphasizes correct alignment, controlled postures or poses, and regulated breathing to help people relax and reduce stress. Controlling breathing helps to quiet the mind. Some forms of yoga involve meditation and developing self-awareness.

Tai chi is an exercise system consisting of stretching and rhythmic movements coordinated with controlled breathing. The postures and movements are practised in a slow, graceful manner. The concentration required for both yoga and tai chi requires a person to relax and forget distressing thoughts.

Guided Imagery

Guided imagery is a technique often used in combination with relaxation strategies for cancer pain and stress. The Canadian Cancer Society (n.d.) outlines techniques for guided imagery for people living with cancer and recommends they consult their health care team for support in using this complementary therapy. (https://www.cancer.ca/en/cancer-information/diagnosis-and-treatment/complementary-therapies/guided-imagery/?region=on). This resource is very helpful not only for people with cancer but also for others, including those who are not ill. Imagery techniques use the person's imagination to stimulate healing mental images designed to promote stress relief. The process involves asking a person to imagine a scene previously experienced as safe, peaceful, or beautiful. Supportive prompts to engage all of the senses deepen the imagery experience. This scene can be used each time the person begins to experience stress. Inspirational music and online videos are also used in connection with guided imagery.

Support Groups

Support groups for people or families struggling with the same health situation or crisis can be extremely helpful in helping them defuse stress and learn coping strategies to self-manage difficult health issues. Examples include bereavement groups, cancer support groups, dementia family groups, and specialized groups for problematic substance use. Psychoeducational groups with supportive interventions include the Canadian Alliance in Mental Illness, cardiac rehabilitation, and health promotion groups for targeted populations.

SIMULATION EXERCISE 17.5 Progressive Relaxation

Purpose

To help students experience the beneficial effects of progressive relaxation in reducing tension

Procedure

This exercise consists of alternately tensing and relaxing skeletal muscles.

1. Sit in a comfortable chair with arm supports. Place the arms on the arm supports, and sit in a comfortable upright position, with legs uncrossed and feet flat on the floor.
2. Close your eyes and take 10 deep breaths, concentrating on inhaling and exhaling.
3. Your faculty or a student member of the group should give the following instructions, and you should follow them exactly:

I want you to focus on your feet and tense the muscles in your feet. Feel the tension in your feet. Hold it, and now let go. Feel the tension leaving your feet.

I would like you to tense the muscles in your calves. Feel the tension in your calves and hold it. Now let go and feel the tension leaving your calves. Experience how that feels.

Tense the muscles in your thighs. Most people do this by pressing their thighs against the chair. Feel the tension in your muscles and experience how that feels. Now release the tension and experience how that feels.

I would like you to feel the tension in your abdomen. Tense the muscles in your abdomen and hold it. Hold it for a few more seconds. Now release those muscles and experience how that feels.

Tense the muscles in your chest. A good way to do this is to take a very deep breath and hold it. (The guide counts to 10.) Concentrate on feeling how that feels. Now let it go and experience how that feels.

I would like you to tense the muscles in your hands. Clench your fists and hold it as hard as you can. Harder, harder. Now release it and concentrate on how that feels.

Tense the muscles in your arms. You can do this by pressing down as hard as you can on the arm supports. Feel the tension in your arms and continue pressing. Now let go and experience how that feels.

I would like to you to feel the tension in your shoulders. Tense your shoulders as hard as you can and hold it. Concentrate on how that feels. Now release your shoulder muscles and experience the feeling.

Feel the tension in your jaw. Clench your jaw and teeth as hard as you can. Feel the tension in your jaw and hold it. Now let it go and feel the tension leave your jaw.

Now that you are in this relaxed state, keep your eyes closed and think of a time when you were really happy. Let the images and sounds surround you. Imagine yourself back in that situation. What were you thinking? What are you feeling?

Open your eyes. Students who feel comfortable in doing so may share the images that emerged in the relaxed state.

Reflective Analysis Discussion

1. What are your impressions in doing this exercise?
2. Do you feel more relaxed after doing this exercise?
3. If applicable, after doing the exercise, in what ways did you feel differently?
4. Were you surprised at the images that emerged in your relaxed state?
5. In what ways do you think you could use this exercise in your nursing practice?

Stress Issues for Nurses: Burnout

Freudenberger (1980) defines *burnout* as "a state of fatigue or frustration brought about by devotion to a cause, way of life, or relationship that failed to produce an expected reward" (p. 13). He refers to burnout as the "overachievement syndrome." Burnout is characterized by emotional exhaustion, depersonalization, and a sense of diminished professional accomplishment. Although burnout shares some characteristics with depression and anxiety, it is a different syndrome, clearly linked to work environments and personal expectations of self and others within that setting.

Nurses face many adverse situations and high-risk conditions that people in other professions do not experience or witness as regularly (Cross, 2015). Over time, prolonged work-related stress takes its toll. Khamisa and colleagues (2013) note that nurses experience a greater vulnerability to burnout because they work in high-stress service environments, helping people cope with serious life and death situations every day. Two related concepts to burnout are compassion fatigue and vicarious trauma. *Compassion fatigue* is defined as a syndrome associated with serious spiritual, physical, and emotional depletion related to caring for those who are seriously ill. It can appear as apathy or indifference toward the suffering of others as the result of overexposure to tragic news stories and images and the subsequent appeals for assistance. **Vicarious trauma** is experienced or realized through imaginative or sympathetic participation in the experience of another. At this time, more research needs to be completed to determine the exact relationships among all the concepts: compassion fatigue, vicarious trauma and burnout. What is known is that all of these phenomena result in negative emotional outcomes for nurses. However, many other factors need to be considered, such as the clinical area of practice, gender, leadership of the area, and so on (Polat et al., 2020; Pirelli et al., 2020; Samad et al., 2020; Zhang et al., 2018).

Burnout develops from combined factors in work-related environments and within the person. Unchecked, it is a progressive syndrome associated with emotional exhaustion and loss of meaning. High achievers and committed nurses who are passionate about their work are more at risk. Burnout begins insidiously, particularly in nurses who strive for perfection. Sources of burnout for nurses include working too many hours or at an accelerated pace with no respite, feeling unappreciated, giving too much to needy people, trying to meet multiple demands of administrators, unrealistic commitment to work demands and loss of balance with other life interests, lack of community with coworkers, and feeling resentment in place of the meaning that work once held.

An excellent resource for nurses to consider when preventing burnout is Self-Care for Nurses, provided by the Registered Practical Nurses Association of Ontario. The resource consists of three modules: Mental Well-being, Emotional Well-being, and Physical Well-being (Registered Practical Nurses Association of Ontario, n.d.).

Fig. 17.3 displays the symptoms of burnout.

Symptoms of Burnout

Khamisa et al. (2013) note typical characteristics of burnout as emotional exhaustion, depersonalization, and a reduced

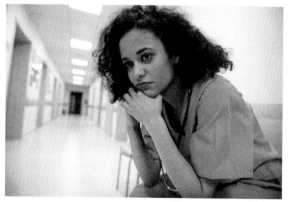

Fig. 17.3 Burnout is a form of occupational stress that compromises performance and professional commitment. Copyright © gpointstudio/iStock/Thinkstock.

sense of competence. Nurses experiencing burnout usually feel disillusioned and lack zest for their work. Other signs include loss of motivation and ideals, boredom or dissatisfaction at work, irritability and cynicism, resentment of expectations, and avoidance of meaningful encounters with people and their families. Headaches, gastric disturbances, skipping meals or eating compulsively on the run, feeling irritated by the intrusion of others, and a lack of balance between a nurse's work and personal life can signal the onset of burnout.

Burnout Prevention Strategies

The ABCs of burnout prevention (Arnold, 2008) are presented in Table 17.3.

Reflecting on the sources of stress in your life puts boundaries on it. Think about your goals and what is important to you. Seek opportunities to talk with trusted coworkers who can offer you the support and sensitivity you need to become aware of what is going on in your life—and what steps you need to recharge of your life so it is more fulfilling and meaningful. Then take the steps to make the needed changes. Self-care is one of the most effective mechanisms for coping with workplace stress (Cross, 2015).

A useful exercise is to imagine yourself a year from now, and ask yourself, "What do I need to do to be happy, a year from now?" Identify the first step you need to take that will move you toward this goal. Then do it!

Identifying realistic, achievable goals that are in line with your personal values is an excellent burnout prevention strategy. Goals should be aligned with purpose and values. Focusing on one thing at a time and finishing one project before starting another has several benefits. Achieving small, related goals promotes self-efficacy and offers hope that more complex goals are achievable.

Give yourself a break! Maintaining a healthy balance between work, family, leisure, and lifelong learning activities enhances personal judgements, satisfaction, and productivity. Actively schedule a time for each of these activities and stick to it. You actually will be a better nurse if you choose a balanced life.

Remember, you always have choices, even if it is to change your attitudes to allow "caring for yourself" as an essential part of providing excellent nursing care. People experiencing burnout lose sight of this fact. Life is a series of choices and negotiations. The choices we make help to create the fabric of our lives. Refusing to delegate work because someone else cannot do it as well as you or not going out to dinner with friends because you have too much work to do are choices you don't have to make.

Detachment from ego is a critical component of burnout prevention. It means that you do not allow emotional involvement in a task or relationship to undermine your

TABLE 17.3 ABCs of Burnout Prevention	
Areas of Focus	**Suggested Strategies**
Awareness	Use self-reflection and conversations with others to sort out priorities and identify parts of life that are out of balance. Recognize and allow feelings.
Balance	Maintain a healthy lifestyle. Balance care of others with self-care and self-renewal needs.
Choice	Differentiate between things you can change and those you cannot. Deliberately make choices that are purpose driven and meaningful.
Detachment	Detach from excessive ego involvement and personal ambition. Share responsibility and credit for care. Use meditation to centre self.
Altruistic egoism	Take scheduled time for self, learn to say no, practise meditation, and develop outside interests that enrich the spirit.
Faith	Burnout is a malaise of the spirit. Trust in a higher power or purpose to centre yourself when you do not know what will happen next.
Goals	Identify and develop realistic goals in line with your personal strengths. Seek feedback and support.
Hope	Hope is nurtured through conversations with others that lighten the burden and a belief in one's possibilities and personal worth in the greater scheme of things.
Integrity	Recognize that each of us is the only person who can determine the design and application of meaning in our lives.

Adapted from Arnold, E. (2008). Spirituality in educational and work environments. In V. Carson & H. Koenig (Eds.), *Spiritual dimensions of nursing practice* (revised ed., pp. 386–399). Templeton Foundation Press.

own quality of life, values, and needs. Someone once asked Mother Teresa how she was able to remain so energetic and hopeful in the midst of the unrelenting suffering she encountered in Kolkata (Calcutta). She replied that it was because she did the best she could and did not worry about the outcome because she could not control it. The same is true for the work that all nurses do. We can control our professional contribution to the care process, but not the outcomes for the people we care for. It is important to pay as much attention to your own personal needs as you do to the needs of others. Although it seems obvious to do so, nurses sometimes consider attention to their own needs as being selfish, especially when the needs of others are worrying. However, one cannot give from an empty cupboard. Replenishing the self actually improves the quality of care a nurse can give to others.

Simulation Exercise 17.6 provides an opportunity to think about your personal potential for burnout and ways to achieve better balance in your life.

Burnout challenges personal integrity when important values are ignored or devalued. When you begin to forget who you are and try to become what everyone else expects of you, you are in trouble. Reclaim yourself! Taking responsibility for yourself as a person *and* as a professional means that you respect yourself and who you are. Take the risk to be all that you are, as well as all that you can be, without worrying about what others think. Seek professional supports such as training, staff retreats, staff support networks, and job rotation to stimulate new ideas and insights. Professional support groups are effective as a means of providing encouragement to nurses in acute settings. Schedule times for fun and self-replenishment.

Case Example: Student Nurse Burnout

Chen Wong, a second-year nursing student, was just starting her practicum on a medical–surgical unit. On the second clinical day, she missed the postconference. When her instructor sought her out and asked for an explanation, Chen said she was far too busy on the unit to attend postconference. The instructor explained that postconference was for supporting each other, applying what was learned, and preparing for the next day. The next day, Chen missed again. The instructor again sought her out and asked if they could have a brief meeting. During the meeting, Chen started to cry. She said she was completely exhausted and since starting this rotation, she was doing research till 4 a.m.. She said she had almost made an assessment mistake, but her buddy nurse

SIMULATION EXERCISE 17.6   Burnout Assessment

Purpose

To help students understand the symptoms of burnout

Procedure

Consider your life over the past year. Complete the questionnaire by answering with a 5 if the situation is a constant occurrence, 4 if it occurs most of the time, 3 if it occurs occasionally, 2 if it has occurred once or twice during the last 6 months, and 1 if it is not a problem at all. Scores ranging from 60 to 75 indicate burnout. Scores ranging from 45 to 60 indicate that you are stressed and in danger of developing burnout. Scores ranging from 20 to 44 indicate a normal stress level, and scores of less than 20 suggest that you are not a candidate for burnout.

1. Do you find yourself taking on or being overwhelmed by other people's problems?
2. Do you feel resentful about the amount or nature of claims on your time?
3. Do you find you have less time for social activities?
4. Have you lost your sense of humour?
5. Are you having trouble sleeping?
6. Do you find you are more impersonal and less tolerant of others than you used to be?
7. Is it difficult for you to say no?
8. Are the things that used to be important to you slipping away from you because you do not have time?
9. Do you feel a sense of urgency and not enough time to complete tasks?
10. Are you forgetting appointments, friends' birthdays?
11. Do you feel overwhelmed and unable to pace yourself?
12. Have you lost interest in intimacy?
13. Are you overeating or have you begun to skip meals?
14. Is it difficult to feel enthusiastic about your work?
15. Do you feel it is difficult to connect on a meaningful level with others?

Creating an Antidote to Burnout

Tally up your scores. Nursing school is a strong breeding ground for the development of burnout (demands exceed resources). To offset the possibility of developing burnout symptoms, do the following:

1. Think about the last time you took time for yourself. If you cannot think of a time, you really need to do this exercise.
2. Identify a leisure activity that you can do during the next week to break the cycle of burnout.
3. Describe the steps you will need to take to implement the activity.
4. Identify the time required for this activity and what other activities will need rearrangement to make it possible.
5. Describe any obstacles to implementing your activity and how you might resolve them.

Reflective Analysis Discussion

1. Was it difficult for you to come up with an activity? If so, why?
2. Were you able to develop a logical way to implement your activity?
3. Were the activities chosen by others helpful to you in any way?
4. How might you be able to use this exercise in your future practice?

---

had corrected her. Now she was checking her work at least three times and could not get all the care done.

1. What is Chen experiencing?
2. How should the instructor manage this situation?
3. What does Chen need to do to be successful in this rotation?

SUMMARY

This chapter focuses on the stress response in health care and supporting people and their families with coping with stress, through nurse–person relationships. Stress can negatively impact outcomes for people in your care, level of satisfaction with care, and compliance with treatment. A fundamental goal in the nurse–person relationship is to empower people and families with the knowledge, support, and resources they need to cope effectively with stress.

Stress is a part of everyone's life. Mild stress can be beneficial, but greater stress levels can be unhealthy. Concurrent and cumulative stresses increase the response level. Theoretical models address stress as a physiological response, as a stimulus, and as a transaction between the person and their environment. Factors that influence the development of a stress reaction include the nature of the stressor, personal interpretation of its meaning, number of previous and concurrent stressors, previous experiences with similar stressors, and availability of support systems and personal coping abilities.

People use problem- and emotion-focused coping strategies to minimize stress. Social support is key to effectively coping with stress. Assessment should focus on stress factors the person is experiencing, the context in which they occur, and identification of coping strategies. Supportive interventions include giving information; opportunities to express their feelings, thoughts, and worries; and anticipatory guidance.

Nurses are at the forefront of health care delivery to people and families experiencing complex health and life issues. They too can experience stress and need support to do their job effectively. Burnout prevention requires recognition and resolution of organizational and personal factors contributing to job-related stress in professional nurses.

👤 ETHICAL DILEMMA

What Would You Do?

The mother of a person with acquired immunodeficiency syndrome (AIDS) does not know her son's diagnosis because her son does not want to worry her and fears her disapproval if she knew that he was gay. The mother asks the nurse if the family should have an oncology consult because she does not understand why, if her son has leukaemia as he says he does, an oncologist is not seeing him. What should the nurse do?

QUESTIONS FOR REVIEW AND DISCUSSION

1. What would you identify as tips for self-care to prevent the development of burnout?
2. Stress is characterized by physical and emotional symptoms of tension. In what ways does stress manifest itself in the behaviours of people you care for?
3. In what ways does stress manifest itself in your behaviour as a student nurse?
4. What are some of the stress management strategies you have tried or observed that seem to work better than others?

REFERENCES

Abela, K., Wardell, D., Rozmus, C. et al. (2020). Impact of pediatric critical illness and injury on families: An updated systematic review. *Journal of Pediatric Nursing, 51*, 21–31. https://doi.org/10.1016/j.pedn.2019.10.013.

Aldwin, C. M. (2010). Culture, coping and resilience to stress. In *Gross national happiness and development—Proceedings of the first international conference on operationalization of gross national happiness*. Centre for Bhutan Studies.

Alsharari, A. F. (2019). The needs of family members of patients admitted to the intensive care unit. *Patient Preference and Adherence, 13*, 465–473. https://doi.org/10.2147/PPA.S197769.

Antoni, M. (2013). Psychosocial intervention effects on adaptation, disease course and biobehavioural processes in cancer. *Brain, Behaviour, and Immunity, 30*(Suppl), S88–S98.

Anxiety Canada. (n.d.). How to do progressive muscle relaxation. https://www.anxietycanada.com/sites/default/files/MuscleRelaxation.pdf.

Arnold, E. (2008). Spirituality in educational and work environments. In V. Carson & H. Koenig (Eds.), *Spiritual dimensions of nursing practice* (Revised ed.) pp. 368–399. Templeton Foundation Press.

Arrogante, O., & Aparicio-Zaldivar, E. (2017). Burnout and health among critical care professionals: The mediational role of resilience. *Intensive and Critical Care Nursing, 42*, 110–125.

Bayuo, J., & Agbenorku, P. (2018). Coping strategies among nurses in the burn intensive unit: A qualitative study. *Burns Open, 2*, 47–52.

Beck, J., & Beck, A. T. (2011). *Cognitive behaviour therapy: Basics and beyond*. Guilford Press.

Bippus, A., & Young, S. (2012). Using appraisal theory to predict emotional and coping responses to hurtful messages. *Interpersonal, 6*(2), 176–190.

Canadian Cancer Society. (n.d.). *Guided imagery*. https://www.cancer.ca/en/cancer-information/diagnosis-and-treatment/complementary-therapies/guided-imagery/?region=on.

Canadian Mental Health Association. (2016). *Stress*. https://cmha.ca/documents/stress.

Canadian Mental Health Association Fort Francis. (n.d). *Social support*. http://www.cmhaff.ca/social-support.

Cannon, W. B. (1932). *The wisdom of the body*. Norton Pub.

Centre for Studies on Human Stress. (2019). *Coping with stress. Coping Strategies*. https://humanstress.ca/stress/trick-your-stress/steps-to-instant-stress-management/.

Cherry, K. (2021). *20 common defense mechanisms used for anxiety*. Verywell Mind. Dotdash Press. https://www.verywellmind.com/defense-mechanisms-2795960.

Cross, W. (2015). Building resilience in nurses: The need for a multiple pronged approach. *Journal of Nursing and Care, 4*, e124–e135.

Freudenberger, H. (1980). *Burn-out: The high cost of high achievement*. Doubleday.

Garcia-Dia, M. J., DiNapoli, J. M., Garcia-Ona, L. et al. (2013). Concept analysis: Resilience. *Archives of Psychiatric Nursing, 27*, 264–270.

Government of Canada. (2008). Mental health—Coping with stress. *It's Your Health*. https://www.canada.ca/en/health-canada/services/healthy-living/your-health/lifestyles/your-health-mental-health-coping-stress-health-canada-2008.html#he.

Graham, H., & Martin, S. (2016). Narrative descriptions of miyo-mahcihoyān (physical, emotional, mental, and spiritual well-being) from a contemporary néhiyawak (Plains Cree) perspective. *Int J Ment Health Syst, 10*, 58. https://doi.org/10.1186/s13033-016-0086-2.

Grover, S., & Ghosh, A. (2014). Somatic symptom and related disorders in Asians and Asian Americans. *Asian Journal of Psychiatry, 7.* 77–79. https://doi.org/10.1016/j.ajp.2013.11.014.

Haugland, T., Veenstra, M., Vatn, M. et al. (2013). Improvement in stress, general self-efficacy and health related quality of life following patient education for patients with neuroendocrine tumors: a pilot study. *Nursing Research and Practice.* https://doi.org/10.1155/2013/695820. Epub 2013.

HealthLinkBC. (2019). *Stress in children and teenagers.* https://www.healthlinkbc.ca/health-topics/ug1832.

Heart and Stroke Foundation & Canadian Mental Health Association. (2013) *Coping with stress.* https://www.heartandstroke.ca/-/media/pdf-files/canada/other/coping-w-ith-stress-en.ashx.

Holmes, T. H., & Rahe, R. (1967). The social readjustment rating scale. *Journal of Psychosomatic Research, 11,* 213–218.

Ishii, K., Mojaverian, T., Masuno, K. et al. (2017). Cultural differences in motivation for seeking social support and the emotional consequences of receiving support: The role of influence and adjustment goals. *Journal of Cross-Cultural Psychology, 48*(9), 1442–1456. https://doi.org/10.1177/0022022117731091.

Jacobson, E. (1938). *Progressive relaxation.* University of Chicago Press.

Jamieson, J., Nock, M., & Mendes, W. (2011). Mind over matter: Reappraising arousal improves cardiovascular and cognitive responses to stress. *The Journal of Experimental Psychology: Genera, 141,* 417–422.

Jaser, S., Faulkner, M., Whittemore, R. et al. (2012). Coping, self-management, and adaptation in adolescents with type 1 diabetes. *Annals of Behavioural Medicine, 43*(3), 311–319.

Khamisa, N., Peltzer, K., & Oldenburg, B. (2013). Burnout in relation to specific contributing factors and health outcomes among nurses: A systematic review. *International Journal of Environmental Research and Public Health, 10*(6), 2214–2240.

Köpsén, S., & Sjöström, R. (2020). Patients' experiences of a stress-management programme in primary care. *Journal of Multidisciplinary Healthcare, 13,* 207–216. https://doi.org/10.2147/JMDH.S235930.

Lavoie, J. (2013). Eye of the beholder: Perceived stress, coping style, and coping effectiveness of discharged psychiatric patients. *Archives of Psychiatric Nursing, 27,* 185–190.

Lazarus, R. S., & Folkman, S. (1991). The concept of coping. In A. Monat & R. S. Lazarus (Eds.), *Stress and coping: An anthology* (pp. 189–206). Columbia University Press. (Reprinted from Stress, *Appraisal, and Coping.* [1984]. Springer Publishing Company, Inc.)

Lee, S., Oh, H., Suh, Y. et al. (2017). A tailored relocation stress intervention programme for family caregivers of patients transferred from a surgical intensive care unit to a general ward. *Journal of Clinical Nursing, 26*(5–6), 784–794. https://doi.org/10.1111/jocn.13568.

Lin, F. Y., Rong, J. R., & Lee, T. Y. (2013). Resilience among caregivers of children with chronic conditions: A concept analysis. *Journal of Multidisciplinary Healthcare, 6,* 324–333.

Marsiglia, F. F., Kulis, S., Garcia Perez, H. et al. (2011). Hopelessness, family stress, and depression among Mexican-heritage mothers in the southwest. *Health & Social Work, 36*(1), 7–18.

McEwen, B. (2012). Brain on stress: How the social environment gets under the skin. *Proceedings of the National Academy of Sciences of the United States of America, 109*(Suppl. 2), 17180–17185.

McEwen, B. S., & Gianaros, P. J. (2011). Stress- and allostasis-induced brain plasticity. *Annual Review of Medicine, 62,* 431–445. https://doi.org/10.1146/annurev-med-052209-100430.

McEwen, B., & Stellar, E. (1993). Stress and the individual mechanisms leading to disease. *Archives of Internal Medicine, 153*(18), 2093–2101. https://doi.org/10.1001/archinte.153.18.2093.

Meyers, D. (2011). *Psychology in everyday life.* Worth Publications.

Moeini, M., Taleghani, F., Mehrabi, T. et al. (2014). Effects of a spiritual care program on levels of anxiety in patients with leukemia. *Iranian Journal of Nursing and Midwifery Research, 19*(1), 88–93.

Pearlin, L., & Schooler, C. (1978). The structure of coping. *Journal of Health and Social Behaviour, 19,* 2–21.

Pirelli, G., Formon, D. L., & Maloney, K. (2020). Preventing vicarious trauma (VT), compassion fatigue (CF), and burnout (BO) in forensic mental health: Forensic psychology as exemplar. *Professional Psychology: Research and Practice, 51*(5), 454–466. https://doi.org/10.1037/pro0000293.

Polat, H., Turan, G. B., & Tan, M. (2020). Determination of the relationship of the spiritual orientation of nurses with compassion fatigue, burnout, and compassion satisfaction. *Perspectives in Psychiatric Care, 56*(4), 920–925. https://doi-org.login.ezproxy.library.ualberta.ca/10.1111/ppc.12513.

Rahmati, M., Khaledi, B., Kahrizi, M. et al. (2017). The effects of spiritual-religious intervention on anxiety level of the family members of patients in ICU ward. *Jentashapir Journal of Health Research, 8*(3), e59148. https://doi.org/10.5812/jjhr.59148.

Ramos, M., Sebastian, R., Stumbo, S. et al. (2017). Measuring unmet needs for anticipatory guidance among adolescents at school-based health centers. *Journal of Adolescent Health, 60*(6), 720–726. https://doi.org/10.1016/j.jadohealth.2016.12.021.

Rao, N., Varambally, S., & Gangadhar, B. (2013). Yoga school of thought and psychiatry: Therapeutic potential. *Indian Journal of Psychiatry, 55*(Suppl. 2), S145–S149.

Registered Practical Nurses Association of Ontario. (n.d.). *RPN practice resources: Self-care for nurses.* https://www.werpn.com/learn/practice-resources/self-care-for-nurses

Reich, J., Zautra, A., & Hall, J. (2010). *Handbook of adult resilience.* Guilford Press.

Samad Dahri, A., Asif Qureshi, M., & Ghaffar Mallah, A. (2020). The negative effect of incivility on job satisfaction through emotional exhaustion moderated by resonant leadership. 3C Empresa. *Investigación y Pensamiento Crítico, 9*(4), 93–123. http://ojs.3ciencias.com/index.php/3c-empresa/article/view/1118.

Schacter, D., Gilbert, D., & Wegner, D. (2010). *Psychology* (2nd ed.). Worth Publications.

Selye, H. (1950). Stress and the general adaptation syndrome. *British Medical Journal, 4667*, 1383–1392.

Sheldon, C., Murphy, M., & Prather, A. (2019). Ten surprising facts about stressful life events and disease risk. *Annual Review of Psychology, 70*, 577–597. annualreviews.org/doi/abs/10.1146/annurev-psych-010418-102857.

Shpancer, N. (2018, February 21). The wisdom of defense mechanisms: Psychological defenses can help manage the internal weather. *Psychology Today*. https://www.psychologytoday.com/ca/blog/insight-therapy/201802/the-wisdom-defense-mechanisms.

Simandan, D. (2010). On how much one can take: Relocating exploitation and exclusion within the broader framework of allostatic load theory. *Health and Place, 16*(6), 1291–1293. https://doi.org/10.1016/j.healthplace.2010.08.009.

Stein, S., & Bartone, P. (2020). *Hardiness: Making stress work for you to achieve your life goals*. John Wiley& Sons.

Thoits, P. (2010). Compensatory coping with stressors. In W. Avison et al. (Eds.), *Advances in the conceptionalization of the stress process*, pp. 23–34. Springer.

Tran, B. X., Giang, C., & Ho, T. (2020). Global mapping of interventions to improve quality of life using mind-body therapies during 1990-2018. *Complementary Therapies in Medicine, 49*, https://doi.org/10.1016/j.ctim.2020.102350.

Wagland, R., Fenlon, D., Tarrant, R. et al. (2015). Rebuilding self-confidence after cancer: A feasibility study of life-coaching. *Support Care Cancer, 23*(3), e651–e659.

Wittenberg-Lyles. E. (2012). *Communication in palliative nursing*. Oxford University Press.

Wolf, A., Moore, L., Lydahl, D. et al. (2017). The realities of partnership in person-centred care: A qualitative interview study with patients and professionals. *British Medical Journal Open, 7*(7), e016491. https://doi.org/10.1136/bmjopen-2017-016491.

Zhang, Y. Y., Zhang, C., Han, X. R. et al. (2018). Determinants of compassion satisfaction, compassion fatigue and burn out in nursing: A correlative meta-analysis. *Medicine, 97*(26), e11086. https://doi.org/10.1097/MD.0000000000011086.

Park, E. R., Traeger, L., Vranceanu, A. M. et al. (2013). The development of a patient-centered program based on the relaxation response: The relaxation response resiliency program (3RP). *Psychosomatics, 54*, 165–174.

Posadzki, P., & Jacques, S. (2014). Tai chi and meditation: A conceptual (re)synthesis. *Journal of Holistic Nursing, 27*(2), 103–114.

Strachan, P., Currie, K., Harkness, K. et al. (2014). Context matters in heart failure self-care: A qualitative systematic review. *Journal of Cardiac Failure, 20*(6), 448–455.

Tay, L., Tan, K., Diener, E. et al. (2013). Social relations, health behaviours, and health outcomes: A survey and synthesis. *Applied Psychology: Health and Well-being, 5*(1), 28–78.

WEBSITE/RESOURCES LIST

childlife.org.

https://www.canada.ca/en/health-canada/services/healthy-living/your-health/lifestyles/your-health-mental-health-coping-stress-health-canada-2008.html#hes.

https://www.childlife.org/the-child-life-profession.

https://cmha.ca/documents/stress.

https://www.healthlinkbc.ca/health-topics/ug1832.

https://humanstress.ca/stress/trick-your-stress/steps-to-instant-stress-management/.

https://brocku.ca/social-sciences/geography/wp-content/uploads/sites/152/Simandan-2010-On-how-much-one-can-take.pdf.

https://www.heartandstroke.ca/-/media/pdf-files/canada/other/coping-w-ith-stress-en.ashx.

https://humanstress.ca/stress/trick-your-stress/steps-to-instant-stress-management/.

https://opentextbc.ca/introductiontopsychology/back-matter/versioning-history/2020.

https://www.patientsafetyinstitute.ca/en/toolsResources/Patient-Engagement-in-Patient-Safety-Guide/Organizations-Supporting-Patient-Engagement/Pages/Canadian-Patient-Organizations.aspx.

https://psychologyfoundation.org/Public/Public/Programs/Stress_Strategies.aspx.

https://www.psychologytoday.com/ca/blog/insight-therapy/201802/the-wisdom-defense-mechanisms.

https://www.camimh.ca.

https://cna-aiic.ca/en/canadian-nurse-home/articles/issues/2019/october-2019/nursing-burnout-we-are-not-doing-enough.

https://www.verywellmind.com/defense-mechanisms-2795960.

https://www.psychologytoday.com/ca/blog/insight-therapy/201802/the-wisdom-defense-mechanisms.

https://www.camh.ca/en/health-info/guides-and-publications/growing-up-resilient.

http://www.cmhaff.ca/social-support.

https://opentextbc.ca/introductiontopsychology/chapter/15-1-health-and-stress/.

https://secure.cihi.ca/free_products/AiB_ReducingPsychological%20DistressEN-web.pdf.

SUGGESTED READING

Boss, P. (2011). *Loving someone who has dementia: How to find hope while coping with stress and grief*. Jossey-Bass.

Bourne, E. J. (2010). *The anxiety and phobia workbook*. New Harbinger.

Fink, G. (2017). Stress: Concepts, definition and history. In *Reference module in neuroscience and biobehavioural psychology*. Elsevier.

Grazzi, L., & Andrasik, F. (2010). Non-pharmacological approaches in migraine prophylaxis: Behavioural medicine. *Neurological Sciences, 31*(Suppl. 1), S133–S135.

Hart, P. L., Brannan, J., & De Chesnay, M. (2014). Resilience in nurses: An integrative review. *Journal of Nursing Management, 22*, 720–734.

http://www.hqontario.ca/Portals/0/modals/qi/en/processmap_
pdfs/resources_links/leading%20practices%20in%20
emergency%20department%20patient%20experience%20
from%20oha.pdf.

https://www.cancer.ca/en/cancer-information/
diagnosis-and-treatment/complementary-therapies/
guided-imagery/?region=on.

https://www.werpn.com/learn/practice-resources/self-care-
for-nurses/.

www.StressStrategies.ca.

18

Communicating With People With Communication Disorders

Olive Yonge

Originating US chapter by *Kathleen Underman Boggs*

OBJECTIVES

At the end of the chapter, the reader will be able to:

1. Describe nursing strategies for communicating with people with communication disorders secondary to visual, auditory, cognitive, or stimuli-related disabilities or that are treatment related.
2. Describe a specific communication disorder advocacy issue for nurses.
3. Access evidence-informed databases for communication disorders and discuss application of these evidence-informed practices and research findings to your clinical practice.

Communication is essential for a full life. When people have difficulty communicating, this affects their relationships with others and their ability to share information, interact with others, and express their wants and needs. One important aspect of life that is affected by difficulty communicating is access to safe health care (Sharpe & Hemsley, 2016). Difficulty communicating leaves people at risk for unsafe situations and preventable adverse events (Yuksel & Unver, 2016). Access to appropriate health care providers occurs less often because people with communication disorders are more likely to forego needed care (Barnett et al., 2017). For some, the underlying problem is related to physiological impairments that make it difficult to communicate their needs. This chapter presents an overview of communication disorders commonly encountered when caring for people. Most nurses will be challenged with caring for people with specialized communication disorders. Consider the following case of Tim Dakota.

Case Example: Tim Dakota

Tim Dakota, age 22 years, is 3 weeks post–traumatic brain injury after a motorcycle accident and has been in your neurological intensive care unit for 2 weeks.

Nurse: Good morning, Mr. Dakota. I am Sue Nance, your nurse for this fine Sunday morning. I am going to give you your bath now. The water will feel a little warm to you. After your bath, your wife will be in to see you. She stayed in the waiting room last night because she wanted to be with you. (No answer is necessary if the person is unable to speak, but the sound of a human voice and attention to his unspoken concerns can be very healing.)

Summary of the strategies this nurse used:
- Called Tim by name
- Introduced self
- Established time (date, time, place would be better)

- Explained procedure before beginning
- Prepared him to see his wife

By arranging for Mr. Dakota to see his wife, the nurse is providing an opportunity for new stimulation, support, and movement.

The United Nations has affirmed the rights of those with communication disorders, among all people with disabilities (1948). In Canada, the voice of patients has been formalized through the Canadian Patient Safety Institute (CPSI). They lobbied to have health care safety content as part of health care providers' curriculum, regardless of the diagnosis (CPSI, 2016). The focus of this chapter is strategies for enhancing communication for people with communication disorders.

BASIC CONCEPTS

"A **communication disorder** is an impairment in the ability to receive, send, process, and comprehend concepts or verbal, nonverbal, and graphic symbol systems" (American Speech-Language Hearing Association [ASHA], 1992). Communication disorders can be congenital or acquired and can be developmental or arise from deafness, blindness or low vision, neurological deficits, or cognitive deficits. They can range from mild to severe. Severe cognitive and sensory deficits interfere with communication, decrease access to health care, and lead to feelings of frustration. Globally, health conditions related to communication disorders are much more prevalent in developing countries. Many of the physical conditions associated with them are preventable or treatable, if only health care were accessible. Worldwide, more than a billion people, or 15% of the population, have some form of disability (World Health Organization [WHO], 2017). One in six people in Canada has a communication disorder. Communication disorders include disorders of speech, language, and hearing (Speech-Language and Audiology Canada [SAC], 2018).

In 2001, the WHO's International Classification of Functioning, Disability, and Health shifted away from a medical diagnosis model to a functional model (i.e., how people with a sensory impairment function in their daily lives). Under this model, a communication disorder definition includes any impairment in body structure or function that interferes with communication, specifically, because of impaired functioning of the brain, with stroke or other neurological cause; one or more of the five senses, such as hearing or vision; or of cognitive processing. Communication disorders can also arise from the kind of sensory deprivation that occurs in some agencies and units, such as in intensive care units (ICUs). The degree of difficulty in communicating is an interaction between the person's type of functional impairment, personal adaptability, and the health care environment (i.e., body factors, personal factors, and environmental factors, as stated in the WHO's model).

Any difficulty sending and receiving information between the person and health care providers may compromise the person's health, safety, health care, and rights to make decisions. When working with people with a communication disorder, you may need to modify communication strategies presented earlier in this textbook. Assess the communication abilities of *every* person in your care—two individuals can have the same communication disorder but have different communication disabilities. As well, each person compensates for their impairment in different ways.

Goal
Our primary nursing goal with someone with a communication disorder is to maximize the person's ability to successfully communicate and interact with the health care system to ensure optimal health and quality of life. Evidence shows us that when a person has difficulty communicating with nurses because of a communication disorder, they can become frustrated, angry, anxious, depressed, or uncertain. Some become so frustrated that they exhibit behavioural problems or even omit needed care. Even when the person does access care, communication disorders interfere with the therapeutic relationship and delivery of optimal care. The person's disorder is one barrier, but other barriers may include staff's negative attitude or inability to adapt their communication.

LEGAL MANDATES
The main federal laws that protect people with disabilities from discrimination include the *Canadian Charter of Rights and Freedoms* and the *Canadian Human Rights Act* (Government of Canada, 2018). The Charter is a set of laws that provide protection to all individuals in Canada as being equal; governments cannot discriminate on the grounds of race, religion, national or ethnic origin, colour, sex, age, or physical or mental disability. The *Canadian Human Rights Act* protects all Canadians when they are employed or receive services from the federal government, First Nations governments, or private companies that are regulated by the federal government (such as banks, trucking companies, broadcasters, and telecommunication companies). Each province and territory also has its own laws and human rights codes. The Council of Canadians with Disabilities (CCD, n.d.) has a human rights committee. Their mandate is to monitor court cases and continuously analyze issues pertaining to human rights for those

with disabilities and make recommendations to the CCD National Council.

Communication Disabilities Access Canada (CDAC) is a national organization that works collaboratively with government, health care, police, and legal and justice services to address social justice and accessibility issues for people with communication disabilities (Communication Disabilities Access Canada, 2021).

HOME-BASED HEALTH CARE

Visiting people with communication disorders in their home allows nurses the time to engage in collaborative negotiations for which there may not have been time during acute care management. Home health nurses can build the infrastructure needed to prevent worsening of disability, as demonstrated in a study of older people by Liebel and colleagues (2012).

TYPES OF DISORDERS

Hearing Loss

Hearing loss is a common problem, with approximately 15% of the world's population reporting it. Globally, approximately 360 million, or 5% of people, have disabling hearing loss, defined as a loss of greater than 35 decibels. More than half of hearing loss is preventable.

Someone with a hearing loss that ranges from mild to severe is considered hard of hearing; someone with a profound hearing loss, with little to no hearing, is considered deaf (WHO, 2017). You may see the word "deaf" (lowercase) or "Deaf" (capitalized); these terms have different meanings. When written in lowercase, *deaf* refers to the audiological condition of deafness; when capitalized, it refers to *Deaf* people, who share and participate in a culture and language of deafness—for example, American Sign Language (Canadian Association of the Deaf [CAD], 2015).

Hearing loss consistently ranks among the top five causes of years lived with a disability. In Canada, an estimated 19% of adults (4.6 million) have at least a mild hearing loss in the speech-frequency range. An even larger percentage of the adult population—35% (8.4 million)—have some degree of hearing loss in the high-frequency range (3, 4, 6 and 8 kHz), which is where age-related hearing loss typically begins. In addition to the aging process, hearing loss may also result from hereditary factors, some chronic conditions, noise exposure, ototoxic substances and medications, as well as other factors. The diminished ability to process acoustic information can impede communication. For example, it can be difficult to hear or understand speech, converse in noisy environments, and identify where sound is coming from (Statistics Canada, 2019; also see Chapter 20). Nurses

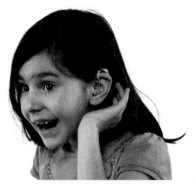

Fig. 18.1 People's sense of hearing alerts them to changes in the environment so they can respond effectively. iStock.com/1001nights

have both a legal and ethical obligation to provide appropriate care. Some people with a hearing loss from birth learn American Sign Language (ASL) as their first language; for these people, English is their second language. Many people who are deaf or hard of hearing use hearing aids or other devices to allow them to communicate; some people with profound hearing loss may have a cochlear implant. Many people who are deaf or hard of hearing learn to speak despite their hearing loss or use a combination of spoken and signed language (CAD, 2015).

People's sense of hearing alerts them to changes in the environment that allow them to respond effectively (Fig. 18.1). The listener hears sounds and words and also the speaker's vocal pitch, loudness, and intricate inflections that accompany the words. Subtle variations can completely change the sense of the message. Combined with the sound and intensity, the organization of the verbal symbols allows individuals to perceive and interpret the meaning of the sender's message. It is sometimes difficult to appreciate the extent of a person's hearing loss because there is often no outward sign that they have difficulty hearing. Even mild to moderate hearing losses can lead to significant functional impairments (George et al., 2012). Most people who are deaf or hard of hearing function well, by using hearing aids or other devices, using oral language, and learning to lipread, or by the use of sign language and interpreters. But some may try to hide their deafness, withdraw from relationships, become depressed, or be less likely to seek information from health care providers.

Children Who Are Deaf or Hard of Hearing

Permanent hearing loss is one of the most common congenital disorders, with an estimated incidence of one to three per thousand live births—far exceeding the combined incidence of other conditions for which newborns are routinely screened, such as congenital hypothyroidism, phenylketonuria, and other inborn errors of metabolism. In the past decade, universal newborn hearing screening (UNHS) has been widely adopted throughout North America, Europe, and in most other developed regions, primarily as a result of technological advances in screening and intervention modalities (Canadian Paediatric Society, 2011). Untreated or delayed hearing loss treatment may be a missed opportunity, as interventions—such as the provision of hearing aids—have been shown to have a positive impact on quality of life (Statistics Canada, 2019).

Older People Who Are Deaf or Hard of Hearing

As we age, we have an increased likelihood for **presbycusis**, or degeneration of ear structures, which is a sensorineural dysfunction that normally occurs with aging.

Vision Loss

Humans rely more heavily on vision than most species do. Globally, vision problems occur in approximately 285 million people; 180 million have vision loss. The majority of these would be treatable if care were accessible (WHO, 2001). The WHO has mounted a call for global action to promote eye care, called "Vision 2020."

Today, an estimated 1.5 million Canadians identify themselves as having vision loss. An estimated 5.59 million more have an eye disease that could cause vision loss (Canadian National Institute for the Blind [CNIB], n.d.). In addition to total loss, visual impairment is defined as at least 3/60 or having less than a 20-degree visual field (McGrath et al., 2016). The majority of these are older than 50 years of age. People who lack vision lose a primary method to decode the meaning of messages. All of the nonverbal cues that accompany spoken communication (e.g., facial expression, gesture, nodding, and leaning toward the person) are lost to those who are blind or have low vision. Even for people with partial vision loss, it is important for you to assess whether the person can read directions, medication labels, and so forth.

Children Who Are Blind or Have Low Vision

Children who are blind or have low vision lack access to visual cues such as the facial expressions and gestures that help to stimulate language development. In Canada, there is not enough evidence to prove that vision screening programs for children are effective (Public Health Ontario, 2016), whereas in the United States, the Preventive Services Task Force (USPSTF) recommends testing children younger than 5 years for amblyopia, strabismus, and visual acuity. Vision testing can be done in preverbal children, and it is recommended that babies have their first eye examination sometime between the ages of 3 and 6 months. Traditional vision screening that requires a verbal child can be done reliably by about age 3 years.

Older People Who Are Blind or Have Low Vision

As we age, the lens of the eye becomes less flexible, making it difficult to accommodate shifts from far to near vision; this is a condition known as **presbyopia**. Macular degeneration has also become a major cause of vision loss in older people.

Language Disorders in Children and Adults

Normal communication allows people to perceive and interact with the world in an organized and systematic manner. People use language to express self-need and to control environmental events. Language is the system people rely on to represent what they know about the world.

There are two main categories of communication disorders: speech disorders, in which the person has difficulty producing the sounds of speech, and language disorders, in which the person has difficulty formulating, expressing and comprehending spoken and written language (ASHA, 1992). People who are unable to speak, even temporarily because of intubation or ventilator dependency, incur feelings of frustration, anxiety, fear, or even panic and need to be given alternative means of communication during that time.

One of the most common language disorders in adults is aphasia. **Aphasia** is a language disorder that results from damage to one or more of the language areas of the brain, most often after a stroke. There are different types of aphasia. Damage to the language area toward the front of the brain causes a nonfluent aphasia; with this type, the person struggles to formulate language and express themselves, verbally and in writing, and usually has less difficulty understanding when they read or listen to others speak. It is important to remember that aphasia does not affect intelligence (Aphasia Nova Scotia, n.d.).

Damage to the language area toward the back of the brain causes a fluent aphasia; with this type, the person's most significant problem is in understanding when others speak or when they try to read. They can speak and write fairly easily, but the content of what they say is affected, and their words often don't make sense. While they may sound confused, they are not—what they mean to say just sounds mixed up. A third type, *global aphasia*, results from a more extensive stroke that includes both of the above language areas and leads to a severe difficulty with both expressive and receptive language, in both spoken and written form. Although people with the different types of aphasia present with different problems, they all have one thing in common: they know what they want to say but have trouble saying it. People with aphasia may have feelings of loss and social isolation. Although there may be no cognitive impairment, they may need extra time to process during a conversation, both to speak and understand others (Aphasia Nova Scotia, n.d.).

Speech Disorders in Children and Adults

Both children and adults can have speech disorders, which can range from very mild to very severe. People with speech disorders have difficulty with speech sounds but not with formulating their ideas, coming up with the right words, understanding others, writing, or understanding what they read. Someone with an articulation disorder has difficulty pronouncing the sounds; this can be a developmental problem from childhood, due to a hearing loss or other causes. Someone with speech apraxia has difficulty organizing the sounds within words, and it might be difficult for other people to understand them. Another speech disorder is stuttering, in which the person repeats sounds or words, prolongs sounds, or has silent blocks. Stuttering usually begins in childhood and, for some people, persists into adulthood. Dysarthria is a speech disorder that makes it difficult to pronounce sounds because of a neurological cause—for example, cerebral palsy, Parkinson's disease, or stroke. Finally, both children and adults can have a voice disorder. Voice disorders can be due to an organic cause (e.g., laryngeal cancer), a functional cause (e.g., yelling or using the voice improperly), or neurological cause (e.g., vocal cord paralysis) (SAC, 2014). People with a severe speech disorder may be completely nonverbal; remember that this does not mean they have difficulty comprehending or have any accompanying cognitive disorder.

Impaired Cognitive Processing

Impaired cognitive processing ability can interfere with communication and lead to anxiety and confusion. Understanding involves receiving new information and integrating it meaningfully with prior knowledge. Individuals with impaired cognitive processing ability have to work harder and require more time for conceptual integration. The responsibility for assessing the ability to understand, give consent, and overcome communication difficulties rests with both social services and health care workers. You need to continually determine the extent of people's understanding and even their ability to understand self-care activities and need for alternative communication aids or devices. For example, although most older people retain their mental acuity, those with impaired cognitive processing may have challenges with correctly taking prescribed medications.

Children With Impaired Cognitive Processing and Developmental Disabilities

Because there is a significant increase in the prevalence of children with impaired cognitive processing and developmental disabilities such as auditory processing disorders (Moore, 2018), traumatic brain injury (Lambregts et al., 2018), and visual impairment (Leung et al., 2018), nurses may be caring for more of them, both in clinical agencies and in the community (Betz, 2012). Atypical communication is often the first behavioural clue to cognitive impairment in young children, which is associated with conditions such as developmental delay, autism spectrum disorder, and mood disorders. As these children grow, they may have subtle or significant difficulties in communication.

Communication Disorders Associated With Some Mental Health Conditions

People with serious mental health disorders may have an associated communication disorder resulting from a range of causes. Take the case of Hilda. She made an appointment with her nurse practitioner because she was having difficulty finding the right words when speaking and remembering what she had read in the newspaper. However, what greatly concerned her was her gradual inability to do crossword puzzles, an activity she had greatly enjoyed. After completing the assessment, the NP suspected Hilda had a neurocognitive disorder. Global incidence of cognitive disorders is unknown, but the WHO estimates that 400 million people are affected, which has made mental health a part of their 2030 goals (WHO, 2017). In any given year, one in five people in Canada personally experiences a mental health problem or disorder. It is estimated that 10–20% of Canadian youth are affected by a mental health disorder, the single most disabling group of disorders worldwide (Canadian Mental Health Association [CMHA], 2013). In addition to illness-related communication disorders, social isolation and difficulty coping may accompany people's difficulty receiving or expressing language.

Some people with mental health disorders have intact sensory channels, but they cannot process and respond appropriately to what they hear, see, smell, or touch. In some forms of *schizophrenia*, there are alterations in the neurotransmitters in the brain, which normally conduct messages between nerve cells and help to orchestrate the person's response to the external environment. Messages have distorted meanings. It is beyond the scope of this text to discuss psychosis in detail, but generally, some people with mental health disorders present with a poverty of speech and limited content. Speech appears blocked, reflecting disturbed patterns of perception, thought, emotions, and motivation. You may notice a lack of vocal inflection and an unchanging facial expression. A "flat affect" makes it difficult to truly understand them. Illogical thinking processes may manifest in the form of illusions, hallucinations, and delusions. Common words assume new meanings known only to the person experiencing them.

Neurocognitive Disorders

The term *dementia*, now referred to as *mild or major neurocognitive disorder* (Ganguli et al., 2011) doesn't actually refer to one, specific disease; rather, it is a symptom of a range of diseases and conditions. Alzheimer's disease is the most common condition that has dementia as a major symptom, followed by vascular dementia. This category also includes Creutzfeldt-Jakob disease, dementia with Lewy bodies, frontotemporal dementia, and others. *Dementia* is an overall term for a set of symptoms caused by these disorders affecting the brain. In 2020, there were over 500000 Canadians living with dementia, and this number is expected to increase to 91200 by 2030. Of those diagnosed, over 65% are women (Alzheimer Society, 2021). On June 17, 2019, Canada passed Bill C-233, which represents a national strategy for Alzheimer's disease and other causes of dementia (Canadian Institute for Health Information [CIHI], 2021). This strategy will help identify research areas and quality of life issues for people with dementia and also address the role of their caregivers. One of the areas of concern for these people is communication. Communication skill training is recommended, especially for family members (Mamo et al., 2017), and for all staff employed in extended care facilities (Fig. 18.2). Some communication strategies for communicating with people with dementia are listed in Table 18.1.

People With Treatment-Related Communication Disorders

Communication is particularly important in nursing situations characterized by sensory deprivation; physical immobility; limited environmental stimuli; or excessive, constant stimuli (Fig. 18.3). Nurses show sensitivity for people in

TABLE 18.1   **Tips for Communicating With People With Dementia**
These suggestions are based on expert opinion (Machiels et al., 2017).
• Gain the person's attention before speaking (face the person).
• Use your active listening skills, especially eye contact.
• Use brief sentences (fewer words).
• Speak clearly and slightly slowly.
• Add nonverbal cues to your message.
• Observe the person for their nonverbal cues.
• Use positive reinforcement (keep messages short and sweet).
• Use familiar objects to give cues, such as holding up a hairbrush when you want to brush the person's hair.
• Use memory books or family photos, especially when the person asks about someone.
• Verify the person's understanding by having them restate (summarize, not just repeat).

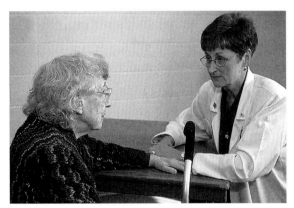

Fig. 18.3 Touch, eye movement, and sounds can be used to support communication with people with aphasia.

bewildering situations, such as emergency departments or ICUs. People in these circumstances may be frightened, in pain, and unable to communicate easily because of intubation or other complications.

People who are immobile, isolated, or intubated, such as in the ICU, often experience absence of stimulation resulting in a gradual decline of cognitive abilities. People with normal intellectual capacity can appear dull, uninterested, and lacking in problem-solving abilities if they do not have frequent interpersonal stimulation (Fig. 18.4).

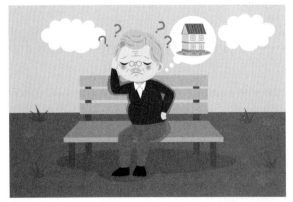

Fig. 18.2 People with dementia may need assistance with cognitive processing. iStock.com/ Lin Shao-hua

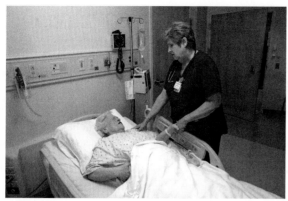

Fig. 18.4 The following are situational factors that affect people's responses to critical care hospital situations:

- Anxiety and fear
- Pain
- Altered stimuli—too much or too little, including unusual noises and isolation
- Sleep deprivation
- Unmet physiological needs such as thirst
- Losing track of time
- Multiple life changes
- Multiple care providers
- Immobility
- Frequent diagnostic procedures
- Lack of easily understood information

When assessing pain in people with communication disorders, it may be difficult to tell if they are accurately answering "yes" or "no." Critical care nurses have validated use of a number of pain assessment graphic assessment scales, such as FACES (Rahu et al., 2015). Never assume that a person who is nonverbal is cognitively impaired (Booker & Haedtke, 2016).

Applications

Communication disorders may be developmental or acquired. The emphasis on person-centred care embodies a need for those with communication disorders to become active participants in their own care.

EARLY RECOGNITION OF COMMUNICATION DISORDERS

Identification of communication disorders is one aspect of your role. For example, if a 4-year-old child fails to speak at all or uses a noticeably limited vocabulary for their age and cannot name objects or follow your directions, would you recognize the need for further assessment? Given this history, you could urge the health team to make a referral for speech and language evaluation by a speech-language pathologist.

ASSESSMENT OF CURRENT COMMUNICATION ABILITIES

Are you assessing each person for communication disorders? Do you tailor a plan of care to help meet identified

---

⟫ DEVELOPING AN EVIDENCE-INFORMED PRACTICE

Access some of the many databases that summarize research to compile "best practice" guidelines for adapting communication, which is especially pertinent for people with communication disorders. Most sites rank the strength of the research evidence from strong to poor. Visit Canadian Assitive Technology (https://canasstech.com/pages/resources) to access all the disability resources in Canada, and the National Institute for Learning Development (https://nildcanada.org/) for the best communication strategies to use, such as using active verbs and short sentences. Another suggestion is to supplement your verbal message with visual aids, such as pictures or written words.

Application to Your Clinical Practice

In a hospital, all staff need to be aware of the person's communication disorder, perhaps by posting a sign or symbol on the door. A speech-language pathologist can provide individualized tips for communication, which can be placed at the bedside or on a whiteboard by the person's bed. Mutual goals involve fostering effective communication with all members of the health team. Nurses with heavy workloads do not always choose to take the time to use communication strategies, sometimes opting just to avoid direct communication, leading to high frustration levels. Even when we are aware of a person's communication disorder, we sometimes lack the ability to communicate effectively. Always let people know when you cannot understand them. Applying communication accommodation theory, nurses can choose to use strategies described in Boxes 18.1, 18.2, and 18.3, in this chapter. A variety of communication aids are available to assist in communication.

communication needs? Provision of alternative communication methods is a legal requirement.

COMMUNICATION STRATEGIES

Using Respectful Terminology

When providing care to people with a communication disorder, it is important to be familiar with the appropriate, respectful terminology related to the person's disability. For some types of disability, "people-first language" is preferred—that is, to name the person with the disorder and then the disorder itself. For example, it is preferable to say "the child with cerebral palsy" rather than "the cerebral palsy child." Other groups, most notably deaf people, have always preferred "identity-first language"—that is, to refer to themselves as "a deaf person" rather than "a person with deafness." Identity-first language is used by some groups as a way of claiming their disability (American Psychological Association, 2019; AutismBC, 2021; Collier, 2012).

The National Center on Disability and Journalism is an excellent source for respectful language around disability (https://ncdj.org/style-guide/). You can also find helpful suggestions for appropriate terminology on websites specific to those disorders—for example, the Canadian Association of the Deaf (http://cad.ca/issues-positions/terminology/), National Association of the Deaf (https://www.nad.org/resources/american-sign-language/community-and-culture-frequently-asked-questions/), Canadian National Institute for the Blind (https://www.cnib.ca/en/sight-loss-info/when-someone-you-know-blind/blindness-etiquette?region=on), and Autism Canada (https://autismcanada.org/wp-content/uploads/2015/04/AC_LanguageDocument-2016-1.pdf).

Strategies for Communicating With People With Communication Disorders

Specific strategies are outlined in Boxes 18.1, 18.2 and 18.3, in this chapter. When communicating with people with communication disorders, you can have the greatest impact by modifying the way you communicate and also by making modifications to the environment. For example, evidence-informed practice suggests that you create a quiet environment, allocate more of your time to facilitate communication, take time to listen, ask yes/no questions, observe nonverbal cues, repeat back comments, effectively use any communication equipment, assign the same staff for care continuity, and encourage family members to be present to assist in communications (Selick et al., 2018).

Sometimes, simple, low-tech solutions are best. A speech-language pathologist can provide a letterboard with letters, numbers, and common words and phrases for the hospital setting that the person can point to. With pen and paper or marker and a whiteboard, the person can try writing or drawing what they are trying to express and the nurse can help by guessing. Writing down key words that the nurse or person has said can help the person keep track of the conversation and gives the person something to point to, to refer back to those words.

Handheld devices such as smartphones and tablets have downloadable applications (apps) that provide picture-to-speech or text-to-speech options and can be used to support verbal communication. Canada has an Accessibility Technology program that co-funds entrepreneurs and researchers in developing innovative assistive and adaptive digital devices and technologies for people with disabilities (Government of Canada, 2019).

An Australian study reported mixed attitudes from nurses regarding the use of assistive devices with people with communication disorders. Nurses expressed concern about their time constraints, device security, and people's conditions and ability to use the devices. On the other hand, they acknowledged that mobile apps could aid in more complex communication than picture boards and could improve communication (Sharpe & Hemsley, 2016).

Strategies for Communicating With People Who Are Deaf or Hard of Hearing

Screening of functional hearing ability is recommended for all people in your care. A finding of hearing loss would provide an opportunity for referral to an audiologist. Consider the age of onset and the severity of the disorder. Hearing loss that begins after the development of speech means that the person has access to word symbols and language skills. Deafness in children can cause developmental delays, which may need to be taken into account in planning the most appropriate communication strategies. Consider that someone might have a hearing loss when people appear unresponsive to sound or respond only when the speaker is directly facing them. Ask whether the person uses a hearing aid and, if so, whether it is working properly.

Strategies for communicating with people who are deaf or hard of hearing depend on the severity of the deafness, but in general, it is best to speak clearly but not shout. Give the person time to respond. Try to avoid background noise and speak in a well-lit area so the person can lipread and watch your facial expressions. Face the person and don't cover your mouth when you speak (SAC, 2018).

During the COVID-19 pandemic beginning in 2020, nurses, people receiving care, and caregivers had to wear masks, which impeded communication, especially for those who read lips. In the community, people who are deaf or hard of hearing found it difficult to remain 2 metres away from a speaker as it would reduce the volume of their

BOX 18.1 Suggestions for Helping People With a Communication Disorder Due to Sensory Loss

- Assess psychological readiness to communicate.
- Introduce yourself and convey respect, an understanding of the person's frustrations, and your willingness to communicate.
- Be concise.
- Always maximize the use of **communication aids**, such as whiteboard and marker, communication boards, pictures, gesture, and electronic communication aids.
- Pick the means of available communication best suited to the person. Multiple pathways using both auditory and visual methods are standard recommendations.
- Always help people to use their assistive equipment (e.g., adjust hearing aids, provide their glasses, use a smartphone for texting).
- Assess the person's understanding of what was said by having them signal or repeat the message.

- Write down important ideas and allow the person the same option to increase the chances of successful communication. Always have a writing pad or smartphone available.
- Arrange for a TTY or relay service or an amplified telephone handset for people who are hard of hearing, if they do not text.
- If the person is unable to hear, rely primarily on visual materials.
- Arrange for closed-captioned television.
- Use text messaging, email, and phone apps.
- Suggest to the person who is deaf or hard of hearing to verbalize speech, even if the person uses only a few words or the words are difficult to understand at first.
- Use an intermediary, such as a family member who knows sign language, to facilitate communication with people who are deaf and who sign.

For People Who Are Deaf or Hard of Hearing
- Tap on the floor or table to get the person's attention via the vibration.
- Communicate in a well-lit room and face the person, so they can focus their attention, see your facial expression, and watch your lips move.
- Choose a quiet, private place; close doors and turn off TVs or radios to decrease environmental noise.
- Use facial expressions, hand signals, and gestures that reinforce verbal content, or request a sign language interpreter, perhaps a family member.
- Speak distinctly, without exaggerating words or shouting. People who are hard of hearing respond best to well-articulated words spoken in a moderate, even tone. Speak only as loudly as you need to.

For People Who Are Blind or Have Low Vision
- Let the person know when you approach by identifying yourself and using a simple touch; always indicate when you are leaving.
- Adapt communication to compensate for lack of nonverbal messaging.
- Adapt teaching for people with low vision by using large print, audio information, or Braille.
- Do not lead or hold the person's arm when walking; instead, allow the person to take your arm.
- Use touch and physical proximity while you are with the person; give the person something substantial to touch in your absence.
- Develop and use signals to indicate changes in pace or direction while walking.

TTY, Teletypewriter.

BOX 18.2 Strategies to Assist People With Cognitive Processing Disorders or Speech and Language Difficulties

- Speak slowly, using simple sentences; ask yes or no questions.
- Talk about one thing at a time, or ask one question at a time; do not rush.
- Give extra time for the person to process what you say and formulate a response; do not interrupt.
- Avoid prolonged, continuous conversations; instead, use frequent, short talks. Present small amounts of information at a time.
- When the person falters in written or oral expression, supply needed compensatory support. Sometimes just giving the person extra time is enough.

- Encourage efforts to communicate.
- Provide regular mental stimulation in a non-taxing way.
- Help people to focus on the faculties still available to them for communication.
- Use visual cues; for print materials, use short, bulleted lists.
- Make referral to a speech pathologist and occupational therapist to help people obtain and use AAC devices.

AAC, Augmentative and alternative communication.

voices and limit their ability to watch the other person's face. If a caregiver has an accent that the person is unaccustomed to, this may also make it difficult for a person who lipreads to understand.

BOX 18.3   Strategies for Communicating With People With Treatment-Related Communication Disorders

- Encourage the person to display pictures or a simple object from home.
- Orient the person to the people, place, and time.
- Ask questions, especially ones the person can answer with a yes or no.
- Frequently provide information about condition and progress.
- Reassure the person that cognitive and psychological disturbances are common.
- Give explanations before procedures by providing information about the sounds, sights, and feelings the person is experiencing.
- Make communication assistive devices available, ranging from paper and pencil, an alphabet board, or communication cards to electronic communication aids.
- Always assess whether your communication was successful by having the person signal back.

Assistive devices such as an amplifier should be made available for someone who is deaf or hard of hearing. Knowing how to operate assistive listening devices, hearing aids, and telephone attachments is important. Some people have hearing aids but do not use them unless family or nurses assist them. Simulation Exercises 18.1 and 18.2 help with understanding what it is like to have a sensory deficit. Refer to Box 18.1 for communication strategies. Consider the case of Timmy.

Case Example: Timmy

Two student nurses were assigned to care for 9-year-old Timmy, who is deaf and nonverbal. They learned from his chart and their supervising nurse that he is able to read lips and uses sign language to communicate; he has normal reading skills. They also spoke to his mother, who recommended that they demonstrate anything they explain to him. When they went into his room for assessment, he was alone, so they didn't have anyone to translate their words into sign language. Instead, they used a pad and paper to communicate with him and also role-played taking vital signs by using some funny facial expressions and demonstrating on a doll.

SIMULATION EXERCISE 18.1   Understanding the Social Model of Disability

Purpose:
To assist students in understanding the move away from seeing disability as primarily a problem related to a person's deficits and thus, seeing it as that person's responsibility to overcome the deficit. In contrast, when a social model is used to determine what is limiting to people with disabilities, the conversation turns to stereotypes and stigma of the person with disabilities, which is alienating.

Procedure:
1. Ask the students to watch the video, Social Model of Disability, here: https://www.youtube.com/watch?v=24KE__OCKMw. The video is 2 minutes and 43 seconds.
2. In groups of three to six, depending on class size, discuss the following questions for 20 minutes:
   a) How have people with disabilities—("dis-abled" giving the impression that they are less able—been portrayed in popular culture?

b) Consider the statement "the person does not have a disability but is disabled by society." What does this mean?
c) What can be done about barriers such as prejudiced opinions and attitudes, restricted access, and systematic exclusion?
d) People with disabilities want opportunities, accessibility, and independence. Give an example of how each has been achieved from your personal experiences.
e) How can health professionals campaign together for equality and human rights?

Reflective Analysis:
After discussing these questions in small groups, discuss as a large class how your findings are addressed in the curriculum thus far.
   Resource that could be assigned as pre reading prior to the simulation:

Barney, K. (2012). Disability simulations: Using the social model of disability to update an experiential educational practice, SCHOLE: *A Journal of Leisure Studies and Recreation Education, 27*(1), 1–11. 10.1080/1937156X.2012.11949361. https://www.nrpa.org/globalassets/journals/schole/2012/schole-volume-27-number-1-pp-1-11.pdf.

SIMULATION EXERCISE 18.2 Sensory Loss: Hearing or Vision

Purpose:
To help raise consciousness regarding loss of a sensory function

Procedure
Watch the video, How do a Blind Person & a Deaf Person Communicate?, here: https://www.youtube.com/watch?v=5ff1tm1AhZg. (Also check out the channel, The Tommy Edison Experience, here: https://www.youtube.com/user/TommyEdisonXP.) This YouTube clip focuses on what it is like to be blind or deaf. He is interviewing Rikki Poynter, who is Deaf and has her own YouTube channel, Youtube.com/Rikkipoynter. Together, they discuss communication strategies to use with people who are hearing impaired or blind.

Discussion
In class, students share observations and answer the following questions.
1. Prior to watching this YouTube clip, what assumptions did you have about people who are deaf or hard of hearing and those who are blind or have low vision?
2. What is the role of the interpreter?
3. What is tactile signing?
4. What is the impact of technology in both Tommy's and Rikki's lives?

Strategies for Communicating With People Who Are Blind or Have Low Vision

Vision assessment is recommended for everyone, routinely. Nurses caring for anyone with vision limitations should perform some evaluation and ensure that if the person wears glasses or needs other equipment that these are available to them. Refer to Box 18.1 for strategies for communicating with people who are blind or have low vision. Use of vocal cues (e.g., speaking as you approach) helps prevent startling. Because people who are blind or have low vision cannot see our faces or observe our nonverbal signals, we need to use words to express what they cannot see in the message. It also is helpful to mention your name as you enter the person's presence. Even people who have limited or partial vision appreciate hearing the name of the person to whom they are speaking. Communication-enhancing equipment for people who are blind or have low vision includes electronic magnifier machines, auditory teaching materials, computer screen readers with voice synthesizers, Braille keypads or cards, and video magnifying machines.

When caring for people with macular degeneration, remember to stand to their side, an exception to the "face the person directly" rule applied with people who are deaf or hard of hearing. People with macular degeneration often still have some peripheral vision. Enhanced lighting and use of light filters to reduce glare may help you communicate with people with reduced vision. With people who are blind or have low vision, the use of touch acts as a social reinforcer and can orient them to your presence. However, use of verbal greetings may better alert people. Vocal tones and pauses that reinforce the verbal content are helpful. Also, let the person know when you are leaving the room. Consider the following case of Ms. Shu.

Case Example: Ms. Shu
You can use words to supply additional information to counterbalance the missing visual cues. Ms. Sue Shu is an older person who is blind and who commented to the student nurse, Ruth, that she felt Ruth was uncomfortable talking with her and perhaps did not like her. Not being able to see Ruth, Ms. Shu interpreted the hesitant uneasiness in Ruth's voice as evidence that Ruth did not wish to be with her. Ruth agreed with Ms. Shu that she was quite uncomfortable but did not explain further. Had Ms. Shu been able to see Ruth's apprehensive body posture, she would have realized that Ruth was quite shy and ill at ease with *any* interpersonal relationship. To avoid this serious error in communication, Ruth might have clarified the reasons for her discomfort, and the relationship could have moved forward.

Orientation to Environmental Hazards for People Who Are Blind or Have Low Vision

When a person who is blind or has low vision is being introduced to a new environmental setting, you should orient them by describing the size of the room and the position of the furniture and equipment. When placing a person's food tray, describe the position of the items, perhaps using a clock face analogy (e.g., "Carrots are at 2 o'clock, potatoes at 11 o'clock"). If other people are present, you could name each person. A good communication strategy is to ask the other people in the room to introduce themselves. In this way, the person can tell whose voice belongs to each person. Avoid any tendency to speak with a louder voice than usual. Speak clearly, but not in an exaggerated manner, as this may be perceived by some as insensitive to the nature of the their disability. Keep your tone of voice natural.

A person who is blind or has low vision may need guidance in moving around in unfamiliar surroundings. For example, surveyed people who were blind or had low vision said they needed assistance getting to and from their bathroom. One way of preserving autonomy is to offer *your* arm to them instead of taking *their* arm. Alert them when there are steps or changes in movement as they are about to occur, to help them in new places or when there are differences in terrain. Some people who are blind or have low vision use wearable navigation systems.

Strategies for Communicating With People With Speech and Language Disorders

Both children and adults can benefit from early intervention to improve communication. Assessment of speech and language is part of the initial evaluation. A speech-language pathologist can conduct an assessment to determine the type of disorder the person has, which will aid in selecting the most appropriate intervention. People with aphasia usually have at least some difficulty with both expressive language—especially difficulty finding words—and receptive language or understanding when others speak. Sometimes, they can find the correct word if given enough time and support, for example, if you give them the start of the word. Others with aphasia have difficulty organizing their words into meaningful sentences or describing a sequence of events. Individuals with receptive language difficulties have trouble following directions, reading information, and relating details to previous knowledge. Even when the person appears not to understand, you should explain in simple terms what is happening. Using touch, gestures, eye movements, and squeezing of the hand should be attempted. If possible, add visual support to the message—for example, by pointing, writing, or drawing a picture. This is especially true for people with global aphasia, who have severe difficulty with both expressing language and understanding when others speak. People appreciate nurses who take the time to respond to communication attempts (Aphasia Institute, n.d.-a).

One of the most effective ways to learn how to communicate is to use the methods taught in the program, Supported Conversation for Adults With Aphasia (SCA™) (Aphasia Institute, n.d.-b). In this method, health care providers learn to use simple communication strategies to help people with aphasia communicate effectively.

Some individuals with aphasia can become frustrated when they are not understood. Struggling to speak causes fatigue. Use short, positive sessions to communicate. Otherwise, they may withdraw as a way of regaining energy and composure. Changes in self-image occasioned by physical changes, the uncertain recovery course and outcome of strokes, shifts in family roles, and the ability to understand others and make themselves understood all make the loss of functional communication particularly agonizing. Make the most of any language skills that are preserved.

Some people with speech and language disorders are able to use alternative means of communication, such as pointing, gesturing, or using pictures, as well as speech-generating electronic devices. Augmentative and alternative communication (AAC) methods have been found to help nurses better communicate with people who are unable to speak. AAC options include communication boards, picture cards, and use of picture pain rating scales, and some people are able to use communication aids. There are also several apps available for smartphone or tablet that allow the person to touch a picture on the screen that will produce the word or phrase aloud (The Ontario Association of Speech-Language Pathologists and Audiologists, n.d.). Refer to Box 18.2 for strategies to use with people with speech and language disorders or cognitive processing disorders.

Strategies for Communicating With People With Certain Mental Health Conditions

When working with people with some mental health disorders, you may face a formidable challenge in trying to establish a relationship. Those with altered reality discrimination have both verbal and nonverbal communication disorders (Fig. 18.5). They rarely initiate contact and approach you directly. They generally respond to questions, but their answers are likely to be brief, and they do not elaborate without further probes. Although the person may appear to rebuff any social interaction, it is important

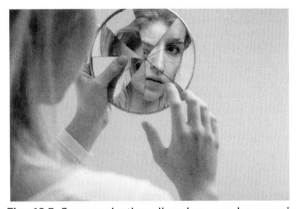

Fig. 18.5 Communication disorders can be associated with some mental health conditions. Source: iStock.com/KatarzynaBialasiewicz/

to keep trying to connect. People with mental health disorders such as schizophrenia are easily overwhelmed by the external environment. It has been demonstrated that people with schizophrenia have the same expressive language difficulties as people with depression. Keeping in mind that their unresponsiveness to words, failure to make eye contact, unchanging facial expression, and monotone voice are parts of the disorder and not a commentary on your communication skills helps you to continue to engage.

If the person is hallucinating or using delusions as a primary form of communication, you should neither challenge their validity directly nor enter into a prolonged discussion of illogical thinking. Often, you can identify the underlying theme they are trying to convey with the delusional statement. For example, when they say, "Voices are telling me to do …," you might reply, "It sounds as though you feel powerless and afraid at this moment." Listening carefully, using an alert posture, nodding to demonstrate active listening, and trying to make sense out of their underlying feelings all model effective communication and help you to understand what they are saying. Simulation Exercise 18.3 may help you to gain some understanding of the communication difficulties experienced by people with schizophrenia.

Strategies for Communicating With People With Treatment-Related Communication Disorders

Communication disorders can stem from sedative medications, mechanical ventilation, isolation in an ICU, or isolation that occurs when older people are in long-term care facilities. A number of studies of communication in intensive care show that people are very dependent on their nurse to institute communication. Specific recommended skills are listed in Box 18.3. A speech pathologist can establish different methods of communication in this environment. Many items such as mobile devices with text-to-speech apps, computers with gaze-controlled programs, pencil and paper or whiteboard and dry-erase marker, and communication boards are useful with people who are temporarily unable to speak because they are on a ventilator. Better communication leads to psychological improvements such as decreased anxiety and depression (Happ et al., 2011; Holden, 2017).

When a person is not fully alert, some nurses may speak in their presence in ways they would not if they thought the person could fully understand what was being said, forgetting that the person can likely still hear. It is not possible to be certain about the person's level of awareness, so it is good practice to never say anything you would not want them to hear. It is also best practice to always call them by name; orient them to person, place, and time; explain all procedures; and use touch. Consider the following case of Mr. Yu.

Case Example: Mr. Yu

Mr. Yu is totally paralyzed and seems unresponsive, immediately after a ruptured blood vessel in his brain. Mrs. Yu tells you he can still blink his eyes. You say, "Mr. Yu, you are in the emergency department of General Hospital. I am your nurse, Kathleen. I need to draw a sample of your blood. Can you feel this? Blink once for yes and twice for no."

For anyone with a communication disorder, convey a caring, compassionate attitude, use alternative communication strategies, and give frequent orienting cues, linking events to routines (e.g., saying, "The X-ray technician will take your chest X-ray right after lunch."). When the person is unable or unwilling to engage in a dialogue, you should continue to initiate communication in a one-way mode.

SIMULATION EXERCISE 18.3 Communicating With a Person With a Communication Disorder Who Has a Major Neurocognitive Disorder

Purpose:
To gain insight into communication disorders associated with people who have a major neurocognitive disorder

Procedure:
Invite a person with a major neurocognitive disorder to class or, if they are unable or it is not appropriate for them to attend class, ask their caregiver(s) to come alone or attend with the person with a major neurocognitive disorder. Prior to coming to class, ask that they plan to identify the strategies that have been helpful to them when communicating with health providers. Also prior to class, ask students to generate questions that will be sent to the person and their caregiver(s).

Reflective Analysis and Discussion:
1. What assumptions did the students make prior to meeting the person and their caregiver(s)?
2. What are the challenges when communicating with the person and their caregiver(s)?
3. How will students change their communication strategies based on the class presentation?

Referrals

Speech-language pathologists can help people with communication disorders. They conduct an assessment and provide recommendations and interventions, including therapy, as appropriate. Part of that intervention involves providing family as well as nurses and other health care providers with strategies to best support the person's communication. As the health team member with the most daily contact with the people you care for, you may be best positioned to know when people with communication disorders are ready for a referral to a speech-language pathologist (SAC, 2021).

ADVOCACY FOR PEOPLE WITH COMMUNICATION DISORDERS

Our nurse role also includes acting as an advocate for people in our care who have communication disorders. Too often, these people are discounted because of their difficulty communicating. Medical treatment decisions may be made without seeking input from them. Appropriate communication aids may be withheld while the person is hospitalized. In the larger community, we need to advocate for community services designed to foster communication, including referrals to speech-language pathologists.

SUMMARY

This chapter discusses the needs of people with communication disorders. Adapting our communication skills and projecting a caring, positive attitude are important in overcoming barriers. Basic issues and applications for communicating with people with speech and language disorders, those who are deaf or hard of hearing, and those who are blind or have low vision, are outlined. Sensory stimulation and compensatory channels of communication are needed for people with sensory deprivation due to hospitalization. People can experience communication isolation and temporary distortion of reality. They need frequent cues that orient them to time and place, as well as sensory stimulation and alternative methods of communication.

All health care providers who come in contact with people with communication disorders need to be aware of strategies to maximize communication. We need to learn how to operate and fit equipment such as hearing aids, because people who are hospitalized often need help with devices. People with mental health disorders have intact sensory systems, but information processing and language are affected by the disorder. It is important to develop a proactive communication approach with people with learning disabilities and those with mental health disorders. Evidence shows that we must be careful not to associate communication disorders with intellectual dysfunction. Our skill in adapting our communication is important.

ETHICAL DILEMMA
What Would You Do?

Working in a health department clinic, the nurse—through a Vietnamese-speaking translator—interviews a 46-year-old married woman about the missing results of her recent breast biopsy for suspected cancer. Because the translator is of the same culture as the person and holds the same cultural belief that suicide is shameful, he chooses to withhold from the nurse information he obtained about a recent suicide attempt. If this information remains hidden from the nurse and doctor, could this adversely affect the person? What ethical principle is being violated?

QUESTIONS FOR REVIEW AND DISCUSSION

As part of our person-centred care expected competencies, evaluate answers for the following situations (https://www.casn.ca).

1. You notice that the people you are caring for on the medical wing at Shangri-La Long-Term-Care Facility are rarely out of their rooms and seem withdrawn. Determine what person-centred interventions might be used to ameliorate stimulation-related communication disorders.
2. Evaluate opportunities for advocacy. Describe one way in which you can advocate for a disorder that is affecting someone's ability to communicate.
3. Create a scenario of your first meeting with a person who is confused as you begin the 3 to 11 p.m. shift in the ICU at General Medical Centres. (Hint: check Box 18.3.)

REFERENCES

Alzheimer Society. (2021). *Dementia numbers in Canada.* https://alzheimer.ca/en/about-dementia/what-dementia/dementia-numbers-canada.

American Psychological Association. (2019). *Disability.* APA Style. https://apastyle.apa.org/style-grammar-guidelines/bias-free-language/disability.

Aphasia Institute. (n.d.-a). *What is aphasia?* Aphasia Institute. aphasia.ca.

Aphasia Institute. (n.d.-b). Communication tools: Communicative access & supported conversation for adults with aphasia (SCA). Aphasia Institute. https://www.aphasia.ca/communication-tools-communicative-access-sca/.

Aphasia Nova Scotia. (n.d.) *What is aphasia?* https://www.aphasianovascotia.ca/what-is-aphasia-1.

AutismBC, (2021). *Autism Q&A: The importance of inclusive language.* AutismBC. https://www.autismbc.ca/blog/inclusive_language/.

Barnett, S. L., Mathews, K. A., Sutter, E. J. et al. (2017). Collaboration with deaf communities to conduct accessible health surveillance. *American Journal of Preventive Medicine, 52*(353), s250–s254.

Betz, C. (2012). Opportunities to create nurse-directed, evidence-based services and programs for children and youth with special health care needs and developmental disabilities. *Journal of Pediatric Nursing, 27*(6), 1–2.

Booker, S. Q., & Haedtke, C. (2016). Assessing pain in nonverbal older adults. *Nursing, 46*(5), 66–69.

Canadian Association of the Deaf. (2015). *Terminology.* http://cad.ca/resources-links/terminology/.

Canadian Institute for Health Information. (2021). *Dementia in Canada: Summary.* https://www.cihi.ca/en/dementia-in-canada/dementia-in-canada-summary.

Canadian Mental Health Association. (2013). *Fast facts about mental health.* Mental Health Commission of Canada. https://cmha.ca/fast-facts-about-mental-illness.

Canadian National Institute for the Blind. (n.d.). Blindness in Canada. https://cnib.ca/en/sight-loss-info/blindness/blindness-canada?region=ab.

Canadian Paediatric Society. (2011). *Position statement: Universal newborn hearing screening.* https://www.cps.ca/en/documents/position/universal-hearing-screening-newborns.

Canadian Patient Safety Institute. (2016). *Report on the integration of the safety competencies framework into health professions education programs in Canada.* Author.

Collier, R. (2012). Person-first language: Noble intent but to what effect? *Canadian Medical Association Journal, 184*(18), 1977–1978. https://www.ncbi.nlm.nih.gov/pmc/articles/PMC3519177/.

Communication Disabilities Access Canada. (2021). *Communication access and social justice.* cdacanada.com.

Council of Canadians with Disabilities. (n.d.) *Human rights.* http://www.ccdonline.ca/en/humanrights/.

Ganguli, M., Blacker, D., Blazer, D. G. et al. (2011). *American Journal of Geriatric Psychiatry, 19*(3), 205–210. https://www.ncbi.nlm.nih.gov/pmc/articles/PMC3076370/.

George, P., Farrell, T. W., & Griswold, M. F. (2012). Hearing loss: Help for the young and old. *The Journal of Family Practice, 61*(5), 268–270.

Government of Canada. (2018). *Rights of people with disabilities.* https://www.canada.ca/en/canadian-heritage/services/rights-people-disabilities.html.

Government of Canada. (2019). *Accessible technology program.* https://www.ic.gc.ca/eic/site/118.nsf/eng/h_00000.html.

Happ, M. B., Garrett, K., Thomas, D. D. et al. (2011). *American Journal of Critical Care, 20*(2), e28–e40. https://www.ncbi.nlm.nih.gov/pmc/articles/PMC3222584/.

Holden, K. (2017). *No longer voiceless in the ICU, 22*(12). https://leader.pubs.asha.org/doi/10.1044/leader.OTP.22122017.40.

Lambregts, S., Smetsers, J., Verhoeven, M. et al. (2018). Cognitive function and participation in children and youth with mild traumatic brain injury two years after injury. *Brain Injury, 32*(2), 230–241. https://doi.org/10.1080/02699052.2017.1406990.

Leung, M., Thompson, B., Black, J. et al. (2018). The effects of preterm birth on visual development. *Clinical and Experimental Optometry, 101*(1), 4–12. https://doi.org/10.1111/cxo.12578.

Liebel, D. V., Powers, B. A., Friedman, B. et al. (2012). Barriers and facilitators to optimize function and prevent disability worsening: A content analysis of a nurse home visit intervention. *Journal of Advanced Nursing, 68*(1), 80–93.

Machiels, M., Metzelthin, S. F., Hamers, J. et al. (2017). Interventions to improve communication between people with dementia and nursing staff during daily nursing care: A systematic review. *International Journal of Nursing Studies, 66*, 37–46.

Mamo, S. K., Nirmalasari, O., Nieman, C. L. et al. (2017). Hearing care intervention for persons with dementia: A pilot study. *American Journal of Geriatric Psychiatry, 25*(1), 91–101.

McGrath, C., Rudman, D. L., Polgar, J. et al. (2016). Negotiating 'positive' aging in the presence of age-related vision loss (ARVL): The shaping and perpetuation of disability. *Journal of Aging Studies, 39*, 1–10.

Moore, D. R. (2018). Editorial: Auditory processing disorder. *Ear and hearing, 39*(4), 617–620. https://doi.org/10.1097/AUD.0000000000000582.

Ontario Association of Speech-Language Pathologists and Audiologists. (n.d.). Augmentative and alternative communication. https://www.osla.on.ca/page/AugmentativeandAlternativeCommunicationAAC.

Public Health Ontario. (2016). *Effectiveness of vision screening programs for children aged one to six years: Systematic review of reviews.* Queen's Printer for Ontario. https://www.publichealthontario.ca/-/media/documents/V/2016/vision-screening-effectiveness.pdf.

Rahu, M. A., Grap, M. J., Ferguson, P. et al. (2015). Validity and sensitivity of 6 pain scales in critically ill intubated adults. *American Journal of Critical Care, 24*(6), 514–524.

Selick, A., Durbin, J., Casson, I. et al. (2018). Barriers and facilitators to improving health care for adults with intellectual and developmental disabilities: What do staff tell us? *Health Promotion and Chronic Disease Prevention in Canada, 38*(10). https://doi.org/10.24095/hpcdp.38.10.01.

Sharpe, B., & Hemsley, B. (2016). Improving nurse-patient communication with patients with communication impairments: Hospital nurses' view on feasibility of using mobile communication technologies. *Applied Nursing Research, 30*, 228–236.

Speech-Language and Audiology Canada. (2014). *Speech and language tip sheet.* https://speechandhearing.ca/wp-content/uploads/2018/03/Speech-and-language-tip-sheet_2014_EN.pdf.

Speech-Language and Audiology Canada. (2018). *Hearing tip sheet.* https://sac-oac.ca/sites/default/files/resources/Hearing%20 tip%20sheet_EN.pdf.

Speech-Language and Audiology Canada. (2021). *What do speech-language pathologists do?* https://www.sac-oac.ca/ public/what-do-speech-language-pathologists-do.

Statistics Canada. (2019). *Unperceived hearing loss among Canadians aged 40 to 79.* https://www150.statcan.gc.ca/n1/ pub/82-003-x/2019008/article/00002-eng.htm.

United Nations. (1948). *Universal declaration of human rights. United Nations.* Mental health disorder.

World Health Organization. (2001). *International classification of functioning, disability, and health.* World Health Organization: Author.

World Health Organization. (2017). *Fact sheets (disability, hearing, vision, mental illness).* www.who/int/mediacentre/ factsheets/; https://www.who.int/news-room/fact-sheets/ detail/disability-and-health; https://www.who.int/news-room/fact-sheets/detail/deafness-and-hearing-loss; https:// www.who.int/news-room/fact-sheets/detail/mental-disorders; https://www.who.int/news-room/fact-sheets/detail/ blindness-and-visual-impairment.

Yuksel, C., & Unver, V. (2016). Use of simulated patient method to teach communication with deaf patients in the emergency department. *Clinical Simulation Nursing, 12,* 281–289.

WEBSITE/RESOURCES LIST

https://alzheimer.ca/cornwall/en/take-action/change-minds/ alzheimers-awareness-month/new-way-looking-impact-dementia-canada).

https://www.canada.ca/en/canadian-heritage/services/rights-people-disabilities.html.

https://canasstech.com/pages/resources.

https://www.casn.ca.

https://cmha.ca/fast-facts-about-mental-illness.

https://cnib.ca/en/sight-loss-info/blindness/blindness-canada? region=ab.

https://cnib.ca/en/documents/position/universal-hearing-screening-newborns.

https://www.doi.org/10.25318/82-003-x201900800002-eng.

https://www.ic.gc.ca/eic/site/118.nsf/eng/h_00000.html.

https://nildcanada.org/.

https://www.patientsafetyinstitute.ca.

https://www.sac-oac.ca/.

https://speechandhearing.ca/brochures-and-backgrounders/.

https://www150.statcan.gc.ca/n1/pub/82-003-x/2019008/ article/00002-eng.htm.

https://www.uspreventiveservicestaskforce.org/uspstf/.

19

Communicating With Children

Olive Yonge

Originating US chapter by *Kathleen Underman Boggs*

OBJECTIVES

At the end of the chapter, the reader will be able to:

1. Identify how developmental levels impact the child's ability to communicate within interpersonal relationships with caregivers.
2. Discuss evidence-informed practice applications for communicating with a child in clinical practice.
3. Describe modifications in communication strategies to meet the specialized needs of children.
4. Describe interpersonal techniques needed to interact with concerned parents of children who are ill.
5. Use a pediatric website to access data for evidence-informed pediatric practice.

This chapter is designed to help you recognize and apply communication concepts related to the nurse–child–family relationship in pediatric clinical situations. Quality person-family–centred care has been associated with improved child health outcomes regardless of income or ethnicity (Bleser et al., 2017). In mastering the Canadian Association of Schools of Nursing (CASN) competency of person-centred care, effective tools need be cognitively, attitudinally, and developmentally appropriate (CASN, 2018). For each of these domains, the child's and family's socioeconomic status and cultural background must be considered.

Communicating with children at different age levels requires modifications of the skills learned in previous chapters. By understanding the child's cognitive and functional level, you are able to select the most appropriate communication strategies. Children undergo significant age-related changes in the ability to process cognitive information and in the capacity to interact effectively with the environment. To have an effective therapeutic relationship with a child, you need to understand the feelings and thought processes from the child's perspective and convey honesty, respect, and acceptance of feelings.

Communicating with parents of children who are seriously ill requires a deliberate effort. Parents need explanations they can understand, need to have established trust with the nurse, and need to feel they have some control over what is happening to their child. This chapter identifies strategies to enhance communication with parents as well as children.

BASIC CONCEPTS

Location

Just as there is a nationwide emphasis on outpatient procedures and home care for adults, the same is true for children.

Attitude

Quality of care studies indicate that, in all settings, children may receive less than half of "best evidence" interventions. Could this be due to overreliance on health care providers' own experience or lack of time to access the latest data and protocols? Major changes in society are mirrored in changing health care for children. Involving children in their own health care decision making is a part of "person-centred care" (Ontario Hospital Association, 2011). Making the child a (limited) partner might lead to better health outcomes than treating the child as a target for our delivery of care.

Cognitive Development

Childhood is very different from adulthood. A child has fewer life experiences from which to draw and is still in the process of developing skills needed for reasoning and communicating. Every child's concept of health and illness must be considered within a developmental framework. Erikson's (1963) concepts of ego development and Piaget's (1972) description of the progressive development of the child's cognitive thought processes together form the theoretical basis for the child-centred nursing interventions described in this chapter. Both theorists say that the child's thought processes, ways of perceiving the world, judgements, and emotional responses to life situations are different from those of the adult. Cognitive and psychosocial developments unfold according to an ordered hierarchical scheme that increases in depth and complexity as the child matures.

Developmentally Appropriate Care

Piaget's descriptions of the stages of cognitive development provide a valuable contribution toward understanding a child's perceptions and communication abilities. Cognitive development and early language development are integrally related. Although current developmental theorists expand on Piaget's theoretical model by recognizing the effects of the parent–child relationship and a stimulating environment on developing communication abilities, his work forms the foundation for the understanding of childhood cognitive development. Piaget observed cognitive development occurring in sequential stages (Table 19.1). The ages are only approximated because Piaget himself was not specific.

Wide individual differences exist in the intellectual functioning of same-age children. Variations also occur across situations, so that the child under stress or in a different environment may process information at a lower level than one under normal conditions. Because two children of the same chronological age may have quite different skills as information processors, we need to assess level of functioning. Language alternatives familiar to one child because of certain life experiences may not be useful in providing health care and teaching with another. Integrating cognitive and psychosocial developmental approaches into communication with children at different ages enhances effectiveness.

Speech and Language Development

Children progress through stages of communication abilities. When an infant uses gestures or cries to get attention to meet a need, this is termed *intentional communication*. This stage continues through age 7 months or so and includes babbling. By 16 months, in the next stage of

TABLE 19.1 Stages of Cognitive Development

Age	Piaget's Stage	Characteristics	Language Development
Birth to 2 years	**Sensorimotor**	Infant learns by manipulating objects. At birth, reflexive communication, then moves through six stages to reach symbolic thinking.	**Presymbolic** Communication largely nonverbal. Vocabulary of more than 4 words by 12 months, increases to >200 words and combines two words around age 2 years.
2–6 years	**Preoperational**	Beginning use of symbolic thinking. Imaginative play. Masters reversibility.	**Symbolic** Actual use of structured grammar and language to communicate. Uses pronouns. Average vocabulary >10,000 words by age 6 years.
7–11 years	**Concrete operational**	Logical thinking. Masters use of numbers and other concrete ideas such as classification and conservation.	Mastery of passive tense by age 7 years and complex grammatical skills by age 10 years.
12+ years	**Formal operational**	Abstract thinking. Futuristic; takes a broader, more theoretical perspective.	Near adultlike skills.

Adapted from Piaget, J. (1972). *The child's conception of the world*. Littlefield, Adams.

symbolic communication, the child uses single words, perhaps combined with gestures, in interactions to get what is wanted. With further development the child enters the *linguistic communication* phase, using two words, then increasing until approximately age 5, when full sentences are used (Brown & Elder, 2015).

INTERPERSONAL

Gender Differences in Communication

Some school-age children are more satisfied if their health care provider is the same sex (Hockenberry & Wilson, 2011; LeBlanc & Bryanton, 2019). Communication by female providers has been viewed as more social and more encouraging. Use of good age-appropriate communication strategies probably outweighs gender as a factor in successful communication with a child, but gender cannot be excluded as a factor affecting communication.

Understanding the Needs of Children Who Are Ill

Difficulties arise in adult–child communication, in part because of the child's limited experience in interpreting subtle nuances of facial expression, inflection, and word meanings. When illness and physical or developmental disabilities occur during formative years, situational stressors are added that affect the way children perceive themselves and the environment. Illness may lead to significant alterations in role relationships with family and peers. You need to assess not only the physical care needs of the child but also the impact of the illness on the child's self-esteem and on relationships with family and friends. Responses to hospitalization vary with the individual child, according to age. Negative responses may include separation anxiety, night terrors, feeding disturbances, or regression to earlier developmental stage behaviour. Things that affect a child's response may include the chronicity of illness, its impact on lifestyle, the child's cognitive understanding of the disease process, and the family's ability to cope with care demands.

Children With Special Health Care Needs

Some children have chronic physical, developmental, behavioural, or emotional conditions that require health services. Years ago, many of these children may not have survived, but today, many are saved by current technology, leaving some with chronic problems. In 2014, approximately 20% of youth aged 12–19 reported having a disability that limited their daily activities. In 2011–2012, 15.3% of children and youth aged 1–19 were living with asthma, while 0.3% were living with diabetes (Clow, 2017). These children and their caregivers typically develop strategies to help them live the best quality of life possible.

Family-Centred Care

In pediatric situations, person-centred care is really family-centred, with attention to family diversity and family processes. Evidence shows relationships between such processes and child health outcomes. If the child needs to be hospitalized, this is a situational crisis for the child and the entire family. Hospitalization is always stressful. Prehospitalization preparation can be done to decrease the child's anxiety. Before elective procedures, many hospitals now offer orientation educational tours to children. There are many good books, available in most public libraries, designed to prepare children for their hospitalization.

Child Coping Strategies

Children who are ill have been shown to successfully develop their own coping strategies (Sposito et al., 2015). For example, they seek cognitive understanding about their disease, employ distractions, and use electronic devices, television, music, and drawing, among other strategies. Hospitalized children have to contend not only with physical changes but with possible separation from family and friends, as well as living in a strange, frightening, and probably painful environment. Usually, having a family member stay with them helps.

Parent Coping Strategies

Parents are reported to have a strong desire to create a sense of normalcy for their child who is ill, even to the point of not revealing or discussing a diagnosis (O'Toole et al., 2016). Parenting a child who is seriously ill has been documented to be very stressful, especially for young parents or those with illness-related perceived financial hardship. Their child's suffering impairs their own coping ability. Nurses are in a position to identify those who are highly stressed. Jones and colleagues (2015), Kodjebacheva and colleagues (2016), Mullen et al. (2015), and others suggest we can help parents to cope by the following:

- Providing emotional support. We need to be accessible and caring and demonstrate continuity of care. Expectations for care and information about treatment need to be clearly communicated, with consistent team members.
- Involving parents in care decisions
- Providing needed information. Written literature needs to be used to supplement our teaching.
- Enabling direct caregiving by the parent. The extent of responsibility the family assumes for basic care of their hospitalized child needs to be negotiated with staff. Some parents prefer to bathe or feed their child themselves.
- Assisting parents to master procedures needed to care for their child, especially those that will be done in the home

- Fostering good, open communication between parents and health team members
- Parents repeatedly express a desire to be present during team rounds. Bedside rounds not only improve communication, they also assist parents in coping.

With children who are chronically ill, the family needs to learn new interactional patterns and coping strategies that take into consideration the meaning of an illness and disability in family life. Caring for a child who is chronically ill demands considerable resources.

APPLICATIONS

Research has contributed to our knowledge of child learning and development. Children are more vulnerable and thus are entitled to extra protection as research subjects. Findings are limited because of overreliance on what parents have told us. Agencies tend to see children as similar, without consideration of differences because of age, gender, race, or culture. To give one example, many of the medicines we use to treat children have been tested only on adults by pharmaceutical companies.

Major sources of stress for parents of children who are critically ill include uncertainty about current condition or prognosis, caring for siblings, lack of control, and lack of knowledge about how to best help their hospitalized child or how to deal with their child's response. Although more nursing research is being conducted on effective communication with both parents and their children who are ill, many of the applications we discuss are based more on experience than on research.

ASSESSMENT

Assessing a child's reaction to illness requires knowing the child's normal patterns of communication. Interactions

---

》 DEVELOPING AN EVIDENCE-INFORMED PRACTICE

Much progress has been made in recognizing pediatric pain, although we continue to undermanage children's pain despite published guidelines (Twycross, 2015). According to Young (2017), a combination of reasons, including the proven falsehood that children do not feel pain or do not have sufficient communication skills to describe pain, while nurses lack adequate methods to assess child pain or fear adverse effects from opioid administration. Findings from a survey of nurses by LaFond and colleagues (2016) confirms these reasons, with the addition of a widespread belief that a nurse must verify child pain with observable physiological markers. Limke, Peabody, and Kullgren (2015) describes an mHealth pilot study using applications (apps) on electronic tablets (iPads) to enable children to self-manage their pain. For example, they use relaxation techniques such as an app titled Breathe2Relax. Several **biofeedback** apps, such as Inner Balance, are also being used on tablets loaned to hospitalized children older than 5 years. Parents and staff are encouraged to coach each child to practise with the apps to manage their pain.

Results
Anecdotal reporting showed unanimous agreement that app use increased parent satisfaction with treatment and taught children new coping skills. Staff said the apps enhanced their ability to teach pain management skills and increased child enthusiasm for practising these skills.

Application to your clinical practice
Although better research is needed to validate effective interventions, this study holds promise. In addition to recognizing that infants and children experience the same or greater pain as do adults with the same disease or undergoing the same procedure, you can provide nonpharmacological interventions that actually help a child manage their pain, such as diaphragmatic breathing. Download a few of the many apps available and try them out. There are many evidence-informed data websites you can use to aid your pediatric practice. The Cumulative Index to Nursing and Allied Health Literature (CINAHL) website has compiled Evidence-Based Care Sheets you can access. For example, they have summarized the best evidence to employ strategies for pediatric pain assessment. They describe research results showing that three-quarters of the children admitted to emergency departments are in pain but that only half of these children receive analgesics. This may be because emergency department nurses are not all using age-appropriate visual pain scales to assess children's pain, even though data show self-reporting is the most reliable tool in children older than age 4 years.

Access CINAHL for application to your practice and then consider the following questions:
1. Which pain assessment scales are available?
2. How much time does it take to use one to assess a child's pain?
3. What reasons do nurses and physicians use to justify not giving pain relief?

are observed between parent and child. The child's behavioural responses to the entire interpersonal environment (including nurse and peers) are assessed. Are the child's interactions age appropriate? Are behaviours organized, or is the child unable to complete activities? Does the child act out an entire play sequence, or is such play fragmented and disorganized? Do the child's interactions with others suggest imagination and a broad repertoire of relating behaviours, or is communication devoid of possibilities? Because children cannot communicate fully with us, we have a special responsibility to assess problems. For example, 25% of the world's adults report having been physically abused as children, and 20% of girls are sexually abused (WHO, n.d.). According to self-reported data from the 2014 General Social Survey on Victimization (GSS), one-third (33%) of Canadians aged 15 and older experienced some form of maltreatment during childhood (Statistics Canada, 2017a).

Once baseline data have been collected, you can plan specific communication strategies to meet the specialized needs of the child (Fig. 19.1). An overview of nursing adaptations needed to communicate effectively with children is summarized in Box 19.1.

Regression as a Form of Childhood Communication

A severe illness can cause a child to show behaviours that are reminiscent of an earlier stage of development. A certain amount of regression is normal. Common behaviours

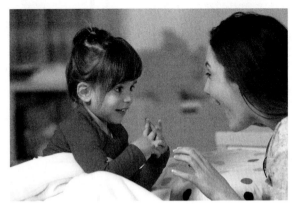

Fig. 19.1 Adapt communication to a child's appropriate developmental level. Copyright © AntonioGuillem/iStock/Thinkstock.

BOX 19.1 Nurse–Child Communication Strategies: Adapting Communication to Meet the Needs of a Child Who Is Ill

- Let the child know you are interested in them; convey respect and authenticity.
- Let the child know how to summon you (e.g., call bell).
- Develop trust through honesty and consistency in meeting the child's needs.
- Use "transitional objects" such as familiar pictures or toys from home.
- Assess:
  Level of understanding
  The child's needs in relation to the immediate situation
  The child's capacity to cope successfully with change
- Observe for nonverbal cues.
- Use *nonverbal* communication:
  Tactile (soothing strokes)
  Kinesthetic (rocking)
  Get down to the child's height; do not tower over them.
  Make eye contact and use reassuring facial expressions.
  Interpret the child's nonverbal cues verbally back to them.
  Instead of conversation, use some indirect, age-appropriate communication techniques (e.g., storytelling, picture drawing, music, and creative writing).

- Use *verbal* communication:
  Use familiar words.
  Use age-appropriate vocabulary.
  Listen without interrupting.
  Use humour and active listening to foster the relationship.
  Use open-ended questions.
  Use "I" statements.
  Help the child to clarify their ideas and feelings ("Tell me more..."; "You got scared when...").
- Respect the child's privacy.
- Accept the child's emotions.
- Help children to understand the difference between thoughts and actions.
- Increase coping skills by providing play opportunities; use creative, unstructured play, medical role play, and pantomime.
- Use alternative, supplementary communication devices for children with specialized needs (e.g., sign language and computer-enhanced communication programs).

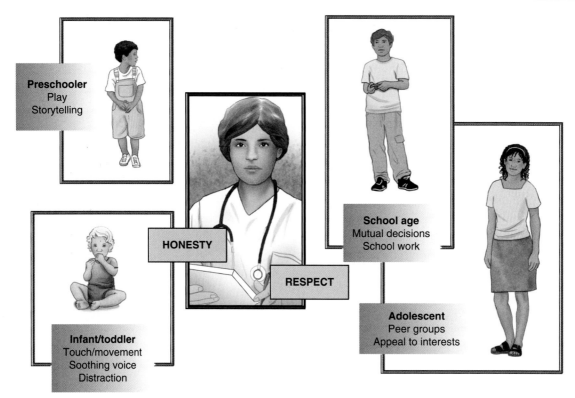

Fig. 19.2 Nursing strategies must be geared toward the developmental level of the child.

in young children include whining, demanding undue attention, withdrawal, or having toileting "accidents." These behaviours might stem from the powerlessness the child feels in attempting to cope with an overwhelming, frightening environment. Reassuring the parent that this is a common response to the stress of illness can be helpful (Fig. 19.2).

Because children have limited life experience to draw from, they exhibit a narrower range of behaviours in coping with threat. The quiet, overly compliant child who does not complain may be more frightened than the child who screams or cries. This should alert you to the child's emotional distress. You need to obtain detailed information regarding the usual behavioural responses of the family and child. Some behaviours that look regressive may be a typical behavioural response for a particular child (e.g., the 2-year-old who wants a bedtime bottle). A complete baseline history offers a good counterpoint for assessing the meaning of current behaviours.

Age-Appropriate Communication

An assessment of vocabulary and understanding is essential in fostering communications. Whenever possible, you should communicate using words that are familiar to the child. Parents are valuable resources in helping to interpret behavioural data. You might assist a child who is having difficulty finding the right words by reframing what he said and repeating it in a slightly different way.

The peers of a child who is ill often have difficulty accepting individual differences created by health deviations. They lack the knowledge and sensitivity to deal with physical changes that they do not understand, as evidenced by "bald" jokes about a child receiving chemotherapy. Children with hidden disorders such as diabetes, some forms of epilepsy, or attention-deficit/hyperactivity disorder seem particularly susceptible to interpersonal distress. For example, it may be difficult for a child with diabetes to regulate their intake of fast foods when all of their friends are able to eat what they want. When peer pressure is at its peak in adolescence, teenagers with newly diagnosed convulsive seizure disorders may find it difficult to tell peers they no longer can ride bicycles or drive cars. Unless the family and nurse provide support, such children have to cope with an indistinct assault to their self-concept alone. A summary of age-appropriate strategies is provided in Box 19.2.

BOX 19.2 Key Points in Communicating With Children According to Age Group

Infants

- Nonverbal communication is a primary mode.
- Infants are biologically "wired" to pay close attention to words. In their first year, infants are able to distinguish all speech sounds.
- Infants are bonded to primary caregivers only. Those older than 8 months may display separation anxiety when separated from parents or when approached by strangers.

Use Kinesthetic Communication

- Use stroking, soft touching, and holding.
- Use motion (e.g., rocking) to reassure the infant. Allow freedom of movement and avoid restraining when possible.
- Learn specifically how the primary caregiver provides care in terms of sleeping, bathing, and feeding, and attempt to mimic these approaches.

Hold Close to Adapt to Limited Vision (20/200 to 20/300 at Birth)

- Encourage the infant's caregivers (parents) to use a lot of intimate space interaction (e.g., 8–18 inches). Mimic the same once trust is established.

Talk with Infants

- Talk with infants in normal conversational tones; soothe them with a crooning voice tone.

Establish Trust

- Have parents give care. Arrange for one or both parents to remain within the child's sight.

Shorten Your Stature

- Sit down on a chair, stool, or carpet to decrease posture superiority, so as to look less imposing.

Handle Separation Anxiety When Primary Caregiver Is Absent

- Establish rapport with the caregiver (parent) and encourage the caregiver to be with the infant, and reassure the infant that staff will be there if the caregiver is away. First, keep at least 2 feet between nurse and infant. Talk to and touch the infant and initially smile often. Provide for kinesthetic approaches; offer self while the infant is protesting (e.g., stay with them, pick them up and rock or walk, talk to them about Mommy and Daddy and how much the infant cares for them).

1- to 3-Year-Olds

- Child begins to talk around 1 year of age; learns nine new words a day after 18 months.
- By age 2, a child begins to use phrases; should be able to respond to "what" and "where" type questions.
- By age 3, a child uses and understands sentences.

Adapt to Limited Vocabulary and Verbal Skills

- Make explanations brief and clear. Use the child's own vocabulary words for basic care activities (e.g., use the child's words for defecate [poop, goodies] and urinate [pee-pee, tinkle]). Learn and use the self-name of the child.
- Rephrase the child's utterances in simple, complete sentences; avoid baby talk. Child should be able to follow simple, two-step directions.

Continue to Use Kinesthetic Communication

- Allow ambulating where possible (e.g., using toddler chairs or walkers). Pull the child in a wagon if the child cannot walk.

Facilitate Child's Struggle With Issues of Autonomy and Control

- Allow the child some control (e.g., "Do you want half a glass or a whole glass of milk?").
- Reassure the child if they display some regressive behaviour (e.g., if the child wets pants, say, "We will get a dry pair of pants and let you find something fun to do.").
- Allow the child to express anger and protest about their care (e.g., "It's okay to cry when you're angry or hurt.").
- Allow the child to sit up or walk as often as possible and as soon as possible after intrusive or hurtful procedures (e.g., "It's all over and now we can do something more fun.").
- Use nondirective modes of conversation, such as reflecting an aspect of appearance or temperament (e.g., "You smile so often.") or playing with a toy and slowly coming closer to and including the child in play.

Recognize Fear of Bodily Injury

- Show hands (free of hurtful items) and say, "There's nothing to hurt you. I came to play (or talk)."

Accept Egocentrism and Possible Regression

- Allow the child to be self-oriented. Use distraction if another child wants the same item or toy rather than expect the child to share. Some children cope with

(Continued)

BOX 19.2   Key Points in Communicating With Children According to Age Group—cont'd.

stress of hospitalization by regressing to an earlier mode of behaviour, such as wanting to suck on a bottle.

Redirect Behaviour to a Verbal Level

- Use a nondirective approach. Sit down and join the parallel play of the child. Reflect messages sent by the toddler (nonverbally) in a verbal and nonverbal manner (e.g., "Yes, that toy does lots of interesting and fun things.").

Deal with Separation Anxiety

- Accept protesting when parent(s) leave. Hug or rock the child, and say, "You miss Mommy and Daddy! They miss you, too." Play peek-a-boo games with the child. Make a big deal about saying, "Now I am here."
- Show an interest in one of the child's favourite toys. Say, "I wonder what it does" folksy. If the child responds with actions, reflect them back.

3- to 5-Year-Olds

- Most children this age can make themselves understood to strangers.
- They speak in sentences but are unable to comprehend abstract ideas.
- Unable to recognize their own anxiety, at this age some will somaticize (i.e., complain only of physical concerns, e.g., stomachache).
- They begin to understand cause-and-effect relationships; they should be able to understand, "If you do ..., then we can ..."
- Can follow a series of up to four directions unless anxious about being hurt.

Use Age-Appropriate, Simple Vocabulary

- Use simple vocabulary; avoid lengthy explanations. Focus on the present, not the distant, future; use concrete, meaningful references. For example, say, "Mommy will be back after you eat your lunch" (instead of "at 1 o'clock").

Behave in a Culturally Sensitive Manner

- In some cultures, a child is unable to tolerate direct eye-to-eye contact, so use some eye contact and attending posture. Sit or stoop, and use a slow, soft tone of voice.

Attempt to Decrease Anxiety about Being Hurt

- Use brief, concrete, simple explanations. Delays and long explanations before a painful procedure increase anxiety.
- Be quick to complete the procedure; give explanations about its purpose afterward. For example, say, "Jimmy, I'm going to give you a shot," then quickly administer the injection. Then say, "There. All done. It's okay to cry

when you hurt. I'd complain too. This medicine will make your tummy feel better." Some experts suggest you create a "safe zone" in the child's bed by doing all painful procedures elsewhere, perhaps in a treatment room.

Use Play Therapy

- Explanations and education can be done using imagination (e.g., puppetry, drama with costumes), music, or drawings.
- Allow the child to play with safe equipment used in treatment. Talk about the needed procedure happening to a doll or teddy bear, and state simply how it will occur and be experienced. Use sensory data (e.g., "The teddy bear will hear a buzzing sound.").

Use Distraction and a Sense of Humour

- Tell silly jokes and laugh with the child.

Allow for Child's Continuing Need to Have Control

- Provide for many choices (e.g., "Do you want to get dressed now or after breakfast?").

5- to 10-Year-Olds

- They are developing their ability to comprehend. Can understand sequencing of events if clearly explained: "First this happens ..., then ..."
- They can use written materials to learn.

Facilitate Child to Assume Increased Responsibility for Own Health Care Practices

- Include the child in concrete explanations about their condition, treatment, and protocols.
- Use draw-a-person to identify what basic knowledge the child has, and build on it.
- Use some of the same words the child uses in giving explanations.
- Use sensory information in giving explanations (e.g., "You're going to smell alcohol in the cast room.").
- Reinforce basic health self-care activities in teaching.

Respect Increased Need for Privacy

- Knock on the door before entering; tell the child when and for what reasons you will need to return to their room.

11-Year-Olds and Older

- They have an increased comprehension about possible negative threats to life or body integrity, yet some difficulty in adhering to long-term goals.
- They continue to use mainly concrete rather than abstract thinking.
- They are struggling to establish their identity and be independent.

BOX 19.2 Key Points in Communicating With Children According to Age Group—cont'd.

Verbalize Issues in Age-Appropriate Ways
- Talk about treatment protocols that require giving up immediate gratifications for long-term gain. Explore alternative options (e.g., tell an adolescent with diabetes who must give up after-school fries with friends that they could save two breads and four fats exchanges to have a milkshake). If you use abstract thinking, look for nonverbal cues (e.g., puzzled face) that may indicate lack of understanding; then clarify in more concrete terms. Use humour or street slang, if appropriate.

Remember That Confidentiality May Be an Issue
- Reassure the adolescent about the confidentiality of your discussion, but clearly state the limits of this confidentiality. If, for example, the child should talk of dying by suicide, be clear that this information needs to be shared with parents and staff.

Foster and Allow a Sense of Independence
- Allow participation in decision making, such as about wearing their own clothes. Avoid an authoritarian or judgemental approach.
- Accept behaviours such as regression, but set limits on injurious behaviour.
- Encourage responsibility for keeping their own appointments, bedtime routines, and administration of their own medications such as insulin.

Assess Sexual Awareness and Maturation
- Demonstrate a willingness to listen. Provide value-free, accurate information.

Updated from material originally supplied by Joyce Ruth, MSN, University of North Carolina Charlotte, College of Health Sciences.

COMMUNICATING WITH CHILDREN WHO ARE PHYSICALLY ILL, IN THE HOSPITAL AND AMBULATORY CLINIC

Overestimating a child's understanding of information about illness results in confusion and increased anxiety, anger, or sadness. Beyond physiological care, children of all ages who are ill need support from every member of the health team—support that they normally would receive from parents. The nurse must provide stimulation to talk, listen, and play. Play is their language, especially because children often have major difficulties verbalizing their true feelings about the treatment experience. As nurses, we adapt our communication to meet the child's needs. Many agencies have play therapists who serve as excellent resources for staff.

COMMUNICATION WITH INFANTS FROM BIRTH TO 12 MONTHS

Cues to assessment of the preverbal infant include tone of the cry, facial appearance, and body movements. Because the infant uses the senses to receive information, nonverbal communication (e.g., touch) is an important tool for the pediatric nurse. Tone of voice, rocking motion, use of distraction, and a soothing touch can be used in addition to or in conjunction with verbal explanations. Face-to-face position, bending or moving to the infant's eye level, maintaining eye contact, and making a reassuring facial expression further help in interactions with infants.

Anticipate developmental behaviours such as "stranger anxiety" in infants between 9 and 18 months of age. Rather than reaching to pick them up immediately, you might smile and extend a hand toward the infant or stroke their arm before attempting to hold them. If the infant is able to understand some words, asking their name and pointing out a pleasant physical characteristic conveys the impression that you see the infant as a unique person. To a tiny infant, this treatment can be synonymous with caring.

COMMUNICATION WITH CHILDREN 1 TO 3 YEARS OF AGE (TODDLERS)

Almost all small children receiving invasive treatment feel some threat to their safety and security, one of Maslow's hierarchies of human needs. This need is exaggerated in toddlers and young children, who cannot articulate their needs or understand why they are ill. To help the child's comprehension, use short phrases rather than long sentences and repeat words for emphasis. Because the toddler has a limited vocabulary, you may need to put into words the feelings that the child who is ill is conveying nonverbally.

Evaluate the Agency Environment

Is it safe? Does it allow for some independence and autonomy? Care in the ambulatory setting is facilitated if a parent or caregiver is present. Agency policies should promote parent–child contact (e.g., unlimited visiting hours, rooming in, or use of various forms of media platforms such as Zoom or Skype, or podcasts of a parent's voice). Familiar objects make the environment feel safer. Use transitional objects such as a teddy bear, blanket, or favourite toy to remind the child who is alone or frightened that the security of the parent is still available even when the parent is not physically present. Distraction is a successful strategy with toddlers in ambulatory settings. Use of stuffed animals, windup toys, or "magic" exam lights that blow out "like a birthday candle" can turn fright into delight. You can wear a small toy bear on your stethoscope and ask the child to help listen for a heart sound from the bear, so the child focuses on the toy, making it easier to listen to the child's heart.

COMMUNICATION WITH CHILDREN 3 TO 5 YEARS (PRESCHOOLERS)

Throughout the preoperational period, young children tend to interpret language in a literal way. For example, the child who is told that he will be "put to sleep" during the operation tomorrow may think it means the same as the action recently taken for a pet dog who was too ill to live. Children do not ask for clarification, so messages can be misunderstood quite easily. Preschool children have limited auditory recall and are unable to process auditory information quickly. They have a short attention span. Verbal communication with the preschool child should be clear, succinct, and easy to understand.

Before the age of 7 years, most children cannot make a clear distinction between fantasy and reality. Everything is "real," and anything strange is perceived as potentially harmful. In the hospital, preschool children need frequent concrete reminders to reinforce reality. Assigning the same caregiver reduces insecurity. Visiting the preschooler at the same time each day and posting family pictures are simple strategies to reduce the child's fears of abandonment. You can link information to activities of daily living. For example, saying, "Your mother will come after you take your nap," rather than "at 2 o'clock" is much more understandable to the preschool child.

Children need to be assessed for misconceptions and troubling problems, preferably using free play and fantasy storytelling exercises. Egocentrism can be a normal developmental process that may prevent children from understanding why they cannot have a drink when they are fasting before a scheduled test. Explanations given a long time beforehand may not be remembered. If something is going to hurt, you should be forthright about it, while at the same time reassuring the child. Simple explanations reduce the child's anxiety. No child should ever be left to figure out what is happening without some type of simple explanation. Reinforce the child's communication by praising the willingness to tell you how they feel. Avoid judging

or censuring the child who yells such things as, "I hate you," or "You are mean for hurting me." Not being able to recognize or communicate anxiety, the child may just complain of a physical symptom, like a headache or stomach ache. Box 19.2 can help you to focus on specific communication strategies with the preschooler who is hospitalized.

Play as a Communication Strategy

The preschooler lacks a suitable vocabulary to express complex thoughts and feelings. Small children cannot picture what they have never experienced. Play is an effective means by which a puzzling and sometimes painful real world can be approached (Fig. 19.3). Play allows the child to create a concrete experience of something unknown and potentially frightening. By constructing a situation in play, the child is able to put together the components of the situation in ways that promote recognition and make it a concrete reality. When the child can deal with things that are small or inanimate, they master situations that might otherwise be overwhelming. Cartoons, pictures, or puppets can be used to demonstrate actions and terminology. Dolls with removable cloth organs help children to understand scheduled operations.

Preschoolers tend to think of their illness, their separation from parents, and any painful treatments as punishment. Play can be used to help children express their feelings about an illness and to role-play coping strategies. Allowing the young child to manipulate syringes and give "shots" to a doll or put a bandage or restraint on a teddy bear's arm allows the child to act out feelings. The child masters fear by becoming "the aggressor." Play can be a major channel for communication. Preschool children develop communication themes through their play and work through conflict situations in their own good time; the process cannot be rushed.

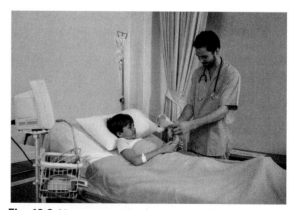

Fig. 19.3 Nurse uses toy bear to explain procedure. iStock.com/Wavebreakmedia

Play materials vary with the age and developmental status of the child. Simple, large toys are used with young children; more intricate playthings are used with older preschoolers. Clay, crayons, and paper become modes of expression for important feelings and thoughts about problems. Play can be your primary tool for assessing preschool children's perceptions about their hospital experience, their anxieties, and their fears. Play can increase their coping ability. Preschoolers love jokes, puns, and riddles—the sillier, the better. Using jokes during the physical assessment, such as "Let me hear your lunch," or "Golly old fashioned. Try Gosh, Could that be a potato in your ear?" helps to form the bonds needed for a successful relationship with the preschool child.

Storytelling as a Communication Strategy

A communication strategy often used with young children is the use of story plots. As early as 1986, Gardner described a mutual storytelling technique. You ask the child to help make up a story. If the child is a little reluctant, you may begin, as described in Simulation Exercise 19.1. At the end of the story, the child is asked to indicate what lesson might be learned from the story. If the child seems a little reluctant to give a moral to the story, you might suggest that all stories have something that can be learned from them. Analyze the themes the child presented, which usually reveal important feelings. Is the story fearful? Are the characters scary or pleasing? The child should be praised for telling the story. The next step in the process is to ask

yourself what would be a healthier resolution than the one the child used. Then suggest an alternative ending. In your version of the story, the characters and other details remain the same initially, but the story contains a more positive solution or suggests alternative answers to problems. The object of mutual storytelling is to offer the child an opportunity to explore different alternatives in a neutral communication process, with a helping person.

COMMUNICATION WITH CHILDREN 6 TO 11 YEARS (SCHOOL AGE)

As children move into concrete operational thinking, they begin to internalize the reasons for illness: illness is caused by germs, or you have cavities because you ate too much candy or did not brush your teeth. In later childhood, most children become better able to work with you verbally. It still is important to prepare responses carefully and to anticipate problems, but the child is capable of expressing feelings and venting frustration more directly through words. Use Simulation Exercise 19.2 to reformulate medical technology into age-appropriate expressions.

Assessment of the child's cognitive level of understanding continues to be essential. Search for concrete examples to which the child can relate rather than giving abstract examples. If children are to learn from a model, they must see the model performing the skill to be learned. School-age children thrive on explanations of how their bodies

---

SIMULATION EXERCISE 19.1   Using a Mutual Storytelling Technique

Purpose:
To give practical experience with the mutual storytelling technique

Procedure:
1. Use the mutual storytelling technique described in the text with a 5- to 8-year-old child in your neighbourhood.
2. Write down the story the child told. Read the story, and suggest alternative endings.
3. Analyze commonalities.

Reflective Analysis:
1. Explain any surprises from the child's story.
2. Describe what you learned about the child when using this technique.
3. Determine any difficulties in engaging the child and explain what techniques you would use next time.
4. After listening to all scenarios, draw conclusions to determine what were the most effective and least effective techniques?

Sample Answer
Nurse: Once upon a time in a land far away, there lived a …
Child: Dragon.
Nurse: A dragon who ate …
Child: Carrots.
Nurse: The dragon ate carrots and slept …
Child: In a cave.
Nurse: One day, he left the cave to go out and find many sweet carrots to eat, but as he walked along he ran into a …
Child: Bike.
Nurse: He was afraid of the bike and so he …
Child: Kicked it and ran away.
Nurse: After he ran away, is there any more to the story?
Child (upset): He got hit with a stick.
Nurse: What is the message to this story? What does it tell us?

SIMULATION EXERCISE 19.2   Age-Appropriate Medical Terminology

Purpose:

To help students think of terminology appropriate to use with children

Procedure:

This activity can be fun if the instructor quickly asks students, going around the room.

Reformulate the following expressions using words a child can understand:

Anaesthesia	Inflammation	NPO
Cardiac catheterization	Injection	Operating room
Disease	Intake and output	Sedation
Dressings	Isolation	Urine specimen
Enema	IV needle	Vital signs
Infection	Nausea	Hydration

Discussion:

Higher-level vocabulary words can be difficult for some children. Try explaining the meaning of the above words.

IV, intravenous; *NPO*, nothing by mouth.

work and enjoy understanding the scientific rationales for their treatment. Ask questions directly to the child, consulting the parent for validation.

Using Audiovisual Aids or Hobbies as a Communication Strategy

Audiovisual aids and reading material geared to the child's level of understanding may supplement verbal explanations and diagrams. Details about what the child will hear, see, smell, and feel are important. For the younger school-age child, expressive art can be a useful method to convey feelings and to open up communication. The older school-age child or adolescent might best convey feelings by blogging or posting on social media or writing a poem or story. Written or digital materials, such as in Cary's case, can assist you in understanding hidden thoughts or emotions.

Case Example: Cary

Ashley, a first-year student nurse, becomes frustrated during the course of her conversation with the child she has been assigned, 11-year-old Cary, who was admitted 5 days ago to the psychiatric unit. Despite a genuine desire to engage him in a therapeutic alliance, he will not talk. Attempts to get to know him on a verbal level seemed to increase rather than decrease his anxiety. The nurse correctly inferred that despite his age, this adolescent needed a more tangible approach. Knowing that he likes cars, Ashley brought in an automotive magazine. Together, they looked at the magazine; the publication soon became their special vehicle for communication, bridging the

gap between inner reality and his ability to express himself verbally in a meaningful way. Feelings about cars gradually generalized to verbal expressions about other situations, and Cary began describing his attitudes about himself. When Ashley left the unit, he asked to keep the magazine and frequently spoke of her with fondness. This simple recognition of his awkwardness in verbal communication and use of another tool to facilitate the relationship had a positive effect.

Mutuality in Decision Making

Children of this age need to be involved in discussions of their illness and in planning for their care. Explanations giving the rationale for care are useful. Involving the child in decision making may decrease fears about the illness, the treatment, or the effect on family life. Videos and written materials may be useful in involving the child in the management phase of care.

COMMUNICATION WITH CHILDREN OLDER THAN 11 YEARS OF AGE (ADOLESCENTS)

An understanding of adolescent developmental principles is essential in working with teens. Adolescence is the time when we clinicians encourage a shift in responsibility for health-related decisions from the parent to the teen. Even teens enjoying good health are forced to deal with new health issues such as acne, menstruation concerns, or sexual activity. The adolescent vacillates between childhood and adulthood and is emotionally vulnerable. The ambivalence of the adolescent period may be normally expressed through withdrawal, rebellion, lost motivation, and rapid mood changes. A teen may look adultlike but, in illness especially, may be unable to communicate easily with care providers. Identity issues become more difficult to resolve when the normal opportunities for physical independence, privacy, and social contacts are compromised by illness or disability. All adolescents have questions about their developing body and sexuality. Teens who are ill have the same longings, but problems may be greater because the natural outlets for their expression with peers are curtailed by the disorder or by hospitalization. Use of peer groups, adolescent lounges (separate from the small children's playroom), and smartphones, as well as provisions for wearing one's own clothes, fixing one's hair, or attending hospital school, may help teenagers to adjust to hospitalization. When the developmental identity crisis becomes too uncomfortable, adolescents may project their fury and frustration onto family or staff. Identifying rage as a normal response to a difficult situation can be reassuring.

Assessment of adolescents should occur in a private setting. Attention to the comfort and space of an adolescent will have a tremendous impact on the quality of the interaction. To the adolescent, the nurse represents an authority figure. The need for compassion, concern, and respect is perhaps greater during adolescence than at any other time in the life span. Often lacking the verbal skills of adults, yet wishing to appear in control, adolescents do well with direct questions. Innocuous questions are used at first, to allow the teenager enough space to check the validity of their reactions to the nurse. In caring for an adolescent in an ambulatory care office or clinic, conduct part of the history interview without the parent present. If the parent will not leave the examination room, find an opportunity to speak privately to the adolescent' Not all have to go to the lab and nor does the nurse walk them there any more. Questions about substance use or sexual activity demand confidentiality.

To assess an adolescent's cognitive level, find out about their ability to make long-term plans. An easy way to do this is the "three wishes question." Ask them to name three things they would expect to have in 5 years. Answers can be analyzed for factors such as concreteness, realism, and goal-directedness.

Some adolescents lack sufficient experience to recognize that life has ups and downs and that things will eventually be better. Suicide is the second leading cause of death in teenagers, and many experts think that the actual rate is greater because many deaths from the number one cause, motor vehicle accidents, may actually be attributed to this cause. Be aware of danger signs such as apathy, persistent depression, or self-destructive behaviour. When faced with a tragedy, adolescents tend to mourn in doses, with wide mood swings. Grieving teens may need periods of privacy but also need the opportunity for relief through distracting activities, music, and games. In communicating with an adolescent who is ill, remember to listen. When adolescents ask direct questions, they are ready to hear the answer. Answer directly and honestly.

Using Hobbies as a Communication Strategy

Adolescents still rely primarily on feedback from adults and from friends to judge their own competency. They may not yet have developed proficiency and comfort in carrying on verbal conversations with adults. They may respond best if the nurse uses several modalities to communicate. Using empathy, conveying acceptance, and using open-ended questions are three useful strategies. Sometimes, more innovative communication strategies are needed.

Dealing With Care Problems

Pain

The major concern is that pain in children is underestimated and inadequately relieved. Lack of adequate pain relief may, in part, be due to fears of oversedating a child but more likely is due to the child's limited capacity to communicate the nature of their discomfort. We need to adapt our pain assessments to be age appropriate. A major transition in pediatric pain management is the shift from the pharmacological intervention model to a biopsychosocial model, which gives us many more intervention strategies to be used instead of or in conjunction with medication.

According to the Canadian Pain Society, one in five Canadian children experiences weekly or more frequent bouts of pain, most often headaches; stomach aches; and muscle, joint or back pain. An estimated 5–8% of children and youth have chronic pain severe enough to interfere with schoolwork, social development, and physical activity. An excellent resource for assessing children who have pain was developed by staff at The Hospital for Sick Children in Toronto. They have assessments for infants to adolescents (SickKids, 2009).

Infants indicate pain with physiological changes (e.g., diaphoresis, pallor, increased heart rate, increased respirations, and decreased oxygen saturation). With children beyond infancy, we use one of the many child-based assessment scales, such as smiley faces or poker chips with toddlers and preschoolers. We also need to instigate protocols for preventing pain associated with treatment. Examples include use of local anesthetics for effective reduction of the pain associated with venipuncture. Effective nonpharmacological interventions for pain include nonnutritive sucking/pacifiers, rocking, physical contact, and swaddling. Use Simulation Exercise 19.3 to develop your own approach to caring for children in pain.

Anxiety

Illness is often an unanticipated event. Uncertainty and even anxiety should be expected when both treatment and outcome are unknown. Young children react to unexpected stimuli, to painful procedures, and even to the presence of strangers with fear. Older children fear separation from parents but also may fear injury, loss of body function, or even a sense of shame for being perceived by friends as different. Many children with chronic health problems experience tension between balancing the restrictions of their treatment regime and their own desires for normal activities (Sparapani et al., 2015). Think of the teen with diabetes who goes to a friend's birthday party and is urged to eat cake! Simulation Exercise 19.4 helps to develop age-appropriate explanations that may reduce anxiety.

Acting-Out Behaviours

Behaviour problems present a special challenge to the nurse. Clear communication of expectations, treatment protocols, and rules is of value. As much as possible, adolescents should be allowed to act on their own behalf in making choices. At the same time, limits need to be set on acting-out behaviour. Limits define the boundaries of acceptable behaviours in a relationship. Initially determined by the parents or the nurse, limits can be developed mutually as an important part of the relationship as the child matures. Determining consequences has a positive value in that it provides the child with a model for handling frustrating situations in a more adult manner.

SIMULATION EXERCISE 19.3   Pediatric Nursing Procedures

Purpose:
To give practice in preparing for painful procedures

Procedure:
Timmy, age 4, is going to have a bone marrow aspiration. (The insertion of a large needle into the hip is a painful procedure.) Answer the following questions:
1. Create a dialogue between nurse and child that will help to prepare the child for a painful procedure.

2. If this is a frequently repeated procedure, how can you make the child feel safe before and after the procedure?
3. How far in advance should you prepare the child?

Reflective Analysis and Discussion:
In a group, critically examine the responses of others. Try to reach consensus on the best practices for pain intervention.

SIMULATION EXERCISE 19.4   Preparing Children for Treatment Procedures

Purpose:
To help students apply developmental concepts to age-appropriate nursing interventions

Procedure:
Students divide into four small groups and role-play interventions in the following situation. As a large group, each small group spokesperson writes the intervention on the board under the label for the age group.

Situation:
Jamie is scheduled to go to the surgical suite later today to have a central infusion catheter inserted for hyperalimentation. This is Jamie's first procedure on the first day of this first hospitalization experience.

Reflective Analysis:
The group focuses on comparing and contrasting interventions across the various age spans to determine age-appropriate nursing interventions.

1. How does each intervention differ according to the age of the child? (Describe age-appropriate interventions for preschooler, school-age child, and adolescent.)
2. What concept themes are common across the age spans? (Consider, for example, education components, assessing initial level of knowledge, assessing ability to comprehend information, readiness to receive information, adapting information to cognitive level of the child.)
3. What formats might be best used for each age group? (Role-play with tools such as dolls, pictures, comic books, educational pamphlets, and peer group sessions.)

Once the conflict is resolved and the child has accepted the consequences of their behaviour, they should be given an opportunity to discuss attitudes and feelings that led up to the need for limits, as well as reaction to the limits set. Serious symptoms such as substance abuse require specialist interventions.

Although communication about limits is necessary for the survival of the relationship, it needs to be balanced with time for interaction that is pleasant and positive. Sometimes with children who need limits set on a regular basis, discussion of the restrictions is the only conversation that takes place between nurse and child. When this is noted, nurses might ask themselves what feelings the child might be expressing through their actions. Putting into words the feelings that are being acted out helps children to trust the nurse's competence and concern. Usually it is necessary for the entire staff to share this responsibility. Box 19.3 presents ideas for setting limits.

More Helpful Strategies for Communicating With Children

Adapting communication strategies presented earlier in this book to interactions with children requires some imagination and creativity. Working with children is rewarding, hard work that sometimes must be evaluated indirectly. For example, George was the primary care nurse who had worked very hard with a 13-year-old girl over a 6-month period while the girl was on a bone marrow transplant unit. He felt bad when, at discharge, the girl stated, "I never want to see any of you people again." However, just before leaving, the nurse found her sobbing on her bed. No words were spoken, but the child threw her arms around George and clung to him for comfort. For this nurse, the child's expression of grief was an acknowledgment of the meaning of the relationship. Children, even those who can use words, often communicate through behaviour rather than verbally when under stress.

Active Listening

The process of active listening takes form initially from watching the behaviours of children as they play and interact with their environments. As a child's vocabulary increases and the capacity to engage with others develops, listening begins to approximate the communication process that occurs between adults, with one important difference: Because the perceptual world of the child is concrete, the nurse's communication should be at the child's developmental level.

Authenticity and Veracity

Sometimes adults ignore children's feelings or else deceive them about procedures, illness, or hospitalization in the mistaken belief that they will be overwhelmed by the truth. Just the opposite is true. Children, like adults, can cope with most stressors as long as they are presented in a manner they can understand and given enough time and support from the environment to cope. Teens rate honesty, attention to pain, and respect as the three most important factors in their quality of care. Never allow any individual, even a parent, to threaten a child. For example, a few parents have been heard to say, "You be good or I'll have the nurse give you a shot." It is appropriate to interrupt this parent to prevent this kind of message.

BOX 19.3   Guidelines for Developing a Workable, Limit-Setting Plan

1. Have the child describe their behaviour.
   Key: Evaluate realistically.
2. Encourage the child to assess their behaviour. Is it helpful for others and them?
   Key: Evaluate realistically.
3. Encourage the child to develop an alternative plan for governing behaviour.
   Key: Set reasonable goals.
4. Have the child sign a statement about their plan.
   Key: Commit to goals.
5. Consequences for unacceptable behaviour are logical and fit the situation.
   Key: Consequences are known.
6. At the end of the appropriate time period, have the child assess their performance.
   Key: Evaluate realistically.
7. Consequences are applied in a matter-of-fact manner, without lengthy discussion.
   Key: Consequences immediately follow the transgression.
8. Provide positive reinforcement for those aspects of performance that were successful.*
   Key: Evaluate realistically.
9. Encourage the child to make a positive statement about their performance.
   Key: Teach self-praise.

*If the child's performance does not meet the criteria set in the plan, return to Step 3 and assist the child in modifying the plan so that success is more likely. If, conversely, the child's performance is successful, help them to develop a more ambitious plan (e.g., for a longer period or for a larger set of behaviours).

Conveying Respect

It is easy for adults to impose their own wishes on a child. Respecting a child's right to feel and to express feelings appropriately is important. Providing truthful answers is a hallmark of respect. When interacting with an older child, using the concept of mutuality promotes respect and should foster more positive and lasting health care outcomes. Confidentiality needs to be maintained unless the nurse judges that revealing information is necessary to prevent harm to the child or adolescent. In such cases, the child needs to be advised of the disclosure.

Providing Anticipatory Guidance to the Child

The nursing profession advocates education for children. The Canadian Paediatric Society (2018) published suggestions for giving caretakers health promotion information at appropriate ages. There is an increased focus on the role a child can assume in being responsible for their own health care. It is never too early to begin. For example, written handouts for incorporating violence prevention can be incorporated into well-child visits.

FORMING HEALTH CARE PARTNERSHIPS WITH PARENTS

Having a child who is ill is stressful for parents. Evidence shows that loss of the ability to act as the child's parent, to alleviate their child's pain, and to offer comfort is more stressful than factors connected with the illness, including coping with uncertainty over the outcome. Studies point to a lack of needed information and support from professionals as being a top stressor. It is essential that we work in partnership with families, especially if we assess risk factors that endanger the child. Most parents want to participate in their child's care during acute hospitalizations but need information, advice, and clarification as to their role (i.e., what is okay to do). They need to feel valued but not pressured into doing tasks they are uncomfortable with or do not want to do. Parents often have questions about discussing their child's illness or disability with others. Telling siblings and friends the truth is important. For one thing, it provides a role model for the siblings to follow in answering the curious questions of their friends. More frustrating to nurses are parents who are critical of the nurse's interventions, displacing the anger they feel about their own powerlessness onto the nurse (Box 19.4). The nurse may be tempted to become defensive or sarcastic or simply to dismiss the comments of the parent as irrational. However, a more helpful response would be to place oneself in the parents' shoes and to consider the possible issues. Asking the parents what information they have or might need, simply listening nondefensively, and allowing the parents to vent some of their frustrations may help to get at underlying feelings. Use of listening strategies is helpful. Sometimes a listening response that acknowledges the legitimacy of the parent's feeling is helpful: "It must be difficult for you to see your child in such pain." These simple comments acknowledge the very real anguish parents experience in health care situations that have few palatable options. If possible, parental venting of feeling should occur in a private setting, out of hearing range of the child. It is very upsetting to children to experience splitting in the parent–nurse relationship. Guidelines for communicating with parents are presented in Box 19.5.

Communicating With Parents of Children With Special Health Care Needs

Many children have a chronic health condition requiring additional services. Caring for these children requires parental time and alters family communication patterns. Studies show these families have less time for communication. Nurses need to provide care and information about the child's condition and time for discussions about balancing family needs with care for this child and suggest strategies for moving the child toward future independence. Refer parents to community resources. We need to recognize that as the child reaches developmental milestones, this can be a time of increased family stress, requiring additional support from us.

Community

Partnering with the family can be the best method you have to address the complex health care needs of children. Parents are the central figures in care planning, especially for children who are chronically ill. We need to help provide information about which community agencies, networks, and professionals will be mobilized to provide care to their child. For example, nurses who have schools in their catchment areas often act as case managers by communicating about the child's needs among parents, care providers, teachers, and other resource personnel. By law in Canada, children with special needs in the educational system are required to have an individualized education program (IEP). A part of this plan may be the health plan for children who need medical intervention or treatment during school time.

Anticipatory guidance in the community. Because the parents usually assume responsibility for the child's care after they leave the hospital, it is essential to encourage their active involvement from the very beginning of treatment. Parents may also need facts about normal development and milestones to expect, as well as information about prevention of illness.

Community Support Groups

Community groups have organized to assist families. Often, information about the groups' meeting times can

---

BOX 19.4   Representative Nursing Problem: Dealing With a Frightened Parent

During the report, the night nurse relates an incident that occurred between Mrs. Smith, the mother of an 8-year-old admitted for possible acute lymphocytic leukemia, and the night supervisor. Mrs. Smith told the supervisor that her son was receiving poor care from the nurses and that they frequently ignored her and refused to answer her questions. While you are making rounds after the report, Mrs. Smith corners you outside her son's room and begins to tell you about all the things that went wrong during the night. She goes on to say, "If you people think I'm going to stand around and allow my son to be treated this way, you are sadly mistaken."

Problem

Frustration and anger caused by feelings of being without power to effect son's hospitalization and possible leukemic condition.

Nursing Goals

Increase the mother's sense of control and problem-solving capabilities; help the mother to develop adaptive coping behaviours.

Method of Assistance

Guiding; supporting; providing an environment that is appropriate to the child's age

Interventions

1. Actively listen to concerns with as much objectivity as possible; maintain eye contact, use minimal verbal activity, allow opportunities for expression of concerns and fears.
2. Use reflective questioning to determine levels of understanding and the extent of information obtained from health team members.
3. Listen for repetitive words or phrases that might serve to identify problem areas or provide insight into fears and concerns.
4. Reassure parents, when appropriate, that their child's hospitalization is indeed frightening and it is alright to be scared; remember to demonstrate interest, and use listening responses (e.g., "It must be hard not knowing the results of all these tests.") to create an atmosphere of concern.
5. Avoid communication blocks, such as giving false reassurance, dictating what to do, or ignoring concerns; such behaviour effectively cuts off therapeutic communication.
6. Keep parents continually informed regarding their child's progress.
7. Involve family in care; do not overwhelm them or make them feel they must give care; watch for cues about readiness "to do more."
8. Acknowledge the effect this illness may have on the family; involve the health team in identifying ways to reduce fears and provide for continuity in the type of information presented to family members.
9. Assign a primary nurse to give care and act as a resource. Identify support systems in the community that might provide help and support.

From M. Michaels, University of Maryland School of Nursing, Baltimore.

BOX 19.5   Guidelines for Communicating With Parents

- Present complex information in informational chunks.
- Repeat information and allow plenty of time for questions.
- Keep parents continually informed of progress and changes in their child's condition.
- Involve parents in determining goals; anticipate possible reactions and difficulties.
- Discuss problems with parents directly and honestly.
- Explore all alternative options with parents.

- Share knowledge of community support; help parents to role-play responses to others.
- Acknowledge the impact of the illness on finances, on emotions, and especially on the family, including siblings.
- Use other staff for support in personally coping with the emotional drain created by working with children who are very ill and their parents.

---

be obtained from health care providers, from the federal, provincial or territorial, or local organization, or online. For parents who cannot travel to meetings, online support groups are available.

Nurse as Advocate for Children in the Community

Because children cannot communicate their needs to policymakers, we need to broaden our advocacy to fight for better child health at local, provincial and territorial, and federal levels. Children's access to health care is affected by their neighbourhood, the level of their parents' education, and problems with referrals. Poverty is associated with poorer child health status, lack of a regular care provider, lack of dental care, and a myriad of other health problems. Part of our advocacy role is to become actively involved in improving access to care and to focus public attention on pediatric health problems. Canadian youth are encouraged to meet federal guidelines for exercise (1 hour per day of moderate to vigorous physical activity [Childhood Obesity Foundation, 2019; Statistics Canada, 2017b]). Child obesity is causing a huge increase in related health problems such as diabetes. Related nursing advocacy interventions include organizing campaigns to eliminate sale of junk food in schools, reinstituting recess and physical education opportunities, and joining community activist groups advocating restructuring of community neighbourhoods to allow for increased exercise, with sidewalks to school and safe bike paths.

SUMMARY

Communicating with children who are ill requires modification of standard communication skills to suit the children's developmental stage. Children's ability to understand and communicate with you is largely influenced by their cognitive understanding, vocabulary level, and limited life experiences. We need to develop an understanding of feelings and thought processes from the child's perspective, and our adaptation of communication should reflect these understandings. Various strategies for communicating with children of different ages are suggested. A marvelous characteristic of children is how well they respond to caregivers who make an effort to understand their needs and take the time to relate to them. Parents of children who are ill are under considerable stress. We need to form a trusting relationship with them and offer open, full communication.

ETHICAL DILEMMA

What Would You Do?

You are caring for Mika Soon, a 15-year-old adolescent. She has confided to you that she is being treated for chlamydia. Her mother approaches you privately and demands to know if Mika has told you if she is sexually active with her boyfriend. Mika is a minor. Are you obligated to tell her mother the truth?

QUESTIONS FOR REVIEW AND DISCUSSION

1. Using the case in the ethical dilemma, describe any interventions you would use with Mika.
2. Evaluate your pain assessment: How does it differ for an infant and a 5-year-old? Use the text to support your answer.

REFERENCES

Bleser, W. K., Young, S. I., & Miranda, P. Y. (2017). Disparities in patient-family-centered care during US children's health care encounters: A closer examination. *Academic Pediatrics*, *17*(1), 17–26.

Brown, A. B., & Elder, J. H. (2015). Communication in autism spectrum disorder: A guide for pediatric nurses. *Pediatrics Nurse*, *40*(5), 219–225.

Canadian Association of Schools of Nursing. (2018). *Entry-to-practice competencies for nursing care of the childbearing family for baccalaureate programs in nursing.* https://www.casn.ca/2018/01/entry-practice-competencies-nursing-care-childbearing-family-baccalaureate-programs-nursing/.

Canadian Paediatric Society. (2018). Medical decision-making in paediatrics: Infancy to adolescence. https://www.cps.ca/en/documents/position/medical-decision-making-in-paediatrics-infancy-to-adolescence.

Childhood Obesity Foundation. (2019). *Statistics.* https://childhoodobesityfoundation.ca/what-is-childhood-obesity/statistics/.

Clow, B. (2017). *Chronic diseases and population mental health promotion for children and youth* (p. 2). Canada: National Collaborating Centres for Public Health. http://nccph.ca/images/uploads/general/04_Chronic_diseases_MentalHealth_NCCPH_2017_EN.pdf.

Erikson, E. H. (1963). *Childhood and society.* Norton.

Hockenberry, M., & Wilson, D. (2011). *Wong's nursing care of infants and children: Multimedia enhanced version* (9th ed.). Elsevier Mosby.

Jones, L., Taylor, T., Watson, B. et al. (2015). Negotiating care in the special care nursery: Parents' and nurses' perceptions of nurse-parent communication. *Journal of Pediatric Nursing*, *30*, e71–e80.

Kodjebacheva, G. D., Sabot, T., & Xiong, J. (2016). Interventions to improve child-parent-medical provider communication: A systematic review. *Social Science and Medicine*, *166*, 120–127.

LaFond, C. M., Vincent, C., Oosterhouse, K. et al. (2016). Nurses beliefs regarding pain in critically ill children: A mixed-methods study. *Journal of Pediatric Nursing*, *31*(6), 691–700.

LeBlanc, M., & Bryanton, K. (2019). Male patients' gender preferences for hospital nurses. *Journal of Nursing Education and Practice*, *9*(9). https://doi.org/10.5430/jnep.v9n9p115.

Limke, C. M., Peabody, M., & Kullgren, K. (2015). Integration of mobile health applications into pain intervention on an inpatient psychology consultation liaison service. *Pediatric Pain Letter, 17*(2), 21–26.

Mullen, J. E., Reynolds, M. R., & Larson, J. S. (2015). Caring for pediatric patients' families at the child's end of life. *Critical Care Nursing, 35*(6), 46–55.

Ontario Hospital Association. (2011). Leading practices in emergency department patient experience. *Prepared for the Ontario Hospital Association by InfoFinders.* http://www.hqontario.ca/Portals/0/modals/qi/en/processmap_pdfs/resources_links/leading%20practices%20in%20emergency%20department%20patient%20experience%20from%20oha.pdf.

O'Toole, S., Lambert, V., Gallagler, P. et al. (2016). Talking about epilepsy: Challenges parents face when communicating with their children about epilepsy and epilepsy-related issues. *Epilepsy and Behavior, 57*, 9–15.

Piaget. J. (1972). *The child's conception of the world.* Littlefield, Adams & Co.

SickKids (The Hospital for Sick Children). (2009). *Tools for measuring pain.* https://www.aboutkidshealth.ca/Article?contentid=2994&language=English#:~:text=One%20behavioural%20tool%20to%20assess,and%20ability%20to%20be%20consoled.

Sparapani, V., Jacob, E., & Nascimento, L. C. (2015). What is it like to be a child with Type 1 diabetes mellitus? *Pediatric Nursing, 41*(1), 17–22.

Sposito, A. M., Silva-Rodrigues, F. M., Sparapani, V. et al. (2015). Coping strategies used by hospitalized children with cancer undergoing chemotherapy. *Journal of Nursing Scholarship, 47*(2), 143–151.

Statistics Canada. (2017a). *Family violence in Canada: A statistical profile, 2015. Juristat.* 85-002-X. https://www150.statcan.gc.ca/n1/daily-quotidien/170216/dq170216b-eng.htm.

Statistics Canada. (2017b). *Directly measured physical activity of children and youth, 2012 and 2013.* Health Fact Sheets. 82-625-X. https://www150.statcan.gc.ca/n1/pub/82-625-x/2015001/article/14136-eng.htm.

Twycross, A. (2015). Pediatric nurses' post-op pain management in hospital settings. *International Journal of Nursing Studies, 52*, 836–863.

World Health Organization. (n.d.). *Child maltreatment.* www.who.int/mediacentre/factsheets/fs150/en/.

Young. V. B. (2017). Effective management of pain and anxiety for the pediatric patient in the emergency department. *Critical Care Nursing Clinics of North America, 29*, 205–216.

WEBSITE/RESOURCES LIST

https://www.canadianpainsociety.ca/.
https://www.canada.ca/en/public-health.html.
https://www.casn.ca.
https://childhoodobesityfoundation.ca/what-is-childhood-obesity/statistics/.
http://www.hqontario.ca/Portals/0/modals/qi/en/processmap_pdfs/resources_links/leading%20practices%20in%20emergency%20department%20patient%20experience%20from%20oha.pdf.
https://www150.statcan.gc.ca/n1/daily-quotidien/170216/dq170216b-eng.htm.
https://www.cps.ca.
http://nccph.ca/images/uploads/general/04_Chronic_diseases_MentalHealth_NCCPH_2017_EN.pdf.
https://www.canada.ca/en/public-health.html.
https://canadianpainsociety.ca.

20

Communicating With Older People

Olive Yonge
Originating US chapter by *Elizabeth C. Arnold*

OBJECTIVES

At the end of the chapter, the reader will be able to:

1. Discuss concepts of normal aging.
2. Identify theoretical frameworks used in communicating with older people and their families.
3. Describe person-centred assessment strategies for older people.
4. Discuss supportive self-management care strategies with older people.
5. Describe person-centred care and communication strategies with people with cognitive impairment.

Older people are the fastest growing segment of the Canadian population. They represent 15.6 % of the population (Government of Canada, 2014). Once-fatal diseases have been replaced with chronic diseases as the major cause of disability and death, as people live longer and healthier lives (Institute of Medicine [IOM], 2008). These disorders require coordinated, long-term care and attention.

This chapter addresses features of the aging process, identifies selected theory frameworks, and discusses how nurses can effectively communicate with older people to promote their health and well-being. The chapter concludes with discussion of dementia and related communication strategies nurses can use with people who have cognitive impairment.

BASIC CONCEPTS

Aging and Age-Related Changes

Aging represents a universal life process characterized by "numerous changes that take place at different levels of the biological hierarchy" (da Costa et al., 2016, p. 90). Age 65 is commonly identified as the beginning of late adulthood (Narang et al., 2013). In part because people are living longer, the term "older person" is broken down into three age cohorts: young old (65–74 years), old-old (75–84 years), and oldest-old (85 years and older) (Moody & Sasser, 2017). Of those older than 65 years, 85% will have at least one chronic disease and 50% will have more than one. Chronological age is only one measurement of old age. Old age is recognized as a significant social and psychological dimension of our lives (Moody & Sasser, p. 3).

Aging is accompanied by changes in appearance and energy levels, diminishing organ functioning, a weaker immune system, sensory losses, and decreased functional capacity related to mobility. As people age, they experience diminished physiological reserve, which affects physical strength, stamina, and flexibility, to varying degrees. It often takes older people more time to recuperate from an injury or illness, as their immune system may not respond as well. Ultimately, the effects of impaired mobility and functional decline may impact a person's ability to independently negotiate their physical environment. Preventing and reducing the major functional losses associated with aging is an essential wellness goal for older people (Gray-Micelli, 2017).

How the aging process influences one's life reflects each person's genetic makeup, personality, motivation, life experiences, level of support, environmental and cultural factors, and engagement with health promotion activities.

Limitations are to some extent preventable or reversible through careful self-management health strategies. Developing the resilience to prevent and effectively self-manage chronic conditions is key to leading a meaningful life as an older person (Ebrahimi et al., 2013).

Psychologically, changes in role responsibilities, and even the meaning of life, can force a re-evaluation of how older people choose to spend their time. As people age, role responsibilities and expectations change; some are desired and embraced. Becoming a grandparent can be an ongoing experience of joy and satisfaction. There is more free time to renew and enjoy friendships, to travel, and to do meaningful volunteer work, contributing to the lives of others. Other age-related changes are not chosen. Limitations in mobility and function, loss of social support through death or retirement, and significant changes in income can be stressful.

Case Example

Before he retired, Pat was a highly paid lawyer, well respected, and very busy. Now retired, he volunteers at his area public library to help young people learn English. He does this twice a week and derives a great deal of pleasure from his new work. Pat is making a difference in the lives of his "students." In the process, his own life has become enriched.

Successful Aging

In Canada, the term *healthy aging* is most commonly used. Healthy aging describes the process of optimizing opportunities for physical, social, and mental health to enable older people to take an active part in society without discrimination and to enjoy independence and quality of life (Government of Canada, 2010). This definition invites older people to take charge of their participation in a personally relevant aging process. Empowering older people to restructure everyday life routines to accommodate and minimize deficits contributes to living a purposeful life, with optimal functioning. Helping older people to enhance security in the home environment and encouraging regular social contacts and connectivity with others are essential supportive interventions for older people. Staying as active as possible, and as engaged in life with supportive relationships, is key to thriving as an older person. Simulation Exercise 20.1, "What Will It Be Like to Be Old?" provides you with an opportunity to explore your personal ideas about aging and what this time of life might mean for you.

Fundamental aspects of successful, active aging includes the autonomy to make decisions. Also important is the capability of coping with daily life in line with personal preference and the capacity to live independently in the community, with little or no assistance from others (Constanca, Ribeiro, & Teixeira, 2012).

Staying actively engaged with chosen life activities and having regular social interactions with others are important dimensions of successful aging (Ebrahimi et al., 2013). Within the community, more nurses play a critical role in helping people embrace new roles that allow them to make these types of creative life choices (Fig. 20.1).

Aging and Health

In Canada, older adults are "living longer and healthier lives than previous generations" (Government of Canada, 2014).

SIMULATION EXERCISE 20.1   What Will It Be Like to Be Old?

Purpose:

To stimulate personal awareness and feelings about the aging process

Procedure:

Think about and write down the answers to the following questions about your own aging process:

- What do you think will be important to you when you are 65 years of age?
- Prepare a list of the traits, qualities, and attributes you hope you will have when you are this age.
- What do you think will be different for you in terms of physical, emotional, spiritual, and social perceptions and activities?
- How would you like people to treat you when you are an older person?

Discussion:

In groups of three to four students, share your thoughts. Have one person act as a scribe and write down common themes. Students should ask questions about anything they do not understand.

- In what ways did doing this exercise give you some insight into what the issues of aging might be for your current age group?
- In what ways might the issues be different for people in your age group and for those who are currently older people?
- How could you use this exercise to better understand the needs of older people in the hospital, long-term care setting, or home?

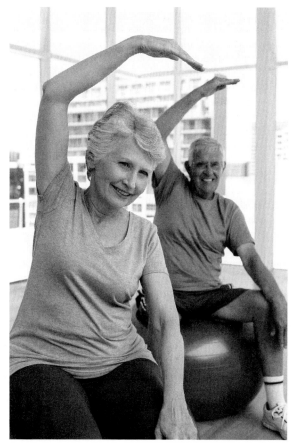

Fig. 20.1 Older people who engage in exercise and other health promotion activities are better able to offset the ills of old age

The life expectancy for women is projected to be 88.8 years and 86.5 years for men. There is also going to be a rapid increase of the number of older adults. By 2030, nearly three quarters of the population will be older adults (Government of Canada, 2014).

Chronic diseases have largely replaced acute infectious conditions as the major source of health care burden (Avolio et al., 2013). Age-related chronic diseases, such as cancer, macular degeneration, glaucoma, cognitive disorders, cardiac and circulatory problems, diabetes, stroke, and degenerative bone loss occur with greater frequency as people live longer. Five functional syndromes associated with aging include falls, urinary incontinence, pressure ulcers, functional decline, and delirium. These are classified as "geriatric syndromes" in the literature (Brown-O'Hara, 2013; Gray-Miceli, 2017).

Barriers to Treatment

Initially described by Dr. Robert Butler in 1969, ageism is still an issue in health care. **Ageism** is defined as discrimination against older people because of their age. In health care, older people can experience discrimination in accessing health care, level of screening, and choice of treatment options. Health care providers are less likely to use extensive diagnostic testing or aggressive treatment with older people, for reasons of age rather than health or function. Kagan (2012) writes, "Discrimination on the basis of chronological age is perhaps the most pervasive unacknowledged prejudice in our society" (p. 60).

Other barriers that older people face include navigating the complexity of an unfamiliar, multifaceted medical system composed of many interacting parts, and working with the current limitations or gaps in services for chronic health care conditions. This obstacle is particularly challenging for people with dementia and their families. After the age of 65, they spend more time in emergency departments and have greater rates of hospitalization (Canadian Institute for Health Information, 2016).

Nurses are in a position to work with people on strategies to prevent falls, which is a major cause of death and disability in older people. It is also helpful to have knowledge of community resources as a basis to recommend community-based strengthening programs such as tai chi, bone builders, and other exercise and general fitness classes for older people.

Health Assessment for Older People

Older people represent a more health conscious and better-informed age group than people in this age group even a decade ago. Many are living into their nineties because of advances in medicine, health screening, technology, and healthy behaviours. They eat better, exercise more, actively engage with life, and take personal responsibility for their health and well-being. Focusing on health promotion and disease prevention enables older people to maintain optimal health and quality of life. They live longer, healthier lives by staying socially connected, increasing their levels of physical activity, eating in a healthy way, taking steps to minimize their risks for falls, and refraining from smoking. There are, however, barriers that block them from adopting these behaviours, such as gender, culture, ability, income, geography, ageism and living conditions (Kelly et al., 2017). Nurses need to be prepared to care for older people in both acute and community-based health care settings (Simulation Exercise 20.2).

SIMULATION EXERCISE 20.2   Quality Health Care for Baby Boomers

Purpose:
To provide an understanding of changes needed to provide quality health care for baby boomers

Procedure:
Break class into groups of four to six students. Allow yourself to go beyond the facts and think about your personal response, and answer the following questions:

- How do you think the influx of baby boomers is affecting health care?
- What types of challenges do you see the health care system facing with the dramatic increase in numbers of older people?
- What are your ideas as future health providers to resolve the health care issues of the care of older people?

SIMULATION EXERCISE 20.3   The Wisdom of Aging

Purpose:
To promote an understanding of the sources of wisdom in older people

Procedure:
- Interview an older person (65 years or older) who, in your opinion, has had a fulfilling life. Ask the person to describe their most satisfying life events, and what they did to accomplish them. Ask the person to identify their most meaningful life experience or accomplishment. Immediately after the interview, write down your impressions, with direct quotes if possible, to support your impressions.
- Reflect on the person's comments and your ideas of what strengths this person had that allowed them

to achieve a sense of well-being and value their accomplishments.

Discussion:
- Were you surprised at any of the older people's responses to the question about most satisfying experiences? Most meaningful experiences?
- On a whiteboard or flip chart, identify the accomplishments that people have identified. Classify them as work-related or people-related.
- What common themes emerged in the overall class responses that speak to the strengths in the life experience of older people?
- How can you apply what you learned from doing this exercise in your future nursing practice?

PSYCHOLOGICAL MODELS AND THEORETICAL FRAMEWORKS

Erikson's Ego Development Model

Erikson's model addresses stage development in later adulthood. With older people, ego integrity becomes the dominant ego strength. **Ego integrity** describes acceptance of "one's one and only life cycle as something that had to be and that by necessity permitted no substitutions" (Erikson, 1980, p. 104). Ego integrity develops through self-reflection and dialogue with others about the meaning of one's life. Nurses can help frame older people's illness stories with recognition of social support and patterns of psychosocial responses, in ways that help them reflect on the personal meaning of life. Nursing strategies encouraging life review and reminiscence groups facilitate the process. Ego despair describes the failure of a person to accept their life as appropriate and meaningful. Left unresolved, despair leads to feelings of emotional desolation and bitterness.

Wisdom is the virtue associated with this stage of ego development. It is a form of "knowing" about the meaning and conduct of life and being willing to share one's wisdom with others (Perry et al., 2015). There are many forms of wisdom; of interest are practical and transcendent wisdom. *Practical wisdom* emphasizes good judgement and the capacity to resolve complex human problems in the real world. *Transcendent wisdom* focuses on existential concerns and self-knowledge, which allows a person to transcend subjectivity, bias, and self-centredness in relation to an issue. Wisdom allows older people to share their understanding of life with those who will follow (Aldwin, Igarashi, & Levenson, 2019). Simulation Exercise 20.3, "The Wisdom of Aging," explores the relationship of life experiences to the development of wisdom.

Theoretical Understandings of Older People

An older person's quality of life correlates with their functional capacity and capacity to meet personal dependency needs (Miller, 2011). A functional consequences framework helps nurses assess people across a continuum of functioning, from high functioning to other older people. This framework emphasizes interventions, which emphasize functional self-management. Activities considered essential to self-regulating functional capacity include self-care, mobility, interaction and relationships with others, cognitive reasoning ability, and engagement with life tasks.

Hierarchy of Needs Theory

Abraham Maslow's (1954) hierarchy of needs theory helps nurses prioritize nursing actions, beginning with basic survival needs. Physiological integrity, followed by safety and security, emerge as the most basic critical issues for older people. These concerns need to be addressed first. For example, Touhy and Jett (2015) note that a person with dementia who is agitated looking for a toilet and not being able to find it will not respond to a nurse's comfort or redirection strategies until the toileting need is met. Love and belonging needs in older people are challenged by increased losses associated with the death of important people in their lives. Esteem needs, especially those associated with meaningful purpose, and independence remain important issues in later life. Maslow believed that self-actualization occurs more often in middle-aged and older people than in younger people (Maslow, 1975).

APPLICATIONS

Self-management is fundamental to the chronic care model (CCM). The concept refers to decisions and behaviours that the person undertakes to independently manage their chronic condition on a day-to-day basis. Successful self-management of chronic disorders requires active partnership by the person and family, in collaboration with health care providers, to achieve desired outcomes. This is accomplished through system-level strategies, use of chronic disease strategies, and using initiatives developed in other countries (Health Council of Canada, 2012).

Guidelines for communication in assessment interviews are found in Box 20.1.

New situations can cause transitory confusion for older people. Heightened anxiety can occur to anyone, but it is even more so for older people with multiple comorbidities.

Older people are aware of stereotypes associated with aging and may be reluctant to expose themselves as inadequate in a new situation. So they wait to see how their comments will be received. Older people may stumble over questions when unusually stressed because of anxiety or needing more processing time. Should this occur, the presence of family members can be helpful in giving the health care team a verbal picture of the person's pre-illness state and normalizing care situations for the person (Happ, 2010).

 DEVELOPING AN EVIDENCE-INFORMED PRACTICE

Purpose

The purpose of the research study was to test the hypothesis that residents who require eating assistance would receive fewer positive mealtime interactions and care practices than those who do not require assistance. Person-centred care (PCC) can improve the mealtime experience for residents in long-term care facilities.

Methods

The study took place in 32 long-term care homes across four Canadian provinces. Mealtime practices were observed by one of eight trained assessors, for 637 randomly selected residents, at three meals on nonconsecutive days. Observation ratings were averaged across the three meals. An Edinburgh Feeding Evaluation in Dementia Questionnaire item determined how often assistance was required (never/rarely, sometimes, or often). A summary score from the Relational/Person-Centred Care in Dining checklist was calculated based on the ratio of positive to negative mealtime specific interactions, with higher scores indicating more positive interactions.

Results

Almost one-quarter (23%) of residents required some level of assistance (11% sometimes and 12% often). Frequency of eating assistance was negatively associated with the ratio of positive to negative mealtime interactions [F(2, 632)=34.72, p=< 0.001; never/rarely=2.3, sometimes=1.6, often=1.5].

Conclusions

Residents requiring more physical eating assistance received fewer positive interactions with staff compared to those requiring no assistance.

Application to Clinical Practice

Eating becomes very important to residents, given they have few pleasures remaining in their lives. This is an area that has not been well studied. The findings from this research highlight the importance of caregivers being more relational and positive when feeding residents.

Adapted from Wu, S., Slaughter, S., Morrison, J. et al. (2017). Person-centred care (PCC) practices and eating assistance in Canadian long-term care facilities. *Innovation in Aging, 1*(Suppl 1), 852–853. https://doi.org/10.1093/geroni/igx004.3069.

BOX 20.1   Communication Guidelines for Assessment Interviews

1. Establish rapport.
2. Use open-ended questions first, followed by focused questions.
3. Ask one question at a time.
4. Elicit the person's perspectives first.
5. Elicit family perspectives, if indicated.
6. Invite ideas and feelings about diagnosis and treatment.
7. Acknowledge feelings and emotions.
8. Communicate a willingness to help.
9. Provide information in small segments.
10. Summarize the problem or condition discussed in the interview.
11. Validate with the person, family, or both, for accuracy.
12. Provide contact information for further questions or concerns.

Older people tend to be more responsive when time is taken to establish a supportive environment before conducting a formal assessment. Sensitive issues such as loneliness, abuse and neglect, caregiver burden, fears about death or frailty, memory loss, incontinence, alcohol abuse, and sexual dysfunction will be discussed only within a trustworthy relationship (Adelman et al., 2000). Continuity of care with one primary caregiver, when possible, helps foster the development of a comfortable nurse–person relationship.

Providing structure for history-taking facilitates communication. Begin by explaining what information is needed and why it is important.

Nurses need to get to know the person as a person rather than categorically as an "older person." Moody and Sasser (2017) maintain that old age "is shaped by a lifetime of experience" (p. 2).

Box 20.1 provides guidelines for communication strategies related to person-centred assessment interviews.

Assessment of older people begins with their story of what brought them to the hospital or health care centre. It is important to understand each person within the context of their biographical narrative (Cenci, 2016). Letting someone share a health history in their own words, with few interruptions, provides information you might otherwise not get.

Asking people to share something about themselves and their life history helps establish rapport and increases the person's comfort level. Listen for the facts, but also pay attention to what the person identifies as their most important concern(s). Look for value-laden psychosocial issues associated with the person's need for medical consultation (e.g., independence, fears about the future, role changes, sensory and cognitive losses, loneliness, and vulnerability) and preferences. These issues can colour an older person's perception of their overall health and well-being.

A person-centred approach to high-quality health care for older people is one that supports a person's dignity and independence. They can be free to engage in self-care without dependence on health care providers (Sundsli

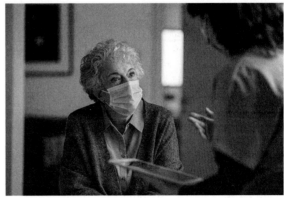

Fig. 20.2 Cognitively intact older people are an important source of information about their health issues. iStock.com/Ridofranz

et al., 2013) (Fig. 20.2). Look for the person's strengths and affirm them. Help people identify their sources of social support, assess their personal and financial resources, and describe their coping strategies. Help family caregivers find community support. Simulation Exercise 20.4, "The Story of Aging," provides a glimpse into the personal life stories of older people.

Accommodating for Sensory Loss

Sensory changes occur with normal aging. Both hearing and vision changes can have a direct and significant impact on communication. Compensatory enhancements are essential to ensuring the person's safety and ability to stay connected with others (Bonder & Dal Bello-Haas, 2018). Because vision and hearing decline are accepted as normal facts of aging, their significance is not always addressed as vigorously as it should be. Sensory impairment can cause major confusion about the meaning of important health messages. Furthermore, people with both sensory impairments and dementia will have greater difficulty communicating (Alzheimer's Society United Kingdom, 2021).

SIMULATION EXERCISE 20.4 **The Story of Aging**

Purpose:
To promote an understanding of older people

Procedure:
1. Interview an older person in your family (minimum age, 65 years). If there are no older people in your family, interview a family friend whose lifestyle is similar to that of your family.
2. Ask this person to describe what growing up was like, what is different today from the way it was when they were your age, what are the important values they held, and if there have been any changes in them over the years. Ask this person what advice they would give

you about how to achieve satisfaction in life. If this person could change one thing about our society today, what would it be?

Discussion:
1. Were you surprised at any of the answers the older people gave?
2. What are some common themes you and your classmates found that related to values and the type of advice older people gave each of you?
3. What implications do the findings from this exercise have for your future nursing practice?

Hearing Loss

Hearing loss affects 10% of all Canadians, 25% of whom are over the age of 45, and 50% of whom are over the age of 65 (Hear-it.org, n.d.). Aside from aging, the causes of hearing loss include drug use, hereditary or genetic factors, smoking, head trauma, malformation of the inner ear, and high noise levels (Connect Hearing, 2021; Statistics Canada, 2016).

There is perhaps nothing more socially isolating than not being able to hear and respond in social situations. Older people with unaided hearing loss have special difficulty in distinguishing sounds from background noises, understanding people talking with accents, and following fast-paced speech. Hearing problems diminish an older person's ability to interact with others, attend concerts and other social functions, and understand medical directions.

Communication difficulties related to hearing are frustrating for both speaker and listener. Difficulties can occur because of environmental factors such as background noise, half-hearing or misinterpreting conversations, or incorrectly manipulating an ear piece (Pryce & Gooberman, 2012). These problems can be overcome with the use of hearing aids and other devices. There are hearing aid programs for people with limited income that can help with financial costs (Canadian Academy of Audiology, n.d.).

Adaptive communication strategies for hearing loss.
- There are proactive strategies redundant to minimize the effects of hearing loss in conversation. By positioning yourself at the same level as the person, the person is more likely to hear what you are saying. Speak distinctly and a little slowly. Enunciate your words without exaggerating them. Repeat what you said if the person looks confused or gives an unusual response. Remember that communication is a two-way street and the most important element is mutual understanding of the conversation.

Other strategies include the following:
- Address the person by name before beginning to speak, to focus attention.
- Maintain eye contact with the person.
- If the person has a "better" ear, sit or stand on that side.
- If your voice is high-pitched, try to speak at a slightly lower pitch.
- Make sure the person can see your facial expression and read your lips to enhance comprehension. Keep the person's view of your mouth unobstructed.
- Help people adjust hearing aids; some may not be able to insert aids correctly to amplify hearing. Make sure hearing aids are turned on. If difficulties persist, check the batteries. people with hearing aids should always have extra batteries readily accessible.
- Keep background noise to a minimum (e.g., radio or television, competing conversations, high-activity locations, children running around, and sudden noises).
- Sometimes you can tell from a vague facial expression or inappropriate response that your message was misheard. Check in with the person frequently. Solicit feedback to monitor how much and what the person has heard.

Age-Related Vision Loss

Vision normally declines as a person ages (Owsley, 2011). Colours become dimmer and images less clear. Brighter lighting and larger print can help. More serious age-related vision problems, such as cataracts, glaucoma, and age-related macular degeneration, can cause blindness in older people, if left untreated. Loss of visual acuity in older people is gradual but progressive, associated with age-related changes in the support structures of the eye and the visual pathway (Mauk, 2010).

Guidelines for effective communication in assessment interviews are found in Box 20.1.

Poor vision has implications for effective communication, safety, and functional ability. Older people with progressive vision loss may miss seeing you shaking your head or nodding, as these are subtle movements. They also may not see slight changes in emotional facial expressions, which can change the meaning of the communication.

Impaired vision can affect a person's ability to perform everyday activities (e.g., dressing, preparing meals, taking medication, driving, handling finances, seeing phone numbers). Poor vision disturbs functional ability to engage in hobbies or leisure activities requiring vision (e.g., reading, doing handiwork, driving, watching television).

Reduced visual acuity, loss of contrast sensitivity, and loss of depth perception create major safety issues related to falls. Vision plays a significant role in postural stability because it provides the nervous system with information regarding the individual's position and movement in relation to the environment (Saftari & Kwon, 2018). Mobility slows as a person ages, and this, combined with decreased vision, can lead to increased risk for falling. Anyone with "balance" issues should avoid ice and uneven terrain.

Adaptive communication strategies for vision loss. Common adaptive devices that older people use for vision are prescription glasses and handheld magnifiers. Nurses can support the independence of people who are blind or have low vision with the following strategies:

- If the person wears glasses, make sure they are clean and in place. (Glasses can be cleaned with a soft cloth and water.)
- Check that the person's vision is assessed on a regular basis and the prescription is updated as the person's vision decreases. Regularly scheduled eye exams are vital. "Mature" eyes undergo age-related structural changes that affect vision.
- Assist older people on steps (particularly on the descent), on curbs, and on uneven terrain.
- Remove all throw rugs.
- Caution older people about slippery or wet floors.
- Verbally note changes in the physical environment that could cause mobility problems *before* people meet them.
- Face the person directly when speaking. It may help them to see your form even when features are indistinct.
- Verbally explain all written information, allowing time for the person to ask questions.
- Provide bright lighting with no glare.
- When using written materials, consider font size (at least14 point) for readability. Use upper and lowercase letters rather than all capitals. Use solid paper, with sharp contrasting writing, and a lot of white space.
- Encourage older people to use audiobooks or electronic readers that can enlarge print. They can use a screen reader on a computer screen.

Older people may require more time to complete verbal tasks or to process unfamiliar information. It also is not uncommon for older people to have trouble with digital communication if they have not been exposed to technology, though more and more, older people are becoming comfortable with it.

Older people are more cautious than younger people. They may hesitate, become flustered, or may not be able to respond as well if they are under time pressure to perform. Otherwise, there should be no significant difference in the cognitive functioning of an older person if they do not have cognitive impairment.

Assessing for Cognitive Changes

Around the world, 50 million people have dementia, and every year there are 10 million new cases. It is estimated that of people over the age of 60 years, 5 to 8% have dementia (World Health Organization, 2020). Approximately 6 to 8% of the population older than 65 years and more than 30% of those who reach the age of 85 years will experience profound progressive cognitive changes associated with dementia (World Health Organization, 2020). Dementia is characterized by working memory loss, particularly for recent events, significant personality changes, and a progressive deterioration in intellectual functioning.

Appraisal of serious cognitive changes is a critical assessment for older people, because it has such a significant effect on their ability to perform activities of daily living (ADLs) (Moody & Sasser, 2017). Performing a mental status assessment early in the interview helps with an accurate diagnosis. The Mini-Mental State Examination (Folstein et al., 1975) measures several dimensions of cognition (e.g., orientation, memory, abstraction, and language). An abnormal score (<26) suggests dementia and the need for further evaluation of cognition. Guidelines for mental status testing are presented in Box 20.2.

COMMON ASSESSMENT ISSUES WITH OLDER PEOPLE

Assessment of Functional Status

The ability to perform ADLs and instrumental activities of daily livings (IADLs) is an essential competency for older people, especially for those who live alone.

Functional status refers to a broad range of purposeful abilities related to physical health maintenance, role performance, cognitive or intellectual abilities, social activities, and level of emotional functioning. Impaired functional status is a determinant of an older person's ability to live independently. Functional status rather than chronological age should be a stronger indicator of disability-related

BOX 20.2   Guide for Mental Status Assessment of Older People

- Select a standardized test such as the Mini-Mental State Examination.
- Administer the test in a quiet, nondistracting environment, at a time when the person is not anxious, agitated, or tired.
- Make sure the person has glasses and hearing aids, if needed, before testing.
- Ask easier questions first and provide frequent reassurance that the person is doing well with the testing.

- Determine the person's level of formal education. For example, if the person never learned to spell, it will be impossible to spell "world" backward. Saying the days of the week backward is a good alternative.
- Document your findings clearly in the person's record, including the person's response to the testing process, so that future comparisons can be made.

needs in older people, as functional impairment is not associated solely with age. Evaluation of functional abilities helps determine the type and level of care an older person requires. Essential ADLs refer to six areas of essential function: toileting, feeding, dressing, grooming, bathing, and ambulation (Miller, 2011).

Pain in Older People

Pain is a common concern of older people, related to an increased number of chronic and acute medical conditions (Horgas, 2017). Moderate, episodic pain associated with chronic disorders associated with aging occurs more frequently than not and needs to be addressed.

More than 50% of older people report persistent pain (Herr, 2013). Pain limits an older person's functional ability and compromises well-being. Although pain is a component of many chronic conditions associated with aging, it should not be considered a normal consequence of aging. Pain in older people is often underreported because people equate pain with being a natural part of the aging process. Furthermore, they may suffer in silence because of the high cost of pain medication, those with cognitive impairments may not be able to effectively communicate their pain, and there may be a cultural expectation to suffer in silence (Registered Nurses' Association of Ontario, 2013). Once the pain has been identified, reducing it to improve function should be a treatment goal (Herr, 2010). There is no more reason for older people to suffer with chronic pain than there is for younger people.

There is a growing awareness in Canada that substance abuse needs to be prevented, managed, and treated. It is now viewed as an illness rather than a character weakness (Health Canada, 2018). Older people are frequently prescribed opioids to control chronic pain, and benzodiazepines for anxiety and insomnia. Neither the prescriber nor the person considers this a potential addictive risk. Chronic coexisting disorders such as depression or dementia can also limit an older person's ability to report and correctly interpret underlying causes of pain. People with cognitive impairment who are agitated are often given benzodiazepines to calm their acute anxiety. For example, undiagnosed depression may present as neck or shoulder pain severe enough to interfere with sleep or activity. Liberal dispensing of analgesics to older people for pain relief without full assessment of the nature of the pain can lead to undesired outcomes. But an alternate system where people can report when their pain interferes with daily functioning, identifying pain levels on a linear scale, can be more of a challenge for older people (Gloth, 2010).

A comprehensive pain assessment for older people should ask the person to do the following:
- Specify the quality and nature of the pain. For example, is it constant, or is it associated with movement or position? Is it aching, burning, pressure, acute, or stabbing? (Some older people will use the word *discomfort* instead of *pain*.)
- Identify when the pain occurs and under what circumstances.
- Identify specific pain patterns and changes in pain intensity.
- Describe how the pain affects the person's physical, psychological, and social functioning.
- Define the area of the body where the pain occurs, whether it is deep or superficial, localized, or radiating.
- Note possible contributing factors such as changes in the person's caregiver, family, or social situation—for example, the death or absence of an important support person.

Assessment of pain in people with cognitive impairment and in those with difficulty communicating is more difficult. It tends to be expressed in behaviour instead of words. Behavioural observation of symptoms suggestive of pain include grimacing, tightened muscles, groaning, crying, agitation, lethargy, and an unwillingness to move. Older people who are socially isolated or depressed can experience greater pain than those who remain connected with a social support system. There is evidence that pain can be effectively measured in people with difficulty communicating using visual means, including certain pain scales—for example, the Abbey pain scale (Nesbitt et al., 2015).

Ask about recent losses and changes. Loss is a recurring issue for older people. Many will suffer losses of people, activities, and functions of importance to them during this life stage. Unlike symptoms of depression in younger people, somatization, with vague physical complaints, is often a presenting sign of depression (Arnold, 2005). Older people, particularly white males, are at higher risk for suicide. Comments reflecting hopelessness, such as "life doesn't hold much for me" or "sometimes I just wish God would take me," should never be taken lightly.

EMPOWERING OLDER PEOPLE: COMMUNICATION STRATEGIES

Promotion of social connectedness is an important dimension of improved health-related quality of life (HRQoL). While older people can experience negative situational stressors, they also possess a lifetime of strengths.

For older people who are cognitively intact, in the community, general nursing care focuses on discussion of supports related to self-management of chronic illness and promoting healthy lifestyles. Sometimes it is simply a lack of information that prevents older people from pursuing possible options. People you provide care for may not be aware of care services for older people: transportation, meals on wheels, sponsored friendly visitors through faith-based institutions, and other initiatives for aging in place. Others know of support services for older people but do not know how to access the available resources in their community. With encouragement, older people may engage in an exercise program, attend seniors' centre activities, or explore a tai chi program combining exercise and meditation. Programs such as bone builders and fall prevention classes often are free for older people in the community.

Studies indicate that many older people experience higher psychosocial well-being compared with their younger counterparts (da Costa et al., 2016). This sounds counterintuitive, but some older people are more likely to seek and enjoy emotionally meaningful activities in the present moment. They may be less competitive and less concerned with high achievement. Many older people appreciate short, frequent conversations. Like everyone else, the need to be acknowledged is paramount to older people's sense of self-esteem.

The *level* of social support people use depends on personal preference; individual, financial, and social resources; plus what older people have at their disposal and are willing and able to use. Asking questions such as, "Can you tell me who visits you?," "Whom have you visited in the last couple of weeks?," or "If you needed immediate help, whom would you call?" are useful ways to introduce the importance of social support as a part of self-management strategies.

Storytelling is a shared experience, reminding people of a valued social identity that goes beyond descriptions of their health. Each time older people tell their story, they remember how they saw themselves as valued, productive members of society. Sharing the story with their nurse tells them they still are valuable. They know someone cares to listen. Nurses can teach and model this communication strategy for use by nursing assistants in long-term settings (Canadian Patient Safety Institute, 2016).

The conversational world for older people may narrow for many reasons: mobility, social isolation, cognitive decline, death of friends, distance, or transportation. Current events to draw from as a means of starting a conversation are not as available, so even cognitively intact older people repeat stories. In addition, family members need empathetic updates and individualized information about their family member that enables realistic decision making with, and for, the person throughout the care experience (Van Vliet et al., 2015).

Each conversation becomes an opportunity to gain insight into the person, such as what the person values, what aspirations and dreams they have fulfilled or not fulfilled, what contributions they value, and what goals they have yet to attain. Focusing on what a person considers important enhances well-being among older people, particularly people who are homebound.

Life Review and Reminiscence

Life review is a useful intervention with older people; it can occur as an individual sharing. Gentle prompts and relevant questions for clarification are usually sufficient to keep the conversation going. Sharing recollections from youth or early adulthood days with a compassionate listener helps older people review their life and re-establish its meaning. Sometimes, telling the story provides useful reasons for older people to resolve longstanding conflicts with important people in their lives (Marquis, n.d.).

Reminiscence

Reminiscence is an empowerment strategy that reminds older people of personal strengths and meaningful goals they have already achieved. Asking simple, concrete questions about the older person's life, where the person grew up, and what was most important to them is a prompt you can use to initiate conversation or when communication stalls. Notice if the person's face seems more animated at any point in the conversation. If so, then comment on it, with simple acknowledgment—for example, "It seems like this was a time that was important to you." Then you can ask for more details.

A specialized group for older people in long-term settings is the reminiscence group (Tarugu et al., 2019). There

BOX 20.3   Working With Older People in Groups

1. Affirm the dignity, intelligence, and pride of group members.
2. Ask group members to introduce themselves and ask how they would like to be called.
3. Make use of humour, but never at the expense of an individual group member.
4. Keep the communication simple, but at an adult level.
5. Ask relevant questions at important points in a person's story.
6. Call attention to the range of life experiences and personal strengths when they occur.
7. Allow group members to voice their complaints, even when nothing can be done about them, and then refocus on the group task.
8. Avoid probing for the release of strong emotions that neither you nor they can handle effectively in the group sessions.
9. Thank each person for contributing to the group and summarize the group activity for that session.

Adapted from Corey, M., & Corey, G. (2013). *Groups for the elderly* (9th ed.). Thompson/Brooks Cole.

is a difference between life review, which explores life events in depth, and reminiscence groups, which focus on sharing important life experiences as simple stories. They follow a structured format, with broad category themes decided on beforehand. Examples include special times in childhood or adolescence, bringing up their children, work experience, and handling of a crisis. The leader guides the group in telling their stories, asking questions, and points out common themes to stimulate further reflections. In the process of remembering critical incidents, people can reconnect with forgotten moments that held meaning for them, thus giving them a sense of continuity with their current circumstances (Marquis, n.d.). Guidelines for group work with older people are presented in Box 20.3.

Encouraging Social and Spiritual Supports

Staying engaged with life and stimulating the mind is essential to the health and well-being of older people (Reichstadt et al., 2010). Older people have the same need for meaningful activity and personal relationships as younger people (Potempa et al., 2010). Age-related changes in eyesight, hearing, and mobility make it more difficult to easily socialize with others. Because older people can lose self-confidence and begin to disengage socially, they may need encouragement to make the additional effort needed to retain social connections. The amount of socialization they engage in depends to some extent on inclination and personality factors; social isolation compromises the health and well-being of older people and may result in premature death and a decrease in the person's sense of well-being (HelpAge Canada, 2021). In many cases, providing social support needs to be proactive due to mobility issues.

For people who have lost their "personal" support system for age-related reasons, a connection with a personal God or spiritual or faith-based community can become an important source of social and spiritual support (Ha-Redeye et al., 2017).

Existential awareness of a shortened life span promotes thinking about death and the meaning of life. Spiritual interventions relevant to the care of older people include instilling hope, prayer, use of spiritual hymns or readings, and talking about the person's spiritual concerns. Helping people cope with unfinished business is an important nursing intervention (Ha-Redeye et al., 2017). In the following case example, note the interaction between social and spiritual connections.

Case Example

Lois visits a person with dementia every week. The woman is mostly nonverbal, with little natural speech. One day, Lois reads her the 23rd Psalm. The woman spontaneously repeats the psalm from a different version, smiling broadly when finished. She could not respond in the present, but she could in the past about something familiar to her.

Supporting Independence

Independence is something most people take for granted as younger adults; it becomes a significant issue for older people and their caregivers, though, especially if they develop chronic conditions (Navarrete-Villanueva et al., 2021).

Nurses need to be sensitive to the often-unexpressed fears of older people around surrendering their independence. For example, an older person awaiting discharge from the hospital told his nurse that he had a bedside commode and no stairs in his home. When the home care nurse visited, there was no commode, and the person's home had a significant number of stairs. When asked about this, he told the nurse he'd been afraid the hospital staff would have insisted he move to a nursing home if he revealed his real circumstances to them. This is a common fear of older people. How could you respond if you were working with this person? Formal support services in the community, meals on wheels, home health aides, medical alerts, and informal family support can be critical factors in enabling older people to remain independent. Nurses can help older people identify and access these supports.

Safety Supports

There often is a delicate balance between the older person's perceived and actual need for safety in health care. Restrictions and supports needed for safety can and should be negotiated, not simply imposed. The personhood of the person should always trump their "patienthood" (Chochinov, 2013).

Interventions to promote quality of life while protecting safety and independence include the following:

- Respecting choices in food selection
- Providing chair risers, walkers, and canes as needed
- Safety modifications in the home (e.g., handrails on stairs, bathtub or shower grip bars, bath bench, scatter rug removal, night lights). Increased frailty may make independent showering a safer option than a bath.
- Including older people in decision making about health care and giving them the information they need to make responsible choices
- Installing home security, health alarm monitors, giving trusted neighbours or relatives keys and emergency phone numbers
- Providing information about low-cost tai chi and other low-impact exercise programs in the community. Inform people about fall prevention programs for people with balance difficulties.

Medication Supports

In general, medications have a stronger effect on the metabolism of older people than younger people, and they take longer to eliminate from the body. Polypharmacy (the use of five or more medications) is a fact of life for many older people, related to multiple chronic conditions. Older people are at risk for medication side effects and drug interactions because of the variety of medications they take, age-related changes in metabolism, metabolic changes, comorbidities, and evolving standards and guidelines (Canadian Medical Protective Association, 2018; Kim, Koncilja, & Nielsen, 2018). Successful self-management of medications requires consistent coordinated and active participation of the person, family, and other health providers to achieve positive health outcomes.

Unmonitored polypharmacy is a major contributor to falls and hip fractures, and medication mismanagement is often a formal reason for hospital or nursing home admissions. Nurses perform important coordinating functions regarding helping older people self-manage their medications and treatments. With limited knowledge of a person's full profile, including over-the-counter medications, dangerous interactions can occur. Important questions you can ask include the following:

- What do you take each medication for?
- How and when do you take it?
- What kind of medical problems are you having? (Gould & Mitty, 2010, p. 294).

Encourage older people and their family members to keep a written list of all medications, including over-the-counter medications and natural remedies, to be shared with each provider. Do not think of herbal supplements only as add-ons; they too can spike interactions if not understood. Use open-ended question, such as "Tell me how you take your medications," rather than asking, "Are you taking your medication as prescribed?" (van Uffelen et al., 2011). Box 20.4 covers key areas for medication assessment.

Ask about medications, including over-the-counter and herbal or natural products. Ask the essential safety questions during initial assessment and during each medical contact or health-related home visit. Reasons for poor self-management of medications include complexity of taking multiple medications, difficulty removing safety tops, using incorrect techniques, improper medication storage, level of health literacy, cost of medications factors, and poor eyesight. Using a teach-back strategy to assess this information is helpful.

BOX 20.4 Areas of Assessment for Medication Self-Management

- List of current and previously taken medications and herbal and over-the-counter medications
- Medications taken episodically for insomnia, pain, intestinal upsets, colds, and coughs
- Allergies (include exact symptoms)
- Determine if the person knows what each medication is for, storage, what to do for missed doses, drug interactions, side effects
- Ability to read medication labels or printed instructions
- Motor difficulties with appropriate medication administration
- Expiration dates, brown bag syndrome (having older person bring all medications in a brown bag for clinic visit observation)
- Determination of family responsibility, and availability if medication administration support is needed

Visually checking medications with the person and talking about how the medication is working with the person or primary caretaker (or both) is essential in home care.

Health teaching helps people establish and maintain appropriate self-management of medications. Simplifying the medication regimen and regular checking of expiration dates enhance medication management and lessen the possibility of adverse reactions. The adage "start low, and go slow" (Miller, 2011), plus regular communication with prescribers, is essential. Careful instruction as to the purpose, dosage, anticipated outcomes, and side effects can increase medication compliance. Establish a system with the person or family for medication administration—for example, prefilled medication dispensers or a medication calendar. Use a teach-back strategy to ensure that instructions are understood and the person or family feels comfortable with their knowledge and capacity to implement administration.

Elder Abuse

Box 20.5 identifies fundamental rights of older people. Elder abuse represents a major threat to the safety and well-being of older people; this term refers to the mistreatment of vulnerable older people, usually at the hands of caregivers, including professional personnel.

The most common form of elder abuse is neglect. Active neglect is deliberate. Passive neglect occurs when people, most notably those with dementia, lack properly

---

> ### BOX 20.5   Fundamental Rights of Older People
>
> Older people need the following:
> - Live in safe and appropriate living environments.
> - Establish and maintain meaningful relationships and social networks.
> - Have equal access to health care, legal services, and social services consistent with their needs.
> - Have the right to make decisions about their care and quality of life.
> - Have their rights, autonomy, and assets protected.
> - Have appropriate information to make reasoned decisions.
> - Have their personal, cultural, and spiritual values, beliefs, and preferences respected.
> - Participate in all aspects of their care plan, including care decisions, to the fullest extent possible.
> - Expect confidentiality of all communication and clinical records related to their care.
> - Be involved in advocacy and the formulation of policies that directly impact their health and well-being.

---

supervised care or essential supports related to implementing instrumental or basic ADLs.

Elder abuse is a difficult problem to identify and treat. Many older people are dependent on their caregivers. For those with diminished mental capacity, a person may not even understand what is happening, let alone take constructive actions to stop the abuse or to use any community services available to them (Employment and Social Development Canada, 2009). Pride, embarrassment, and a desire to protect family members can all prevent vulnerable older people from wanting to prosecute a family member for abuse or neglect. If the nurse identifies abuse or neglect, it must be reported to appropriate social and legal protective services.

Advocacy Support

Fundamental rights of older people in health care settings are identified in Box 20.5. Nurses have an important role in explaining treatment to people and their families, helping them frame questions for physicians and hospitalists and arranging for continuity of care with community agencies (see also Chapter 25). Role modelling is an indirect form of advocacy, which nurses provide in institutional settings. Treating older people with respect, not becoming impatient with primitive behaviours, and providing excellent care is noted by family and nonprofessionals. Holding health care providers accountable for maintaining quality care is a nursing responsibility.

HEALTH PROMOTION FOR OLDER PEOPLE

Health-damaging behaviours such as poor nutrition, inactivity, alcohol misuse, and tobacco use contribute heavily to the onset of disability in older people. Budib and colleagues (2020) discovered through their research that older people had improved functionality and independence when provided with an integrated health promotion approach to address their common risk factors and comorbidities. Older people benefit from health promotion activities tailored to their stage of life. It is never too late to practise good nutrition; engage in healthful exercise such as strength training, walking, and yoga; connect with social relationships on a regular basis; and improve safety factors. Most urban communities have groups specifically for older people (Fig. 20.3).

At the same time, healthy older people have special needs. Health requirements change as a person ages; their nutrition, exercise, sleep, and other health needs are different from those of younger people. Health promotion strategies need to be modified to meet the unique requirements of older people (Golinowska et al., 2016). Box 20.6 describes five key focus areas for older people: social connection, physical activity, healthy eating, falls prevention, and tobacco control.

Nurses can engage older people in health promotion activities by appealing to their interests and by incorporating cultural values in the presentation. Examples of relevant activities can include the following:

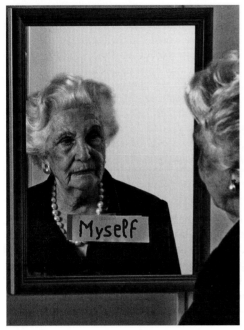

Fig. 20.3 One of the most disabling chronic conditions experienced by older people is Alzheimer's disease. iStock.com/Syldavia/iStock

- Preparing examples of healthy ethnic food (e.g., "soul cooking the healthy way")
- Assigning blocks of time for preventive screening, specifically for older people
- Combining multiple prevention services into one clinical visit

Health Teaching

Moody and Sasser (2017) notes that health teaching for older people is critical if they are to master the tasks of old age and maintain their health. Healthy older people's learning capabilities remain intact, given extra time to think about how they want to handle a situation. The sensitive nurse observes the person before implementing teaching, to be able to match teaching strategies to the individual learning needs of each person. Four aspects of successful aging—fall prevention, adequate nutrition, socialization, and medication management—lend themselves to health teaching formats.

Simulation Exercise 20.5 provides an opportunity to think about health teaching for older people.

It is a common error to assume that all older people lack the capacity to understand instructions, as many are cognitively intact. Health care providers often direct instruction to the older person's younger companion or family member, even when the person has no cognitive impairment. This action invalidates the person and diminishes self-worth. Mauk (2006) identifies simple modifications to reduce age-related barriers to learning when teaching older people. Suggestions include the following:
- Explain why the information is important to the person.
- Use familiar words and examples in providing information.

BOX 20.6 Healthy Aging in Canada

A discussion brief, "Healthy Aging in Canada: A New Vision, a Vital Investment" outlines the vision and focus for promoting healthy aging in Canada. The vision is to build: "A society that:
- Values and supports the contributions of older people
- Celebrates diversity, refutes ageism and reduces inequities
- Provides age-friendly environments and opportunities for healthy choices that enhance independence and quality of life"

These healthy aging strategies focus on five key areas:
1. Social Connectedness: Develop policies, services and programs to remove barriers that restrict or limit social engagement.
2. Physical Activity: Make physical activity more accessible and attractive to older people.
3. Healthy Eating: Develop healthy eating and nutrition policies to address factors that affect older people's food choices, nutritional needs, determinants of nutrition status, and vulnerability to deficiencies.
4. Falls Prevention: Implement effective combinations of interventions to prevent falls, across the country.
5. Tobacco Control: Develop interventions specifically for older people to help people quit smoking and document what works.

Adapted from Healthy Aging and Wellness Working Group. (2006). Healthy aging in Canada: A new vision, a vital investment. A discussion brief prepared for the federal, provincial and territorial committee of officials (seniors). https://www.phac-aspc.gc.ca/seniors-aines/alt-formats/pdf/publications/public/healthy-sante/vision/vision-eng.pdf.

SIMULATION EXERCISE 20.5   Health Promotion Teaching for Older People

Purpose:
To provide a health teaching segment for an older person

Procedure:
1. Develop a step-by-step mini teaching plan related to fall prevention for a cognitively intact older person.
   a. Consider what person-centred information you will need from the person to effectively provide individualized content.
   b. Identify specific content you will need to include in your presentation.
   c. Describe teaching strategies you will use.
   d. What accommodations will you need to make?
   e. How will you evaluate the person's understanding of the material?

2. Implement the teaching plan.
3. Share your experience with other students in groups of three to six students.

Discussion:
1. Were there any similarities or differences in themes or the person's responses to the teaching session?
2. Were you surprised at anything you found that differed in preparing for the teaching session versus what occurred during the session?
3. If you had to provide education to the person on another topic relevant to them, what would you do differently, if anything?
4. What did you learn from doing this exercise that you could use in future practice with older people?

- Draw on the person's experiences and interests when creating an action plan.
- Make teaching sessions short enough to avoid tiring the person and frequent enough for continuous learning support.
- Speak slowly, naturally, and clearly.

Two other suggestions to enhance communication to effect positive behaviour changes are the following (World Health Organization, 2015):

- Manage emotional distress. If managed successfully it will be a stimulus for behaviour change.
- Consider the older person's social support. It may deter or enhance behavioural changes in the person.

COMMUNICATING WITH OLDER PEOPLE WITH COGNITIVE IMPAIRMENT

The term *dementia* refers to a progressive deterioration of cognitive functioning and intellect that interferes with daily living. The term does not refer to a specific disease but to a collection of symptoms that fall under the categories of mild and major neurocognitive disorder, as described by the *Diagnostic and Statistical Manual of Mental Disorders, fifth edition (DSM-5)* (American Psychiatric Association, 2013). When a person has dementia, many people tend to focus on the cognitive and behavioural deficits and overlook the psychosocial, emotional, and spiritual personality components that make up the whole person (MacKinlay, 2012).

Symptoms of cognitive impairment and communication difficulties in older people can appear similar to those in people suffering from depression, delirium, and dementia, so accurate diagnosis is important. Communicating with a person with dementia requires a different set of strategies

from those used for people with depression. Table 20.1 identifies important differences between the three disorders in older people. Secondary clinical depression and delirium can be superimposed on dementia, making a difficult situation even more challenging. Simulation Exercise 20.6 provides an opportunity to distinguish between dementia, delirium, and depression, using a case study.

Supporting Adaptation to Daily Life

Box 20.7 outlines early cognitive changes seen with dementia. Memory loss is a consistent finding. Structure and consistency in the environment are important themes to consider. In the early stages, nurses can help people develop reminder strategies such as making notes to themselves and using coloured labels, alarms, or calendars. Focusing on what the person can do, rather than on their deficits, taps into the functions still available to the person and decreases feelings of hopelessness (Alzheimer Society of Canada, 2016).

Apraxia, defined as the loss of the ability to take purposeful action even when the muscles, senses, and vocabulary are intact, is a common feature of dementia. The person appears to register a command but acts in ways that suggest they have little understanding of what was said. In the following case example, the caregiver observes the person's difficulty. Notice how her response supports his ability to function.

Case Example

The care staff member noticed I.A.'s restlessness as he struggled to figure out which shoes to put on. I.A. began looking around with darting eyes, quickly

TABLE 20.1 Sorting Out the Three D's: Delirium, Dementia, Depression

Disorder	Delirium	Disorders With Dementia	Depression
Onset	Acute, over hours, days	Insidious, over months, years	Relatively rapid, over weeks to months
Acuity	Acute symptoms, medical emergency	Chronic symptoms, progresses slowly	Episodic symptoms, coincides with losses
Course	Short term; resolves with identification of cause, treatment	Gradual, progressive deterioration, memory loss	Self-limiting; recurrent symptoms; often resolves with treatment
Duration	Lasts hours to weeks, resolves with treatment	Progressive and irreversible, ends in death	At least 2 weeks, may last months to years, responds to treatment
Alertness or consciousness	Fluctuates, intervals of lucidity and confusion, worse at night	Clear, stable during day, sundowning syndrome	Clear, thinking may appear slowed; decreased alertness because of lack of motivation
Attention	Trouble focusing, short attention span, fluctuates	Usually unaffected	Minimal deficit, difficulty concentrating
Orientation	Disoriented to time and place, but not to person	Impaired as disease progresses; inability to recognize familiar people or objects, including self	Selective disorientation
Memory	Recent and immediate impaired	Impaired memory for immediate/recent events; unconcerned about memory deficits	Selective impairment, concerned about memory deficits
Thinking	Incoherent, global disorganization	Impoverished, inability to learn, trouble with word finding	Intact, negative themes
Perception	Gross distortions; illusions, visual, tactile hallucinations	Prone to hallucinations as disease progresses	Intact, but coloured by negative themes
Speech	Incoherent, disorganized, loud, belligerent	Impoverished, tangential, repetitive, superficial, confabulations	Quiet, decreased, can be irritable; language skills intact
Sleep/wake cycle	Disturbed; changes hourly	Disturbed; day/night reversal	Disturbed; early morning waking, hypersomnia during day
Contributing factors	Underlying medical cause; toxicity, fever, tumor, infection, drugs	Degenerative disorder associated with age, cardiovascular deficits, substance dependence	Significant or cumulative loss; drug toxicity, diabetes, myocardial infarction

Adapted from Arnold, E. (2005). Sorting out the three D's: Delirium, depression, dementia. *Holistic Nursing Practice, 19*(3), 99–104.

shifting his gaze from here to there. The care staff member said, "I'm sorry. I have put two pairs of shoes here and it's confusing. Please put these on." I.A. looked relieved, put on the shoes, and moved to a table where the care staff member placed a box that had many small articles brought from I.A.'s company. The care staff member said, "Would you help us, president?" I.A. smiled and said, "Okay ... I can see you need help here," as he began to organize the articles into piles. He did not wander on that day (Ito et al., 2007, p. 14).

SIMULATION EXERCISE 20.6   Distinguishing Between Dementia, Delirium, and Depression in Older People

Purpose:

To differentiate between the 3 D's

Mrs. S. is a recently widowed 78-year-old woman, living alone in a seniors' apartment complex in a suburban community. Her son and his wife live nearby and visit weekly. Over the last month, the family has noticed that Mrs. S. "has not been herself." Once a meticulous dresser, she shows no current interest in dressing and grooming. She has had difficulty keeping doctor's appointments and getting medications refilled. When approached by the family regarding her change in behaviour, Mrs. S. says that she "doesn't know—if I could just get a good night's sleep, I would feel better."

Discussion

1. What distinguishing alterations in cognition does Mrs. S. exhibit to suggest depression or dementia?
2. What additional questions would you like to ask to support your observations?
3. What screening tools are appropriate?
4. What approaches would you suggest for communicating with Mrs. S.?
5. Identify ways to improve Mrs. S.'s ability to function safely and independently.
6. What sources of support can you identify to help Mrs. S. and her family cope?

Developed by Spellbring, A. M., PhD, RN, FAAN, February 9, 2010.

BOX 20.7   Signs of Early Cognitive Changes With Dementia

- Difficulty remembering appointments
- Difficulty recalling the names of friends, neighbours, and family members
- Using the wrong word when talking
- Jumbling words: mixing up or missing letters in words when talking
- Not following the conversations of friends or coworkers
- Not understanding an explanation or story
- Difficulty recalling whether a task was just completed the day or week before
- Difficulty keeping up with all the steps to a task
- Difficulty planning and doing an activity such as a board meeting or family reunion
- New difficulty filling out complicated forms such as income tax forms
- Changes in behaviour: restless, quick to get angry, constant hunger (especially for sweets), quiet or withdrawn, and so forth
- Buying items and forgetting they have the same items at home
- Struggling with work or home tasks that used to be routine and easy
- Loss of interest in meeting with friends or doing activities

---

Supporting Communication

Difficulty with purposeful communication is a hallmark of dementia. The person's loss is a gradual process initially, so many people can maintain superficial conversation, with empathetic support. Dementia affects basic receptive (decoding and understanding) and expressive (conveying information) forms of communication. People with dementia can also have aphasia, which means difficulty expressing themselves, finding the right words, understanding the words heard, reading, and writing (Alzheimer Society of Canada, 2016). Dementia influences the person's capacity to think abstractly and solve problems. Although people may speak in fragments, they are still capable of interacting with prompts, especially when given your full attention.

Difficulty with word retrieval can reflect impairment in attention and short-term memory. People may stop mid-sentence and look confused. They may ask for help with a word or continue with phrases that have little to do with the intended conversation (Mace & Rabins, 2017).

Providing *verbal cues* helps older people with short-term memory impairment. Nurses can support people by suggesting a missing word or providing a simple meaning. Check with the person that your interpretation is accurate. Sometimes you can grasp what the word might be from its context.

Case Example

In a conversation with her nurse, Carol Buret could not retrieve the word "Halloween." Instead, she said, "When people dress in costumes." The nurse said, "You mean like Halloween?" The person said yes, and the conversation continued.

You also can ask the person to point to an object or describe something similar if you do not understand what the person is referencing.

Short-term memory allows people to follow a conversation when the topic changes. People with cognitive impairment have difficulty with short-term memory, so topic transitions can be difficult (McCarthy, 2011). Restate ideas using simple words, and sequence and validate the meaning of a person's response. Using words directly applicable to daily routines, such as "before lunch," can anchor the person's recognition of time frames better than saying a specific time such as 11 a.m.

Use plain language and simple questions that can be answered with yes or no. Keep in mind that the person is acutely aware of your body language and may consider it as a measure of your acceptance. Your goal is to try to make each conversation a "person-centred" verbal connection. Box 20.8 summarizes communication guidelines for communicating with people with cognitive impairment.

People with cognitive impairment often have trouble following instructions consisting of multiple steps. Breaking instructions into single steps helps them master tasks that otherwise are beyond their comprehension. Keep the conversation simple and focused only on one step at a time. Give the subsequent step only after the person has completed the first instruction.

Case Example

A young woman in a dementia support group for family members spoke of a meaningful experience with her grandmother. As she went to make a tuna fish sandwich for her grandmother, she decided to involve her in the process. She gave her grandmother step-by-step verbal instructions (e.g., "Get the tuna fish out of the cabinet." "Now, get the knife from the drawer.") Her grandmother was able to do all of the steps, with structured guidance. As the granddaughter was spreading the mayonnaise, her grandmother said, "Now don't forget the onions." It was a priceless moment of connection for the granddaughter.

Do not explain why or what will happen if the directions are not followed. Scolding usually worsens confusion. Unlike children, who can learn from a mistake, people with dementia cannot. If the person does not do a task or follows directions incorrectly, keep the words simple. Proactively state a next step in pleasant calm tones, for example, "Let's see if we can …" (followed by a one-step directive).

People with dementia often retain many of their social skills, even when their cognitive memory significantly declines, especially in the early stages (Mace & Rabins, 2017). Asking older people with mild to early moderate cognitive impairment about their past life experiences is a way to connect verbally with those who might have difficulty telling you what they had for breakfast 2 hours ago. Remote memory (recall of past events) is retained longer than memory for recent events. For the person, the experience of connecting with another person is more important than having an in-depth conversation. Giving a compliment helps. Family members can be encouraged to reminisce with people with dementia. Even if the person cannot

---

BOX 20.8   Do's and Don'ts for Communicating With Older People With Dementia

Communication Do's

- Simplify environmental stimuli before beginning to converse.
- Look directly at the person when talking.
- Ask the person what they would like to be called.
- Try to identify the emotions behind the person's words or behaviour.
- Identify and minimize anything in the environment that creates anxiety for the person.
- Watch your body language; convey interest and acceptance.
- Repeat simple messages slowly, calmly, and patiently.
- Give clear, simple directions, one at a time, in a step-by-step manner.
- Direct conversation toward concrete, familiar objects.
- Communicate with touch, smiles, calmness, and gentle redirection.
- Structure the environment and routines to allow freedom within limits.
- Use soft music or hymns when the person seems agitated.

Communication Don'ts

- Don't argue or reason with the person; instead, use distraction.
- Avoid confrontation.
- Don't use slang, jargon, or abstract terms.
- If attention lapses, don't persist. Let the person rest a few minutes before trying to regain their attention.
- Don't focus on difficult behaviour; look for the underlying anxiety and redirect.
- Avoid hand restraints if at all possible.
- Avoid small objects that could be a choking hazard.

respond verbally, sometimes behaviours will show through facial expression or garbled words an appreciation for the connection. Sometimes this occurs when least expected.

Case Example

Mary was visiting her sister with dementia. She had travelled from Alberta to Ontario to visit her. Her sister was unresponsive to her, and Mary was upset that she did not seem to realize that she was her sister. A few days after Mary returned home, her sister told the nurse, "You know, my sister Mary was here last week." Things register with people with dementia that are not always apparent. This is important information to share with family members.

Touch

Touch is something people with dementia can no longer ask for, create for themselves, or tell another of its meaning. Touching a person is a way of being with them (Petty et al., 2020). Touch is a form of communication that immediately acknowledges the person with dementia's stress, calms a person who is agitated, and provides a sense of security, particularly if accompanied by a smile or a compliment and a gentle approach. As dementia progresses, informal and professional caregivers can use gentle touch to gain a person's attention, guide a person toward an activity, or simply as an expression of caring.

In general, people with dementia appreciate the use of touch. But to some, it can be frightening, particularly if you move in too fast. Before using touch, make sure that the person is open to it. You can usually tell when a person thinks you are entering their personal space by looking at the person's body language and facial expression. Touch, used in direct care such as putting lotion on dry skin, giving back rubs, and warming cold hands or feet, can be meaningful to the person. When a person is no longer able to recognize familiar caregivers by name, nurturing touch provides a touchstone with the physical reality of someone who cares about the person.

Reality Orientation Groups

People experiencing memory loss may forget exactly where they are, what time it is, who they are with, and in the later stages, even who they are, particularly if they are in a new setting. Using simple prompts in conversation can decrease anxiety and promote interpersonal comfort. Helping people focus on their immediate personal environment and providing visual prompts (clocks, calendars, name ID on room doors, and photos) connect the person with their personal environment. Calling the person by name, putting the names of caregivers on white boards, and repeating information about time or place also strengthens recognition.

Reality orientation groups are used with older people experiencing moderate cognitive impairment. These groups keep people in touch with time, place, and person. The group leader introduces the topic for the day and then goes around the group for individual responses. Topics can include landmarks in the dining room; routes to the dining room or bathroom; the date, time, and weather; what people would like to wear; and so on. Reality orientation groups may be conducted daily or weekly, with three to four people (Chiu et al., 2018).

Validation Therapy

Validation therapy describes a therapeutic communication process used in later stages of dementia. Developed by Naomi Feil, validation therapy recognizes that a person with dementia is responding to a different reality related to time, place, and person (Maki, 2018). Rather than confronting people with dementia with "facts"—that people they knew or places they have lived are no longer available to them—focus on the personal meaning events and people hold for the person. For example, you might say, "Tell me about Chris," or "What was it like living on M street?"

Attending to the Special Needs of People with Dementia

Catastrophic Reactions

Older people with memory loss lack the cognitive ability to develop alternatives. They may emotionally overreact to situations and can have what look like temper tantrums in response to real or perceived frustration. These behavioural outbursts are called **catastrophic reactions**. Usually, there is something in the immediate environment that precipitates the reaction—fatigue, multiple demands, overstimulation, misinterpretations, or an inability to meet expectations are often contributing factors (Mace & Rabins, 2017). Keep in mind that the emotion may be appropriate, even if the way it is expressed is not. Warning signs of an impending catastrophic reaction include agitation or restlessness, body stiffening, verbal or nonverbal refusals, and general uncooperativeness. Instead of focusing on the behaviour, try to identify and eliminate the cause(s) (Bendigo Health, n.d.).

You can use distraction to move the person away from the offending stimulus in the environment—for example, with a simple statement like, "I really need your help over here," or use postponement. Or, for example, you can say, "We'll do that later; right now, it's time to go out on the porch," while gently leading the person away. Direct confrontation and an appeal for more civilized behaviour usually serve to escalate, rather than diminish, the episode. Your tone of voice in supplying the distraction is important. A calm, kind tone gets the best results.

Sundowning

Sundowning is a term used to describe agitated behavioural symptoms that people with dementia usually experience later in the day. Common behaviours include fretfulness, anxiety, and demanding behaviours. Days and nights may be reversed. This behaviour can be very difficult for family members because their sleep is disturbed. Keeping the person active during the day helps. Small doses of medication are used to alleviate symptoms. Caution is needed to avoid oversedating the person and to prevent medication buildup, which can occur because medications are metabolized more slowly in older people.

Legal Issues

People with dementia in early stages can still make simple decisions, if they are supported and are patiently respected.

Decisional capacity refers to the capability of a person to do the following:

- Understand and process information about diagnosis, prognosis, and treatment options.
- Weigh the benefits, burdens, and risks of the proposed options.
- Apply a set of personal values to the analysis.
- Arrive at a decision that is consistent over time.
- Communicate the decision (Farber Post & Boltz, 2016, p. 44).

If a person is unable to make a cogent decision about the type of application of personal health care, they can designate a medical **power of attorney** to make realistic health decisions, including "do not resuscitate" decisions.

Mental competence represents a medicolegal determination, related to injury, disease, or intellectual disability of a person's ability to manage their personal legal affairs. By contrast with decisional capacity, *mental incompetence* occurs when a person lacks the capacity to negotiate legal tasks such as making a will, entering into a contract, or making certain legal decisions.

The time to execute legal documents to people's rights is *before* they become unable to cognitively assign decision-making authority to someone they trust. People in the early stages of a mild or major neurocognitive disorder usually have sufficient mental competence to participate in legal decisions regarding their health care and finances. The criterion is that the person has to understand what they are signing and be in agreement with the course of action as it is presented in the document. Later, as the person loses significant cognitive capacity, this same person may be unable to lawfully execute legal documents.

Consultation with a lawyer regarding wills, power of attorney, and living wills should be accomplished while the person is still legally competent. Once cognitive capacity is lost, a court procedure is necessary to establish a conservatorship or guardianship. This action is costly and emotionally painful for most families because it requires legally certifying the person as incompetent.

Advocating for the Person with Major Neurocognitive Disorders

Before an older person needs a power of attorney, advanced directive, co-decision making, living trust or will, these need to be legally completed. If, in the power of attorney document, a guardian is not mentioned but needed, the court will appoint a guardian for an older person. If a person dies without a will or personal directive, their decision makers will need to contact a lawyer who specializes in this area. Each province and territory has its own laws regarding these matters (Government of Canada, 2018).

Nurses should refer the person's family members to a support group through the local Alzheimer Society. These support groups provide a place to talk about the challenges of caring for their family members. *All Things Consoled*, written by award-winning Canadian author, Elizabeth Hay (2018), tells a poignant story of the failing of her older parents and what this meant to her.

CARING FOR PEOPLE WITH ADVANCED DEMENTIA

Major neurocognitive disorders are associated with progressive disease; people gradually lose control over body functions and the capacity to handle even simple tasks. Meaningful verbal communication terminates. Attempts to communicate through behaviour are primitive and not easily understood.

Is the self still there? The answer is yes, but as dementia progresses, people have increasingly limited ways to connect with their environment and people in a meaningful way (Fig. 20.3). Touch, smiling, and gentle, kind approaches are meaningful. Just think what it would be like if you could no longer communicate with words. Family members often speak of two deaths they experience with a family member with dementia—the death of self and the actual death.

Rabins et al. (2016) identifies care of the person with dementia as consisting of four pillars:

1. Treating the disease
2. Treating the symptoms
3. Supporting the person
4. Supporting the caregiver (p. 100).

Since dementia attacks short-term memory first, talking or asking questions about past memories may stimulate conversations that otherwise would not be available to the person with a neurocognitive disorder in the early to middle stages.

Treatment goals for people with advanced dementia should emphasize dignity, quality of life, and supportive comfort strategies (Rabins et al., 2016). Table 20.2 identifies

TABLE 20.2   Symptoms of Dementia With Suggested Behavioural Communication Interventions

Dementia Symptom Pattern	Suggested Intervention
Agitation	• Identify and remove cause • Assess for physical problems • Reduce stimuli, suggest a walk • Use simple repetitive activities: folding towels, rolling socks • Use soothing music • Look for patterns that trigger agitation
Aggression: grabbing, hitting	• Recognize that the person is frightened • Decrease stimuli, move person to a quiet place • Do not take the person's behaviour personally • Respect and enlarge the person's personal space • Identify and minimize cause • Make eye contact; speak in a calm voice • Acknowledge frustration; do not reprimand • Check medications
Withdrawal: decreased socialization, apathy, social isolation	• Use simple activities • Find simple socialization opportunities and support the person's involvement
Refusal or resistance to suggestions	• Drop the topic or activity and reintroduce it later
Disturbed motor activity: wandering, pacing, raiding garbage cans, shadowing caregiver	• Keep the environment safe • Remove garbage • Use medical alert bracelets • Label drawers, room (photos help) • Use locks on doors at home
Sleep disturbances: day/night sleep reversal, calling out, moaning in sleep	• Keep active during the day • Toilet the person as needed during night, without conversation • Control wandering at night; lead back to bed; avoid use of restraints
Hallucinations, delusions, illusions	• Respond to the emotion, not content • Reduce stimuli • Use good, nonglare lighting • Use distraction (e.g., walk, do simple activity) • Use touch, reassurance, postponement
Disinhibition: inappropriate speech, touching, improper body exposure, entering other people's space	1. Do not reprimand 2. Respond to the emotion 3. Redirect person to other activities
Incontinence: urine, feces, eliminating in wrong places	1. Check for bladder infection, fecal impaction 2. Note elimination pattern; establish corresponding toileting timetable 3. Schedule toileting at frequent intervals 4. Toilet before bedtime 5. Take person to bathroom, verbally cue 6. Use washable clothing, Velcro closings on the gowns
Swallowing difficulty: choking, stuffing mouth, not swallowing	1. Cut food into small pieces, offer small quantities of liquid at one time 2. Check medications for size, modify as needed 3. Sit with person while eating 4. Verbally cue to chew and swallow
Agnosia: difficulty recognizing familiar things (e.g., prosopagnosia is difficulty recognizing faces, including one's own)	1. Remove or cover mirrors if person is frightened by self-image 2. Verbally identify familiar people and their relationship to the person

common neuropsychiatric symptoms associated with advanced dementia, with suggested behavioural communication interventions.

SUMMARY

Statistics reveal that older people constitute the fastest growing population group in Canada (Government of Canada, 2014). Aging is a universal life process with distinctive features. Typically, older people experience a progressive decline in sensory and motor functions but, with appropriate supports, they can expect to live longer and enjoy a better quality of life than in previous generations.

Erikson's theory of psychosocial development identifies ego integrity versus despair as the central maturational crisis of old age. People who believe that their lives have purpose and meaning, and that they have few or no regrets about a well-lived life, demonstrate the ego strength of integrity. Supportive communication and empowerment strategies assist people in maximizing their health and well-being.

This chapter presents current understanding about the course of dementia and discusses related communication strategies with people and their families. Differential assessment of depression, delirium, and dementia is important, as symptoms can appear similar. Communication strategies with people with dementia emphasize verbal supports. Helping people tell their story, promoting autonomy, using a proactive approach in conversations, acting as an advocate, and treating older people with dignity are essential. Health promotion activities that take into account the unique needs and cultural values of older people are more likely to be successful. As a primary provider in long-term care and in the community, the nurse is in a unique role to support and meet the communication needs of older people.

👤 ETHICAL DILEMMA

What Would You Do?

Mrs. Allan is an accomplished, 82-year-old woman, living alone. She treasures her independence. While she realizes she is having difficulties managing her housework, she is in a quandry because she does not want to leave her home or lose her independence. Her daughter is worried about her and wants her to move to an assisted living facility. During your initial assessment for a recent fall, Mrs. Allan confides that while she does have "some" memory lapses, she can't bear the idea of what assisted living will mean for her independence and quality of life. She asks you to keep her confidence. You can understand Mrs. Allan's concerns but you also know that keeping silent may not be in her best interest. How could you balance the ethical concept of beneficence with the concerns of the person in your care? What would you do?

QUESTIONS FOR REVIEW AND DISCUSSION

1. What are some examples of ageism that affect older people?
2. How is ageism perpetuated?
3. From an advocacy perspective, how could you as a nurse help create a more positive image of older people?

REFERENCES

Adelman, M., Greene, M., & Ory, M. (2000). Communication between older patients and their physicians. *Clinics Geriatric Medicine, 16*(10), 1–24.

Aldwin, C. M., Igarashi, H., & Levenson, M. R. (2019). Wisdom as self-transcendence. In R. J. Sternberg & J. Glück (Eds.), *The Cambridge handbook of wisdom* (pp. 122–143). Cambridge University Press. https://doi.org/10.1017/9781108568272.007.

Alzheimer Society of Canada. (2016). *Day to day series— Communication.* https://alzheimer.ca/sites/default/files/files/national/brochures-day-to-day/day_to_day_communications_e.pdf.

Alzheimer's Society United Kingdom. (2021). *Dementia and sensory impairment: communicating.* https://www.alzheimers.org.uk/about-dementia/symptoms-and-diagnosis/symptoms/communicating-someone-sensory-impairment.

American Psychiatric Association. (2013). *Diagnostic and statistical manual of mental disorders* (5th ed.). Author.

Arnold, E. (2005). Sorting out the 3 D's: Delirium, dementia, depression: Learn how to sift through overlapping signs and symptoms so you can help improve an older patient's quality of life. *Holistic Nursing Practice, 19*(3), 99–104.

Avolio, M., Montagnoli, S., Marino, D. et al. (2013). Factors influencing quality of life for disabled and nondisabled elderly population: The results of a multiple correspondence analysis. *Current Gerontology and Geriatrics Research,* 258–274.

Bendigo Health. (n.d.). *Catastrophic reactions: Preventing and managing catastrophic reactions. Loddon Mallee regional dementia management strategy.* http://www.dementiamanagementstrategy.com/Pages/ABC_of_behaviour_management/Management_strategies/Catastrophic_reactions.aspx.

Bonder, B. R., & Dal Bello-Haas, V. (2018). *Functional performance in older adults* (4th ed.). FA Davis.

Brown-O'Hara, T. (2013). Geriatric syndromes and their implications for nursing. *Nursing, 43*(1), 1–3.

Budib, M. B., Zulim, M. I., de Oliveira, V. M. et al. (2020). Integrated continuous care: Collaborating with the elderly functionality. *Bioscience Journal, 36*(1). https://doi.org/10.14393/BJ-v36n1a2020-42308.

Canadian Academy of Audiology. (n.d.) *Advocacy.* https://canadianaudiology.ca/what-we-do/advocacy/.

Canadian Institute for Health Information. (2016). *Dementia in hospitals. Seniors with dementia more likely to be hospitalized, stay longer in emergency department.* https://www.cihi.ca/en/dementia-in-canada/dementia-across-the-health-system/dementia-in-hospitals.

Canadian Medical Protective Association. (2018). *Safe prescribing: Risks for older patients.* 8-28-E. https://www.cmpa-acpm.

ca/en/advice-publications/browse-articles/2018/safe-prescribing-risks-for-older-patients.

Canadian Patient Safety Institute. (2016). *Patient stories.* https://www.patientsafetyinstitute.ca/en/toolsResources/Member-Videos-and-Stories/Pages/default.aspx.

Cenci, C. (2016). Narrative medicine and the personalization of treatment for elderly patients. *European Journal of Internal Medicine, 32,* 22–25.

Chiu, H.-Y., Chen, P.-Y., Chen, Y.-T. et al. (2018). Reality orientation therapy benefits cognition in older people with dementia: A meta-analysis. *International Journal of Nursing Studies, 86,* 20–28. https://doi.org/10.1016/j.ijnurstu.2018.06.008.

Chochinov, H. M. (2013). Dignity in care: Time to take action. *Journal of Pain and Symptom Management, 46,* 756–759.

Connect Hearing. (2021). *Understanding hearing loss.* https://www.connecthearing.ca/hearing-loss/deafness/.

Constanca, P., Ribeiro, O., & Teixeira, L. (2012). Active ageing: An empirical approach to the WHO model. *Current Gerontology and Geriatrics Research, 382–972.* https://doi.org/10.1155/2012/382972.

da Costa, J. P., Vitorino, R., Silva, G. M. et al. (2016). A synopsis on aging—Theories, mechanisms and future prospects. *Ageing Research Reviews, 29,* 90–112. https://doi.org/10.1016/j.arr.2016.06.005.

Ebrahimi, Z., Wilhelmson, K., Moore, C. et al. (2013). Health despite frailty: Exploring influences on frail older adults experiences of health. *Geriatrics Nursing, 34,* 289–294.

Employment and Social Development Canada. (2009). *Elder abuse: It's time to face the reality.* Cat. No. NS4-61/2009. ISBN: 978-0-662-06370-4. https://www.canada.ca/en/employment-social-development/campaigns/elder-abuse/reality.html#f.

Erikson, E. (1980). *Identity and the life cycle.* Norton.

Farber-Post, L., & Boltz, M. (2016). Health care decision making. In M. Boltz, E. Capezuti, T. Fulmer, et al. (Eds.), *Evidence based geriatric nursing protocols for best practice* (5th ed., pp. 43–49). Chapter 4.

Folstein, M., Folstein, S., & McHugh, P. R. (1975). Mini-mental state: A practical method for grading cognition state of patients for the clinician. *Journal of Psychiatric Research, 12,* 189–198.

Gloth, F. (2010). *Handbook of pain relief in older adults* (2nd ed.). Humana Press.

Golinowska, S., Groot, W., Baji, P. et al. (2016). Health promotion targeting older people. *BMC Health Services Research, 16,* 345. https://doi.org/10.1186/s12913-016-1514-3.

Gould, E., & Mitty, E. (2010). Medication adherence is a partnership, medication compliance is not. *Geriatric Nursing, 31,* 290–298.

Government of Canada. (2010). *The Chief Public Health Officer's Report on the state of public health in Canada 2010—Canada's experience in setting the stage for health aging.* https://www.canada.ca/en/public-health/corporate/publications/chief-public-health-officer-reports-state-public-health-canada/annual-report-on-state-public-health-canada-2010/chapter-2.html.

Government of Canada. (2014). *Action for seniors report. Profile of seniors in Canada.* https://www.canada.ca/en/employment-social-development/programs/seniors-action-report.html.

Government of Canada. (2018). *Financial consumer agency of Canada.* https://www.canada.ca/en/financial-consumer-agency/services/estate-planning/will-estate-planning.html.

Gray-Miceli, D. (2017). Impaired mobility and functional decline in older adults. Evidence to facilitate a practice change. *Nursing Clinical North America, 52,* 469–487.

Happ, M. B. (2010). Individualized care for frail older adults: Challenges for health care reform in acute and critical care. *Gerontological Nursing, 31*(1), 63–65.

Ha-Redeye, O., Latif, R., & Pirzada, K. (2017). *Integrating religious and cultural supports into quality care in the last stages of life in Ontario: Improving the last stages of life.* Law Commission of Ontario. https://www.lco-cdo.org/wp-content/uploads/2015/05/Latif-et-al-Final1.pdf.

Hay, E. (2018). *All things consoled.* McClelland & Stewart.

Health Canada. (2018). *Background document: Public consultation on strengthening Canada's approach to substance use issues.* https://www.canada.ca/en/health-canada/services/substance-use/canadian-drugs-substances-strategy/strengthening-canada-approach-substance-use-issue.html.

Health Council of Canada. (2012). *Self-management support for Canadians with chronic health conditions: A focus for primary health care.* p. 6. https://www.selfmanagementbc.ca/uploads/HCC_SelfManagementReport_FA.pdf.

Hear-it.org. (n.d.). *Hearing loss in North America.* https://www.hear-it.org/three-million-canadians-suffer-from-hearing-loss.

HelpAge Canada. (2021). *Social isolation and loneliness.* https://helpagecanada.ca/resources/social-isolation-and-loneliness/.

Herr, K. (2010). Pain in the older adult: An imperative across all health care settings. *Pain Management Nursing, 11*(Suppl. 2), S1–S10.

Herr, K. (2013). *Retooling pain assessment for older adults.* Presentation at the American Pain Society, 32nd Annual Scientific Meeting. New Orleans: LA.

Horgas, A. (2017). Pain assessment in older adults. *Nursing Clinical North America, 5*(3), 375–378.

Institute of Medicine. (2008). *Retooling for an aging America: Building the health care workforce.* National Academies Press.

Ito, M., Takahashi, R., & Liehr, P. (2007). Heeding the behavioral message of elders with dementia in day care. *Holist Nursing Practice, 21*(1), 12–18.

Kagan, S. (2012). Gotcha! Don't let ageism sneak into your practice. *Geriatric Nursing, 33*(1), 60–62.

Kelly, M. E., Duff, H., Kelly, S. et al. (2017). The impact of social activities, social networks, social support and social relationships on the cognitive functioning of healthy older adults: A systematic review. *Systematic Reviews Journal, 6,* 259. https://doi.org/10.1186/s13643-017-0632-2.

Kim, L., Koncilja, K., & Nielsen, C. (2018). Medication management in older adults. *Cleveland Clinic Journal of Medicine, 85*(2), 129–135.

Mace, N., & Rabins, P. (2017). *The 36-hour day: A family guide to caring for people with Alzheimer's disease, other dementias, and memory loss* (6th ed.). Johns Hopkins University.

MacKinlay, E. (2012). Resistance, resilience, and change: The person and dementia. *Journal of Religion, Spirituality & Aging, 24,* 80–92.

Maki, Y. (2018). A reappraisal of the evidence of non-pharmacological intervention for people with dementia. *Journal of Geriatric Care and Research, 18*(5), 1–2.

Marquis, I. (n.d.) *Using memories as therapy*. Research Perspectives. University of Ottawa. https://research.uottawa.ca/perspectives/using-memories-therapy.

Maslow, A. (1954). *Motivation and personality*. Harper & Row.

Maslow, A. (1975). *Motivation and personality*. Harper & Row.

Mauk, K. L. (2006). Healthier again: Reaching and teaching older adults. *Holist Nursing Practice, 20*(3), 158.

Mauk, K. L. (2010). *Gerontological nursing: Competencies for care.* Jones & Bartlett.

McCarthy, B. (2011). *Hearing the person with dementia: Person centered approaches*. Jessica Kingsley.

Miller, C. (2011). *Nursing for wellness in older adults*. Wolters Kluwer.

Moody, H., & Sasser, J. (2017). *Aging: Concepts and controversies* (9th ed.). Pine Forge Press.

Narang, D., Kordia, K., Meena, J. et al. (2013). Interpersonal relationships of elderly within the family. *International Journal of Social Sciences & Interdisciplinary Research, 2*(3), 132–138.

Navarrete-Villanueva, D., Gómez-Cabello, A., Marín-Puyalto, J. et al. (2021). Frailty and physical fitness in elderly people: A systematic review and meta-analysis. *Sports Medicine, 51,* 143–160. https://doi.org/10.1007/s40279-020-01361-1.

Nesbitt, J., Moxham, S., Ramadurai, G. et al. (2015). Improving pain assessment and management in stroke patients. *British Medical Journal Quality Improvement Reports, 4*(1), u203375. w3105. https://www.ncbi.nlm.nih.gov/pmc/articles/PMC4645684/#.

Owsley, C. (2011). Aging and vision. *Vision Research, 51*(13), 1610–1622. https://doi.org/10.1016/j.visres.2010.10.020.

Perry, T. E., Ruggiano, N., Shtompel, N. et al. (2015). Applying Erikson's wisdom to self-management practices of older adults: Findings from two field studies. *Research on Aging, 37*(3), 253–274. https://doi.org/10.1177/0164027514527974.

Petty, S., Dening, T., Griffiths, A. et al. (2020). Meeting the emotional needs of hospital patients with dementia: A free listing study with ward staff. *The Gerontologist, 60*(1), 155–164. https://doi.org/10.1093/geront/gny151.

Potempa, K., Butterworth, S., & Flaherty-Robb Gaynor, W. (2010). The healthy ageing model: Health behaviors for older adults. *Collegian, 04*(008), 51–55.

Pryce, H., & Gooberman, R. (2012). There's a hell of a noise: Living with a hearing loss in residential care. *Age Ageing, 41,* 40–46.

Rabins, P., Lyketsos, C., & Steele, C. (2016). *Practical dementia care* (3rd ed.). Oxford University Press.

Registered Nurses' Association of Ontario. (2013). *Assessment and management of pain* (3rd ed.). Registered Nurses' Association of Ontario. https://rnao.ca/sites/rnao-ca/files/AssessAndManagementOfPain_15_WEB-_FINAL_DEC_2.pdf.

Reichstadt, M., Sengupta, G., Depp, C. et al. (2010). Older adults' perspectives on successful aging. Qualitative interviews. *American Journal of Geriatric Psychiatry, 18*(7), 567–575.

Saftari, L., & Kwon, O. (2018). Ageing vision and falls: A review. *Journal Physiological Anthropology, 37,* 11. https://doi.org/10.1186/s40101-018-0170-1.

Statistics Canada. (2016). *Hearing loss of Canadians, 2012 to 2015.* https://www150.statcan.gc.ca/n1/pub/82-625-x/2016001/article/14658-eng.htm.

Sundsli, K., Espnes, G. A., & Söderhamn, O. (2013). Lived experiences of self-care among older physically active urban-living individuals. *Clinical Interventions in Aging, 8,* 123–130. https://doi.org/10.2147/CIA.S39689.

Tarugu, J., Pavithra, R., Vinothchandar, S. et al. (2019). Effectiveness of structured group reminiscence therapy in decreasing the feelings of loneliness, depressive symptoms and anxiety among inmates of a residential home for the elderly in Chittoor district Jayanthi. *International Journal of Community Medicine and Public Health, 6*(2), 847–854. https://doi.org/10.18203/2394-6040.ijcmph20190218.

Touhy, T., & Jett, K. (2015). *Ebersole and Hess' healthy aging: Human needs and nursing response* (9th ed.). Elsevier.

van Uffelen, J. G., Heesch, K. C., Hill, R. L. et al. (2011). A qualitative study of older adults' responses to sitting-time questions: Do we get the information we want? *BMC Public Health, 11,* 458. https://doi.org/10.1186/1471-2458-11-458.

Van Vliet, E., Lindenberger, E., & Van Weert, J. (2015). Communication with older, seriously ill patients. *Clinical Geriatric Medicine, 31,* 219–230.

World Health Organization. (2015). *Ageing and life-course. Health promotion for older people: not business as usual.* https://www.who.int/ageing/features/health-promotion/en/.

World Health Organization. (2020). *Dementia. Key facts.* https://www.who.int/news-room/fact-sheets/detail/dementia.

WEBSITE/RESOURCES LIST

https://www150.statcan.gc.ca/n1/pub/82-625-x/2016001/article/14658-eng.htm; https:/.

https://www150.statcan.gc.ca/n1/pub/11-402-x/2008/70000/ceb70000_000-eng.htm.

https://alzheimer.ca/sites/default/files/files/national/brochures-day-to-day/day_to_day_communications_e.pdf.

https://www.alzheimers.org.uk/about-dementia/symptoms-and-diagnosis/symptoms/communicating-someone-sensory-impairment.

https://www.canada.ca/en/employment-social-development/campaigns/elder-abuse/reality.html#f.

https://www.canada.ca/en/employment-social-development/programs/seniors-action-report.html.

https://www.canada.ca/en/health-canada/services/substance-use/canadian-drugs-substances-strategy/strengthening-canada-approach-substance-use-issue.html.

https://www.canada.ca/en/public-health/corporate/publications/chief-public-health-officer-reports-state-public-health-canada/annual-report-on-state-public-health-canada-2010/chapter-2.html.

https://canadianaudiology.ca/what-we-do/advocacy/.

https://www.cihi.ca/en/dementia-in-canada/dementia-across-the-health-system/dementia-in-hospitals.

https://www.cmpa-acpm.ca/en/advice-publications/browse-articles/2018/safe-prescribing-risks-for-older-patients.

https://www.connecthearing.ca/hearing-loss/deafness/.

http://www.dementiamanagementstrategy.com/Pages/ABC_of_behaviour_management/Management_strategies/Catastrophic_reactions.aspx.

https://content.oma.org//wp-content/uploads/patient-centredcare.pdf.

https://www.hear-it.org/three-million-canadians-suffer-from-hearing-loss.

https://www.homecareontario.ca/home-care-reports/other-home-care-publications/aging-senior.

https://journals.plos.org/plosone/article?id=10.1371/journal.pone.0205857.

https://www.lco-cdo.org/wp-content/uploads/2015/05/Latif-et-al-Final1.pdf.

https://medicine.jrank.org/pages/227/Canada-Health-Care-Coverage-Older-People-Use-health-services-by-older-Canadians.htm.

http://www.ncoa.org/.

https://www.patientsafetyinstitute.ca/en/toolsResources/Member-Videos-and-Stories/Pages/default.aspx.

https://research.uottawa.ca/perspectives/using-memories-therapy.

https://rnao.ca/sites/rnao-ca/files/Assessment_and_Management_of_Pain_in_the_Elderly_-_Learning_Package_for_LTC.pdf.

https://www.selfmanagementbc.ca/uploads/HCC_Self ManagementReport_FA.pdf.

https://www.who.int/ageing/features/health-promotion/en/.

https://www.who.int/news-room/fact-sheets/detail/dementia.

21

Communicating With People in Crisis

Olive Yonge

Originating US chapter by *Pamela E. Marcus*

OBJECTIVES

At the end of the chapter, the reader will be able to:
1. Define *crisis* and related concepts.
2. Discuss theoretical frameworks related to crisis and crisis intervention.
3. Identify and apply structured crisis intervention strategies in the care of people experiencing a crisis state.
4. Apply crisis intervention strategies to mental health emergencies.
5. Discuss crisis management strategies in disaster and mass trauma situations.

The purpose of this chapter is to describe communication strategies nurses can use with people and their families experiencing a crisis situation. The chapter describes the nature of crisis and identifies its theoretical foundations. The application section provides practical guidelines nurses can use with people in crisis and during mental health emergencies and disaster management.

BASIC CONCEPTS

Definitions

Crisis

A *crisis* is a time-limited response to a life event that overwhelms a person's usual coping mechanisms. It occurs as a response to situational, developmental, biological, psychological, sociocultural, or spiritual factors" (Registered Nurses' Association of Ontario [RNAO], 2017). The COVID-19 pandemic created a great deal of stress for many people, from locally to globally, ranging from friends and family becoming ill and dying to mass unemployment, as countries enforced social distancing and restrictions of people gathering.

People in a **crisis state** experience an actual or perceived overwhelming threat to self-concept, an insurmountable obstacle, or a loss that conventional coping measures cannot handle. Unabated, the resulting tension continues to increase, creating majour personality disorganization and a crisis state.

The word *crisis* comes from the Greek root word *krinen*, meaning "to decide," and in Latin, crisis means the turning point of a disease" (Vroomen et al., 2013, p. 10). Personal responses to crisis can be adaptive or maladaptive. Nurses can help people with restorative coping strategies to lessen the damaging impact of crisis. Successfully working through a crisis has the potential to strengthen people's coping responses and encourage a sense of self-efficacy. Maladaptive responses can result in the development of acute or chronic psychiatric symptoms.

Crisis State. A crisis state is *not* a mental health disorder, although individuals with mental health disorders can experience a crisis state associated with their disorder. Crisis is a complex concept, which can defy easy cause-and-effect explanations. Given that a crisis state represents a personal response, two people experiencing the same crisis event will respond differently to it. Understanding someone's personal response to a crisis rather than an objective crisis stressor is critical to successful crisis intervention.

Individuals in crisis feel vulnerable. Crisis intervention strategies are designed to help support people experiencing crisis to achieve psychological homeostasis. A favourable outcome depends on the person's combined interpretation of the crisis, perception of coping ability, resources, and level of social support (Loughran, 2011). If the person does not seek help and comes out of the crisis state by use of defence mechanisms, there is the possibility of a lowered functioning level and possibly psychosis or even death (RNAO, 2017).

Types of Crisis

Developmental Crisis

A crisis is classified as developmental or situational. Erikson's (1982) stage model of psychosocial development forms the basis for exploring the nature of developmental crises. Developmental crises can occur as individuals negotiate developmental, age-related milestones in their lives—for example, becoming a parent or retiring from long-term employment. Normative psychosocial crises are used as benchmarks for assessing signs and symptoms of developmental crisis. When a situational crisis is superimposed on a normative developmental crisis, the crisis experience can be more intense. For example, a woman losing a spouse at the same time as she is going through menopause can experience a more intense impact.

Situational Crisis

A situational crisis refers to an unusually stressful life event that exceeds a person's resources and coping skills. Examples include unexpected illness or injury, rape, a car accident, the loss of a home or spouse, or being laid off from a job. A disaster or adventitious (unexpected, unplanned, or random) crisis results from events that are not part of everyday life. These crises may threaten survival, like the COVID-19 pandemic. Experiencing or witnessing such events can also overwhelm a person's ability to cope (RNAO, 2017). A situational crisis is described as being in response to events that are external and unanticipated, such as a loss or change of a job, death of someone close, financial troubles, exacerbation of a chronic condition, or the experience of sudden illness (Jakubec, 2014). How successfully a person responds to a crisis can depend on the following:

- Previous experience with crises, coping, and problem solving
- Perception of the crisis event
- Level of help or obstruction from significant others
- Developmental level and ego maturity
- Concurrent stressors

Loughran (2011) emphasizes determining how the individual involved in the incident identifies the crisis. It may be that the person does not recognize the event as a crisis, whereas others may perceive the same occurrence as having crisis proportions. To provide individual care, it is important to determine the type of crisis and whether the individual is experiencing the events as a crisis. Box 21.1 explains the signs and symptoms of crisis.

Behavioural Emergencies

James and Gilliland (2013) state that a **behavioural emergency** occurs "when a crisis escalates to the point that the

---

BOX 21.1   Signs and Symptoms of Crisis

Signs and Symptoms of Crisis	
Inability to meet basic needs	Incoherence
Decreased use of social support	Depression
Inadequate problem solving	Self-hatred
Inability to attend to information	Feels strange
Isolation	Perceived lack of control
Denial	Weeping
Exaggerated startle response	Grief/sadness
Hypervigilance	Irritability
Panic attacks	Being on guard or jumpy
Feeling numb	Physical symptoms (e.g., shaking, headaches, fatigue,
Confusion	loss of appetite, aches and pains)

Sources: Adapted from Registered Nurses' Association of Ontario. (2017). *Crisis intervention for adults using a trauma-informed approach: Initial four weeks of management* (3rd ed.). Author. https://rnao.ca/sites/rnao-ca/files/bpg/Crisis_Intervention_FINAL_WEB.pdf; Jakubec, S. L. (2014). Crisis and disaster. In J. H. Halter, C. L. Pollard, S. L. Ray et al. (Eds.), Canadian psychiatric mental health nursing (pp. 491–507). Saunders; World Health Organization, War Trauma Foundation & World Vision International. (2013). *Psychological first aid: Facilitator's manual for orienting field workers.* World Health Organization. https://apps.who.int/iris/handle/10665/102380.

situation requires immediate intervention to avoid injury or death" (p. 8). Examples include any type of violent interpersonal behaviour, psychotic crisis, suicide, or homicide. A behavioural emergency describes any type of thinking or behaviour that places an individual in an immediate potentially injurious or lethal situation. A behavioural emergency is when there is violent behaviour that is not yet managed. The behaviours are a result of unmet health, functional, or psychosocial needs that can be managed by addressing the conditions that produced them (Emanuel et al., 2013). In addition to assessing the person's risk characteristics, it is important to evaluate the environmental features and other factors that can either increase or decrease suicidal risk. When this person is discharged from the hospital, the family and the person should be provided suicide prevention information, for example, the number to a crisis hotline.

Case Example: COVID 19 Pandemic

The pandemic that started in Wuhan, China spread to North America mainly through international travel. By March 2020, Canadian government officials at the federal and provincial and territorial levels were having urgent meetings to determine how the spread of the virus could be contained. At the same time, researchers from all disciplines began lobbying for funding to research vaccines, attitudes towards the pandemic, and how to develop effective personal protective equipment, and health care agencies started to plan staffing levels, what resources they had available, extra shelters for people who were infected, protocols to keep front-line workers safe, and so on. The media began a campaign to educate the public about all aspects of COVID-19, from what it was to how people could keep themselves safe. The key components for intervention were masking with a medically approved mask, staying 2 metres from others not in their place of dwelling, washing hands very frequently (the virus dissolves with use of soap or alcohol-based hand sanitizer and vigorous handwashing) and not touching one's eyes, nose, and mouth without handwashing first. The virus mainly locates itself in the nose and throat and then descends into the lower lungs. The effects of the pandemic have been devasting for those who died in isolation, populations of older people housed in facilities that contributed to the spread, those who had existing health issues, and those who lived in poverty or had multiple residents in a dwelling. Young adults and even children were also not spared from death. Front-line health care workers also became infected and some of them died. Some people with COVID developed significant post-pandemic health issues (Center for Addiction and Mental Health [CAMH], 2021; Ottawa Public Health, 2021)

This pandemic is relatively unprecented, as it is the first global pandemic of the social media age (Galea, 2020). However, lessons can be learned from another, smaller, pandemic, severe acute respiratory syndrome (SARS). Hawryluck et al. (2004) surveyed 129 quarantined Torontonians during the SARS outbreak. They found symptoms of post-traumatic stress disorder (PTSD) in 28.9% of the respondents—longer durations of quarantine increased the prevalence of PTSD symptoms. Symptoms of depression were observed in 31.2% of respondents. Quarantine measures undertaken during the SARS epidemic led to mental health problems, including increased depression, anxiety, and stress symptoms (Brooks et al., 2020). These same findings will be present for the current pandemic. Those at risk for mental health disorders will be people with low incomes, those with pre-existing mental health conditions, people with chronic conditions, those who live alone, and older people (Luchetti et al., 2020; Parlapani et al., 2020). Another group of people who are at risk is those who contracted the virus and developed a post-virus syndrome as a result. These people are called "long haulers" and have symptoms such as extreme fatigue, uncertainty, joint pain, persistent chest pain, shortness of breath, and anxiety. Since the treatment is unknown, they also have a sense of helplessness. Cities across Canada are starting clinics to assist them in recovering from their symptoms, mainly by giving them support (https://www.healthing.ca/diseases-and-conditions/coronavirus/covid-long-haulers-i-dont-know-if-im-ever-gonna-be-back-to-normal).

Crisis Intervention

Crisis intervention is an immediate and short-term emergency response to mental, emotional, physical, and behavioural distress. Crisis interventions help to restore an individual's equilibrium to their biopsychosocial functioning and minimize the potential for long-term trauma or distress (Vertava Health, 2020).

Crisis intervention strategies should be adapted to fit each person's preferences, beliefs, values, and individual circumstances. The goals of crisis intervention are rapid resolution of the crisis, enhancement of coping skills, and promotion of a sense of control and self-efficacy (RNAO, 2017). As a nurse, you cannot always change the nature of a crisis situation, but you can help defuse a person's emotional reaction to it with compassionate, professional support and guidance.

Crisis intervention is a time-limited treatment. Four to six weeks is considered the standard time frame for crisis resolution. Interventions should be present-focused and action-oriented. The emphasis is on immediate problem solving and strengthening the personal resources of the people involved and their families. Nurses function as advocates, resources, partners, and guides in helping people resolve crisis situations, usually as part of a larger crisis intervention team.

THEORETICAL FRAMEWORKS

Lindemann (1944) and Caplan (1964) developed the most widely used models of crisis and crisis intervention. Lindemann's study of bereavement provides a frame of reference for understanding the stages involved in resolving emotional crisis and bereavement. His findings suggest, "proper psychiatric management of grief reactions may prevent prolonged and serious alterations in the person's social adjustment, as well as potential medical disease" (p. 147).

Caplan broadened Lindemann's model to include the concepts of developmental crisis and personal crisis. Although the focus of crisis intervention is on secondary prevention because the crisis state is already in motion, Caplan's model of preventive psychiatry starts in the community. He introduced practical crisis intervention strategies—for example, crisis telephone lines, training for community workers, and early response strategies. He viewed nurses as key service providers in crisis intervention.

Caplan discusses a crisis response pattern. He identifies a person's initial response to a crisis state as *shock*, with varied emotions and responses, ranging from anger, laughing, hysterics, crying, and acute anxiety to social withdrawal.

An extended period of adjustment follows the state of shock, with a period of *recoil*, which can last from 2 to 3 weeks. Behaviour appears normal to outsiders, but people describe nightmares, phobic reactions, and flashbacks of the crisis event.

Restoration or reconstruction describes the final phase of crisis intervention. This phase involves developing a plan and taking constructive actions to resolve the crisis situation. If successfully negotiated, the person returns to a pre-crisis functional level, which is the desired clinical outcome. Maladaptive coping strategies, such as drug or alcohol use, violence, or avoidance prevent restoration and place the person at risk for further problems. Simulation Exercise 21.1 is designed to help you to understand the nature of crisis.

Nursing Model

The nursing model developed by Aguilera (1998) approaches crisis intervention from a balancing perspective, between a crisis situation and a person's capacity to resolve it. The model proposes that a crisis state develops because of a distorted perception of a situation or because the person lacks the resources to cope successfully with it. Balancing factors include a realistic perception of the event, the person's internal resources (beliefs or attitudes), and the person's external (environmental) support. These factors can minimize or reduce the impact of the stressor, leading to resolution of the crisis.

Absence of adequate situational support, lack of coping skills, and a distorted perception of the crisis event can result in a crisis state, leaving individuals and families feeling overwhelmed and unable to cope. Interventions are designed to increase the balancing factors needed to restore a person to pre-crisis functioning.

SIMULATION EXERCISE 21.1   Understanding the Nature of Crisis

Purpose

To help students understand crises, in preparation for assessing and planning communication strategies in professional crisis situations

Procedure

1. Describe a crisis you experienced in your life. There are no right or wrong definitions of a crisis, and it does not matter whether the crisis would be considered a crisis in someone else's life.
2. Identify how the crisis changed your roles, routines, relationships, and assumptions about yourself.
3. Apply a crisis model to the situation you are describing.

4. Identify the strategies you used to cope with the crisis.
5. Describe the ways in which your personal crisis strengthened or weakened your self-concept and increased your options and your understanding of life.

Discussion

1. What did you learn from doing this exercise that you can use in your clinical practice?
2. Having done this simulation, what will you do differently and what will you do the same the next time you have a crisis?
3. Reflecting on this crisis, who has taught you how to manage crises in the past?

DEVELOPING AN EVIDENCE-INFORMED PRACTICE

Purpose

The researchers examined the moral experiences of children related to conflict and crisis management and the related use of restraint and seclusion in a Canadian child mental health setting.

Method

A participatory, hermeneutic (method of interpretation of texts, interviews, and observations of others) framework was used. Researchers using this method use an interpretive process and are informed by the social, historical, and cultural contexts. Over 5 months, data was collected on 12 children with diagnoses such as attention-deficit/hyperactivity disorder, oppositional defiant disorder, disruptive mood dysregulation disorder, and conduct disorder, with many children having multiple diagnoses. Twelve of the 24 children in the day program participated. Data was collected mainly through participant observation, including field notes combined with interviews with seven children as key informants and a review of key clinical documents. Interviews lasted between 15 minutes and 1.5 hours and ranged from one to four interviews with each child.

Findings

The participants saw value in using restraints and seclusion, especially if another child was being aggressive to them or engaging in self-injury. However, when they were restrained, they were more negative, especially if they did not understand why they were being restrained. Most believed restraint was a form of punishment. Children believed developing a relationship with staff was more helpful in the case of a crisis than the use of punishment.

Application to Your Clinical Practice

It is paramount that in settings such as these, staff consider the effectiveness of understanding and applying the principles of the nurse–person relationship. The children understood the ineffectiveness of using standardized protocols for crisis management. They asked that they be consulted as to what would be helpful for them in case of a potential crisis. The results of this study demonstrate the importance of considering children's perspectives. Nurses on the unit viewed the use of restraint and seclusion differently from children and did use them as a way to "teach" children what is considered good or bad behaviour, which was ethically suspect. This study reinforced the importance of finding out people's perspectives in informing better and more effective practices for nurses and nursing students.

Adapted from Montreuil, M., Thibeault, C., McHarg, L. et al. (2018). Children's moral experiences of crisis management in a child mental health setting. *International Journal of Mental Health, 27*(5), 1440–1448. https://doi.org/10.1111/inm.12444.

APPLICATIONS

The goal of crisis intervention is to return the person to their previous level of functioning. Achievement of this goal is evidenced by:

- Stabilization of distress symptoms
- Reduction of distress symptoms
- Restoration of functional capabilities to pre-crisis levels
- Referrals for follow-up support care, if indicated (Vertava Health, 2020)

STRUCTURING CRISIS INTERVENTION STRATEGIES

Roberts (2005) provides a seven-stage sequential blueprint for clinical intervention, which can be used to structure the crisis intervention process in nurse–person relationships. This model is compatible with the nursing process sequence of assessment, planning, implementation, and evaluation.

Step 1 (Assessment): Assessing Lethality and Mental Status

Initially, assessment should focus on determining the severity of a person's current danger potential—both to self and to others. Box 21.2 outlines some of the risk factors for those needing assistance and for caregivers.

The Public Services Health & Safety Association (PSHSA) has developed five risk assessment toolkits to help health care organizations protect staff while meeting legal responsibilities for ensuring safe and healthy workplaces and assessing the risk level for dangerous behaviour from people in their care. The toolkits are as follows:

1. Workplace Violence Risk Assessment
2. Individual Client Risk Assessment
3. Flagging
4. Security
5. Personal Safety Response System

The Violence Assessment Tool (VAT) assesses the person's immediate risk of violence. The VAT contains (1) risk indicators, (2) behaviours observed, (3) overall risk rating, and (4) triggers

---

BOX 21.2   Risk Factors for People Needing Assistance and for Caregivers

Risk Factors for People Needing Assistance
- Stressors related to being ill and factors surrounding the illness (unable to work, having to secure child care, uncertainty of prognosis)
- Ability to navigate health care system
- Other issues aside from the illness (e.g., substance use)
- Unmanageable pain
- Behavioural or cognitive impairments
- History of violence

Risk Factors for Caregivers
- Not knowing the person's underlying conditions (e.g., substance use)
- Staffing shortages
- Not knowing a person's propensity for violence
- Strain on the staff due to high acuity levels
- Caregivers experiencing verbal or physical abuse from those they are trying to care for

---

BOX 21.3   Workplace Violence Toolkit

The Canadian Federation of Nurses Unions produced a toolkit to provide a "one-stop shop" for relevant resources for workplace violence and to share and spread the implementation of best practices related to violence prevention and return to work programs in jurisdictions across Canada. The toolkit contains four valuable sections:
1. What Workplace Violence Looks Like—defines various types of workplace violence, has an interactive map of provincial and territorial legislation for each type of violence; highlights front-line stories of health care providers, and contains relevant media clips organized by year.
2. Workplace Violence Research—statistics, legal resources by province and territory, and available research by publication year.

3. Making Change—examples and links to campaigns and public materials, information on collective bargaining agreement language, and case studies of best practices, current standards, and landmark reports.
4. Getting Started—workplace champions, violence prevention training, and guides related to policies and resources for effective implementation of workplace violence prevention strategies.

   This toolkit is an online hub for resources, research, information, tools, and best practices related to violence in health care workplaces that is updated frequently and is available at https://nursesunions.ca/.

---

and contributing factors. It is intended to be used in acute care, long-term care, community care, and emergency care.

Box 21.3 presents an overview of the elements of the VAT, a field-expedient tool for initial assessment of a potential behavioural emergency, developed by the PSHSA. Health care providers and crisis intervention teams (CITs) use this tool and others to assess people with potentially dangerous behaviours. CITs are a collaboration between law enforcement officers and mental health providers that assist individuals in the community who are exhibiting a mental health crisis (Browning et al., 2011; Davis, 2014a, 2014b).

Individuals with psychosis and those under the influence of drugs who are severely agitated or temporarily out of control for medical reasons require immediate triage to stabilize their physical and mental conditions. Crisis states complicated by delirium or nonlethal self-harm necessitate high-priority medical attention before addressing crisis intervention issues. For example, researchers Kouyoumdjian et al. (2019) found that out of 547 adults with mental health disorders living in Toronto, Ontario, 55.8% had interacted with police in the previous year.

Step 2: Establishing Rapport and Engaging the Person in Crisis

Once the initial triage assessment of a person in crisis is completed, the nurse performs a more comprehensive crisis appraisal. This assessment should be specific to the person's current state and circumstances. People in crisis look to health providers to structure interactions. Introduce yourself briefly, and quickly orient the person to the purpose of the crisis questions and how the information will be used, including information about race; religion; age; marital status; medical, education, or employment history; and financial information. The **Personal Information Protection and Electronic Documents Act (PIPEDA)** requires confidentiality (Office of the Privacy Commissioner of Canada, 2021). If people expect family members to give or receive information to health providers when the person is not present, the person needs to sign a consent form.

People experiencing a crisis state require a compassionate, flexible, but clearly directive, calm approach from nurses. Place the person in a quiet, lighted room with no shadows, away from the mainstream of activity. Avoid the use of touch, as the person may be supersensitive to any form of unexpected response from a health provider. If there is a need to restrain a person temporarily, explain what is happening simply and directly. Use fewer rather than more words to explain. Utilize a clear, concrete communication style, with an emphasis on attending to the person's needs.

Only a minimum number of people should be involved with the person, until they are emotionally stabilized. If the person is unable to cooperate, for safety reasons, more than one professional may be needed to stabilize the situation. Depending on the nature of the crisis and the person's responses, a trusted family member may be included.

Speak calmly and use short, clear, direct phrases and questions. James and Gilliland (2013) advocate the use of closed-ended questions in the early stages of crisis intervention, related to safety issues, requesting specific information, and eliciting a commitment to immediate action needed to stabilize the crisis situation.

Careful, accurate listening skills are essential. It is important to discover the person's perception of the crisis—how it developed, how it impacts the person's life, and so on. One way to ask assessment questions can be as follows:

"Is this the first time you have experienced a crisis like this?
Have you had other crises? What were they like?
How did you understand what was happening to you?
How did you problem-solve these crises?"

Questions to assess the person's perception of their emotional coping strength are important. James (2008) suggests asking questions such as, "How were you feeling about this before the crisis got so bad?" "Where do you see yourself headed with this problem?" (p. 51).

Use reflective listening responses to identify feelings (e.g., "It sounds as if you are feeling very sad [angry, lonely] right now."). You can help people focus on relevant points by repeating a phrase, asking for validation or clarification to focus the discussion. Family and significant others can provide essential data related to the person's current crisis state (e.g., documenting changes in behaviour, ingestion of drugs, or medical history) if the person is unable to do so.

Simulation Exercise 21.2 offers an opportunity to understand reflection as a listening response in crisis situations.

Step 3 (Assessment): Identifying Major Problems

Keep the focus on the here and now. Questions should be short and relevant to the crisis.

Request more specific details (e.g., ask who was involved, what happened, and when it happened) if this information is needed.

Ask about the feelings associated with the immediate crisis.

Responses to the person should be brief, empathetic, and clearly related to the person's story.

Note changes in expression, body posture, and vocal inflections as people tell their story and at what points they occur. Be alert for any escalation of agitation or verbal outbursts. If the person shows signs of agitation, ask what would be helpful right now. Ask the person if they need a brief break from talking about the crisis. What thoughts may help the person feel better; such as thinking about a favourite prayer, song, or story? The break may assist the person to gather their emotional resources to further cope with the crisis.

Identify central emotional themes in the person's story (e.g., powerlessness, shame, stigma, hopelessness) to provide a focus for intervention. The following actions will assist in de-escalating the crisis:

- Proceed slowly, with a calm tone and direct communication.
- Affirm the person's efforts and offer encouragement.

SIMULATION EXERCISE 21.2 Using Reflective Responses in a Crisis Situation

Purpose
To provide students with a means of appreciating the multipurpose uses of reflection as a listening response in crisis situations

Procedure
Have one student role-play a person in an emergency department situation involving a common crisis (e.g., fire, heart attack, motor vehicle accident). After this person talks about the crisis situation for 3 to 4 minutes, have each student write down a reflective listening response that they would use with the person in crisis. Have each student read their reflective response to the class. (This can also be done in small groups of students if the class is large.)

Discussion
1. Were you surprised at the variety of reflective themes found in the students' responses?
2. In what ways could differences in the wording or emphasis of a reflective response influence the flow of information?
3. In what ways do reflective responses validate the person's experience?
4. How could you use what you learned from doing this exercise in your clinical practice?

- Summarize content often, and ask for validation so that you and the person are on the same page, with a comprehensive understanding of major issues.
- Periodically ask the person to summarize thoughts.
- Check for personal reservations about part or the entire care plan.

Identifying Feelings

People can have difficulty putting crisis emotions into words because of high anxiety. Nurses can help people clarify important feelings with observations about the person's responses (e.g., "I wonder if because you think your son is using drugs [precipitating event], you feel helpless and confused [person's emotional response] and don't know what to do next [person's behavioural reaction].". "Does that capture what is going on with you?") Checking in with a person helps to ensure that your interpretations represent the person's truth.

People in crisis tend to develop tunnel vision (Dass-Brailsford, 2010). Often, they feel there is no solution. Losing sight of personal assets and potential reserves, which could be used to defuse the crisis, some people are frightened by the intensity of their emotional reactions. People appreciate hearing that most people experience powerful and conflicting feelings in crisis situations. The message you want to get across is "You are not alone, and together we can come up with a plan to deal with this difficult situation." Global reassurance is not helpful, but specific supportive comments that recognize the person's efforts can help to de-escalate a crisis event to workable proportions.

Affirming Personal Strengths

When combined with social support and community resources, professional, **compassionate witnessing** of the situation and calling attention to personal strengths can significantly enhance coping skills. For example, financial resources and knowledge about accessing health care services are critical assets people lose sight of in crisis situations. Reinforce personal strengths as you observe them or as the person identifies them. Simulation Exercise 21.3 provides an opportunity to experience the value of personal support systems in crisis situations.

Providing Explicit Information

Being truthful about what is known and unknown and updating information as you learn about it helps build trust with people in crisis. Even with unknowns, people cope better when uncertainty is briefly acknowledged rather than not mentioned. Explain what is going to happen, step by step. Letting people know as much as possible about progress, treatment, and the consequences of choosing different alternatives allows people to make informed decisions and reduces the heightened anxiety associated with a crisis situation.

Step 4 (Planning): Exploring Alternative Options and Partial Solutions

Step 4 strategies focus on broadening the person's perspective by looking at partial solutions. Breaking tasks down into small, achievable parts empowers people. Proposed strategies should accommodate both the immediate problems and resources.

It is important to encourage the person to make autonomous choices rather than give advice. You can assist people in discussing the consequences, costs, and benefits of choosing one action versus another (e.g., "What would happen if you chose this course of action as compared with

---

SIMULATION EXERCISE 21.3   Personal Support Systems

Purpose
To help students appreciate the breadth and importance of personal support systems in stressful situations

Procedure
All of us have support systems we can use in times of stress (e.g., friends, family, coworkers, clubs, faith-based institutions, recreational groups).
1. Identify a support person or system you use or could use in a time of crisis.
2. Reflect on why you would choose this person or support system.
3. What does this personal support system or person do for you (e.g., listen without judgement; provide honest, objective feedback; challenge you to think; broaden

your perspective; give unconditional support; share your perceptions)? List all relevant reasons.
4. What factors go into choosing your personal support system (e.g., availability, expertise, perception of support)? Which is the most important factor?

Discussion
1. What types of support systems were most commonly used by class or group members?
2. What were the most common reasons for selecting a support person or system?
3. After doing this exercise, what strategies would you advise using for enlarging a personal support system?
4. What applications do you see in this exercise for your nursing practice?

…?" or "What is the worst that could happen if you decided to …?"). Making choices helps people re-establish control. Even a small decision encourages people to become invested in the solution-finding process and hopeful about finding a resolution to a crisis situation.

Involving Immediate Support Systems and Community Resources

Accessing immediate social support and available community resources provides a buffer and can act as a source of information and a sounding board for individuals in a crisis state. Support networks provide practical advice and a sense of security. They are a source of encouragement that can reaffirm a person's worth and help defuse anxiety associated with the uncertainty of a crisis situation. In addition to inquiring about the number and variety of people in the person's support network, find out, "Who does the person and family trust?" and "Who would the person be most comfortable telling about their situation?" It is helpful to learn when the person or family last had contact with the identified person. In crisis situations, many people and their families temporarily withdraw from natural support systems and may need encouragement to reconnect.

Step 5 (Planning): Develop a Realistic Action Plan

Crisis intervention "is action-oriented and situation focused" (Dass-Brailsford, 2010, p. 56). Formulating a realistic action plan starts with prioritizing identified problems and related essential action steps. An effective crisis plan should have a practical, here-and-now, therapeutic, short-term focus and should reflect the person's choices about best options (Loughran, 2011, p. 89). Stabilizing the person through guidance, careful listening, and developing small viable plans helps to defuse the sense of helplessness in a crisis situation.

Focus on the Present

Help people think in terms of short-term intervals and immediate next steps (e.g., "What can you do with the rest of today just to get through it better?"). Examples include getting more information, gathering essential data, taking a walk, calling a family member, or taking time for self. When people begin to take even the smallest step, they gain a sense of control, and this stimulates hope for future mastery of the crisis situation. Thinking about crisis resolution as a whole is counterproductive.

Incorporate Previously Successful Coping Strategies

Looking at past coping strategies can sometimes reveal skills that could be used in resolving the current crisis situation. Ask, "What do you usually do when you have a problem?" or "To whom do you turn when you are in trouble?"

Explore the nature of tension-reducing strategies that the person has used in the past (e.g., aerobics, calling a friend, participating in a hobby, walking in nature). If the person seems immobilized and unable to give an answer about usual coping strategies, you can offer prompts, such as, "Some people talk to their friends, meditate, practice yoga …" Usually, with verbal encouragement, people begin to identify successful coping mechanisms, which can be built on, for use in resolving the current crisis.

Step 6 (Implementation): Developing an Action Plan

Developing Reasonable Goals

Crisis offers people an opportunity to discover and develop new self-awareness about things that are important to them. Developing realistic goals is a critical component of crisis intervention. This process includes becoming aware of choices, letting go of ideas that are toxic or self-defeating, and making the best choice among the viable options. Goal-directed activities should reflect the person's strengths, values, capabilities, beliefs, and preferences. Tangible, achievable goals give people and their families hope that they can get to a different place with resolving their crisis. Goals with meaning to the person are more likely to be accomplished.

Designing Achievable Tasks

Help people choose tasks that are within their capabilities, circumstances, and energy level. Achievable tasks can be as simple as getting more information or making time for self. You can suggest, "What do you think needs to happen first?" or "Let's look at what you might be able to do quickly." Engaging people in simple problem solving reduces crisis-related feelings of helplessness and hopelessness. Problem-solving tasks that strengthen the person's realistic perception of the crisis event, incorporate a person's beliefs and values, and integrate social and environmental supports offer the best chance for success. Loughran (2011) suggests that helping people tap into and use their personal resources to achieve goals facilitates crisis resolution and provides individuals with tools for further personal development.

Providing Structure and Encouragement

People need structure and encouragement as they perform the tasks that will move them forward. Setting time limits and monitoring task achievement is important. Resolving a crisis state is not a straightforward movement. There will be setbacks. People need ongoing affirmation of their efforts. Supportive reinforcement includes validation of the struggles that people are coping with, anticipatory guidance regarding what to expect, and discussion of ambivalent feelings, uncertainty, and fears surrounding the process. Comparing progressive functioning with baseline admission presentations helps nurses and people they work with mutually evaluate progress, foresee areas of necessary focus, and monitor progress toward treatment goals.

Providing Support for Families

Crisis intervention strategies should include support for family members. A crisis affects family dynamics, such that each family member is coping with some sort of emotional fallout brought about by the person's crisis. Additionally, there may be issues requiring family response to an unstable home environment created by the person's absence or an inability to function in their previous roles. There may be legal or safety issues that family members also have to address (Bluhm, 1987).

Individual family members experience a crisis in diverse ways, so different levels of information and support will be required. Bluhm (1987) suggests picturing the family as "a group of people standing together, with arms interlocked. What happens if one family member becomes seriously ill and can no longer stand? The other family members will attempt to carry the person, each person shifting weight to accommodate the additional burden" (p. 44). Giving families an opportunity to talk about the meaning of the crisis for each family member, and offering practical guidance

about resources they can use to support the person and take care of themselves, are important strategies nurses can use with families.

Step 7 (Evaluation): Developing a Termination and Follow-Up Protocol

People should receive verbal instructions, with written discharge or follow-up directives and phone numbers to call for added help or clarification. Although acute symptoms subside with standard crisis intervention strategies, many people will need follow-up for residual clinical issues.

People need to be encouraged to mobilize community resources to provide essential support. Some people are reluctant to use social services, medications, or mental health services, even in the short term, because of the stigma they feel about their use (Coleman et al., 2017). Others are cautious about the need for follow-up. Nurses can help people and their families sort out their concerns, assess their practicality, and develop viable contacts. If indicated, nurses can facilitate the referral process by sharing information with community agencies and by giving people enough information to follow through on getting additional assistance. Having written referral information available regarding eligibility requirements, location, and accessibility can make a difference in the person's interest and adherence. Simulation Exercise 21.4 provides an opportunity to practise crisis intervention skills.

SIMULATION EXERCISE 21.4 Interacting in Crisis Situations

Purpose

To give students experience in using the three-stage model of crisis intervention

Procedure

1. Break the class up into groups of three. One student should take the role of the person in crisis and one the role of the nurse; the third student functions as the observer.
2. Using one of the following role-plays or one from your current clinical setting, engage the person, and use the crisis intervention strategies presented in this chapter to frame your interventions.
3. The observer should provide feedback.

This exercise can also be handled as discussion points rather than a role-play, with small-group or class feedback as to how students would have handled the situations.

Role-Play

Kainat is a 23-year-old graduate student who has been dating Dan for the past 3 years. They plan to marry within the next 6 months. Last summer, she had a brief affair with another graduate student while Dan was away but never told him. She is seeing you in the clinic, having just found out that she has herpes from that encounter.

Wase is a 59-year-old woman who is postmenopausal and has been admitted for diagnostic testing and possible surgery. She has just found out that her tests reveal a malignancy in her colon with possible metastasis to her liver. You are the nurse responsible for her care.

Bill's mother was admitted last night to the ICU, with sepsis. She is on life support and intravenous antibiotics. Bill had a close relationship with his mother earlier in his life, but he has not seen her in the past year. You are the nurse for the shift but do not yet know her well.

Discussion

1. After completing this exercise, what would you want to do differently when communicating with the person in crisis?
2. What was the effect of using the three-stage model of crisis intervention as a way of organizing your approach to the crisis situation?

MENTAL HEALTH EMERGENCIES

Mental health emergencies present significant challenges for nurses. Whether encountered in the community or with people admitted to an emergency department, these people often present as a danger to themselves or others. They present with chaotic distress behaviours that are not under the person's control.

In addition to mental health emergencies, nurses should be aware of the presentation of co-occurring disorders. A person with a co-occurring disorder presents with both a mental health disorder and a substance use disorder. Often, these people will stop taking their prescribed psychotropic medications and instead self-medicate with other, nonprescribed medications (sometimes from other family members or friends) or illicit drugs or alcohol. People may feel that their psychiatric symptoms have subsided or even gone away for a while when they self-medicate. The problems arise with the propensity of overdose and the possibility of going into drug-induced delirium (also known in the law enforcement field as "excited delirium") or other somatic effects (e.g., cardiac problems) or drug-induced effects (e.g., difficulty driving, impulsive behaviour). Nurses should be aware that these people may present at the emergency department seeking legitimate care for their symptoms or may present to obtain medications (e.g., narcotics, benzodiazepines) that they are either out of or use regularly, which in turn can counter or repress their psychiatric symptoms (Davis, 2014b; Vierheller & Denton, 2014).

One of the most significant mental health emergencies that Canadians are facing is the opioid crisis. Opioids produce a feeling of well-being and euphoria; these drugs can be obtained through licit or illicit channels. A person who has a great deal of pain welcomes the relief from consuming them. Popular opioids are codeine, fentanyl, morphine, and oxycodone. Fentanyl is the most problematic drug because it is highly potent and increases the risk of death; between 2016 and 2018, there were 11500 deaths from opioid overdoses in Canada (Canadian Centre on Substance Use and Addiction [CCSA], 2021). This number has increased significantly every year. To better understand the scope of the crisis in Canada, view the interactive map from Health Canada's National Report: Apparent Opioid-Related Deaths in Canada, (Government of Canada, 2021). Note the high numbers of death related to opioids and other illicit drugs in British Columbia. Some of the reasons for opioid misuse and consequent deaths are: public misunderstanding of addictive risk; availability of illicit opioids (including from family and friends); frequent opioid prescribing for pain relief; and risk factors such as genetics, trauma, poverty, and food and housing insecurity. The most immediate and effective treatment is the administration of naloxone, which is widely available in a kit and obtained as a free resource from pharmacies and other agencies associated with helping those with addictions. It is an opioid antagonist and counteracts the life-threatening depression of the central nervous and respiratory systems. Although traditionally administered by emergency response personnel, naloxone can be administered by minimally trained laypeople. Naloxone is used if a person is hard to wake up, has pinpoint pupils and cold clammy skin, and is not breathing normally. The effects of naloxone last 20 to 90 minutes but may wear off and a second dose may be required. The kit has syringes and needles, a nasal adapter for the syringes and a separate nasal spray. Each kit contains two doses. Naloxone may be injected in the muscle, in a vein, under the skin, or sprayed into the nose. The person should be assessed after receiving the drug to ensure there are no opioids left in their system (HealthLinkBC, 2020).

Mental health emergencies require an immediate coordinated response designed to alleviate the potential for harm and restore basic stability. Examples of a mental health emergencies include suicidal, homicidal, or threatening behaviour; self-injury; severe drug or alcohol impairment; and highly erratic or unusual behaviour associated with serious mental health disorders. Unpredictability, acute emotions, and acting-out behaviours increase the intensity of mental health emergencies. Myer and Conte (2006) describe a triage assessment system (TAS) for mental health crises that can help nurses understand a person's responses across three domains: affective, behavioural, and cognitive. The research on this tool is very positive. All three response domains are interrelated, but Myer and Conte suggest that clinicians first focus on the person's affective reaction—for example, anger, fear, or sadness. Box 21.4 provides de-escalation tips for use with people presenting in the community with mental health emergencies.

To avoid retraumatizing individuals with mental health disorders who are already experiencing a chaotic, distressed state, especially acute anxiety, model respect while communicating with them. People with mental health disorders respond best to respectful, calmly presented suggestions rather than commands.

It is helpful to provide additional personal space for individuals who have experienced a crisis and who have a mental health disorder. Keep communication calm, short, compassionate, and well defined. Do not indicate that you feel threatened or argue the logic of a situation. Avoid intimidating the person but set reasonable limits. Proceed slowly with purpose. Avoid sudden movements. Whenever possible, offer simple choices with structured coaching. People experiencing a psychiatric emergency usually require medication for stabilization of symptoms and close supervision.

BOX 21.4   De-escalation Tips for Mental Health Emergencies

De-escalation Tips

Following are some suggestions that can be used by nurses to de-escalate people's responsive behaviours and implement person-preferred interventions to assist them to cope.

1. Always identify yourself.
2. Talk and think calm.
3. Ask people how they are doing or what's going on.
4. Ask people if they are hurt (assess for medical problems).
5. Ask people if they were having some difficulty or what happened before they got upset.
6. Remember why the person is in the hospital.
7. Find a staff member that has a good rapport and relationship with the person and have them talk to the person. Let the person know you are there to listen.
8. Offer medication if appropriate.
9. Help people remember and use coping mechanisms they identified on the Patient Reported Therapeutic Interventions Survey.
10. If a person screams and swears, reply with a calm nod, say okay, and don't react.
11. Use a team or third-party approach. If the person is wearing down one staff member, have another take over (10 minutes of talking might avoid a restraint incident).
12. Reassure people and maintain professional boundaries (tell people you want them to be safe, that you are there to help them).
13. Allow quiet time for people to respond—silent pauses are important.
14. Ask the person, if they would be willing to talk to you (repeat requests, persistently, kindly).
15. Respect needs to communicate in different ways (recognize possible language or cultural differences as well as the fear, shame, and embarrassment the person may be experiencing).
16. Empower people. Encourage them with every step they take toward calming themselves.
17. Make it okay to try to talk over the upsetting situation even though it may be very painful or difficult.
18. Acknowledge the significance of the situation for the person.
19. Ask the person how else you can help.
20. Ask the person's permission to share important conversations with other caregivers for ongoing discussion.

From: RNAO. (n.d.). De-escalation Tips. *Nursing Best Practice Guidelines*. https://bpgmobile.rnao.ca/node/849.

Types of Mental Health Emergencies

Violence

Violence is a mental health emergency that creates a critical challenge to the safety, well-being, and health of the person and others in their environment. Nurses should always assume an organic component (e.g., drugs, alcohol, psychosis, or delirium) underlying the aggression in people presenting with disorganized, impulsive or violent behaviours, until it is proven otherwise (Penterman & Nijman, 2011).

The person's body language offers clues to escalating anxiety, through pacing, inability to have a conversation, difficulty sitting still, excessive talking, using a raised volume of voice, clenching fists, threatening gestures, or darting eye movements. Table 21.1 presents indicators of increasing tension as precursors to violence. Common contributing factors are a history of violence, childhood abuse, substance use, neurodevelopmental disorders, problems with impulse control, and psychosis, particularly when accompanied by command hallucinations.

Treatment of people who are violent consists of immediately providing a safe, nonstimulating environment for the person. Often, the possibility of aggression is reduced if the person is taken to an area with less sensory input. The person should be checked thoroughly for potential weapons and physically disarmed, if necessary. Short-term medication usually is indicated to help defuse potentially harmful behaviours. The nurse should briefly identify why the medication is being given, and then carefully monitor the person for physical and behavioural responses.

Sexual Assault

Sexual assault is a serious form of interpersonal victimization, which violates the core of self in ways that are probably only second to murder. The person's subjective stress is intense and long-lasting. In the immediate aftermath of a sexual assault, everything should be done to help the person feel safe and supported. The person should be taken to a private room and not be left alone. Evidence, if it is to be collected, requires that the person not shower or douche prior to being examined. Larger emergency departments have a sexual assault nurse examiner (SANE) program, staffed by a specially trained nurse who provides first-response medical care and crisis intervention (James & Gilliland, 2013; Nova Scotia, 2019).

TABLE 21.1 Behavioural Indicators of Potential Violence

Behavioural Categories	Potential Indicators
Mental status	Confused
	Paranoid ideation
	Disorganized
	Poor impulse control
Motor behaviour	Agitated, pacing
	Exaggerated gestures
	Rapid breathing
Body language	Eyes darting
	Prolonged (staring) eye contact or lack of eye contact
	Spitting
	Pale or red (flushed) face
	Menacing posture, throwing things
Speech patterns	Rapid, pressured
	Incoherent, mumbling, repeatedly making the same statements
	Menacing tones, raised voice, use of profanity
	Verbal threats
Affect	Belligerent
	Labile
	Angry

Anderson, K., & Jenson, C. (2019). Violence risk–assessment screening tools for acute care mental health settings: Literature review. *Archives of Psychiatric Nursing, 33*(1), 112–119. https://doi.org/10.1016/j.apnu.2018.08.012Get rights and content.

Adapting psychological first aid (PFA) to people who have been raped and sexually assaulted is a helpful, comprehensive, action-oriented intervention (Eifling & Moy, 2015; Forbes et al., 2011). PFA consists of eight core actions:

1. Contact and engagement
2. Safety and comfort
3. Stabilization
4. Information gathering
5. Practical assistance
6. Connection with social supports
7. Information on coping support
8. Linkage with collaborative services

In a sexual assault situation, there should be no blaming or conjecture about the role in the attack of the person who was assaulted. Sexual assault is always an act of violence and control. It is not a voluntary sexual act, even if the perpetrator and person assaulted are known to each other. Follow-up referral to a mental health professional can help the person cope with stress symptoms, shame, and the intrusive thoughts that frequently develop after the assault.

Psychosis

An acute psychotic break represents a serious mental health behavioural emergency. People with psychosis or delirium have disorganized thinking, reduced insight, and limited personal judgement. People experiencing *command hallucinations*, defined as auditory hallucinations that direct the person to carry out an act, are at a higher risk for suicide and aggression. Medication is almost always indicated to manage acute psychotic symptoms, and one-to-one supervision is required (Randall et al., 2017). Allow the person sufficient space to feel safe, and never try to subdue a person by yourself. Remain calm and positive. Use fewer rather than more words. An open expression, eye contact, a calm voice, and simple concrete words invite trust. Do not use touch, as it can be misinterpreted.

Suicide

Suicide is the ninth leading cause of death in Canada. For every person who dies by suicide, there are: 5 self-inflicted injury hospitalizations, 25–30 suicide attempts, and 7–10 people profoundly affected by suicide loss (Government of Canada, 2016). *Suicide* is defined as any self-injurious behaviour that results in the death of an individual. Suicide is classified as a behavioural emergency. The World Health Organization (WHO) describes death by suicide as a public health priority (WHO, 2016). The Joint Commission (2017) identifies suicide as a **sentinel event** and calls for appropriate screening in behavioural care units, medical–surgical units, and emergency departments, to avert a death. People turn to suicide as an option in times of acute distress, when under the influence of drugs, or when they believe there are no other alternatives. Impulsivity and hopelessness often go together with suicidal behaviours. Behavioural indicators of escalating suicidal ideation include a noteworthy change in behaviour, often characterized by a burst of energy. Examples of changes in behaviour of an individual who died by suicide include:

- A father gave away all of his deceased wife's jewelry 2 weeks before his death.
- An 18-year-old young man went door-to-door in his neighbourhood, apologizing for his past erratic behaviour, 3 days before he shot himself.

- An outpatient with a chronic mental health disorder shared personal information and talked extensively in group therapy for the first time the week before he jumped off a bridge.

Impact of Suicide on Others

An individual who dies by suicide creates long-lasting effects for families, friends, coworkers, and the larger community. Individuals who are experiencing suicidal thoughts are often hesitant to talk about their feelings, due to stigma and hopelessness. They can be quite isolative or hard to engage in meaningful relationships. It is hard for family members or friends to know how to respond. People who talk about harming themselves are not necessarily at less risk, but there is more opportunity to prevent suicide. Every suicidal statement, however indirect, should be taken seriously. Even with people who indicate that they are "just kidding," the fact that they have verbalized the threat places them at greater risk.

Passive suicidal wishes and actions, such as not taking medications, not practicing safer sex, drinking too much, driving too fast, and not caring if they are in an accident warrant exploration. Pay attention to statements such as "I don't think I can go on without …," "I sometimes wish I could just disappear," or "People would be better off without me," as they are examples of suicidal ideation. Such statements require further clarification (e.g., "You say you can't go on without … Can you tell me more about what you mean?"). Nurses should be careful to use sensitive terminology around suicide. A good example of appropriate terms can be found on the website for the Canadian Association of Mental Health at https://www.camh.ca/-/media/files/words-matter-suicide-language-guide.pdf.

Nurses should ask directly:

"Do you have any thoughts of hurting yourself?" (include frequency and intensity of thoughts). Do you have a plan? Individuals with a detailed plan and the means to carry it out are at greatest risk for suicide. If the person answers yes, you should assess the lethality of the plan and inquire about the method and the person's knowledge and skills about its use, along with the accessibility of the means to facilitate the suicide attempt.

You should also ask the following questions if you have any concerns about suicidal intent:

- Have you ever rehearsed the plan for suicide? What was that like? How did you interrupt the rehearsal?
- What do you hope to accomplish with the suicide attempt? (look for hopelessness, including severity and duration)
- Have you thought about when you might do this? (immediate versus chronic thinking)
- Have you ever attempted suicide in the past? What happened? What type of care did you receive? How was it helpful?
- Has anyone in your family ever attempted or died by suicide?
- Who are you able to turn to when you are in trouble? (social support)
- What thoughts or activities help you to interrupt thoughts of suicide?

Risk Factors

People with mental health disorders, particularly depression, bipolar disorder, schizophrenia with command hallucinations, panic disorder, and comorbidity with substance use are more at risk for suicide than other people. Although psychiatric diagnosis is a risk factor for suicide, many people who have died by suicide have no previous psychiatric history and no evidence of prior suicide attempts (Rittenmeyer, 2012). The WHO (2017) identified individuals who are unable to deal with life stresses, experience a break-up of a relationship, or experience chronic pain or illness as having a possibility of an impulsive suicide attempt. Individuals who are isolated or experienced conflict, disaster, violence, abuse or loss are also at risk (WHO, 2017).

The highest suicide rates are committed by those aged 40 to 59. However, suicide ranks second as a leading cause of death for people aged 15 to 34. Males are far more likely to die by suicide than females (Navaneelan, 2017).

Women attempt three times to every one of the reported nonfatal attempts by men. Other high-risk factors include the following:

- Previous attempts or family history of suicide
- Family history of child abuse
- History of alcohol and substance use
- Major physical illness
- Social isolation, lack of social support
- Recent major loss
- History of trauma
- A sense of hopelessness
- Local epidemics of suicide
- Easy access to lethal means
- Not obtaining help due to stigma
- Within the first few weeks of discharge from a psychiatric hospital
- Within 72 hours of discharge from a hospital, including the emergency department (Joint Commission International, 2020; Government of Canada, 2016)

Stabilization of symptoms and safety of the person are the most immediate concerns with people experiencing a suicidal crisis. Possible weapons (e.g., mirrors, belts, knitting needles, scissors, razors, medications, clothes hangers) should be removed.

Explain in a calm, compassionate manner the reason why the items should not be in the person's possession and where they will be kept. People need to be assured that the items will be returned when the danger of self-harm is resolved. Connectedness with others is considered a key protective factor in suicide prevention (Rodgers, 2017).

Death by suicide occurs more frequently when a person is hospitalized than one would suppose. People experiencing intense pain, a terminal prognosis, substance use, or a recent bereavement are at higher risk. People have greater access to potentially lethal means to die by suicide, and health providers do not immediately think of suicide in medical health situations. The Joint Commission International has determined that 1089 deaths from suicide occurred between the years 2010 to 2014 within 72 hours of discharge from a hospital setting, including the emergency department. This has been attributed to the health care staff not completing a comprehensive assessment for suicide (Joint Commission International, 2020). Documentation of a suicidal risk assessment, interventions, and the person's responses is essential. Included in the documentation should be quotes made by the person, details of observed behaviour, a review of identified risk factors, and the person's responses to initial crisis intervention strategies. The names and times of anyone you notified and contacts with family should be documented. Protective measures, such as individuals who the person can call in a time of crisis, ways the person can reduce their desire to die, and available telephone numbers for help, are important to assess and document. The Joint Commission International requires that any death that is not consistent with a person's disease process, or any permanent loss of function occurring as a consequence of an attempted suicide in a hospital, be reported as a sentinel event (Joint Commission International).

Most psychiatric inpatient settings and emergency departments have written suicide precaution protocols that must be followed when someone presents with suicidal ideation. People exhibiting high-risk behaviours require constant, one-to-one staff observation; a person who is potentially suicidal should never be left alone. Monitoring of people who are suicidal ranges from constant 1:1 observation to 15- or 30-minute observational checks. Less restrictive checks can include supervised bathroom visits, unit restriction or restriction to public areas, and supervised sharps. Nursing staff need to be familiar with indications, policies for appropriate pharmacological intervention, seclusion, restraints, and body and belongings searches (Nova Scotia, 2019).

The frequency and type of observation is dependent on the suicidal assessment of the person.

Consistent with a high risk for suicidal behaviour is a sense of hopelessness, lack of meaningful connection with others, and the feeling of being a burden to others. Acceptance of the person is a critical element of rapport. Nurses need to explore their own feelings about suicidal behaviours as the basis for understanding the person in danger of self-injury.

Suicidal ideation waxes and wanes, so careful observation is critical even after the acute crisis has subsided.

Competencies for Registered Psychiatric Nurses in Canada

Entry-level registered psychiatric nurses in Canada have a specialized body of knowledge of mental health and mental health disorders. Listed below are their competencies (Registered Psychiatric Nurse Regulators of Canada, 2014):

- Nurses have a strong foundation in communication, psychology, sociology, mental health and illness, developmental and intellectual disability, psychiatric nursing theory, research and ethics.
- They integrate the foundation of knowledge, skills and theories from nursing and other disciplines into psychiatric nursing practice.
- They have foundational knowledge from the biological and nursing sciences, and they possess a range of general medical and surgical nursing competencies.
- They apply critical thinking, problem solving, clinical reasoning and judgment into their professional practice.
- Psychiatric nursing education programs prepare entry-level Registered Psychiatric Nurses to practise safely, competently and ethically in a variety of practice settings, in situations of health and illness, and with diverse populations of individuals, families, groups and community
- They enter practice with competencies that are transferable across practice settings, even though their psychiatric nursing education program may not have exposed them to all practice environments or client types.
- They practise autonomously, and continue to consolidate theoretical and experiential learning through collaboration, mentoring and support from the interprofessional team.
- They practise collaboratively and assume leadership roles.
- They practise as a self-regulated profession and practise according to federal/provincial/ territorial legislation and regulation.

Assessments should be repeated whenever changes in behaviour are noted and again before discharge. The person and nurse should develop a safety planning intervention (Stanley & Brown, 2012). This document is not a contract for safety but rather a collaborative plan that empowers the person to determine ways to reduce the drive to die by suicide. The safety planning intervention helps the person to identify the following:

- Warning signs of suicide
- Internal coping strategies: the person identifies what they can do to interrupt thoughts about suicide
- People or social settings that can assist the person to distract from the drive to die by suicide
- People in the person's life that can be called to assist the person to maintain safety
- Professionals or agencies that the person can call during a crisis; available 24/7/365 (Crisis Services Canada, 2021) and 1-800-273-8255 for veterans (National Suicide Prevention Lifeline, 2021; Sadek, 2019)
- Ways to make the environment safe by removing all available means to die by suicide

The nurse and the person should discuss these items together. Following each discussion, the person should write down the relevant safety plan information that was discussed so the person can refer to this safety plan at a later date. The safety planning intervention should begin after the person has had an assessment for suicidal intent, and it should be revisited by the nurse after each assessment.

Crisis Intervention Teams and Co-Response Teams

In the community, police and nurses or social workers with special training are important professionals to assist in behavioural health emergencies (Canadian Mental Health Association [CMHA], 2009) Community-based Crisis Intervention Teams (CITs) offer a successful model of collaborative interventions between specially trained law enforcement officers and mental health care providers designed to treat rather than incarcerate people with mental health disorders with comorbid behavioural emergencies (Davis, 2014a, 2014b) and symptoms (Watson & Fulambarker, 2012). A professional co-responder such as a registered nurse will have specialized knowledge in the assessment of medical conditions particularly when there is more than one presenting condition like drug use and diabetes. They are also able to set priorities, which results in life-saving interventions. The combined knowledge of the criminal and health care systems that each responder brings to an intervention, is invaluable in obtaining timely help for the person. Emergency nurses and paramedics are important stakeholders and collaborators with CIT-trained law enforcement officers (Ellis, 2011; Ralph, 2010).

There are over 3 000 CIT programs internationally, while only a small number of CITs operate in Canada, primarily in Halifax, Toronto, Hamilton, and some divisions of the Ontario Provincial Police (Koziarski, 2018). According to Koziarski, the co-response team model is more prevalent in Canada than elsewhere. York Region, in Ontario, has created a Co-Response Mental Health Unit to provide on-scene mental health assessment, consultation, and support to their regional police service and paramedics, including a mental health support worker. Of the CIT programs, cities have created unique programs to meet their unique needs. The city of Toronto has instituted mobile CITs, which are partnerships between Toronto Police Services and participating area hospitals, where a mental health nurse and a specially trained officer are paired to respond to situations involving a person experiencing a mental health crisis. Vancouver has Community Response Units specialized to work with youths. They operate several "cars" and teams to provide specialized services and support to Vancouver youth. Of these, Car 87—Mental Health Car—is not just for youths. It is a partnership between the Vancouver Police Department and Vancouver Costal Health's Access and Assessment Centre's Crisis Response Team. A constable is teamed with a registered nurse or registered psychiatric nurse to provide on-site assessment and intervention for people living with a mental health disorder. (Toronto Police Service, n.d; Vancouver Police Department, n.d). In Newfoundland and Labrador, the RCMP partnered with provincial health officials to create Mobile Crisis Response teams consisting of a registered nurse or other mental health worker and an officer, and together, they have responded to over 5000 mental health–related calls since 2018 (Northcott, 2020). These are a few examples of the growth and development of unique team partnerships between multiple agencies to assist in behavioural health crisis situations.

People experiencing mental health emergencies may perceive necessary medical procedures as being intrusive and threatening. It is important to adhere to a nursing principle that, before starting any procedure, you should tell the person exactly what you are going to do and why the procedure is necessary, with a request to cooperate. If the person refuses, do not insist, but explain the reason for doing the procedure in a calm, quiet voice. If you can help people regain a sense of control, they are more likely to cooperate with you. Your movements should be calm, firm, and respectful.

DISASTER MANAGEMENT

Disaster and Mass Trauma Situations

A *disaster* is defined as "a great or sudden misfortune" (Canadian Oxford Dictionary, n.d.). Recent years have borne witness to more natural disasters, terrorism, and war than the world has seen in many decades. Terrorist attacks spontaneously occur in many areas, and the threat of nuclear war from adversarial nations has heightened attention and tension. Terrorist attacks have stimulated a fresh awareness of the need for community and national planned responses to disaster events. These events can happen anywhere and at any time to innocent masses of people.

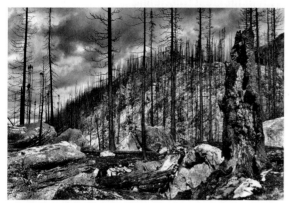

Fig. 21.1 Each year in Canada, an average of 8600 wildfires burn 2.5 million hectares of land, threatening communities and homes and requiring the evacuation of residents. Reducing the threat to communities requires understanding both biophysical risk and the social aspects of wildfire risk management. This photo shows damage from the Excelsior wildfire in Maligne Valley, Jasper National Park. Photo: iStock.com/IanChrisGraham.

In Canada, we experience wildfires, avalanches, earthquakes, floods, landslides, hurricanes, and tornadoes (see Fig. 21.1). In fact, we are ranked the country with the second-most number of tornadoes, behind the United States (Government of Canada, 2019). Examples of some traumas that Canadians have endured included the following: On April 23, 2018, in Toronto, Ontario, a young man drove a rented van onto a sidewalk filled with pedestrians and killed 10 people and injured another 15 (Humphreys et al., 2018). On May 1, 2016, a fire started outside of Fort McMurry, Alberta, and burned until August 2, 2016. The fire caused 80000 people to flee, destroyed 2400 buildings and caused an estimated $3.8 billion in insured damage (The Canadian Press, 2017). Between April 18 and 19, 2020, a denturist killed 22 people in Nova Scotia. He dressed in an RCMP uniform and drove a car that looked very similar to a police car, making it possible to randomly kill many unsuspecting people (CBC News, 2020).

Mass trauma events are events such as wars, political violence, torture, and natural disasters; these events raise important mental health, human rights, and political issues. There are millions of people around the world who are suffering the debilitating psychological effects of wars, armed conflicts, torture, and natural disasters (see Table 21.2). Canada has a long history of supporting refugees fleeing countries destabilized by conflict or lacking resources to live. The Canadian Mental Health Commission has provided resources and coordination across Canada to assist refugees (Agic et al., 2016). The approach to assisting

TABLE 21.2	Canadian Emergency Response System
Threat	• Presence of a hazard and an exposure pathway by inhalation, ingestion, or skin absorption results in the need for measurement (e.g., of air quality, food samples, blood samples) • Natural (e.g., floods, avalanches, landslides) • Human-induced (e.g., pollution, dam failures, factory explosions) • Accidental trauma (e.g., train derailment) results in human injury or death • Intentional (e.g., mass shootings, wars, torture)
Legislation	• *Emergency Management Act*: federal level; lead is Minister of Public Safety Canada • Each province and territory has emergency management legislation under the umbrella of the *Emergency Management Act*
Response Activities	• Situational awareness: communication, synthesizing information, liaising with stakeholders and contacts at all levels of government • Risk assessment: impact on environment, critical infrastructure, and the economy • Planning: mitigate risks and development of a response, i.e., deploying hazard plans, contingency plans, and action plans • Logistics: provide required personnel, goods, transportation, etc.
Public Communications	• Dissemination of clear, factual information that will assist in minimizing the threat

Adapted from the Government of Canada. (2011). *National emergency response system*. https://www.publicsafety.gc.ca/cnt/rsrcs/pblctns/ntnl-rspns-sstm/ntnl-rspns-sstm-eng.pdf.

refugees in Canada has been reducing risk factors, offering culturally sensitive services, sensitizing Canadians to the needs of different cultures, from immigration officers to health personnel, and communicating the message that everyone is responsible to help newcomers integrate into society.

Planning for Disaster Management

In Canada, the National Emergency Response System is responsible for setting forth recommendations related to creating an effective disaster plan (Public Safety Canada, 2018a). Community-based governments and businesses, first responders, hospitals, and health providers are expected to be actively involved in community disaster planning. Around the globe, tsunamis in Indonesia, earthquakes occurring in rapid succession in China, Iceland, and South America, the threat of nations developing nuclear weapons, pandemics like COVID-19 and SARS remind us of the need for a global approach to emergency preparedness. The Sendai Framework was adapted by the United Nations (UN) to promote a prevention-based approach to international disasters. The emphasis in the Sendai Framework is on early warning when a disaster may take place; predicting the event and needs for prevention of casualties; recovery after the disaster; and rehabilitation once recovery of the disaster takes place. The Sendai Framework goals will be implemented and utilized between the years of 2015 and 2030 (Aitsi-Selmi & Murray, 2016).

Strategies for creating and sustaining community-wide emergency preparedness are published by The Joint Commission International (2020). These plans include the following:

- Exploring ethical considerations, including legal authority and environmental concerns
- Education and information sharing
- Provider and community engagement
- Development of clinical processes and operations, performance improvement
- Hospital care, outpatient care, Emergency Medical Services (EMS), public health, and public safety
- Local, provincial and territorial, and federal government emergency-management standards stress promotion of adaptive function (Joint Commission International, 2020)

Disaster planning can act as a deterrent to terrorist activity and as an immediate resource in a disaster situation. Disaster management requires providing immediate physical and emotional first aid.

The all-hazards risk approach is a set of actions required to mitigate the effects of emergencies. Irrespective of the nature of the event, they are essentially all the same, thereby permitting an optimization of scarce planning, response, and support resources. An all-hazards approach incorporates natural and man-made hazard threats, including traditional emergency management events such as flooding and industrial accidents, as well as national security events such as acts of terrorism and cyber events (Public Safety Canada, 2018b).

Critical Incident Debriefing

Disasters, deliberate violence, and terrorist attacks are random events that produce permanent changes in people's lives and shake their perception of being in charge of their lives. Critical incident stress management (CISM) is used to help people who have witnessed or experienced a crisis event to externalize and process its meaning. Guided sharing of the crisis experiences by those most impacted by it can be healing. CISM may be done on an individual basis, if indicated by the incident. The debriefing allows the people involved in a traumatic situation to achieve a sense of psychological closure. The debriefing team also teaches participants about the nature of distress reactions and offers helpful hints to reduce their effects (Everly & Mitchell, 2017).

Critical Incident Stress Debriefing Process

A specially trained professional generally leads the debriefing. The leader introduces the purpose of the CISM and assures the participants that everything said in the session will be kept confidential. People are asked to identify who they are and what happened from their perspective, including the role they played in the incident. After preliminary factual data are addressed, the next step is to explore feelings. The leader asks participants to recall the first thing they remember thinking or feeling about the incident. Participants are asked to discuss any stress symptoms they may have related to the incident. The final discussion focuses on the emotional reactions associated with the critical incident. This part of the session is followed by psychoeducational strategies to reduce stress. Any lingering questions are answered, and the leader summarizes the high points of the critical incident debriefing for the group (Everly & Mitchell, 2017).

Critical incident debriefings are used with families witnessing a tragedy involving a family member, for children and adolescents dealing with the death of a classmate, mass murders, robberies, and environmental disasters. A **critical incident stress debriefing** offers people an opportunity to externalize a traumatic experience through being able to vent feelings, discuss their role in the situation, develop a realistic sense of the big picture, and receive peer support in putting the crisis event in perspective (Everly & Mitchell, 2017).

Critical Incident Debriefing for Health Care Providers

The COVID-19 pandemic was a trigger for post-traumatic stress disorder (PTSD). There is not yet any current data indicating the incidence or prevalence of PTSD in Canada, but there will be a significant increase due the anxiety of managing people who are infected, those dying from COVID-19, and front-line workers becoming infected and some colleagues dying (Public Health Agency of Canada, 2020).

Health care providers who assist or witness critical incidents can be vulnerable to experience "secondary traumatization" similar to that experienced by direct survivors of the incident. The providers can experience PTSD and display symptoms of anxiety and depression. Principles of critical incident debriefing can also be applied to strengthen the emotional coping skills of staff working in clinical settings on units with frequent or unexpected loss. Support for nurses, first responders, and emergency health care providers includes the use of employee assistance programs (EAPs). In Canada, we have a national action plan for public health safety workers (Public Safety Canada, 2019). Box 21.5 "outlines the seven phases of formal critical incident stress debriefing (CISD) designed to promote the emotional processing of crisis events and support positive coping mechanisms for future experiences" (RNAO, 2017, p. 84).

Community Response Patterns

The Joint Commission International (2020) explicitly portrays disaster management and emergency preparedness as a community responsibility. When disaster strikes, the existence and function of the community are significantly impaired. Initially, people are confused and stunned. Emotions vary as the extent of the impact is realized. The closer the person is to the crisis event, the more intense the impact. The immediate concern is protection of self and those closest to them. By preparing for a disaster, the community is more resilient and able to recover faster (Zukowski, 2014).

Disaster Management in Health Care Settings

All hospitals are required to form disaster committees composed of key departments within the hospital, including nursing. Nurses interested in emergency volunteer activities should become aware of credentialing requirements to ensure their participation as part of a national emergency volunteer system for health care providers. Hospital and community disaster planning must be coordinated so that all phases of the disaster cycle are covered. Designated hospital personnel must receive training to carry out triage at the emergency department entrance. Protocols should contain the capability to relocate staff and people seeking care to another facility if necessary, and a plan must be in place detailing mechanisms for equipment resupply. Policies regarding notification, maintenance of accurate records, and establishment of a facility control centre are required (Joint Commission International, 2020).

BOX 21.5 Critical Incident Stress Debriefing (CISD) Steps

The following table outlines the seven phases of formal critical incident stress debriefing (CISD), designed to promote the emotional processing of crisis events and support positive coping mechanisms for future experiences.

Phase 1: Introductory Phase
Facilitator introduces themselves, confidentiality is carefully explained, and the person is urged to talk if they wish.

Phase 2: Facts Phase
The person is asked to describe what happened during the incident, from their own perspective. This may include stating who they are, where they were, and what they heard, saw, smelled, and did. This helps to give a total picture of what happened.

Phase 3: Feeling and Thoughts Phase
The person describes their first thoughts about the event. The discussion becomes more personal.

Phase 4: Emotions
The person discusses their emotional reactions. This phase can be combined with Phase 3 (Feeling and Thought Phase).

Phase 5: Assessment and Symptom Phase
Physical and psychological symptoms are noted and discussed.

Phase 6: Teaching Phase
The facilitator and person discuss stress reaction and responses and coping strategies.

Phase 7: Re-entry Phase
The person asks questions, wraps up any loose ends, answers outstanding questions, provides final reassurances, and makes a plan of action. Team leaders summarize what has occurred, provide team members with contact information, and draw the debriefing to a close.

From Registered Nurses' Association of Ontario. (2017). *Crisis intervention for adults using a trauma-informed approach: Initial four weeks of management* (3rd ed.). Author. p. 84. https://rnao.ca/sites/rnao-ca/files/bpg/Crisis_Intervention_FINAL_WEB.pdf.

Citizen Responders

Unsolicited citizen responders play a large role in sudden onset, large-scale disasters. Emergency plans should anticipate the presence of unsolicited individuals who respond to the disaster, wishing to assist. As part of a comprehensive community disaster plan, an infrastructure for coordinating their efforts should be developed. Public education related to the citizen role in disaster management is essential.

HELPING CHILDREN COPE WITH TRAUMA

In Canada, 1.4% of children have experienced trauma. If the child lives in poverty or has a parent with a mental health disorder or a criminal record, they are four times as likely to experience trauma as a child without these disadvantages (Children's Health Policy Centre, 2011). Pre-existing exposure to traumatic events and lack of social support increase vulnerability. Children do not have the same resources when coping with traumatic events as adults do. It is not unusual for children to demonstrate regressive behaviours as a reaction to crisis. While helping the child work through the emotional aspects of a trauma, be sure to utilize language appropriate to the child's level of development and cognitive ability. Assess how the child perceives the stressor, and determine the child's self-perception of how they are able to problem-solve (Pfefferbaum et al., 2012).

Children will look for cues from key adults in their lives and tend to mirror their adult caregivers, so it is essential to communicate calmly and with confidence. More than anything else, children need reassurance that they and the people who are important to them are safe. Encourage the family to maintain regular routines. Parents need to provide children with opportunities both to talk about the crisis and to ask questions. Repetitive questions are to be expected. This often reflects the child's need for reassurance. Offering factual information helps dispel misperceptions.

HELPING OLDER PEOPLE COPE WITH TRAUMA

Reducing anxiety is especially important for older people who have experienced a disaster. Even the most capable older person can appear confused and vulnerable in a disaster situation. Actions nurses can take include the following:
1. Initiate contact and take the older person to as safe a place as possible.
2. Speak calmly and provide concrete information, in simple terms, about what is happening and what you need the person to do.
3. Assess the person for mobility, and provide assistance where needed.

4. Older people may need warmer clothing because of compromised temperature regulation.

Functional limitations associated with compromised physical mobility, diminished sensory awareness, and pre-existing health conditions create special issues for older people impacted by a disaster. They have more injury and greater disaster-related deaths than adults in other age groups. Within the older population, special attention should focus on those who require medical or nursing care and those receiving services, care, or food from health, social, or volunteer agencies.

Disaster management for older people needs to be proactive (Johnson et al., 2015). The following core actions can make a difference in helping older people weather a disaster event successfully. Proactive planning includes working with people as follows:
- Identify a support network that can be used in an emergency situation. Facilitate connections with social support systems and community support structures. Have this information readily available for use in an emergency situation.
- Older people with a disability should wear tags or a bracelet to identify their disability. Keeping extra glasses and hearing aid batteries on hand and identifying any assistive devices is essential.
- Identify the closest special needs evacuation centre.
- Develop a written list of all medications, with any special directions—for example, crushing pills, hours of administration, and dietary restrictions.
- Identify physicians and social support contacts, including someone apart from people in the local area who can be contacted.

Other actions, such as ensuring the person's safety, meeting mobility needs, and medication administration need special attention during the course of actual disaster management.

SUMMARY

Crisis is defined as an unexpected, sudden turn of events or set of circumstances requiring an immediate human response. People experience a crisis as overwhelming, traumatic, and personally intrusive. It is an unexpected life event challenging a person's sense of self and their place in the world. The most common types of crisis are situational and developmental crises. Most health crises are situational. Crisis can be private, involving one person, or public, involving large numbers of people.

Theoretical frameworks guiding crisis intervention include Lindemann's (1944) model of grieving and Caplan's (1964) model, based on preventive psychiatry concepts.

Aguilera's (1998) nursing model explores the role of balancing factors in defusing the impact of a crisis state. Erikson's (1982) model of psychosocial development provides a framework for exploring developmental crises.

Crisis intervention is a time-limited treatment, which focuses on the immediate crisis and its resolution. Roberts' (2005) seven-stage model, used to guide nursing interventions, consists of assessing lethality, establishing rapport, dealing with feelings, defining the problem, exploring alternative options, formulating a plan, and follow-up measures. The goal of crisis intervention is to return the person to their pre-crisis level of functioning.

Mental health emergencies require immediate assessment interventions and close supervision. The most common types of mental health emergencies are violence, suicide, and psychotic breaks. Guidelines for communication with people experiencing mental health emergencies (e.g., violence, suicide) focus on safety and rapid stabilization of the person's behaviour. CITs represent a new model of collaboration between local law enforcement and mental health services designed to treat rather than punish individuals experiencing mental health emergencies in the community (Davis, 2014a; Watson & Fulambarker, 2012).

As the world becomes more dynamically unstable, nurses will need to understand the dimensions of disaster management and develop the skills to respond effectively in disaster situations. Disaster management is a special kind of crisis intervention applied to large groups of people. The Joint Commission International requires hospitals to develop and exercise disaster-management plans at regular intervals. CISM is a crisis intervention strategy designed to help those closely involved with disasters process critical incidents in health care, thereby reducing the possibility of symptoms occurring.

👤 ETHICAL DILEMMA

What Would You Do?

Sara Murdano is only 20 years old when she arrives at the intensive care unit (ICU), but this is not her first hospital admission. She has previously been treated for depression. She states that she is determined to die by suicide because she has nothing to live for and that it is her right to do so because she is no longer a minor. As she describes her life to date, you cannot help but think that she really does not have a lot to live for. How would you respond to this person from an ethical perspective?

QUESTIONS FOR REVIEW AND DISCUSSION

1. What would you identify as the essential knowledge, skills, and attitudes required of a nurse confronted with a person who is at high risk for a suicide attempt?
2. What questions would you ask Sara to determine her level of risk and protective measures?
3. How would you apply The Joint Commission International safety standards in the emergency department?
4. What would you document regarding Sara's assessment and interventions?

REFERENCES

Agic, B., McKenzie, K., Tuck, A. et al. (2016). *Supporting the mental health of refugees to Canada*. Mental Health Commission of Canada. https://www.mentalhealthcommission.ca/sites/default/files/2016-01-25_refugee_mental_health_backgrounder_0.pdf.

Aguilera, D. (1998). *Crisis intervention: Theory and methodology* (7th ed.). Mosby.

Aitsi-Selmi, A., & Murray, V. (2016). Protecting the health and well-being of populations from disasters: Health and health care in the Sendai framework for disaster risk reduction 2015–2030. *Prehospital and Disaster Medicine*, 31(1), 74–78. https://doi.org/10.1017/S1049023X15005531.

Bluhm, J. (1987). Helping families in crisis hold on. *Nursing*, 17(10), 44–46.

Brooks, S., Webster, R., Smith, L. et al. (2020). The psychological impact of quarantine and how to reduce it: Rapid review of the evidence. *The Lancet*, 395, 912–920. https://doi.org/10.1015/S0140-6736(20)30460-8.

Browning, S. L., Van Hasselt, V. B., Tucker, A. S. et al. (2011). Dealing with individuals who have mental illness: The crisis intervention team (CIT) in law enforcement. *British Journal of Forensic Practice*, 13(4), 235–243. https://doi.org/ezproxy.pgcc.edu/10.1108/14636641111189990.

Canadian Centre on Substance Use and Addiction. (2021). *Opioids*. https://www.ccsa.ca/opioids.

Canadian Mental Health Association. (2009). *Crisis intervention team*. https://cmha.bc.ca/wp-content/uploads/2016/07/CIT-summary.pdf

Canadian Oxford Dictionary. (n.d.) Disaster. In *Canadian Oxford Dictionary*. Retrieved from https://www.oxfordreference.com/view/10.1093/acref/9780195418163.001.0001/acref-9780195418163.

Caplan, G. (1964). *Principles of preventive psychiatry*. Basic Books.

CBC News. (2020). *Nova Scotia mass killings: What we know and what we don't know*. April 19, 2020. https://www.cbc.ca/news/canada/nova-scotia/mass-killings-what-we-know-what-we-don-t-1.5537918.

Centre for Addiction and Mental Health. (2021). Mental health and the COVID-19 pandemic. https://www.camh.ca/en/health-info/mental-health-and-covid-19.

Children's Health Policy Centre. (2011). Helping children overcome trauma. *Children's Mental Health Research Quarterly, 5*(3). Children's Health Policy Centre, Simon Fraser University. https://childhealthpolicy.ca/wp-content/uploads/2012/12/RQ-3-11-Summer.pdf.

Coleman, S. J., Stevelink, S. A. M., Hatch, S. L. et al. (2017). Stigma-related barriers and facilitators to help seeking for mental health issues in the armed forces: A systematic review and thematic synthesis of qualitative literature. *Psychological Medicine, 47*(11), 1880–1892. https://doi.org/ezproxy.pgcc.edu/10.1017/S0033291717000356.

Crisis Services Canada. (2021). *The Canada suicide prevention service.* https://www.crisisservicescanada.ca/en/.

Dass-Brailsford, P. (2010). *Crisis and disaster counseling: Lessons learned from hurricane Katrina and other disasters.* Sage Publications.

Davis, S. (2014a). *CIT Teams* [unpublished manuscript].

Davis, S. (2014b). *De-escalation tips in crisis situations.* In Montgomery County. Rockville, MD: MD Police Department.

Eifling, K. M. D., & Moy, H. P. M. D. (2015). Evidence-based EMS: Psychological first aid. *EMS World, 44*(7), 32–34. https://ezproxy.pgcc.edu/login?url=https://search-proquest-com.ezproxy.pgcc.edu/docview/1708156049?accountid=13315.

Ellis, H. A. (2011). The crisis intervention team—A revolutionary tool for law enforcement: The psychiatric-mental health nursing perspective. *Journal of Psychosocial Nursing and Mental Health Services, 49*(11), 37–43. https://doi.org/ezproxy.pgcc.edu/10.3928/02793695-20111004-01.

Emanuel, L. L., Taylor, L., & Hain, A. (Eds.), (2013). *The patient safety education program—Canada Curriculum.* © PSEP-Canada. https://www.patientsafetyinstitute.ca/en/education/PatientSafetyEducationProgram/PatientSafetyEducationCurriculum/Documents/Module%2013d%20Seclusion%20and%20Restraint.pdf.

Erikson, E. (1982). *The life cycle completed.* Norton.

Everly, G. S., & Mitchell, J. T. (2017). Critical incident stress management (CISM): A practical review. ICISF. https://icisf.org/a-primer-on-critical-incident-stress-management-cism/.

Forbes, D., Lewis, V., Varker, T. et al. (2011). Psychological first aid following trauma: Implementation and evaluation framework for high-risk organizations. *Psychiatry, 74*(3), 224–239. https://doi.org/ezproxy.pgcc.edu/101521psyc2011743224.

Galea, S. (2020). *Mental health in a time of pandemic.* https://www.psychologytoday.com/us/blog/talking-about-health/202003/mental-health-in-time-pandemic.

Government of Canada. (2016). *Suicide in Canada: infographic.* https://www.canada.ca/en/public-health/services/publications/healthy-living/suicide-canada-infographic.html.

Government of Canada. (2019). *Natural hazards. Services and information.* https://www.canada.ca/en/services/policing/emergencies/hazards.html.

Government of Canada. (2021). *Opioid- and stimulant-related harms in Canada.* https://health-infobase.canada.ca/substance-related-harms/opioids-stimulants/maps.

Hawryluck, L., Gold, W. L., Robinson, S. et al. (2004). SARS control and psychological effects of quarantine, Toronto, Canada. *Emerging Infectious Diseases, 10*(7), 1206–1212. https://doi.org/10.3201/eid1007.030703.

HealthLinkBC. (2020). Take-home naloxone kits for opioid overdose. https://www.healthlinkbc.ca/health-topics/abs2222.

Humphreys, A., Blackwell, T., & Brean, J. (2018). 'Pure carnage' as van hits pedestrians in Toronto: 10 dead, 15 injured and man arrested. *National Post* May 8, 2018. https://nationalpost.com/news/canada/newsalert-toronto-police-say-a-van-has-hit-up-to-10-people-extent-of-injuries-unknown.

Jakubec, S. L. (2014). Crisis and disaster. In J. H. Halter, C. L. Pollard, & S. L. Ray (Eds.), *Canadian psychiatric mental health nursing* (pp. 491–507). Saunders.

James, R. (2008). *Crisis intervention strategies* (8th ed.). Thompson Brooks/Cole.

James, R., & Gilliland, B. (2013). *Crisis intervention strategies* (7th ed.). Thomson Brooks/Cole.

Johnson, H. L., Ling, C. G., & McBee, E. C. (2015). Multidisciplinary care for the elderly in disasters: An integrative review. *Prehospital and Disaster Medicine, 30*(1), 72–79. https://doi.org/ezproxy.pgcc.edu/10.1017/S1049023X14001241.

Joint Commission. (2017). *Sentinel events: Comprehensive accreditation manual for behavioral health care (CAMBHC)* E-dition, July 1, 2017b. https://www.jcrinc.com/?_ga=2.94685660.1542418870.1631935698-568943722.1618081436.

Joint Commission International. (2020). *JCI navigator.* https://www.jointcommissioninternational.org/en/.

Kouyoumdjian, F., Wang, R., Mejia-Lancheros, C. et al. (2019). Interactions between police and persons who experience homelessness and mental illness in Toronto, Canada: Findings from a prospective study. *The Canadian Journal of Psychiatry, 64*(10), 718–725. https://doi.org/10.1177/0706743719861386.

Koziarski, J. (2018). Policing mental health: *An exploratory study of crisis intervention teams and co-response teams in the Canadian context* [Unpublished master's thesis]. University of Ontario Institute of Technology. https://ir.library.dc-uoit.ca/bitstream/10155/932/1/Koziarski_Jacek.pdf.

Lindemann, E. (1944). Symptomatology and management of acute grief. *American Journal of Psychiatry, 101*, 141–148.

Loughran, H. (2011). *Understanding crisis therapies: An integrative approach to crisis intervention and post traumatic stress.* Jessica Kingsley Publishers.

Luchetti, M., Lee, J. H., Aschwanden, D. et al. (2020). The trajectory of loneliness in response to COVID-19. *The American Psychologist, 75*(7), 897–908. https://doi.org/10.1037/amp0000690.

Myer, R., & Conte, C. (2006). Assessment for crisis intervention. *Journal of Clinical Psychology, 62*(8), 959–970.

National Suicide Prevention Lifeline. (2021). *Veterans.* https://suicidepreventionlifeline.org/help-yourself/veterans/.

Navaneelan, T. (2017). Statistics Canada. Health at a glance. Suicide rates: An overview. Catalogue no. 82-624-X. https://www150.statcan.gc.ca/n1/pub/82-624-x/2012001/article/11696-eng.htm.

Northcott, P. (2020). *Mobile response teams help people in crisis. Royal Canadian Mounted Police.* https://www.rcmp-grc.gc.ca/en/gazette/mobile-response-teams-help-people-crisis.

Nova Scotia. (2019). *Expansion of sexual assault nurse examiner program.* https://novascotia.ca/news/release/?id=20191009001.

Office of the Privacy Commissioner of Canada. (2021). The Personal Information Protection and Electronic Documents Act (PIPEDA). https://www.priv.gc.ca/en/privacy-topics/privacy-laws-in-canada/the-personal-information-protection-and-electronic-documents-act-pipeda/.

Ottawa Public Health. (2021). *Mental health and COVID-19.* https://www.ottawapublichealth.ca/en/public-health-topics/mental-health-and-covid-19.aspx.

Parlapani, E., Holeva, V., Nikopoulou, V. A. et al. (2020). Intolerance of uncertainty and loneliness in older adults during the COVID-19 pandemic. *Frontiers in Psychiatry, 11* https://doi.org/10.3389/fpsyt.2020.00842.

Penterman, B., & Nijman, H. (2011). Assessing aggression risks in patients of the ambulatory mental health crisis team. *Community Mental Health Journal, 47*(4), 463–471. https://doi.org/ezproxy.pgcc.edu/10.1007/s10597-010-9348-7.

Pfefferbaum, B., Noffsinger, M. A., & Wind, L. H. (2012). Issues in the assessment of children's coping in the context of mass trauma. *Prehospital and Disaster Medicine, 27*(3), 272–279.

Public Health Agency of Canada. (2020). *Federal framework on posttraumatic stress disorder: Recognition, collaboration and support.* https://www.canada.ca/en/public-health/services/publications/healthy-living/federal-framework-post-traumatic-stress-disorder.html.

Public Safety Canada. (2018a). *National emergency response system.* https://www.publicsafety.gc.ca/cnt/rsrcs/pblctns/ntnl-rspns-sstm/index-en.aspx.

Public Safety Canada. (2018b). *Federal policy for emergency management.* https://www.publicsafety.gc.ca/cnt/rsrcs/pblctns/plc-mrgnc-mngmnt/index-en.aspx.

Public Safety Canada. (2019). *Supporting Canada's public safety personnel: An action plan on post-traumatic stress injuries.* https://www.publicsafety.gc.ca/cnt/rsrcs/pblctns/2019-ctn-pln-ptsi/index-en.aspx.

Ralph, M. (2010). The impact of crisis intervention team programs: Fostering collaborative relationships. *Journal of Emergency Nursing, 36*(1), 60–62.

Randall, J., Chateau, D., Bolton, J. M. et al. (2017). Increasing medication adherence and income assistance access for first-episode psychosis patients. *PLoS One, 12*(6), e0179089. https://doi.org/ezproxy.pgcc.edu/10.1371/journal.pone.0179089.

Registered Nurses' Association of Ontario. (2017). *Crisis intervention for adults using a trauma-informed approach: Initial four weeks of management* (3rd ed.). Author. https://rnao.ca/sites/rnao-ca/files/bpg/Crisis_Intervention_FINAL_WEB.v2.pdf.

Registered Psychiatric Nurse Regulators of Canada. (2014). *Registered psychiatric nurse entry-level competencies.*

http://www.rpnc.ca/sites/default/files/resources/pdfs/RPNRC-ENGLISH%20Compdoc%20%28Nov6-14%29.pdf.

Rittenmeyer, L. (2012). Assessment of risk for in-hospital suicide and aggression in high dependency care environments. *Critical Care Nursing Clinics of North America, 24,* 41–51.

Roberts, A. (2005). *Crisis intervention handbook: Assessment, treatment and research.* Oxford University Press.

Rodgers, P. (2017). Suicide prevention resource center: *Understanding risk and protective factors for suicide: A primer for preventing suicide.* www.sprc.org/library_resources/items/understanding-risk-and-protective-factors-suicide-primer.

Sadek, J. (2019). *A clinician's guide to suicide risk assessment and management.* Switzerland AG: Springer Nature. https://doi.org/10.1007/978-3-319-77773-3.

Stanley, B., & Brown, G. (2012). Safety planning intervention: A brief intervention to mitigate suicide risk. *Cognitive and Behavioural Practice, 19,* 256–264. http://www.suicidesafety-plan.com; www.sciencedirect.com.

The Canadian Press. (2017, September 1). Devastating Fort McMurray wildfire declared out 15 months later. *CBC News.* https://www.cbc.ca/news/canada/edmonton/fort-mcmurray-fire-beast-extinguished-out-1.4271604.

Toronto Police Service. (n.d.). *Mental health: Mobile crisis intervention team (MCIT).* http://www.torontopolice.on.ca/community/mcit.php.

Vancouver Police Department. (n.d). *Youth community response unit.* https://vpd.ca/police/organization/investigation/investigative-support-services/youth-services/community-response.html.

Vertava Health. (2020). *What is a crisis intervention?* https://vertavahealth.com/addiction-treatment/intervention/crisis/.

Vierheller, C. C., & Denton, M. (2014). When mental health and medicine collide: Maintaining safety in the emergency department. *Journal of Nursing Education and Practice, 4*(2), 49–55. https://doi.org/10.5430/jnep.v4n2p49.

Vroomen, J. M., Bosmans, J. E., van Hout, H. P. et al. (2013). Reviewing the definition of crisis in dementia care. *BMC Geriatrics, 13*(10). https://doi.org/10.1186/1471-2318-13-10.

Watson, A., & Fulambarker, A. (2012). The crisis intervention team model of police response to mental health crises: A primer for mental health practitioners. *Best Practice Mental Health, 8*(2), 71–77.

World Health Organization. (2016). *Preventing suicide: A community engagement toolkit. Pilot version 1.0.* http://www.who.int/mediacentre/factsheets/fs398/en/.

World Health Organization. (2017). *Suicide.* https://www.who.int/news-room/fact-sheets/detail/suicide.

Zukowski. R. S. (2014). The impact of adaptive capacity on disaster response and recovery: Evidence supporting core community capabilities. *Prehosp Dis Med, 29*(4), 380–387. https://doi.org/10.1017/S1049023X14000624.

SUGGESTED READING

Davis, S. (2015). *Field expedient tool to assess dangerousness in self and others.* In Montgomery County, Rockville, MD: MD Police Department.

WEBSITE/RESOURCES LIST

https://www.addictioncampuses.com/addiction-treatment/
intervention/crisis/2020.

https://www.canada.ca/en/public-health/services/publications/
healthy-living/federal-framework-post-traumatic-stress-
disorder.html.

https://www.canada.ca/en/public-health/services/publications/
healthy-living/suicide-canada-infographic.html.

https://www.canada.ca/en/services/policing/emergencies/hazards.
html.

https://www.cbc.ca/news/canada/edmonton/fort-mcmurray-
fire-beast-extinguished-out-1.4271604.

https://www.crisisservicescanada.ca/en/.

https://www.jointcommissioninternational.org/en/.

https://nationalpost.com/news/canada/newsalert-toronto-police-
say-a-van-has-hit-up-to-10-people-extent-of-injuries-
unknown.

https://novascotia.ca/news/release/?id=20191009001.

https://novascotia.cmha.ca/wp-content/uploads/2019/01/AClinic
ian'sGuidetoSuicideRiskAsse.pdf.

https://www.patientsafetyinstitute.ca/en/education/PatientSafety
EducationProgram/PatientSafetyEducationCurriculum/
Documents/Module%2013d%20Seclusion%20and%20
Restraint.pdf.

https://www.priv.gc.ca/en/privacy-topics/privacy-laws-in-canada/
the-personal-information-protection-and-electronic-
documents-act-pipeda/.

https://www.publicsafety.gc.ca/cnt/rsrcs/pblctns/2019-ctn-pln-ptsi/
index-en.aspx.

https://rnao.ca/sites/rnao-ca/files/Assessment_and_Care_of_
Adults_at_Risk_for_Suicidal_Ideation_and_Behaviour_0.
pdf.

https://rnao.ca/sites/rnao-ca/files/bpg/Crisis_Intervention_FINAL_
WEB.pdf.

http://www.rpnc.ca/sites/default/files/resources/pdfs/RPNRC-
ENGLISH%20Compdoc%20%28Nov6-14%29.pdf.

https://suicidepreventionlifeline.org/help-yourself/veterans/.

https://www150.statcan.gc.ca/n1/pub/82-624-x/2012001/
article/11696-eng.htm.

https://www.thechronicleherald.ca/news/provincial/nova-scotia.

22

Communication Approaches in Palliative Care

Olive Yonge

Originating US chapter by *Elizabeth C. Arnold*

OBJECTIVES

At the end of the chapter, the reader will be able to:

1. Discuss the concept of loss.
2. Identify theory-based concepts of grief and grieving.
3. Describe the nurse's role in palliative care.
4. Discuss key issues and approaches in end-of-life (EOL) care.
5. Identify cultural and spiritual needs in EOL care.
6. Describe supportive strategies for children who are dying or have a person close to them who is dying.
7. Discuss strategies to help people achieve a good death.
8. Identify stress issues for nurses in EOL care.

The purpose of this chapter is to introduce palliative care approaches that nurses can use to effectively communicate with people and their families in the last stage of life. The chapter identifies selected theoretical frameworks related to loss, stages of dying, and the process of grief and grieving. The application section highlights communication and care issues nurses face in providing people and their families with palliative care. Helping clinicians recognize and cope with the high stress of providing quality EOL care is also addressed.

BASIC CONCEPTS

Loss, Grief, and Bereavement

The *Canadian Oxford Dictionary* defines *loss* as "the act or an instance of losing; the state of being lost; the fact of being deprived of a person by death, estrangement, etc." Important losses occur as part of everyone's personal experience. Anything or anyone in whom we invest time, energy, or a part of ourselves creates a sense of loss when it is no longer available to us. When people "suffer the loss" of someone or something important to them, there is a loss of their sense of "wholeness," and a break in the person's expected life story (Sen, 2015). The passage of time never fully erases this sense of loss.

The feelings associated with each loss differ only in the intensity with which one experiences them. Mark Twain noted, "Nothing that grieves us can be called little; by the eternal laws of proportion a child's loss of a doll and a king's loss of a crown are events of the same size" (Twain, n.d.). Only the person experiencing the loss can appreciate the unique void and strength of feelings that each loss entails. Some losses are gradual; others occur concurrently or sequentially. There is no right or wrong way to experience grief. Feelings and thoughts about grief are unique to that person (Canadian Mental Health Association, 2016).

One loss can precipitate other losses. For example, someone with Alzheimer's disease doesn't simply lose memory. Accompanying cognitive deficits are accumulating losses of role, communication, independence, and gradual loss of identity. Simulation Exercise 22.1 is designed to help you understand the dimensions of personal loss.

SIMULATION EXERCISE 22.1   The Meaning of Loss

Purpose
To consider personal meaning of losses

Procedure
Consider your answers to the following questions:
- What losses have I experienced in my life?
- How did I feel when I lost something or someone important to me?
- How was my behaviour affected by my loss?
- What helped me the most in resolving my feelings of loss?
- How has my experience with loss prepared me to deal with further losses?

- How has my experience with loss prepared me to help others deal with loss?

Discussion
1. In the larger group, discuss what gives a loss its meaning.
2. What common themes emerged from the group discussion about successful strategies in coping with loss?
3. How does the impact of necessary losses differ from that of unexpected, unnecessary losses?
4. How can you use in your clinical work what you have learned from doing this exercise?

Multiple Losses

Acknowledging differences between single and multiple loss helps people put the enormity of multiple losses into perspective (Wilson et al., 2020). Older people typically experience the deaths of friends and family members with greater frequency than younger people do. Others lose multiple friends due to illnesses such as cancer or mental health disorders such as depression, as well as natural or man-made disasters. A car accident can wipe out an entire family or group of friends.

Multiple losses intensify the grief experience and it usually requires more time to resolve grief feelings. From a communication perspective, helping people focus on one relationship at a time instead of trying to address the losses together works best. Otherwise, bereavement can be overwhelming. Patience with oneself is critical to successfully working through difficult emotions associated with multiple losses. Bereavement takes time, and one should not rush the process.

DEATH: THE FINAL LOSS

Death represents a tangible loss in that the *physical* presence of the lost person can never be replaced. More than a biological event, death has spiritual, social, and cultural features that help people make sense of its meaning. Regardless of the primary medical diagnosis of the person who died, people who grieve that person's death experience many different emotions, ranging from anger or sadness to a sense that the person who died was at peace about a life well lived, with few regrets as they approach death.

For some people, a significant family member is snatched away in an instant. For others, there are precious, time-limited opportunities to say goodbye and to find a sense of closure. Being able to actively participate in helping a loved one achieve the peace of having a good death is comforting. Sharing in an end-of-life (EOL) process with a loved one is meaningful, especially if family members receive support with the process. The memory of this time together is critically important to those left behind.

Death is a normal part of the life order for everyone. It is not a failure. No one can tell you how it will be for you, based on their experience. Pashby (N. Pashby, personal communication, 2015), an expert hospice nurse, states that most people identify fear of pain, losing control, and dying alone as their principal fears. Nurses are an important resource in providing practical support and offering meaningful presence to people and families coping with life-limiting illnesses.

THEORETICAL FRAMEWORKS

Elisabeth Kübler-Ross (1969), a psychiatrist, was not a researcher but observed those who were dying and created and described five stages of grief: denial, anger, bargaining, depression, and acceptance (Keegan & Drick, 2011). Unfortunately, these stages have been used inappropriately. Not every person who is dying experiences each stage or necessarily experiences them in the same sequence or in any sequence. Some people remain in the denial stage until the very end of their illness. Their right to do so should be respected. Furthermore, Dr. Kübler-Ross believed there was a stage missing and asked David Kessler, her student and a thenatologist (a person who studies death and dying), to develop the sixth stage of grief which was finding the meaning of grief for the people who are still living (Kessler, 2019). She also noted that she had not focused on grieving—just grief—and thus while she was dying, she and Kessler co-wrote *On Grief and Grieving* (Kübler-Ross & Kessler, 2005). Her work is included in this chapter because she identified a language that could be used to talk about grief.

Denial

Kübler-Ross (1969) characterizes the denial stage as the "No, not me" stage. Nurses should be sensitive to the person's need for denial.

Anger

Anger is characterized as the "Why me?" stage. This stage can produce feelings about the unfairness of life or anger with God. Feelings often get projected on those closest to the person. Family members need support to recognize that the anger is not a personal attack (although sometimes it feels that way to the family member).

Bargaining

Kübler-Ross refers to the bargaining stage as the "Yes, me, but … I need just a little more time." Bargaining is not a futile exercise. Sometimes the extra energy a person gets by focusing on living long enough to attend a graduation, a birth, or a wedding is meaningful to all involved in making it happen. By supporting hope and avoiding challenges to the person's reality, the nurse facilitates the process of living while dying.

Depression

The "Yes, me" stage of dying is expressed through depressive feelings and mood swings. You can help family members understand that this is a "normal" response to anticipating loss. Review of significant life events and relationships helps people consider unfinished business that could be reworked. Serving as an empathetic listening witness to the pain that people and their families experience in this stage helps them work through it.

Acceptance

The acceptance stage is characterized by an acknowledgment of an inevitable end to physical life. There is a gradual detachment from the world; the person experiences being almost "void of feeling" (Kübler-Ross, 1969, p. 124). Ideally, people experience a personal sense of peace and letting go. To outsiders, the person is straddling between two world realities: the organic and the existential.

Meaning

Kessler (2019) believes that each person must find meaning in the loss of a loved one, to heal. One of the most effective ways of doing this is to have grief witnessed. This happens through rituals, such as attending a funeral or memorial.

Meaning is also found in the gathering of mourners, who create a sense of community. The goal is to honour loved ones who have died and to transform personal grief into a peaceful experience.

Grief

Eric Lindemann (1994/1944) pioneered the concept of grief work based on interviews with bereaved people suffering a sudden tragic loss. He described patterns of grief and identified physical and emotional changes associated with significant loss. Lindemann observed that grief can occur immediately after a loss, or it can be delayed. He summarized three components of support: (a) open, empathetic communication, (b) honesty, and (c) tolerance of emotional expression as being important in grieving. When the symptoms of grief are exaggerated over a period of time, or absent, it is considered pathological or complicated grief. People experiencing complicated grief may require psychological treatment to resolve their grief and move into life again.

Engel's Contributions

George Engel's (1964) concepts built on Lindemann's work. He described three sequential phases of grief work: (a) shock and disbelief, (b) developing awareness, and (c) restitution.

In the shock and disbelief phase, a newly bereaved person may feel alienated or detached from normal—"literally numb with shock; no tears, no feelings, just absolute numbness" (Lendrum & Syme, 1992, pp. 24–25). Seeing or hearing the lost person or sensing their presence is a temporary, altered sensory experience related to the loss, which should not be confused with psychotic hallucinations.

The developing awareness phase occurs slowly as the void created by the loss fully enters consciousness. People experience a loss of energy—not the kind that requires sleep but rather recognizing that one lacks the functional energy to engage fully in normal everyday responsibilities.

The restitution phase is characterized by adaptation to a new life without the deceased person. There is a resurgence of hope and a renewed energy to fashion a new life. With successful grieving, the loss is not forgotten, but the pain diminishes and is replaced with memories that enrich and give energy to life.

Case Example

"Throughout the year following my mother's death, I was aware of a persistent feeling of heaviness—not physical heaviness, but emotional and spiritual. It was as if a dark cloud hung over my heart and soul. I tired easily, with little energy to do anything but the most essential activities, and even those frequently received perfunctory attention. My usual pattern of 'sleeping like a log' was disrupted, and in its place, I experienced uneasy rest that left me feeling as if I had never closed my eyes" (Anonymous).

Listening, identifying feelings, and having an empathetic willingness to repeatedly hear the person's story without needing to give advice or interpretation offer presence without demands.

Contemporary Models

Doughty et al. (2011) describe a number of theories, including making meaning construction as a central issue in grief work. The past is not forgotten; instead, there is a continuous spiritual connection with the deceased person, which illuminates different features of self and possibilities for fuller engagement with life. Features of past experiences with the loved one are transformed and rewoven into the fabric of a person's life in a new form. The concept of a **palliative approach** to care represents an integrative model that can guide the care of people at any stage of chronic illness, dispelling the myth that palliative care is only for EOL.

Stroebe and Schut (2010) from the Netherlands developed the dual process model of coping with bereavement. A person who is grieving oscillates between a loss and restorative orientation. In the loss-orientation mode, the person feels all the emotions of grief that other theorists have proposed. However, there are secondary losses such as having to solely manage a business or do housework. These losses give the person who is bereaved something else to focus on and provide small breaks from the loss-orientation. A bereaved person moves back and forth (oscillation) between these two orientations.

GRIEF AND GRIEVING

The concept of **grief** describes a holistic, adaptive process that a person goes through following a significant loss. Grief is an adaptive process that is different for each person (Jeffreys, 2011). There is an ebb and flow to the intense feelings that a death or significant loss stimulates in those who remain. Awareness of the loss creates recurring, wavelike feelings of memories and sadness. People describe it as "feeling unexpectedly punched in the gut." Intense feelings are particularly inclined to surface when the person grieving is alone, for example, while driving. Certain situations, holidays, and anniversaries, particularly during the first few years, make feelings of grief more poignant.

Case Example

"I would think I was doing okay, that I had a handle on my grief. Then, without warning, a scent, a scene on television, an innocuous conversation would flip a switch in my mind, and I would be flooded with memories of my mother. My eyes would fill up with tears as my fragile composure dissolved. My grief lay right under the surface of my awareness and ambushed me at times and in places not of my choosing" (Anonymous).

Over time, grief feelings usually diminish in intensity, but there is no magic time frame. Grief over the loss of a child can be particularly pervasive, sometimes lasting a lifetime. Variables affecting the intensity and time frame for the grieving process after a death include the following:

- "Cultural beliefs and rituals
- Nature of relationship with the deceased person
- Previous losses
- Spiritual and religious background
- Support system available" (Keegan & Drick, 2011, p. 113)

As people work through their grief, they are more open to the spiritual continuance of a relationship with the deceased person, occurring as cherished memories or supportive remembrances of "what the deceased person might say or do in the situation." These shared moments provide an affirming spiritual union with the deceased person and a personal knowing of self in relationship. They offer a unique legacy, which will continue to influence the behaviours of future generations.

John Thomas (2011) describes his sense of successfully making the journey through grief with a stronger sense of self. He states, "I want to be known as one who:

- Is identified with life and love rather than loss and grief.
- Walks with the stride of renewal rather than the shuffle of grief.
- Still embraces life knowing that the pain of loss is intense.
- Has one foot planted firmly in this life and is developing an equally firm footing in the spiritual realm.
- Is confident about the future without needing a tangible GPS.
- Can be alone without being lonely.
- Faced grief head-on, and reached a deeper core of self, faith, and spirituality.
- Has much to give in many arenas living a life that honors my past, and shares the blessings derived from it …" (Thomas, pp. 202–203).

PATTERNS OF GRIEVING

Acute Grief

Acute grief occurs as "somatic distress that occurs in waves with feelings of tightness in the throat, shortness of breath, an empty feeling in the abdomen, a sense of heaviness and lack of muscular power, and intense mental pain" (Lindemann, 1994/1944, p. 155). Acute grief is intense, and the emotional pain can be beyond imagination. It lasts a short time, and gradually subsides, as the bereaved person begins to re-engage in meaningful activities (Zisook et al., 2010).

People who survived a suicide attempt are at a disadvantage, made worse by their reluctance to discuss death details because of shame or perceived stigma. Survivors usually need more support, but often, they get less because people are uncomfortable about suicide or do not know how to talk about it with those most intimately involved (Harvard Women's Health Watch, 2009). Suicide survivor support groups can offer the specialized help that many survivors need after a suicide (Andriessen et al., 2019).

Anticipatory Grief

Anticipatory grief is an emotional response that occurs before the actual death, around a family member with a degenerative or terminal disorder. A person thinking about their own death also can experience anticipatory grief. Grief symptoms are similar to those experienced after death but are often coloured by ambivalent feelings.

Case Example

Marge's husband, Albert, was diagnosed with Alzheimer's disease 5 years ago. Albert is in a nursing home, unable to care for himself. Marge grieves the impending loss of Albert as her mate. At the same time, she would like a life of her own. Her "other feelings" of wishing it could all be over cause her to feel guilty. Simulation Exercise 22.2 helps you explore grief from a personal perspective.

Chronic Sorrow

Chronic sorrow is the ongoing grief that accompanies nonfinite losses; grief is ongoing because the loss is also ongoing (Harris, n.d.). Many parents of children with a physical, developmental, emotional, or chronic disorder experience chronic sorrow. Families need nurses to affirm their coping efforts and acknowledge the legitimacy of their sadness. Providing timely support for families when there is an exacerbation of symptoms can make the situation more manageable.

Complicated Grieving

Complicated grieving represents an intense expression of grief, which lasts significantly longer and is emotionally incapacitating. A history of depression, substance abuse, death of a parent or sibling during childhood, prolonged conflict or dependence on the deceased person, or a succession of deaths within a short period predispose a person to complicated grief. Statements such as "I never recovered from my son's death" or "I feel like my life ended when my husband died" can alert the nurse to potential complicated grief.

Complicated grief can also present as an absence of grief in situations where it would be expected, for example, a marine who displays no emotion over the deaths of war comrades. When deaths and important losses are not mourned, the feelings do not just disappear; they reappear in unexpected ways, sometimes years later. Simulation Exercise 22.3 provides a personal opportunity to reflect on the relevance of memories in significant relationships.

SIMULATION EXERCISE 22.2 A Personal Grief Inventory

Purpose
To provide a close examination of one's history with grief

Procedure
Complete each sentence and reflect on your answers:
   The first significant experience with grief that I can
      remember in my life was _____.
   The circumstances were _____.
   My age was _____.

The feelings I had at the time were_____.
The thing I remember most about that experience was

   _____.
I coped with the loss by _____.
The primary sources of support during this period
   were _____.
What helped most was _____.
The most difficult death for me to face would be

   _____.

Adapted from Carson, V. B., & Arnold, E. N. (1996). *Mental health nursing: The nurse-patient journey*, (p. 666). WB Saunders.

SIMULATION EXERCISE 22.3   Reflections on Memory Making in Significant Relationships

Purpose

To provide students with an opportunity to see the value of memory making as a strategy for facilitating the grieving process

Procedure

1. Write a letter to someone who has died or is no longer in your life. Before writing the letter, reflect on the meaning this person had for you and the person you have become.
2. In the letter, tell the person what they meant to you and why you miss them.
3. Tell the person what you remember most about your relationship.

4. Tell the person anything you wished you had said but didn't when the person was in your life.

With a partner, each student should share their story without interruption. When the student finishes sharing their story, the listener can ask questions for further understanding.

Discussion

1. What was it like to write a letter to someone who had meaning in your life and is no longer available to you?
2. Were there any common themes?
3. In what ways was each story unique?
4. How could you use this exercise in your care of people who are grieving?

⟫ DEVELOPING AN EVIDENCE-INFORMED PRACTICE

Historically, people died at home, but as new hospitals were built and rooms were assigned for palliative care, people started dying in hospitals. However, another trend is emerging and people are requesting to die at home. The researchers sought to determine if the numbers were significant.

Methods

Recent individual-anonymous population-level inpatient Canadian hospital data were analyzed to answer two questions: (1) what proportion of deaths in provinces and territories across Canada are occurring in hospital now? and (2) who is dying in hospital now?

Results

In 2014–2015, 43.9% of all deaths in Canada (excluding Quebec) occurred in hospital. However, considerable cross-Canada differences in end-of-life hospital utilization were found. Some cross-Canada differences in hospital decedents were also noted, although the most common demographic to die in hospital were older males, and they died during a relatively short hospital stay after being admitted from their homes and through the emergency department, after arriving by ambulance.

Implications for Clinical Practice

Since the number is approaching 50% of deaths occurring at home, this has implications for the workload of nurses working in home care. It also means families will be drawing more on community resources like Meals on Wheels to support them while caring for their dying family member.

Adapted from Wilson, D., Shen, Y., Errasti-Ibarrondo, B. et al. (2018). The location of death and dying across Canada: A study illustrating the socio-political context of death and dying. *Societies, 8*, 112.

APPLICATIONS

Palliative Care: Nursing Care at the End of Life
Structure and Process of Palliative Care

Palliative care is person-centred care, with an emphasis on care of people with diagnosed, progressive, life-limiting health conditions (Sawatzky, 2016). Those providing care in palliative care emphasize support rather than curative actions, with comfort measures increasing and curative activities diminishing as the person prepares for the EOL. Treatment goals progress from disease control to maintaining a good quality of life, and comfort, and control of pain and other symptoms. Health care providers can greatly assist people and their families to make difficult decisions and be better prepared for what's coming. This includes preparing advance directives, which includes medical care preferences in case a time comes when they are no longer competent to make decisions on end-of-life interventions or treatments (Canadian Institute for Health Information, 2018).

Palliative care is unique in that it considers care for the person *and* the family as a single integrated care unit. As a person's life-limiting condition progresses, palliative care supports "living while dying" as comfortably as is possible, as displayed in Fig. 22.1. Symptom management for the person and practical support for the family as they negotiate the last stage of life becomes the priority. Unlike hospice, people admitted to palliative care services can still receive active treatment for their disease process, to control symptoms and improve quality of life (Canadian Institute for Health Information, 2018). Primary dimensions of palliative care identified by the World Health Organization (WHO) are presented in Box 22.1 (Al-Mahrezi & Al-Mandhari, 2016).

The overarching goal of palliative care is to help people improve function and quality of life, regardless of stage of disease or the presence of other treatments, and to prevent or relieve suffering (Kogan et al., 2017). Palliative care

strategies are designed to help people who are critically ill and their families understand the dying process as a part of life, and to maximize a person's quality-of-life options in the time left to them.

The basic axiom for palliative care is to follow what people want for themselves, based on their needs and personal preferences (Canadian Institute for Health Information, 2018). After a person's death, palliative care personnel offer bereavement support for family members.

Nursing Initiatives: End-of-Life Care

There are statements in the Canadian Nurses Association's (CNA) Code of Ethics that outline the nurse's role in relation to end-of-life care. Nurses are to ensure they have the person's informed consent to provide nursing care, and as well, they are to support the person if they want to refuse or withdraw consent at any time. Nurses are to relieve pain and suffering and to help the person live and die with dignity. "When a person receiving care is terminally ill or dying, nurses foster (comfort, alleviate suffering, advocate for adequate relief of discomfort and pain, and assist people in meeting their goals of culturally and spiritually appropriate care" (p. 13). This includes providing "a palliative approach to care for the people they interact with across the lifespan and the continuum of care, support for the family during and following the death, and care of the person's body after death" (p. 13) (Canadian Association of Schools of Nursing [CASN], 2011; Canadian Nurses Association, n.d.-a, n.d.-b)

Nurses have been at the forefront of developing guidelines for quality EOL care for many years, beginning with the original work of Dame Cicely Saunders, Florence Wald,

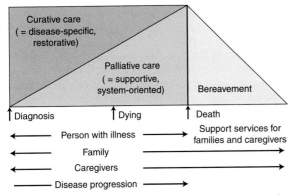

Fig. 22.1 Model of Curative and Palliative Care for Progressive Illness

---

BOX 22.1   Key Facts of Palliative Care

- Palliative care improves the quality of life of people and their families who are facing challenges associated with life-threatening illness, whether physical, psychological, social, or spiritual. The quality of life of caregivers improves as well.
- Each year, an estimated 40 million people are in need of palliative care; 78% of them live in low- and middle-income countries.
- Worldwide, only about 14% of people who need palliative care currently receive it.
- Unnecessarily restrictive regulations for morphine and other essential controlled palliative medicines deny access to adequate palliative care.

- Adequate national policies, programs, resources, and training on palliative care among health providers are urgently needed in order to improve access.
- The global need for palliative care will continue to grow as a result of the ageing of populations and the rising burden of noncommunicable diseases and some communicable diseases.
- Early delivery of palliative care reduces unnecessary hospital admissions and the use of health services.
- Palliative care involves a range of services delivered by a range of professionals that all have equally important roles to play—including physicians, nurses, support workers, paramedics, pharmacists, physiotherapists, and volunteers—in support of the person and their family.

From World Health Organization. (2020). *Fact Sheets: Palliative Care.* https://www.who.int/news-room/fact-sheets/detail/palliative-care.

and others. In 1991, the Canadian Hospice Palliative Care Association was established. Its purpose was to advance and advocate for quality end-of-life/hospice palliative care in Canada; its work includes public policy, public education, and awareness (Canadian Hospice Palliative Care Association, 2021).

Palliative Care Team Approaches

Palliative care is a team effort designed to "assess and manage people's and families' care needs across physical, psychological, social, spiritual, and information domains" (Bruera & Yennurajalingam, 2012, p. 268). An interdisciplinary palliative care team usually consists of nurses, physicians, social workers, and clergy specially trained in palliative care. People are enrolled in palliative care, which operates as a 24-hour resource providing comprehensive, holistic services to people and their families in hospitals, people's homes, nursing homes, and other community settings. The therapeutic focus in palliative care is on the person's comfort, pain control, management of physical symptoms, and easing the psychosocial and spiritual distress experienced by people and their families as they come to terms with coping with a life-limiting illness. In addition to practical, spiritual, and supportive care for people and their families, team members provide education and consultation about EOL care for hospital staff. Palliative comfort care can be used concurrently with disease-modifying treatment. The level of comfort care increases according to the person's needs and wishes. The goal is to give the person and their families a greater sense of control. The position statement issued by the CNA states that the palliative approach for nurses uses palliative care principles (i.e., dignity, hope, comfort, quality of life, relief of suffering) with people facing chronic, life-limiting conditions at all stages, not just at the end of life (Canadian Nurses Association, n.d.-a, n.d.-b). Furthermore, the CNA document lists the following values and responsibilities for nurses: to provide safe, compassionate, competent and ethical care; promote health and well-being; promote and respect informed decision making; preserve dignity with death; provide support for the family during and following the death; maintain privacy and confidentiality; promote justice; and be accountable.

Nurses play a pivotal role as professional coordinators, direct providers of care, and advocates for the person's autonomy, dignity, and control in EOL care. They are in a key position to help the family maintain its integrity, to support their efforts in managing the process of living while dying, and in preparing families for the death of their loved one. The palliative care model is displayed in Fig. 22.1.

Pain assessment. Pain is a complex phenomenon, with sensory, emotional, cognitive, and behavioural dimensions (Wilkie & Ezenwa, 2012). Pain is a subjective experience, assessed verbally with the person or observed in the person's behaviour (or both) (see Fig. 22.2). The Wong–Baker FACES Pain Rating Scale is a tool that can be used with children aged 3 and older, for pain assessment only. Nurses perform screenings for pain, focused on the following:

- Onset and duration of pain
- Location of the pain
- Character of the pain (sharp, dull, burning, persistent, changes with movement, direct or referred)
- Intensity—using a 0–10 numerical rating scale, with 0 being no pain and 10 being unbearable pain (use the Wong–Baker FACES Pain Rating Scale for children and people with limited health literacy or who have difficulty communicating)
- History of substance dependence (needed to determine potential crossover tolerance)
- Aggravating factors such as difficulty breathing or turning
- Relief factors such as distraction with visitors, food or fluids, reassurance

Small children usually cannot meaningfully measure nor directly communicate their pain level. Instead, look for behavioural indicators of pain such as abrupt changes in activity, crying, inability to be consoled, listlessness or unwillingness to move, rubbing a body part, wincing, or facial grimacing (Registered Nurses' Association of Ontario [RNAO], 2013). See Box 22.2, Validated Behavioural Pain

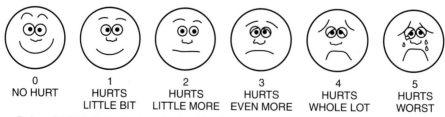

0	1	2	3	4	5
NO HURT	HURTS LITTLE BIT	HURTS LITTLE MORE	HURTS EVEN MORE	HURTS WHOLE LOT	HURTS WORST

Fig. 22.2 Wong–Baker FACES Pain Rating Scale. Used with permission, Wong-Baker Foundation. (2016). www.WongBakerFaces.org. (Original work published in Wong, D. L., Rentfro, A. R., & McCampbell, L. (1998). *Whaley & Wong's nursing care of infants and children*. Elsevier.)

BOX 22.2 Validated Behavioural Pain Assessment Tools* for Children

Measure	Indicators/ Components	Considerations
**Revised FLACC (r-FLACC)	Facial expression, leg movement, activity, cry, and consolability	• Initially developed as FLACC and intended for use in children aged 2 months to 8 years but has been used in children aged 0–18 years • Later amended to r-FLACC, to include pain behaviours common to people with cognitive impairments; has been used in children aged 4-21 years who are cognitively impaired • Validated for procedural and postoperative pain • Each category is scored on a 0–2 scale, which results in a total score between 0 and 10 • Well established evidence of reliability and validity; however, inconsistent ability to detect change demonstrated with FLACC • Simple to use, score and interpret • High feasibility • Cannot be used in people who are paralyzed; some preliminary data suggests it may be useful with people who are ventilated; important to note that consolability requires (a) an attempt to console, and (b) a subjective rating of response to that intervention, which complicates the scoring
• ***Noncommunicating Children's Pain Checklist—Revised (NCCPC-R)	• Vocal, social, facial expressions, activity, body and limbs, physiological and eating/ sleeping	• Designed for children aged 3–18 years who are unable to speak due to cognitive impairments or disabilities • Designed to be used without training, by parents and caregivers • Intended for use in any setting • Completion of the score based on a 2-hour observation period of the child • For post-operative pain, the Non-communicating Children's Pain Checklist—Postoperative Version should be used

*Note: Screening tools for the presence/absence of pain but NOT pain intensity

**Malviya, S., Voepel-Lewis, T., Burke, C. et al. (2006). The revised FLACC observational pain tool: Improved reliability and validity for pain assessment in children with cognitive impairment. *Pediatric Anesthesia, 16*(3), 258–265; Merkel, S., Voepel-Lewis, T., Shayevitz, J. et al. (1997). The FLACC: A behavioral scale for scoring postoperative pain in young children. *Pediatric Nursing, 23*(3), 293–297; von Baeyer, C. L., & Spagrud, L. J. (2007) Systematic review of observational (behavioral) measures of pain for children and adolescents aged 3 to 18 years. *Pain, 127*(1–2), 140–150. https://doi.org/10.1015/j.pain.2006.08.014; Voepel-Lewis, T., Malviya, S., Tait, A.R. et al. (2008). A comparison of the clinical utility of pain assessment tools for children with cognitive impairment. *Anesthesia and analgesia,* 106(1). https://doi.org/10.1213/01.ane.0000287680.21212.d0; van Herk, R., van Dijk, M., Baar, F. P. et al. (2007). Observation scales for pain assessment in older adults with cognitive impairments or communication difficulties. *Nursing research, 56*(1), 34–43. https://doi.org/10.1097/00006199-200701000-00005; Voepel-Lewis, T., Zanotti, J., Dammeyer, J. A. et al. (2010). Reliability and validity of the Face, Legs, Activity, Cry, Consolability Behavioral tool in assessing acute pain in critically ill patients. *American Journal of Critical Care: An Official Publication, American Association of Critical Care Nurses, 19*(1), 55–62. https://doi.org/10.4037/ajcc2010624.

***Breau, L. M., McGrath, P. J., Camfield, C. S. et al. (2002). Psychometric properties of the non-communicating children's pain checklist—revised. *Pain, 99*(1–2), 349–357. https://doi.org/10.1016/s0304-3959(02)00179-3; Registered Nurses' Association of Ontario. (2013). Appendix J. *Assessment and management of pain* (3rd ed.). Registered Nurses' Association of Ontario, pp. 91–92. https://rnao.ca/sites/rnao-ca/files/AssessAndManagementOfPain_15_WEB-_FINAL_DEC_2.pdf.

Assessment Tools for Children—this is a resource that health providers can use to assess for the presence or absence of pain but not the pain intensity.

The same is true for people with cognitive impairment related to delirium, dementia, or changes in consciousness—it might be only through their behaviour changes, particularly when associated with agitation, that you can tell that they are in pain. Observation of behavioural distress indicators is particularly important with older people.

Estimates of older people with significant pain range from greater than 40%. Some are able to evaluate their pain, using the suggestions above, but those with even mild cognitive changes may not be able to do so accurately when stressed.

Chronic pain related to cancer, diabetic neuropathy, osteoporosis, or arthritis may not readily respond to pain medication. Pain in older people can be underrecognized and therefore undertreated. The key is to have early interventions for pain to avoid future pain (Guido, 2010; Noroozian et al., 2018). Care providers can assume that people cannot tolerate strong pain medications, or that their pain is due to chronic, persistent conditions that will not be as responsive. Misperceptions about addiction and medication strength can result in inadequate pain management for children and people with mentally health disorders (RNAO, 2013).

Pain Assessment and Management

Pain assessment and management control is an essential component of quality palliative care, and the Canadian Pain Society (2020) views the treatment of pain as a basic human right. The Joint Commission International (2020), and Veterans Canada (Vets Canada, n.d.) identify pain as the fifth vital sign to be assessed with standard vital signs (temperature, pulse, respiration, and blood pressure). Standards for pain management established by the Joint Commission (2010) require that every inpatient be routinely assessed for pain, with documentation of appropriate monitoring and pain management.

People needing palliative care often experience moderate to severe levels of pain. This often leads to increased functional impairment, depression, impaired sleep, decreased appetite and social isolation (RNAO, 2013). Having appropriate pain control for moderate-to-severe pain usually requires the use of opioids. Misperceptions about pain-relieving opioids are a major, unnecessary barrier to adequate pain control. According to Pashby (N. Pashby, personal communication, March 2014), nurses need to educate people and their families about pain control, including the differences between pain associated with disease progression and adverse effects related to opioids. For example, some people do not want to take opioids for fear of "feeling loopy" or not being able to think clearly.

Everyone, including addicts, is entitled to appropriate and adequate pain management of severe pain. There is a fundamental difference between taking essential medication for pain control on a prescribed scheduled basis, and addictive use. People who are addicted may require larger doses of pain medication because of cross-tolerance. Other barriers include a belief that suffering should be tolerated (stoicism) or that pain is an unavoidable part of the dying process. Limited capacity to accurately describe pain intensity, or seeing pain as a weakness, also represent obstacles (Aronowitz et al., 2021).

Families sometimes attribute signs and symptoms of approaching death—such as increased lethargy, confusion, and declining appetite—to side effects of opioids. This is not usually true. With or without pain medication, people who are actively dying become less responsive as death approaches. Although they may experience drowsiness with initial dosing, this side effect quickly disappears. Once people and families understand the mechanisms and goals of pain control and are assured that the person will not die from the medication or become addicted from appropriate pain control, most will support its use in palliative care. People approaching death can experience "breakthrough" pain, which occurs episodically as severe pain spikes. When breakthrough pain occurs, rescue medications, which are faster acting, can be used. Touch and light massage are helpful adjuncts for pain relief. *The bottom line is that no person should suffer from preventable pain* (RNAO, 2013).

KEY ISSUES AND APPROACHES IN END-OF-LIFE CARE

Self-Awareness

Self-awareness is a critical foundation for effective palliative nursing practice. Nurses must be aware of their personal feelings about death and previous EOL experiences, including attitudes, expectations, and feelings about death and the process of dying. Nurses are not immune to fears of being alone at the time of death, or of feeling stress when helping people cope with unrelenting pain. You may find it difficult to maintain a balance between your own sensitivity to a person's death and providing the empathy and support needed by people and their families. Self-awareness about death and dying issues is critical in palliative care.

As the body begins to shut down in preparation for imminent death, the gold standard for EOL care is to restrict nutritional support (Kim & Seo, 2016). However, a teaspoon of ice chips and mouth care can be a comfort measure. The person's preferences often change over time. Care directives often must be revisited, especially if there is a change in prognosis and the potential for quality of life diminishes significantly (Guido, 2010).

Supporting End-of-Life Decision Making

EOL is a continuum experienced as a series of transitions from diagnosis to death (Schüklenk et al., 2011). People and their families face difficult, irreversible decisions in the last phase of life. Preference decisions related to discontinuation of fluids, antibiotics, blood transfusions, and ventilator support require a clear understanding of a complex care situation. These are emotional issues with adaptive components for families. Much more than simple clinical explanation is needed (Adams et al., 2013). Families need support in meeting the adaptive challenges EOL decisions present, which cannot be resolved with technical intervention or clear-cut solutions (Canadian Nurses Association, n.d.-a, n.d.-b).

EOL decisions should be transparent, meaning that all parties involved in the decisions should fully understand the implications of those decisions. For example, to make an informed decision about the use of life supports for people who are terminally ill, people and their families need to know whether further treatments will enhance or diminish quality of life, their potential impact on life expectancy, and whether the treatment is known to be effective or is an investigative treatment.

Family members need to understand the potential implications of choosing one option over another. Making unrealistic hypothetical choices without carefully considering the longer-term potential impact on quality of life and financial considerations helps no one. For example, keeping a person in a permanent unconscious condition alive on a ventilator can be harmful to the person—and family. This and other futile "curative" treatments can cause needless pain and physical symptoms. Additionally, they can create noteworthy quality-of-life issues, health care cost issues, and unnecessary anxiety for people and their families.

Ethical and Legal Issues

People and their families must consider a number of legal issues as people approach the EOL. Below is information about the legal protections people need related to finances and choices about medical care.

Advance Directives

On February 24, 2020, the Minister of Justice and Attorney General of Canada introduced *An Act to amend the Criminal Code (medical assistance in dying)* in Parliament, which proposes changes to Canada's law on medical assistance in dying (Government of Canada, 2020). This document notes who can provide assistance and who can help provide assistance; it outlines the protections of the providers and how people can access this service. Participants have two options. A medical practitioner or nurse practitioner directly administers a substance causing death; this is known as "clinician-administered medical assistance in dying." Or a drug is prescribed for the person to take, which is known as "self-administered medical assistance in dying" (Dying With Dignity Canada, 2020).

Advance directives specify a person's right to participate in and direct personal health care decisions, including do not resuscitate (DNR) directives. This information should be documented and made available for review by caregivers directly involved in the person's care. An advance directive is not permanently binding; if the person chooses to later revoke the document, they can do so. Timing is important. Advance directives completed too far in advance or too close to death may not truly reflect the person's goals or preferences (Billings & Bernacki, 2014; Government of Canada, 2018).

The nurse's role is to provide the person with full information about risks and benefits of prolonging life and to serve as an advocate in support of the person's right to make decisions about treatment and care (Canadian Nurses Association, 2015). Given that nurses are the most constant care providers, they best understand the wishes of the person, be it to prolong life through heroic measures or that they be allowed to die (Canadian Nurses Association). When people are making decisions competently, they should be key decision makers. If a person is not competent, or is unable to articulate their wishes, a responsible family member or significant person can be designated to legally assume the responsibility of surrogate spokesperson. Here, the conversation can start with asking the family "What would this person prefer under the circumstances if the person was able to speak for himself?" (Adams et al., 2013).

Durable Power of Attorney for Health Care

People who are competent can choose to appoint a surrogate decision maker (durable power of attorney for health care) in the event that they cannot make important health decisions on their own behalf. This designation includes the surrogate's authority to accept or refuse treatment on the person's behalf.

Some people have neither power of attorney for health nor advance directives. Box 22.3 provides guidelines for talking with families about care options at EOL when an advance directive or durable power of attorney is not in effect.

Communication in End-of-Life Care

Communication skill is equal to or supersedes clinical skill in EOL care. Everyone experiences a death differently; it is the uniqueness of each person's experience that the nurse

---

BOX 22.3   Talking With Families About Care Options

If neither durable power of attorney nor written directive is in effect, nurses can facilitate the process by helping to do the following:

- Determine who should be approached to make decisions about care options.
- Determine whether any key members are absent. (Try to keep those who know the person best in the centre of decision making.)
- Find a quiet place to meet where each family member can be seated comfortably.
- Sit down and establish rapport with each person present. Ask about the relationship each has with the person and how each feels about the person's current condition.

- Try to achieve a consensus about the person's clinical situation, especially prognosis.
- Provide a professional observation about the person's status and expected quality of life—survival versus quality of life. Ask what each of them thinks the person would want.
- Should the family choose comfort measures only, assure them of the attention the person will receive to their comfort and dignity.
- Seek verbal confirmation of understanding and agreement.
- Attention to the family's emotional responses is appropriate and appreciated.

Adapted from Lang, F., & Quill, T. (2004). Making decisions with families at the end of life. *American Family Physician, 70*(4), 720.

---

attempts to tap into and facilitate discussion of through conversation. Conversations with people and their families provide nurses with insights about personal values and preferences regarding EOL care and provide a forum to answer difficult questions in a supportive environment. There is some evidence that if clinicians discuss the person's preferences, and if they are documented, they are more likely to be fulfilled (Cox et al., 2011).

The quality of the relationship between nurse, person, and family members is a key factor contributing to creating an environment to support a good death. Nurses who work in this area, now considered a highly valued specialty, enhance the quality of life of those who are dying and their families, regardless of the person's age (Canadian Nurses Association, n.d.-a, n.d.-b). EOL interactions help people find meaning, achieve emotional closure, and provide the best means for helping people and their families make complex life decisions. Understanding the person's and family's perceptions of their EOL experience is essential. One area that is highly significant is the person's right to refuse life-saving treatment through a do-not-resuscitate (DNR) order. By filling out a DNR order, a person is communicating that they do not want to receive emergency life-saving measures, such as cardiopulmonary resuscitation (CPR), in the event that they become critically ill or suffer a catastrophic injury (Dying With Dignity Canada, 2019a).

Personal reflections are critical sources of assessment data. Once rapport is established, Pashby (N. Pashby, personal communication, 2015) suggests nurses can ask people how they learned of their diagnosis. She notes that a terminal diagnosis is usually a "technicolour moment" that the person remembers vividly and appreciates talking about. Other questions such as, "What has changed for you since the diagnosis?" or "What is it like for you now?" provide

additional data. Giving voice to the experience helps people to consider its personal meaning and provides the nurse with a more complete picture of each person's distinctive concerns and goals.

Most people know intuitively when their time is getting shorter, but the exact time frame may not be apparent until very close to death. It is not unusual for a person to ask in the course of conversation, "Am I going to die?" or "How much longer do you think I have?" Before answering, find out more about the origin of the question. A useful listening response is, "What is your sense of it?" Box 22.4 provides guidelines for communicating with people in palliative care.

Communicating With Families

Family members have different levels of readiness to engage in discussions about the dying process. It is "normal" for an impending death to have a different impact on each family member because each has had a unique relationship with the person who is dying. Conversations with families need not be long, but regularity is important.

Common concerns include discontinuing life support; conflicts among family members about care; tensions between the person and family, or the physician and family about treatment; where death should occur (home, hospital, hospice); and if or when hospice should be engaged. The clear goal of palliative care is to improve people's quality of life through the management of their symptoms, whether medical, emotional, spiritual, or psychosocial" (Fox, 2014, p. 40).

Creating Family Memories

People and their families need to talk about things other than the disease process and treatments. Nurses can help make this happen. There are spiritual stories, cultural

---

BOX 22.4 Guidelines for Communicating With Someone Who Is Dying

Avoid automatic responses and trite reassurances.

- Each death is a unique, deeply personal experience for the person and should be treated as such.
- Avoid destroying hope. Reframe hope to what can happen in the here and now.
- Let the person lead the discussion about the future. Be comfortable with focusing on the here and now. (This discussion is not a one-time event; openings for discussion should be encouraged as the person's condition worsens.)
- Relate on a human level. Show humour as well as sorrow.
- Use your mind, eyes, and ears to hear what is said as well as what is not said.

- Respect the individual's pattern of communication and ways of dealing with stress. Support the person's desire for control of their life to whatever extent is possible.
- Maintain a sense of calm. Use eye contact, touch, and comfort measures to communicate.
- Do not force the person to talk. Respect the person's need for privacy, be sensitive to their readiness to talk, and let them know that you will be available to listen.
- Humility and honesty are essential. Be willing to admit when you do not know the answer.
- Be willing to allow the person to see some of your fears and vulnerabilities. It is much easier to open up to someone who is "human and vulnerable" than to someone who appears to have all the answers.

---

stories, funny stories, developmental stories, narratives of advocacy, and family stories. Each reinforces the bonds and affirms the depth of meaning a family holds with a person who is dying. The moments of laughter, foibles, and shared experiences are connections that need to be remembered.

Case Example

Evelyn was an 83-year-old woman diagnosed with terminal lung cancer. During a guided imagery exercise, the nurse asked her to recall a time when she felt relaxed and happy. Evelyn described in vivid detail being with her family at a picnic near a lake, many years ago. When her family came to visit that night, Evelyn related the story again, and the entire family talked about their parts in the remembered event. It was one of their last conversations, one that reinforced family bonds in the initial telling and later as her family remembered Evelyn after her death. Later, her daughter made a special point of letting the nurse know how important sharing this story had been to the person and family.

Providing Information

Nurses are key informants about the person's status and changes in the person's condition. There are fundamental differences in the level of information an individual or family will desire. The response of the person should determine the content and pace of sharing information. Talking with families about care details and potential outcomes should happen often overall, but even more frequently when the person's health status begins to decline or show a change.

Ideally, one nurse serves as the primary contact for the person and family and acts as a liaison between providers and people in their care. This nurse keeps other health team members informed of new issues and shares their input into planning and evaluation of care with the family. Using precise language, giving full and truthful information about the person's condition, and admitting to uncertainty, when it exists, are important dimensions of EOL information giving.

Family Conferences

Family conferences are effective tools to alleviate family anxiety about the dying process, reduce unnecessary conflict between family members, and assist family members with important decision-making processes. It is through these conferences that the effectiveness of the collaborative practice of an interdisciplinary team is realized. Due to representation and the expertise of many disciplines, the team can work toward meeting the physical, emotional, psychosocial, cultural, and spiritual needs of the person and their family (Canadian Nurses Association, n.d.-a, n.d.-b).

The team approach prevents fragmentary and inconsistent care. The person, too, can inform themselves and others around them to identify the best things that can be done to protect them and their choices and can even appoint a substitute decision maker who understands their wishes and would carry them out (Dying With Dignity Canada, 2019b).

Getting everyone's input is important as a source of information, explanation, and support for the person. Formal family meetings held with the palliative care team provide an essential opportunity for providing the same information to all involved family members at the same time, thereby ensuring full disclosure, with opportunities to ask questions (Canadian Nurses Association, n.d.-a, n.d.-b).

Much more than simple clinical explanation is needed. If an essential family member cannot be physically present, having that person available by phone may be the next best option. What is helpful in many situations is to have one family person identified as the point of contact for follow-up issues. Nurses are invaluable resources in clarifying meanings with people or individual family members after the conference.

ADDRESSING CULTURAL AND SPIRITUAL NEEDS

Incorporating Cultural Differences

Canada's population is diverse, composed of many ethnic backgrounds, languages, cultures, and lifestyles. A guiding principle in Health Canada's Palliative Framework is being inclusive, ensuring underserviced populations are taken into consideration, and guaranteeing universal access to palliative care. Indigenous peoples in Canada have requested that there be culturally appropriate palliative care for their communities. It is important to ensure that cultural diversity is respected through the development of new tools and resources like mygrief.ca or kidsgrief.ca, which include age-specific needs (Government of Canada, 2018).

Asking people and their families directly about their cultural values and issues as a starting point helps ensure cultural safety for them. Chovan, Cluxton, and Rancour (2015) note, "The transition from life to death is as sacred as the transition experienced at birth" (p. 49). The dying process, grief, and death itself herald a spiritual crisis— a crisis of faith, hope, and meaning for many people. Spiritual pain occurs when a person's sense of purpose is challenged or one's existence is threatened. When this happens, it is called *spiritual distress* (Horst, 2019). For many cultures, spirituality is significantly embedded in a person's culture, and many cultures have special rituals at EOL. A simple question such as, "Can you tell me about how your family, culture, and spiritual beliefs view serious illness or treatment?" provides a framework for discussion. When cultural differences are considered, it is important to avoid stereotyping, as each person's interpretation of their culture is unique. Once cultural needs are identified, every effort should be taken to honour their meaning to people and their families, by incorporating them in care (see Chapter 7). Box 22.5 presents cross-cultural variations found in palliative and EOL care.

Attending to Spiritual Needs

It is not unusual for people who have previously declined spiritual interventions to desire them as they move into the final phase of life. Spiritual beliefs and religious rituals provide a tangible vehicle for individuals and families to express and experience meaning and purpose. Religious practices and rituals relevant to EOL can be important to people, even if they no longer formally practise the religion. Facilitating these practices touches the person's inner core and helps them move toward a peaceful death They often want to talk about their spiritual beliefs to help them cope with dying. Their quality of life is improved when their spiritual needs are addressed (Horst, 2019).

Nurses can ask the person and family if they would like a visit from an appropriate clergy, faith leader, spiritual elder, or hospital chaplain. They too can ask the person if there is anything they should know about the person's spiritual or religious beliefs. They can offer to sit and listen to the person as they talk about their spiritual needs.

When individuals frame their spirituality from an existential perspective, it is appropriate to explore spirituality sources in terms of meaningful relationships. Asking a question such as "Can you tell me about the relationship you had with someone you loved who has died?" helps start the conversation. A follow-up question relates to how the person feels about the person now. The value of this intervention is that it emphasizes that the person's life held meaning for this other person. This line of

---

BOX 22.5 **Cross-Cultural Variations in End-of-Life Care**

- Emphasis on autonomy versus collectivism
- Attitudes toward advance directives
- Decision making about life support, code status guidelines
- Preference for direct versus indirect disclosure of information
- Individual versus family-based decision making about treatment
- Disclosure of life-threatening diagnoses
- Provider's choice of words in verbal exchanges
- Reliance on physician as the ultimate authority
- Specific rituals or practices performed at time of death
- Role of religion and spirituality in coping and afterlife
- Views about suffering

Adapted from Searight, H., & Gafford, J. (2005). Cultural diversity at the end of life: Issues and guidelines for family physicians. *American Family Physician, 71*(3), 515–522.

questioning indirectly tells the person that they too will be remembered after death (N. Pashby, personal communication, 2015).

People benefit from telling stories about how they view their life, and to validate its meaning. A life review helps people consider the deeper values and purpose of their lives, the experience of joy and sorrow. As one person stated, "I lived my life as best I could. I have no regrets." A follow-up listening response to help the person put into words what they reflect on might be, "Tell me more about this."

EOL is a time for people and their families to explore spiritual questions, to find meaning in the experience of dying and to look for ways to express deep caring (Horst, 2019). The most important intervention nurses can provide is to actively and respectfully listen to each person's search for clarity about their spirituality, with compassion and a desire to understand. Helping people think through spiritual preferences and assisting them in identifying resources that can give them strength, courage, purpose, and encouragement to cope with their situation is highly valued. Providing explicit attention to inclusion of appropriate spiritual advisors, prayer, and scripture reading can be helpful to people who are faith-based and families coping with a terminal condition.

Spiritual issues that trouble people relate to forgiveness, unresolved guilt issues, expressions of love, saying goodbye to important people, and existential questions about the meaning of life and the hereafter, and concern for their family (Baird, 2010). Nurses need to take an honest look at their own spirituality. Self-awareness allows nurses to enter the person's spiritual world from an authentic position, without imposing personal values and beliefs.

PALLIATIVE CARE FOR CHILDREN

It is not the natural order of things for a child to die. People are supposed to live into adulthood. When a child is diagnosed with a life-limiting condition, the effect on parents is devastating; it influences role functioning, friendships, and treatment of siblings (Canadian Cancer Society, 2021a). Children are such an integral part of their parents' identity that issues of parental protectiveness, guilt, responsible caregiving, balancing family demands, and the helplessness parents feel should be part of the discussion. In addition to providing appropriate medications for symptom management to make the child more comfortable, the following interventions are supportive to children with a life-limiting illness.

1. Encourage visits from family and friends.
2. Involve and inform the child of everything that is going on, with developmentally appropriate language and content.
3. Encourage the family to keep the child's life as normal as possible.
4. Suggest ways to enhance family functioning, with attention paid to making special time for siblings and involving them in care discussions.
5. Arrange respite for parents and encourage special parent times.
6. Encourage families to maintain or adapt cultural, family, and religious traditions.
7. Encourage families to seek emotional support: support groups, extended family, friends.

Parents are a major anchoring force for children. They need to be recognized as the expert and a primary advocate for their child. A nurse can take the time to explore with the parents how they conceptualize quality of life for their child, and what is important for the nurse to know about the child's preferences. Nurses can identify situations in which there is a mismatch between a child's condition and a parent's understanding of that. This is important information that needs to be shared with the palliative care multidisciplinary team. By observing the child, nurses can begin to note preferences. Children also value being asked about likes and dislikes. There should be no surprises. You need to talk with the child and the parents about each procedure, in language they can understand. Giving a child a sense that the nurses and parents are on the same page provides security and comfort. Critical to parent satisfaction is the knowledge that everything possible was done for their child; that they received accurate, timely information and support; and that preventable suffering was not permitted.

Grief Issues

Children grieve within the context of the family, but they do not grieve in the same ways. Nurses can help parents talk with their children about the impending death of a significant person in their lives. Encourage parents to explain what is happening in a concrete, direct way, using clear, concrete language suitable to the child's developmental level. Questions should be answered directly and honestly at the child's developmental level of comprehension, free of medical jargon. This type of discussion should *not* be a one-time event, and parents may need to be proactive in initiating the conversation.

Sometimes a family will want to exclude young children from contact with or knowledge about a person who is likely to die soon. Sometimes it is a judgement call as to whether visitation is a good idea. Drawing a picture or sending a note card is another way for a child to connect with a relative who is critically ill if visitation is not an option. With preparation, adolescents can benefit from being allowed to visit with people who are terminally ill.

Case Example

Brendan and his grandfather had a close relationship. Earlier in life, they would stroke each other's thumbs as part of a "special handshake." Now, at 15, his grandfather was close to death and unresponsive. As Brendan sat next to him, stroking his thumb in the remembered way, he felt sure that his grandfather had squeezed his hand more than once. It was a weak squeeze, but it was a meaningful connection for Brendan.

Death of a significant person is difficult for children because they have neither the cognitive development nor the life experiences to fully process its meaning. A child younger than 5 years has no clear concept of what death means.

Until children reach the formal operations stage of cognitive development, they can have fantasies about the circumstances surrounding the death and their part in it.

How a Child Grieves

Children do not express their grief in the same way adults do. Unpredictable acting-out behaviours, withdrawal, anger, fear, and crying are common responses. One minute, the child may be playing, the next he is angry or withdrawn. Preschoolers may repeatedly ask when someone close to them will be coming home even if parents tell them that person has died. Developmentally, they do not understand the permanence of death. Elementary school children accept the permanence of death but view it in a concrete manner.

Case Example

A short time after 5-year-old Aidan's grandfather died, he asked his grandmother where his grandfather had gone. She told him that grandpa died and was in heaven, to which Aidan said, "Oh no, Grandma, he's in that brown box in the ground."

The Canadian Cancer Society identifies common concerns children may have about the death of someone important to them (Canadian Cancer Society, 2021b):
1. Did I cause the death to happen?
2. Is it going to happen to me?
3. Who is going to take care of me?

Parents can create opportunities for children to ask these questions. Asking the child about potential concerns can elicit a conversation that will not happen otherwise. When nurses and parents speak to the child, they need to be cautious about using the words "bad" and "good" to describe cancer cells. The child may believe that they were bad to have bad cancer cells. It is better to use the phrase "cells that are sick" and to openly use the word "cancer." This will help decrease misunderstandings (Canadian Cancer Society, 2021b).

Maintaining daily routines in the child's life after the death of a parent or primary caregiver is critical. Children need to know that they are safe and will be taken care of by the remaining adults in their life. If changes are needed, children should have the opportunity to discuss the reasons for them and time to absorb this information, if at all possible.

Adolescents are particularly vulnerable to unresolved grief. They are often expected to act grown up and model the grieving process for younger siblings. It is unfair to have this expectation. Adults expect adolescents to grieve a death more as an adult than a child, but they lack the life experience to do so.

Sometimes, adolescents will not openly ask questions because they do not want to interfere with parental grief. They may not know how to frame important questions, or they are not sure of the reaction. Any or all of these feelings are normal. Nurses can help parents to gently and proactively offer lead-ins to relevant concerns. Even if the child cannot respond at the moment, having an adult reach out can be very meaningful to a child or adolescent.

At the other extreme, the remaining parent may be unable to fully connect with a child's grief because their own grief is overwhelming. Expectations that an adolescent will step up to the plate and perform household duties or child care are common. Without a place to talk about their feelings, an adolescent may bury feelings that are necessary to process for healing. Adolescents need physical contact, reassurance, and many relevant discussions about the person who has died. If parents are unable to provide the level of communication an adolescent needs, nurses can help them with appropriate referrals.

ACHIEVING QUALITY CARE AT END-OF-LIFE

Death is a deeply personal experience. The Institute of Medicine (2014) defines a **good death** as "one that is free from avoidable distress and suffering for patients, families, and caregivers; in general accord with patients' and families' wishes; and reasonably consistent with clinical, cultural, and ethical standards" (p. 82). Pain and symptom relief, transparent decision making, preparation for death, affirmation of the whole person, and the sense of contributing to others are identified in other research (Steinhauser et al., 2000). In the example below, a nurse helps a person who is terminally ill achieve a sense of spiritual completion.

Case Example

George was in the last stages of his end-of-life journey. He had repeatedly refused to have spiritual visits and had no desire for the sacrament of the living (a religious rite in the Catholic church). His nurse said the priest was close by in the hospital, and asked him if he would like to receive communion. He answered, "Yes, but nothing else." The priest gave him communion, after which the person asked him to hear his confession and requested the last rites. This would not have happened without the collaborative efforts of this nurse's advocacy. After the priest left, George told his nurse, "You always seem to know what to do and when to do it—thank you."

Simulation Exercise 22.4 provides you with the opportunity to personally think about what constitutes a good death.

What to Expect: Anticipatory Guidance

Dying is a normal life process and most family members feel privileged to be present. But, as death approaches, communication becomes more challenging. Anticipatory guidance and nursing presence become important interventions. Family members look to the nurse for information about the dying process, and for emotional support. Nurses have a great deal of knowledge about dying, given the frequency with which they assist people and families through the process. They have the competencies required to manage the complexity of the situation (RNAO, 2011). Unsupported, the process of watching someone die can be a frightening experience for the family.

Family members appreciate anticipatory guidance about what is happening and what to expect, with concrete suggestions about ways to connect with their loved one. With some people, the dying process is swift. With others, there is a gradual downward spiral. Common symptoms include long periods of sleeping or coma, decreased urinary output (dark urine), changes in vital signs, disorientation, restlessness and agitation, dyspnea (breathlessness), Cheyne–Stokes breathing, picking at bed clothes, plus skin temperature and colour changes. All of these changes are normal findings as a person prepares to leave this world. People experience profound weakness when they are dying, such that they cannot independently complete even basic hygiene.

You can help family members understand that as death approaches, there are significant changes in the person's capacity to connect with others or to participate in conversation. Physically touching the person can be comforting as can holding the person's hand.

It is the person's right to stop life-sustaining measures, which means food and hydration. This stoppage may hasten death and is known as voluntarily stopping eating or drinking (VSED).

When attempted by a person who is terminally ill or very weak, VSED usually leads to death within 10 to 14 days. However, even with VSED, death can take longer for people who are younger and more physically robust (Dying With Dignity Canada, 2016). This is a natural part of the body's effort to shut down; it is important to not force food. Giving very small amounts of ice chips or using glycerin mouth swabs can keep the person comfortable. The extremities may become colder to touch and appear mottled. This also is normal. Oxygen can help with breathing and usually is available even in-home settings if the person has hospice care. The person's comfort should be the number one consideration. The Canadian Cancer Society website provides an excellent description of typical changes in the person when death is near and offers a clear outline of what caregivers can do to provide comfort to the person (Canadian Cancer Society, 2021c).

A nurse's calming presence is perhaps the most important form of communication and emotional support for people who are dying and their families (Fig. 22.3). Most people cannot carry on an in-depth conversation as death approaches. Flexibility in allowing family and significant

---

SIMULATION EXERCISE 22.4 What Makes for a Good Death?

Purpose
To help students focus on defining the characteristics of a good death

Procedure
1. In pairs or small groups, think about, write down, and then share briefly examples of a "good" and a "not-so-good" death that you have witnessed in your personal life or clinical setting.

2. What were the elements that you thought contributed to it being a "good" or "not-so-good" death?

Discussion
Were there any common themes found in the stories as to what constitutes a "good" death? How could you use the findings of this exercise in helping people achieve a "good" death?

others open access to the person can reduce family anxiety and can be comforting for all concerned. At the same time, as people approach death, it becomes an effort for the person to respond to family and friends. Telling the family that it is their presence that matters and to use gentle touch or simple words without expecting much verbal communication in return is a helpful intervention. Box 22.6 identifies family communication needs when death is imminent.

Case Example

"I remember standing next to my mom's bed. We had gone to her room to pay our last respects. A young nurse stood near to me and reached out gently and touched my shoulder. Softly she said, 'I'll just stay here with you in case you need something.' When I

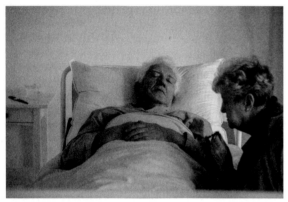

Fig. 22.3 Nurses can facilitate meaningful family "presence" at life's ending, even when verbal communication is limited. iStock.com/KatarzynaBialasiewicz

looked at her, I saw eyes brimming with tears and a profound sadness on her face. Her presence meant so much; I was grateful for her open expression of sorrow. It confirmed the pain we were all experiencing" (Anonymous).

Family members often find it difficult to leave a person who is dying, even when it would be in their best interest to take a short respite. Assuring family members that the nurse will check on the person frequently and will call the family immediately if change occurs gives families permission to take a brief respite from the person's bedside.

Caring for the Person After Death

Respect for the dignity of the person continues after death. If the family is present at the time of death, allowing uninterrupted private time with the person before initiating post-mortem care is important. If the family is not present, all excess equipment and trash should be removed from the room. The nurse can offer presence and emotional support as they escort the family into the room. Some families will want privacy; others will appreciate having the presence of the nurse or chaplain; regardless, family preference should be honoured.

The nurse needs to create a peaceful atmosphere by providing soft lighting, chairs for the family, and tissues. The person's head should be elevated at a 30-degree angle, in a natural position. Hair should be combed, exposed body parts cleaned, and dentures replaced if possible. It is important for the nurse to allow the family as much time as they need with the person. The nurse can obtain signatures to release the person to the funeral home *after* the family has spent some time with the person.

BOX 22.6   Imminent Death: Family Communication Needs

- Honest and complete answers to questions; repetition and further explanation if needed
- Updates about the person's condition and changes as they occur
- Clear, understandable explanations delivered with empathy and respect
- Frequent opportunities to express concerns and feelings in a supportive, unhurried environment
- Information about what to expect—physically, emotionally, spiritually—as death approaches
- Discussion of whom to call, legal issues, memorial or funeral planning

- Conversation about cultural and religious rituals at time of and after death
- Appreciation of the conflicts that families experience when the illness dictates that few options exist; for example, a frequent dilemma at end of life is whether life support measures are extending life or prolonging the dying phase
- Short private times to be present or minister to the person
- Permission to leave the person who is dying for short periods with the knowledge that the nurse will contact the family member if there is a change in status

STRESS ISSUES FOR NURSES IN PALLIATIVE CARE SETTINGS

Nurses become invested in the care and comfort of people and their families facing immediate death; it is an emotional time for everyone involved. **Disenfranchised grieving** is a term applied to the grief nurses can experience after the death of a significant person in their care. It is a very deep loss that others may not understand. Nurses may feel unheard and unsupported. Unlike the people they care for, who live through one loss at a time, nurses can experience several losses a week while caring for people who are terminally ill and their families (Toth, 2017).

Nurses can experience **compassion fatigue**—a syndrome associated with serious spiritual, physical, and emotional depletion related to caring for people—which can affect the nurse's ability to care for other people. Nurses can experience exhaustion, frustration, anger, depression, and trauma and then may experience a secondary trauma related to the negative consequences of fear and work-related trauma (Wu et al., 2016). Unrelieved compassion fatigue can result in burnout and a nurse's decision to leave nursing.

Case Example

Barbara was a new graduate, selected as a nursing intern on a research oncology unit, providing care for children who were seriously ill, on an oncology unit. She had a degree in another field and an excellent job but had always wanted to pursue nursing. Her original preceptor left the hospital and was replaced by an efficient nurse without much empathy. The stress of weekly deaths, severe symptomatology, and lack of empathetic support led Barbara to leave nursing entirely after less than a year and return to her former position.

Developing Self-Compassion

All nurses, but particularly those working on high-intensity units, need to actively pursue ways to experience self-compassion. Self-compassion encourages nurses to balance care for others with care for self. Reflecting on the meaning of connections with people who are dying, and becoming aware not only of your personal strengths but also your limitations, are essential forms of the self-awareness needed for self-compassion. Regular self-reflection allows you to know yourself and gives you more options in relating to people you care for, their families, and other members of the health care team (Wittenberg-Lyles et al., 2013). It gives the nurse a sense of empowerment, improves critical thinking, and, improved quality of care and

outcomes for the people they care for (College of Nurses of Ontario, 2015). Support groups for nurses in which they can successfully address and resolve the secondary stress of continuously caring for people who are terminally ill and some of the ethical issues involved with that care are helpful to nurses. See also the strategies presented in Chapter 17, related to burnout prevention.

SUMMARY

This chapter describes the stages of death and dying, as well as the theory frameworks of Eric Lindemann and George Engel, for understanding grief and grieving. Palliative care is discussed as a philosophy of care and an emerging discipline focused on making EOL care a quality life experience. A good death is defined as a peaceful death experienced with dignity and respect; one that wholly honours the person's values and wishes at the EOL. Nurses can offer compassionate communication, presence, and anticipatory guidance to ease the grief of loss.

Nursing strategies are designed to help people cope with the secondary psychological and spiritual aspects of having a terminal illness such that they achieve the best quality of life in the time left to them. Talking with people about advance directives is a professional responsibility of nurses, and it reduces unnecessary conflict among family members at this critical time in a person's life. Talking with children about terminal illness or death of a relative, or in coping with a terminal diagnosis themselves, should take into consideration the child's developmental level. Questions should be answered honestly and empathetically.

As death approaches, nurses can help families understand the physiological changes signalling the body's natural shutdown of systems. Providing support for clinicians is considered a quality indicator in EOL care. When not addressed, the disenfranchised grief that nurses experience with providing EOL care to multiple people can lead to compassion fatigue, burnout, and moral distress.

ETHICAL DILEMMA
What Would You Do?

Francis Dillon has been on a ventilator for the past 3 weeks. He is not competent to make decisions, and he is not able to communicate. Although he has virtually no chance of recovery, his family refuses to take him off the ventilator because "there is always the chance that he might wake up." What do you see as the ethical issues, and how would you, as the nurse, address this problem?

QUESTIONS FOR REVIEW AND DISCUSSION

1. Describe your most challenging EOL experience. How did you cope with it?
2. What does the concept "quality of life" mean in EOL care?
3. How do you care for yourself when working with people who are seriously ill, and what would you recommend to avoid burnout?

REFERENCES

Adams, J., Bailey, D., Anderson, R. et al. (2013). Adaptive leadership: A novel approach for family decision making. *Journal of Palliative Medicine, 16*(3), 326–329.

Al-Mahrezi, A., & Al-Mandhari, Z. (2016). Palliative care: Time for action. *Oman Medical Journal, 31*(3), 161–163. https://doi.org/10.5001/omj.2016.32.

Andriessen, K., Krysinska, K., Hill, N. T. M. et al. (2019). Effectiveness of interventions for people bereaved through suicide: A systematic review of controlled studies of grief, psychosocial and suicide-related outcomes. *BMC Psychiatry, 19*(49). https://doi.org/10.1186/s12888-019-2020-z.

Aronowitz, S., Compton, P., & Schmidt, H. (2021). Innovative approaches to educating future clinicians about opioids, pain, addiction and health policy. *Pain Management Nursing, 22*(1), 11–14. https://doi.org/10.1016/j.pmn.2020.07.001.

Baird, P. (2010). Spiritual care interventions. In B. R. Ferrell & N. Coyle (Eds.), *Oxford textbook of palliative nursing* (3rd ed., pp. 663–671). Oxford University Press.

Billings, J. A., & Bernacki, R. (2014). Strategic targeting of advance care planning interventions: The goldilocks phenomenon. *JAMA Internal Medicine, 174*(4), 620–624.

Bruera, E., & Yennurajalingam, S. (2012). Palliative care in advanced cancer patients: How and when? *The Oncologist, 17*, 267–273.

Canadian Association of Schools of Nursing. (2011). *Palliative and end-of-life care: Entry-to-practice competencies and indicators for registered nurses.* https://casn.ca/wp-content/uploads/2014/12/PEOLCCompetenciesandIndicatorsEn.pdf.

Canadian Cancer Society. (2021a). *Your child has cancer. Coping when your child has cancer.* https://www.cancer.ca/en/cancer-information/cancer-type/childhood-cancer-information/your-child-has-cancer/?region=on.

Canadian Cancer Society. (2021b). *Talking to your child about their cancer. Coping when your child has cancer.* https://www.cancer.ca/en/cancer-information/cancer-type/childhood-cancer-information/talking-to-your-child-about-their-cancer/?region=on.

Canadian Cancer Society. (2021c). *End-of-life care. Coping when your child has cancer.* https://www.cancer.ca/en/cancer-information/cancer-type/childhood-cancer-information/palliative-care/end-of-life-care/?region=ab.

Canadian Hospice Palliative Care Association. (2021). *Strategic Plan 2019–202: Caring for Canadians at the end of their lives.* https://www.chpca.ca/wp-content/uploads/2019/12/strategic_plan_2019-2022_-_en.pdf.

Canadian Institute for Health Information. (2018). *Access to Palliative Care in Canada.* Canadian Institute for Health Information. https://www.cihi.ca/sites/default/files/document/access-palliative-care-2018-en-web.pdf.

Canadian Mental Health Association. (2016). *Grieving.* https://cmha.ca/documents/grieving.

Canadian Nurses Association. (n.d.-a). *The palliative approach to care and the role of the nurse.* https://www.cna-aiic.ca/~/media/cna/page-content/pdf-en/the-palliative-approach-to-care-and-the-role-of-the-nurse_e.pdf.

Canadian Nurses Association. (n.d.-b). *Palliative and end-of-life care.* https://www.cna-aiic.ca/en/policy-advocacy/palliative-and-end-of-life-care.

Canadian Nurses Association. (2015). *Ethics in practice. Respecting choices in end-of-life care: Challenges and opportunities for RNs.* [Research paper]. https://canadian-nurse.com/~/media/canadian-nurse/files/pdf%20en/respecting-choices-in-end-of-life-care.pdf.

Canadian Pain Society. (2020). https://www.canadianpainsociety.ca.

Chovan, J., Cluxton, D., & Rancour, P. (2015). Principles of patient and family assessment. In B. Ferrell & N. Coyle (Eds.), *Textbook of palliative nursing* (4th ed.). Oxford University Press.

College of Nurses of Ontario. (2015). Practice reflection: Learning from practice. March 3, 2015. http://www.cno.org/globalassets/4-learnaboutstandardsandguidelines/prac/learn/teleconferences/practice-reflection--learning-from-practice.pdf.

Cox, K., Moghaddam, N., Almack, K., et al. (2011). Is it recorded in the notes? Documentation of end-of-life care and preferred place to die discussions in the final weeks of life. *BMC Palliative Care, 10*(18), 1–9.

Doughty, E. A., Wissel, A., & Glorfield, C. (2011). Current trends in grief counseling. http://counselingoutfitters.com/vistas/vistas11/Article_94.pdf.

Dying With Dignity Canada. (2016). *End-of-life considerations.* https://www.dyingwithdignity.ca/other_end_of_life_options.

Dying With Dignity Canada. (2019a). *End-of-life considerations.* https://www.dyingwithdignity.ca/other_end_of_life_options.

Dying With Dignity Canada. (2019b). *Make an advance care plan.* https://www.dyingwithdignity.ca/download_your_advance_care_planning_kit.

Dying with Dignity Canada. (2020). *Navigating a request.* https://www.dyingwithdignity.ca/navigating_a_request.

Engel, G. (1964). Grief and grieving. *American Journal of Nursing, 64*(7), 93–96.

Fox, M. (2014). Improving communication with patients and families in the intensive care unit: Palliative care strategies for the intensive care unit nurse. *Journal of Hospice & Palliative Nursing, 16*(2), 93–98.

Government of Canada, (2018). *Framework on palliative care in Canada.* Health Canada. https://www.canada.ca/en/health-canada/services/health-care-system/reports-publications/palliative-care/framework-palliative-care-canada.html#exec.

Government of Canada. (2020). *Government of Canada reintroduces proposed changes to medical assistance in dying legislation.* https://www.canada.ca/en/department-justice/news/2020/10/government-of-canada-reintroduces-proposed-changes-to-medical-assistance-in-dying-legislation.html.

Guido, G. (2010). *Nursing care at the end of life*. Pearson.

Harris, D. (n.d.). *Overview of grief*. [PowerPoint slides]. King's University College Thanatology Program. King's College, University of Western Ontario. https://www.swpalliativecare. ca/Uploads/Documents/Overview%20of%20Grief.pdf.

Harvard Women's Health Watch. (2009). *Left behind after suicide*. www.health.harvard.edu.

Horst, G. (2019). *Spirituality and life-limiting illness*. Canadian Virtual Hospice. http://www.virtualhospice.ca/en_US/Main+ Site+Navigation/Home/Topics/Topics/Spiritual+Health/ Spirituality+and+Life_Limiting+Illness.aspx.

Institute of Medicine. (2014). *Dying in America: Improving quality and honoring individual preferences near the end of life*. National Academy Press.

Jeffreys, J. (2011). *Helping grieving people—When tears are not enough: A handbook for care providers* (2nd ed.). Brunner-Routledge.

Joint Commission. (2010). *The approaches to pain management: An essential guide for clinical leaders* (2nd ed.). Joint Commission Resources.

Joint Commission International. (2020). *JCI Navigator*. https:// www.jointcommissioninternational.org/en/.

Keegan, L., & Drick, C. (2011). *End of life: Nursing solutions for death with dignity*. Springer.

Kessler, D. (2019). *Finding meaning: The sixth stage of grief*. Scribner.

Kim, S., & Seo, M. (2016). Description of good patient care at end of life. *Applied Nursing Research, 32*, 245–246.

Kogan, M., Cheng, S., Rao, S., et al. (2017). Integrative medicine for geriatric and palliative care. *Medical Clinics of North America, 101*, 1005–1029.

Kübler-Ross, E. (1969). *On death and dying: What the dying have to teach doctors, nurses, clergy, and their own families*. Scribner.

Kübler-Ross, E., & Kessler, D. (2005). *On grief and grieving*. Scribner.

Lendrum, S., & Syme, G. (1992). *Gift of tears: A practice approach to loss and bereavement counseling*. Routledge.

Lindemann, E. (1994). Symptomatology and management of acute grief. *The American Journal of Psychiatry, 151*(Suppl. 6), 155–160. (Original work published 1944).

Noroozian, M., Raeesi, S., Hashemi, R., et al. (2018). Pain: The neglect issue in old people's life. *Open Access Macedonian Journal of Medical Sciences, 6*(9), 1773–1778. https://doi. org/10.3889/oamjms.2018.335.

Registered Nurses' Association of Ontario. (2011). *End-of-life care during the last days and hours*. Clinical Best Practices and Guidelines. Registered Nurses' Association of Ontario. https://rnao.ca/sites/rnao-ca/files/End-of-Life_Care_During_ the_Last_Days_and_Hours_0.pdf.

Registered Nurses' Association of Ontario. (2013). Appendix J. *Assessment and management of pain* (3rd ed.). Registered Nurses' Association of Ontario, pp. 91–92. https://rnao.ca/ sites/rnao-ca/files/AssessAndManagementOfPain_15_WEB-_ FINAL_DEC_2.pdf.

Sawatzky, R. (2016). Conceptual foundations of a palliative approach: A knowledge synthesis. *BMC Palliative Care, 15*, 5.

Schüklenk, U., Van Delden, J., Downie, J. et al. (2011). *Bioethics, 25*(Suppl 1), 1–4. https://doi.org/10.1111/j.1467-8519.2011.

01939.x. https://www.ncbi.nlm.nih.gov/pmc/articles/ PMC3265521/.

Sen, K. (2015). The restoration of wholeness. *Integral Review, 11*(1), 55–64.

Stroebe, M., & Schut, H. (2010). The dual process model of coping with bereavement: A decade on. *OMEGA: Journal of Death and Dying, 61*(4), 273–289. https://doi.org/10.2190/OM.61.4.b.

Thomas, J. (2011). *My saints alive: Reflections on a journey of love, loss and life*. CreateSpace Independent Publishing Platform.

Toth, T. (2017). Recognizing and treating disenfranchised grief. *Insights Magazine*. Winter 2017. https://bc-counsellors.org/ wp-content/uploads/2018/01/Recognizing-and-Treating-Disenfranchised-Grief-Tricia-Toth-Winter-2017.pdf.

Twain, M. (n.d.). Mark Twain quotations, newspaper collections, & related resources. www.twainquotes.com.

Vets Canada. (n.d.). Help for Canadian veterans. Veterans emergency transition services. https://vetscanada.org/.

Wilkie, D., & Ezenwa, M. (2012). Pain and symptom management in palliative care and at end of life. *Nursing Outlook, 60*(6), 357–364.

Wilson, D., Rodríguez-Prat, A., & Low, F. (2020). The potential impact of bereavement grief on workers, work, careers, and the workplace. *Social Work in Health Care, 59*(6), 1–16.

Wittenberg-Lyles, E., Goldsmith, J., Ferrell, B., et al. (2013). *Communication in palliative nursing*. Oxford University Press.

Wu, S., Singh-Carlson, S., Odell, A., et al. (2016). Compassion fatigue, burnout, and compassion satisfaction among oncology nurses in the United States and Canada. *Oncology Nurses Forum, 43*(4), E161–E169. https://doi.org/10.1188/16.ONF. E161-E169.

Zisook, S., Simon, N., Reynolds, C., et al. (2010). Bereavement, complicated grief and DSM. *The Journal of Clinical Psychiatry, 71*(8), 1097–1098.

SUGGESTED READING

Bruera, E., & Yennurajalingam, S. (2011). *Oxford American handbook of hospice and palliative medicine*. Oxford University Press.

Dahlin, C. (2010). Communication in palliative care: An essential competency for nurses. In B. R. Ferrell & N. Coyle (Eds.), *Oxford textbook of palliative nursing* (3rd ed., pp. 663–671). Oxford University Press.

Davies, B., Contro, N., Larson, J., et al. (2010). Culturally sensitive information sharing in pediatric palliative care. *Pediatrics, 4*, e859–e865.

Hui, D., De La Cruz, M., Mori, M., et al. (2013). Concepts and definitions for "supportive care", "palliative care" and "hospice care" in the published literature, dictionaries, and textbooks. *Supportive Care in Cancer, 21*(3), 659–685.

Jevon, P. (2010). *Caring of the dying and deceased patient: A practical guide for nurses*. Wiley-Blackwell.

National Cancer Institutes of Health. (2011). *Grief, bereavement, and coping with loss*. Author. http://cancer.gov/cancertopics/ pdq/supportivecare/bereavement/HealthProfessional.

Neimeyer, R., Currier, J., Coleman, R., et al. (2011). Confronting suffering and death at the end of life: The impact of religiosity, psychosocial factors and life regret among hospice patients. *Death Studies, 35,* 777–800.

Noroozian, M., Raeesi, S., Hashemi, R., et al. (2018). Pain: The neglected issue in old people's life. *Open Access Macedonian Journal of Medical Sciences, 6*(9), 1773–1778. https://doi.org/10.3889/oamjms.2018.335.

Noyes, J., Hastings, R., Lewis, M., et al. (2013). Planning ahead with children with life-limiting conditions and their families: Development, implementation and evaluation of "My Choices." *BMC Palliative Care, 12*(5), 1–17.

Perrin, K., Sheehan, C., Potter, M., et al. (2012). *Palliative care nursing: Caring for suffering patients.* Jones and Bartlett Learning.

Puntillo, K., Nelson, J., Weissmann, D., et al. (2013). Palliative care in the ICU: Relief of pain, dyspnea, and thirst—A report from the IPAAL—ICU Advisory board. *Intensive Care Medicine*(2), 235–248. https://doi.org/10.1007/s00134-013-3153-z.

Sherman, D. (2010). Culture and spirituality as domains of quality palliative care. In M. Matzo & D. W. Sherman (Eds.), *Palliative care nursing: Quality care at the end of life* (pp. 3–38). Springer.

Steinhauser, K. E., Clipp, E., McNeilly, M., et al. (2000). In search of a good death: Observations of patients, families, and providers. *Annals of Internal Medicine, 132*(10), 825–832.

Thomas, J. (2010). My saints alive: A journey of life, loss, and love. [Unpublished manuscript].

Walczak, A., Butow, P., Bu, S., et al. (2016). A systematic review of evidence for end of life communication interventions: Who do they target, how are they structured and do they work? *Patient Education and Counseling, 99,* 3–16.

World Health Organization (WHO). (2016). *WHO definition of palliative care.* Geneva: WHO. http://www.who.int/cancer/palliative/definition/en/.

WEBSITE/RESOURCES LIST

https://bc-counsellors.org/wp-content/uploads/2018/01/Recognizing-and-Treating-Disenfranchised-Grief-Tricia-Toth-Winter-2017.pdf.

https://www.canada.ca/en/health-canada/services/health-care-system/reports-publications/palliative-care/framework-palliative-care-canada.html#exec.

https://canadian-nurse.com/~/media/canadian-nurse/files/pdf%20en/respecting-choices-in-end-of-life-care.pdf.

https://www.canadianpainsociety.ca.

https://www.cancer.ca/en/cancer-information/cancer-type/childhood-cancer-information/palliative-care/end-of-life-care/?region=ab.

www.capc.org.

https://casn.ca/wp-content/uploads/2014/12/PEOLCCompetenciesandIndicatorsEn.pdf.

https://www.chpca.ca.

www.chpcc.org.

https://www.cihi.ca/sites/default/files/document/access-palliative-care-2018-en-web.pdf.

https://cmha.ca/documents/grieving.

https://www.cna-aiic.ca/~/media/cna/page-content/pdf-en/the-palliative-approach-to-care-and-the-role-of-the-nurse_e.pdf.

https://www.cna-aiic.ca/en/policy-advocacy/palliative-and-end-of-life-care#sthash.uhSsBMXY.dpuf.

http://www.cno.org/globalassets/4-learnaboutstandardsandguidelines/prac/learn/teleconferences/practice-reflection--learning-from-practice.pdf.

http://www.cpsa.ca/management-chronic-non-cancer-pain-older-adults/.

https://www.dyingwithdignity.ca/get_the_facts_assisted_dying_law_in_canada.

https://www.dyingwithdignity.ca/other_end_of_life_options.

www.hpna.org.

https://www.jointcommissioninternational.org/en/.

https://www.ldoceonline.com/dictionary/loss.

https://www.ncbi.nlm.nih.gov/pmc/articles/PMC4852088/.

www.nhpco.org

https://www.researchgate.net/profile/Grace_Reynolds/publication/304069423_Compassion_Fatigue_Burnout_and_Compassion_Satisfaction_Among_Oncology_Nurses_in_the_United_States_and_Canada/links/586557e308aebf17d397f402/Compassion-Fatigue-Burnout-and-Compassion-Satisfaction-Among-Oncology-Nurses-in-the-United-States-and-Canada.pdf.

https://rnao.ca/sites/rnao-ca/files/AssessAndManagementOfPain_15_WEB-_FINAL_DEC_2.pdf.

https://www.swpalliativecare.ca/Uploads/Documents/Overview%20of%20Grief.pdf.

www.virtualhospice.ca.

http://www.virtualhospice.ca/en_US/Main+Site+Navigation/Home/Topics/Topics/Spiritual+Health/Spirituality+and+Life_Limiting+Illness.aspx.

https://www.who.int/news-room/fact-sheets/detail/palliative-care.

23

Role Relationship Communication Within Nursing

Olive Yonge
Originating US chapter by *Kathleen Underman Boggs*

OBJECTIVES

At the end of the chapter, the reader will be able to:

1. Discuss professional role relationships among nurses in health care.
2. Distinguish among the professional nursing role opportunities.
3. Describe the components of professional role socialization in nursing.
4. Construct a model of safe, supportive work environments they would work in.
5. Discuss the advocacy role in nurse–person relationships.
6. Apply evidence-informed role research to clinical practice situations.

This chapter presents an overview of role relationships within professional nursing and their implications for professional communication, education, and practice. Being clear about your professional role is essential for meaningful functional relationships with others. Empirical evidence shows effective communication among members of the team reduces the potential for error and the consequences of error, aiding us in providing safe care (Amodo et al., 2017). Applications address the process of professional nursing socialization, role development, mentorship, and communication with all team members. Leadership competencies are discussed. Chapter 24 will address communication in interdisciplinary teams.

BASIC CONCEPTS

Role

Role is a multidimensional psychosocial concept defined as a traditional pattern of behaviour and self-expression performed by or expected of an individual within a given society. People develop social, work, and professional roles throughout life. Some roles are conferred at birth (ascribed roles), and some are attained through circumstance during a lifetime (acquired roles). Personal ascribed role performance standards reflect social, cultural, gender, and family expectations.

Clinical practice blends your knowledge, skills, and attitudes with caring for people. Professional and work relationships have distinctive expectations for your role participation as a member of the organization. These expectations influence communication content and style of presentation (MacArthur et al., 2016). Work relationships have tangible and intangible structural elements that define communication. For example, nurses communicate differently with their peers, supervisor, those they supervise, and the people they care for. Institutional norms also have an effect on the enactment of professional roles and vary according to the work environment.

The ability to accurately interpret and negotiate role relationships in a work setting helps nurses to communicate more effectively.

Professionalism and Work Environment

A nurse's professional relationships and work environment play a big part in satisfaction. Job dissatisfaction contributes to high turnover rates at a time when there is a worldwide nursing shortage (World Health Organization [WHO], 2010). Even in developed countries, new graduates leave their jobs and even the profession in high numbers. Job attrition is cited as running between 15% and greater than 60% in various countries, as cited by numerous articles (Phillips et al., 2015; Shatto et al., 2016). Could creating a supportive workplace with open communication and respect promote better retention?

Professionalism in Nursing

Professional nurses comprise the largest professional group of health care providers. They spend more sustained professional time with people and their families than any other hospital care professional. Nursing roles have steadily evolved to include current expectations for nurses to assume leadership roles, provide primary care, and act as first-line providers in implementing health care reform initiatives.

Professional Nursing Roles

Nurses who provide direct care to people are expected to exhibit competent care skills and also show competency in their communication skills. Contemporary professional nursing roles reflect the increasing complexities of health care, globalization, changing demographic characteristics and diversity of the people they care for, and the exponential growth of health information technology.

The bedside nurses' role consists of delivery and organization of care for multiple people. This role includes quality control issues, problem solving, education, and coordination of communication among the many health team members (McKenna et al., 2017). There is a strengthened focus on health promotion and disease prevention, and self-management of chronic disorders also echoes new economic realities and provider availability. Fig. 23.1 identifies the core professional role competencies required of contemporary nurses, identified by the Institute of Medicine (IOM, 2011). To deliver high-quality, safe, person-centred care, the focus is on collaboration (Farrell et al., 2015), a hallmark of role

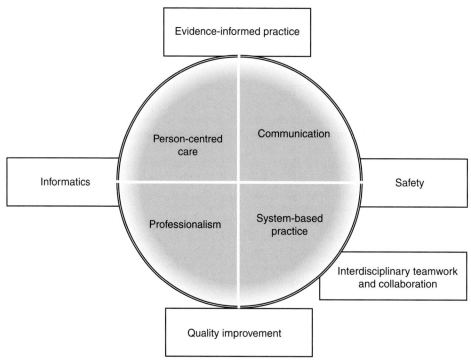

Fig. 23.1 Professional nursing role: Core competencies for health providers. Modified from the Institute of Medicine. (2011). *The future of nursing: Leading change, advancing health.* Author.

competence. We need to know our own role so we can work together smoothly. Read the case of Ms. Feather for an example of person-centred care.

Case Example: Ms. Feather

As a home care nurse, you make a home visit to Ms. Feather, who has diabetes and multiple health issues. She lives in a rural area, with no transportation since the bus service from the nearest city was discontinued. Her primary physician reports that she does not follow the Canadian Diabetic Association diet the nutritionist prescribed using Telehealth. You discover that her only source of food is a fast food place on a nearby highway. Given that you live in the same town, you know about food sources like the food bank and the community garden initiative. You suspect part of Ms. Feather's poor eating habits are due to eating alone and needing more support from others in the community. The town has a small hospital and, since you have at least 10 people on your caseload with diabetes, you ask the administrator if you can run a monthly diabetes awareness and support clinic. Diet is only one aspect of this illness; the people also need to know about foot care, issues with vision, appropriate exercises, and so on. The administrator quickly grasps that you are providing an intervention that could result in decreased need for hospitalization and suggests that the clinic be run weekly. The hospital will provide the space and even provide diabetic-based healthy snacks to be used for teaching purposes and to help people maintain their blood glucose levels.

The scope of practice for professional nurses continues to expand to include health screening and promotion, risk reduction, and disease prevention strategies. Nurses increasingly provide care as part of interdisciplinary health care teams, in hospitals and the community. All nurses are expected to advocate for health care transformation and to take a leadership role in addressing environmental, social, and economic determinants of health. Nurses are assuming public advocacy roles to inform policymakers, educators, and other health care providers about health-related issues. Nurses also provide leadership and coordination in health care improvement through education and participation in research. Simulation Exercise 23.1 is designed to help you look at the different role responsibilities of practising nurses.

Technology

Competency in use of technology is a goal for the Canadian Association of Schools of Nursing (CASN, 2012), and technology permits swift transactions, universal access, and levels of portability unanticipated 20 years ago. Defining aspects of caring and communication with people in your care are supported, not led, by technology. Nurses are more responsible than ever to devise communication strategies that preserve the caring aspects of nursing. Chapters 26 and 27 provide in-depth discussions of communication and technology use issues.

Leadership

Hesburgh's (1971) description of leadership, and its relationship to caring, still holds true:

> The mystique of leadership, be it educational, political, religious, commercial or whatever, is next to impossible to describe, but wherever it exists, morale flourishes, people pull together toward common goals, spirits soar, order is maintained, not as an end in itself, but as a

---

SIMULATION EXERCISE 23.1 Professional Nursing Roles

Procedure:

Ask a nurse whom you admire if you can have a 20-minute interview related to their role development as a registered nurse in clinical practice.

Ask the following questions:

1. What are the different responsibilities involved in their job?
2. What training and credentials are required for the nurse's position?
3. What is the type of population they encounter in their work?
4. What are the most difficult and rewarding aspects of the job?
5. Why did the nurse choose a particular area or role in nursing?
6. What opportunities does the nurse see for the future of nursing?
7. You are also encouraged to add your own explorative questions.

Discussion

1. Describe anything that surprised you during the interview.
2. Compare similarities and differences in the results of your interview with those of your classmates.
3. Create a scenario from what you have learned that you can implement in a future professional experience.

means to move forward together. Such leadership always has a moral as well as intellectual dimension; it requires courage as well as wisdom; it does not simply know, it cares (p. 764).

Role Clarity

Professional role clarity is an essential quality for working with health care teams. If nurses are not clear about their professional roles, it is difficult for them to communicate their value as health care providers to other professionals. Yet, a 2017 study found that new graduates still lack knowledge about their role (McKenna et al., 2017). Role clarity about professional competencies is necessary to support safety initiatives for people in your care that lead to improved outcomes. Influencing change and making difficult decisions become easier when nurses have a clear vision of their professional role because they are better able to stimulate confidence in others.

Competency

Competency is defined as "a set of capabilities, skills, aptitude, expertise, and experience" (Rick, 2014). In addition to development of technical nursing skills, technology, and communication skills, collaborative skills are needed to become a positive force in team-based health care.

New Differentiated Practice Roles

The IOM (2011) mandate to increase the number of professional nurses in advanced practice roles makes a strong statement in health care reform. An empowering aspect of the nurse role is the opportunity to evolve roles, change specialties of care, move into advanced roles, or take on new administrative roles. Nurses must put forth the value of nurses as skilled health care providers. Evolved scopes of practice and professional standards serve as the foundation for practice accountability and decision authority in contemporary nursing practice.

Advanced Practice Nurses

An **advanced practice nurse** (APN; also referred to as an APRN) is a licensed, skilled practitioner holding a minimum of a master's degree in a clinical specialty, with the expert knowledge base, complex decision-making skills, and clinical competencies required for expanded specialty practice. Various countries have established many roles for APNs, including nurse practitioners, clinical nurse specialists, certified nurse midwives, nurse anaesthetists, and others. Specialized training allows APRNs to diagnose and independently manage care, including prescriptive authority for some. In addition to clinical roles, APRNs function in research, educational, and administrative roles. A significant issue yet to be completely resolved is a lack of

consistency across provinces and territories that has lessened but still exists surrounding role responsibilities and scope of practice of APRNs.

The Clinical Nurse Specialist (CNS) and Nurse Practitioner (NP)

Nurses working in advanced practice roles like clinical nurse specialists (CNSs) or nurse practitioner **nurse practitioners (NPs)** levels meet the complex health needs of Canadians in a wide variety of settings and contribute to the development of a sustainable, efficient, and effective health system. A CNS is a registered nurse with advanced nursing knowledge and skills in making complex decisions, who holds a master's or doctoral degree in nursing with expertise in a clinical nursing specialty. They first emerged as a speciality in the 1970s but as the cuts to health care started in the 1980s and 1990s, many were laid off. An NP is a registered nurse with additional educational preparation and experience who possesses and demonstrates the competencies to autonomously diagnose, order, and interpret diagnostic tests, prescribe pharmaceuticals, and perform specific procedures within their legislated scope of practice. NPs gained formal recognition in the 1970s, when this role was recommended to provide care to isolated populations.

Education programs were started, but a perceived oversupply of physicians in urban areas, a lack of enabling legislation, and problems related to remuneration resulted in a lack of interest in promoting this role. However, interest was rekindled in the 1990s by health care reform, an increased demand for access to primary health care, and the need for integrated care. Formal legislation and regulation for NPs started in 1998, and all the provinces and territories now have it. The supply of NPs in Canada has more than tripled from 1 393 in 2007 to 5 274 in 2017 (Canadian Nurses Association [CNA], 2021a).

The Doctor of Nursing Practice

In 2004, the doctor of nursing practice (DNP) as a terminal practice degree for professional nurses was introduced in the United States. The complexity of the nation's health care environment served as a major impetus for promoting transitions to practice doctorates, as did the need to position nursing professionally on par with other majour health professions, all of which offer practice-focused doctorates. The curriculum combines advanced nursing practice skill proficiency with a solid foundation in the clinical sciences, evidence-informed practice methods, system leadership, information technology, health policy, and interdisciplinary collaboration (American Association of Colleges of Nursing [AACN], 2004). Canada has been slow to follow. Currently, only the University of Toronto has introduced a doctor of nursing (DN) option for students, and they admitted their first class in September 2021. The focus of the program is preparing nurses for leadership roles in health care settings, policy, or nursing education, whereas the PhD program prepares nurses for careers as research scientists in academia and other research-intensive environments (Bloomberg Faculty of Nursing, 2021).

The PhD-Prepared Nurse Researcher

Doctoral research degree programs in nursing have grown substantially in developed countries. These nurses are prepared to conduct original research, to be primary investigators seeking substantial grants, working not only in university settings but in many health care corporations.

Trends in Education That Develop Communication Skills

Experiential learning

Experiential learning is defined as active participation in learning scenarios, with self-reflection to analyze learning components. Contemporary health care education depends on experiential learning for developing both technical care skills and communication proficiency. Its competency-based goal is to provide students with the knowledge, skills, and attitudes needed to effectively collaborate and improve the quality of health care. Students use case study analyses, role play, exercise activities, computer simulations, standardized models, and so on. The most vital part of the experiential learning process is the final activity of reflection analysis to recap what was learned and strategize about how to correct mistakes made.

Clinical Simulations

Problem-based learning scenarios provide innovative opportunities for students to analyze and find solutions in a safe, controlled environment. Clinical simulation is a preferred learning strategy because it allows interdisciplinary students to give close attention to all aspects of the clinical environment and to actively problem solve solutions from a collaborative team perspective. Students construct and develop "live" understanding of interdisciplinary health team functioning through shared reflection on their actions and interactions with each other in collectively meeting identified person-centred goals.

Interdisciplinary Courses

Interdisciplinary education is defined as educational occasions when two or more professions learn from and about each other to improve collaboration and the quality of care. Introducing interdisciplinary coursework early in the curriculum helps students to understand nursing roles and communication across other professionals. It gives some insight into the "mindset" of other professionals and encourages a pattern of collaboration. Generally, teams in health care are characterized as an "interprofessional collaborative," with the first term alluding to an integration of two or more professional cultures operating in a transdisciplinary manner and the second encompassing concepts of sharing, partnership, interdependency, power, and process (Canadian Patient Safety Institute, 2021a; Schot et al., 2020). Students gain first-hand understanding of the professional values held by other disciplines. In clinical scenarios, the decision-making process with team approaches is more complex than with single discipline methods, acknowledging and respecting that the unique expected behaviours and skill sets of each health discipline fosters understanding. Frequent communication is essential to good results.

Examples of shared interdisciplinary electives include ethics, death and dying, culture, quality improvement (QI), genomics, emergency preparedness, gerontology, health policy, and legal issues. Clinical simulation courses open to students from multiple health disciplines provide unique opportunities for students in the health care professions to work together in the clinical management of complex disease health conditions.

Case Example

Three final-year, baccalaureate nursing students and four third-year medical students plus their preceptors undertook preceptorships concurrently, in a semi-rural acute care setting in Alberta, Canada. The goal of the pilot project was to emphasize interprofessional (IP) collaboration and team building. The researchers collected data through midpoint and endpoint semi-structured interviews and two focus groups. The data were coded and analyzed using Glaserian grounded theory.

The participants reported that they had enhanced knowledge of each others' scope of practice, resulting in increased confidence in working with other disciplines and fully understanding the meaning of IP teamwork. Given that the setting was in a rural area, the medical and nursing students continued embracing interprofessional collegiality beyond the clinical setting. The success of this initiative was based on preparing the medical and nursing students for an IP experience before the clinical rotation and providing modules for them to learn more together about the meaning of IP and the nature of rural work. There were a few issues with logistics, turf consciousness, and expectations for students to take initiative and be self-reliant. However, overall, the pilot was a tremendous success and the program has continued, with many more students requesting rural placements.

Adapted from Jackman, D., Yonge, O., Myrick, F. et al. (2016). A rural interprofessional educational initiative: What success looks like. *Online Journal of Rural Nursing and Health Care* 16(2), 5–26. DOI:10.14574/ojrnhc.v16i2.417.

APPLICATIONS

Professional Role Socialization

Professional role socialization is a complex, continuous, interactive educational process through which student nurses acquire the knowledge, skills, attitudes, norms, values, and behaviours associated with the nursing profession (deSwardt et al., 2017; Strouse & Nickerson, 2016). Beginning nurses acquire their professional identity. Role identity is thought to mitigate the negative effects of stress, helping them avoid "burnout" (Sun et al., 2016). Transmission of the cultural value system inherent in the nursing profession is seen as the key element in role socialization. For example, beginners learn that nurses value their autonomy and the people in their care (Thomas et al., 2015). Building on Leininger's ideas (1991) about the culture of nursing, there is a process of mastering the knowledge, skills, and attitudes on role. Although greater understanding of the transition process is needed, we know that role modelling by academics and especially by expert clinicians is vital (Baldwin et al., 2014).

Acquiring the Profession's Culture

Acquiring the profession's culture involves internalizing the values, standards, and role behaviours associated with professional nursing. As students begin to try out new professional behaviours, they receive feedback and support for their efforts from clinical staff, faculty, and the people in their care. Positive feedback empowers students by acknowledging their clinical judgements and encourages them to perform successfully.

Academic Role Models as Socializing Agents

Initially, nursing students are absorbed in learning basic knowledge and skills. They depend on textbooks, instructors, and simulation labs to help them. As students become comfortable with foundational nursing knowledge, they interact with clinical staff. With increased experience, students begin to trust their reasoning in making clinical judgements.

Clinical Nurses as Socializing Agents

Nursing faculty, clinical preceptors, and nursing mentors serve as important socializing agents, helping students learn the values, traditions, norms, and competencies of the nursing profession (Felstead & Springett, 2016).

 DEVELOPING AN EVIDENCE-INFORMED PRACTICE

Purpose
The researchers wanted to understand the weight management approaches used by primary care providers working in team-based settings and how they determined the most suitable approach for a person.

Methods
A total of 20 primary care providers (13 nurse practitioners and 7 family physicians), working in 6 multidisciplinary clinics in Ontario, were interviewed. A descriptive, qualitative design was used, incorporating content analysis and NVivo qualitative software.

Results
The 20 primary care providers most frequently referred to onsite programming and determined that the most suitable weight management approach based on people's preference, motivation, and so on. The pharmacological approach was underutilized due to perceived adverse side effects and cost to people in the study.

Conclusions
Given the availability of onsite resources, it was easy to refer people. If they did not follow through, it was viewed as their choice.

Application to Your Clinical Practice
The finding of this research study demonstrates the importance of team-based care for people. They are more likely to be referred and given resources if their primary caregiver is aware and in close proximity to the resources.

Adapted from Aboueid, S., Jasinska, M. & Bourgeault, I. (2018). Current weight management approaches used by primary care providers in six multidisciplinary healthcare settings in Ontario. *Canadian Journal of Nursing Research, 50*(4), 169–178. https://doi.org/10.1177/0844562118769229.

Clinical Preceptors

In a formalized, goal-directed clinical orientation relationship, the **clinical preceptor** is an experienced nurse, chosen for clinical competence and charged with supporting, guiding, and participating in the evaluation of student or new graduate clinical competence on a one-to-one basis. Perhaps designated by employers or by virtue of being on a career ladder, clinical preceptors model professional behaviours, give constructive feedback, and promote clinical thinking in the novice nurse or nursing student (Oosterbroek et al., 2017).

Mentors

Mentoring describes a commitment to help another nurse become the best professional they can be. Mentors are expert nurses who act as advisors for less experienced nurses, generally over a long time period. They can be a sounding board for career option discussions and for providing guidance in looking at the whole picture while considering what will fit in with our personal responsibilities. Every nurse should seek out a career mentor, someone whose experience can help to guide their career (Yonge et al., 2012).

Orientation

Accrediting agencies now recommend formal "orientation" programs to orient and guide new graduate nurses, suggesting that to be effective, such programs need to be at least a year in length. The programs combine some didactic instruction with clinical guidance by one or more preceptors. Expectations about profession communication skills and agency goals, rules and communication styles are imparted (MacArthur et al., 2016). The attitudes, actions, and directed support of the preceptor encourages students to adopt clinically appropriate professional behaviours. On the other hand, a clinical mentor who does not follow good communication strategies, such as the tools provided by the TeamSTEPPS program (Canadian Patient Safety Institute, 2021a, 2021b), can negate all that the mentored nurse has learned in the classroom (Amodo et al., 2017). In addition to clinical preceptors, other informal socializing agents include the people in their care, families, and peers. These people promote understanding of the professional nursing role from a consumer perspective.

Employment Transition

Transitioning to a new role is always stressful, even for experienced nurses. Personality traits that include resilience and inquisitiveness aid this transition. The Bauer and Erdogan (2011) "socialization model" as well as organizational theories have been applied to understand what makes a nurse effectively transition from student to novice nurse to competent practitioner (Phillips et al., 2015).

Internationally, several authors developed models designed to describe the role transition process all new nurses undergo during their first year of work (Benner, 1984/2001; Duchscher & Kramer, 2012). In her classic work discussing the theory–practice gap and subsequent "reality shock," Benner describes five developmental stages of formative role development in professional nursing. Based on the Dreyfus and Dreyfus model (1980) of skill acquisition, each developmental stage demonstrates increasing proficiency in implementing the professional nursing role: novice, advanced beginner, competence, proficiency, and expert.

1. Novice. The first stage is referred to as the *novice stage.* Initially, students have limited or no nursing experience to perform required nursing tasks. Novice nurses need structure and exposure to the objective foundations upon which to base their nursing practice. They tend to compare clinical findings with the textbook picture because they lack the practice experience to do otherwise. Theoretical knowledge and confidence in the expertise of more practiced nurses and faculty serve as guides to practice. Schoessler and Waldo's model (2006) suggests that in the first 3 months of employment, the new graduate nurse struggles to develop organizational skills, master technical skills, and deal with coping with mistakes or the fear of making them.

2. Advanced beginner. In this stage, nurses understand the basic elements of practice and can organize and prioritize clinical tasks. Although clinical analysis of health care situations occurs at a higher level than strict association with the textbook picture, the advanced beginner is able to only partially grasp the unique complexity of the situation of each person in their care. Preceptors can make a difference in helping new nurses cope with the uncertainty of new clinical situations and to hone their skills. They act as a "guide by the side" in helping new nurses gain nursing proficiency (Dracup & Bryan-Brown, 2004). The people in the new nurse's care are also an important resource. For example, they can help us to develop a greater appreciation for the complexity of social, psychological, and physical aspects of chronic disease as a result of their interactions. By paying close attention to the people they care for, and what seems to work best, advanced beginner nurses learn the art of nursing. In the Schoessler and Waldo model, this time is referred to as a "neutral zone," the phase in which communication with others, including physicians or people they care for, is still problematic, while feeling more comfortable with organization and knowledge. After the first year and before 18 months, the new nurse enters a "new beginning" phase of feeling comfortable with nursing activities.

3. Competence. The competence stage occurs 1 to 2 years into nursing practice. The competent nurse is able to easily manage the many contingencies of clinical nursing (Benner, 1984/2001). Nurses begin to practise the "art" of nursing. They view the clinical picture from a broader perspective and are more confident about their roles in health care.

4. Proficiency. The proficiency stage occurs 3 to 5 years into practice. Nurses in this stage are self-confident about their clinical skills and perform them with competence, speed, and flexibility. The proficient nurse sees the clinical situation as a whole, has well-developed psychosocial skills, and knows from experience what needs to be modified in response to a given situation (Benner, 1984/2001).

5. Expert. This last stage of expert nurses is marked with a high level of clinical skill and the capacity to respond authentically and creatively to people's needs and concerns. Expert nurses "have confidence in their own ability and rarely panic in the face of a breakdown" (Benner, 1984/2001, p. 115). They can recognize the unexpected and work creatively with complex clinical situations. Expert nurses demonstrate mastery of technology, sensitivity in interpersonal relationships, and specialized nursing skills in all aspects of their caregiving. Being an expert nurse is not an end point; nurses have the professional and ethical responsibility to continuously upgrade and refine their clinical skills through professional development and clinical skill training. Table 23.1 identifies behaviours associated with the different levels of Benner's model.

Continuing Education

Professional development represents a lifelong commitment to excellence in nursing and requires regular upgrading of skills. Standard means of continued professional development include relevant continuing education presentations, staff development modules, conference

TABLE 23.1   Benner's Stages of Clinical Competence

Nurse Competency Level	Description of Behaviours
Advanced beginner	• Enters clinical situations with some apprehension • Sees task requirements as central to the clinical context, whereas other aspects of the situation are seen as background • Requires knowledge application to meet clinical realities • Perceives each clinical situation as a personal challenge • Is typically dependent on standards of care, unit procedures
• Competent	• Focuses more on clinical issues in contrast to tasks • Can handle familiar situations • Expects certain clinical trajectories on the basis of their experience with particular people they've cared for • Searches for broader explanations of clinical situations • Has enhanced organizational ability, technical skills • Focuses on managing people's conditions
• Proficient	• Responds to particulars of clinical situations in a broader way • Requires an experiential base with past populations they've cared for • Understands people's transitions over time • Learns to gauge involvement with people and their families to promote appropriate caring
• Expert	• Has increased intuition regarding what are important clinical factors and how to respond to them • Engages in practical reasoning • Anticipates and prepares for situations while remaining open to changes • Performs care in a "fluid, almost seamless" manner • Bonds emotionally with people and their families, depending on their needs • Sees the big picture, including the unexpected • Works both with and through others

From Norman, V. (2008). Uncovering and recognizing nurse caring from clinical narratives. *Holistic Nursing Practice, 22*(6), 324–335, with permission.

attendance, academic education, specialized training, and research activities. Professional development also occurs through informal means such as consultation, professional reading, experiential learning, giving presentations, and self-directed learning activities such as Internet-based modules. The CNA and regulators in the provinces and territories all expect nurses to engage in continuing education (CNA, 2021b). These education methods offer unique opportunities to access new information and to network, share expertise, and learn different perspectives from others in the field.

Strategic Career Planning

Serious career plans should reflect careful appraisal of values, skills, interests, and different career possibilities. Mentors can be helpful in this area.

Role Relationships Within Nursing

It is inevitable that you will encounter some communication and collaboration problems with nurse colleagues. If managed appropriately, these difficulties can become opportunities for innovative solutions and improved relationships. A number of strategies discussed in Chapter 24 are useful in dealing with fellow nurses.

Peers

The nurse–person relationship occurs within the larger context of your professional relationships with coworkers. Issues will arise. However, if we ignore relationship problems, others may unconsciously "act out" and undermine care. Historically, newly hired staff nurses encountered as much "hazing" as they received support. Bullying is discussed in Chapter 24. Occasionally you may have to work with a peer with whom you develop a "personal conflict." Stop and consider what led up to the current situation. Most often, it is due to the accumulation of small annoyances that occur over time. The best method of approaching this situation is to verbalize occurrences rather than ignoring them until they become a major problem. Avoid "the blame game," and discuss in a private, calm moment what you both can do to make things better. Modelling positive interactions may assist in resolution. Holding an "intervention" or "crucial conversation" discussion is needed.

Whenever there is covert conflict among nurses, it is the person in your care who ultimately suffers the repercussions. Sanner-Stiehr and Ward-Smith (2014) describe a case whereby a very experienced nurse is offered a position in the ICU. Since she has never worked in the ICU, her preceptor is cold and, worse, indifferent to her. No one models positive interactions or holds an intervention. Finally, she is set up by her preceptor to give a medication the wrong way and then blamed by the doctor for compromising the patient. The level of trust people being cared for have in the professional relationship is compromised until the staff conflict can be resolved. Getting accepted and building congenial working relationships take time and some energy.

Supervisors

Negotiating with people in authority can be stressful, even threatening, because such people have control over your future as a staff nurse or student. Supervision implies shared responsibility in our overall goal of providing safe, high-quality care to people in our care. The wise supervisor is able to promote a nonthreatening environment in which all aspects of professionalism are allowed to emerge. In the supervisor–nurse relationship, conflict may arise when performance expectations are unclear or when the nurse is unable to perform at the desired level. Communication of expectations often occurs after the fact, within the context of employee performance evaluations. Effective management means these job expectations are known from the first day. Frequent feedback and performance reviews are used to let you know about areas needing improvement, as part of an ongoing, constructive relationship. When a supervisor gives constructive criticism, it should be in a caring, nonthreatening manner.

Supervision of Staff

Use of open communication techniques already discussed is effective in supervising others. If a problem occurs, use the same communication techniques described in Chapter 14: state your concern, state expectations, and mention outcomes that will occur if the problem behaviour persists. There are two categories of personnel you as a staff nurse might be responsible for supervising: unlicensed and licensed personnel.

Unlicensed Assistive Personnel

Our nursing workload demands have given rise to employment of several types of unlicensed personnel, such as health care aides. Although we are ultimately responsible for the quality and safety of care given under our supervision, we delegate less complex tasks to assistants. **Delegation** is defined as the transfer of responsibility for the performance of an activity from one individual to another while retaining accountability. Whether delegating to a peer or unlicensed assistive personnel (UAP), the nurse is only transferring a task, not responsibility for care (Saskatchewan Registered Nurses Association, 2015). Delegation can free up a nurse to attend to more complex care needs. In the current health care environment, some UAPs possess minimal knowledge or experience skills, whereas others have excellent abilities. Refer to your licensure organization for guidelines.

Licensed Nurses

There are several categories of nurses who have a more limited scope of practice and may require supervision. In some countries, these nurses are known as **licensed practical nurses (LPNs)**, nursing assistants (NAs), **unregulated care providers (UCPs)**, registered practical nurses (PNs) and, in the four western provinces, there are **registered psychiatric nurses (RPNs)**. For the latter category, depending on the agency they are working in, RPNs may be fully independent practitioners. Role overlap, lack of clear distinctions in roles, power factors, and pay inequality still lead some to struggle with maintaining collegial relationships (Limoges & Jagos, 2015). Appropriate use of delegation can facilitate meeting these challenges. More often than not, novice nurses are inadequately prepared for the demands of delegation (College of Nurses of Ontario, 2018).

Case Example: Monica Lewis, RN

After receiving the report of her assignments for people to provide care to, Monica Lewis assigns a newly hired unregulated care provider (UCP), Sally, to provide routine care (morning bath, assistance with breakfast) to several people assigned to her, including Ms. Jones, who was admitted yesterday for exacerbation of her type 2 diabetes mellitus. Monica completes a head-to-toe health assessment on Ms. Jones. She then turns to Sally and asks her to give Ms. Jones foot care. Sally admits she has never given foot care to a person with diabetes but knows

that she has to be very careful not to cut the nails or the skin because typically people with diabetes have impaired circulation. Monica had assumed all UCPs underwent training on principles and administration of foot care.

Inherent in effective delegation is an adequate understanding of the skills and knowledge of UAPs, as well as abiding under the legal act of each province and territory. These acts clearly state what can and what cannot be delegated and to what type of personnel these actions can be delegated. The employing agency and the nurse need to reinforce the UAP's knowledge base, assess current level of abilities, oversee tasks, and evaluate outcomes. This is a costly process both in time and energy. Simulation Exercise 23.2 should help you to consider the principles of delegation.

Self-Awareness

Self-awareness is defined as the capacity to accurately recognize emotional reactions as they happen and to understand your responses to different people and situations. Self-awareness helps nurses work from their strengths and cope more effectively to minimize personal weaknesses in interactions with others. Developing self-awareness allows nurses to make higher-quality decisions because decisions are more likely to be based on facts than personal feelings.

It is not always easy to be completely honest about one's personal weaknesses, values, and beliefs. However, this level of self-awareness is a crucial component of effective

---

SIMULATION EXERCISE 23.2   Applying Principles of Delegation

Purpose:
To help students differentiate between delegating nursing tasks and evaluating outcomes

Procedure:
Divide the class into two groups. Reflect on the following case study of a typical day for the charge nurse in an extended-care facility. Group A is to describe the nursing tasks they would delegate to assistants and the instructions they would give. Group B is to describe the responsibilities of the professional nurse related to the delegated work.

Reflective analysis and discussion: identify goals.

Case:
Anne Marie Roach, RN, is the day shift charge nurse at Shadyside Extended Care Facility. Today, the unit census is 24, and her staff includes four nursing assistants (NAs)

and two licensed practical nurses who are allowed to administer oral medications. The NAs are qualified to give morning baths; assist with feeding; obtain and record vital signs, intake, and output; do finger sticks for blood glucose readings; turn and reposition people who are confined to their beds due to mobility challenges; and assist the others to ambulate. They also change wound dressings for the three people needing this care. Of the residents, 12 are confined to their beds, requiring full baths and feeding assistance. The remaining 12 need some assistance with morning care and ambulation to the dining room. Nine residents need glucose levels taken; seven have weakness due to stroke. All residents are at risk for falls. The night shift reported all residents' conditions as stable. Now it is time to make today's assignments.

Reflective Analysis
Discuss and evaluate group responses.

professional leadership development. Self-awareness directly affects self-management and how we respond professionally to others. Professional self-awareness promotes recognition of the need for continuing education, the acceptance of accountability for one's own actions, the capacity to be assertive with professional colleagues, and the capability of serving as an advocate for the people in your care when the situation warrants it, even if it is uncomfortable to do so.

Nurses Have Rights

In addition to significant responsibilities, as a nurse, you have rights in your professional relationships with colleagues and people you provide care for (see Box 23.1).

Think about your professional collegial relationships and your dual professional commitment to self and others. How can you balance your legitimate responsibilities to yourself and your responsibilities to people you care for and your coworkers?

Transformational Leadership

Leadership plays a pivotal role in setting expectations regarding scope of practice, collaboration, optimal interdisciplinary teamwork, and empowered knowledge partnerships in professional nursing practice. Transformational leadership requires engaging the hearts as well as the minds of those in the workforce. The transformational leader is self-actualized; stays focused on group processes; influences others in a warm, trusting climate; inspires trust; challenges the status quo; and empowers others. Simulation Exercise 23.3 provides an opportunity to examine nurse leadership behaviours.

Strong nursing leadership is the driving force for creating an empowering work environment that fosters positive outcomes for nurses and people in their care (Boamah, 2018). Transformational leadership qualities include a clear vision and commitment to excellence, with a willingness to take reasonable risks and consult with others, and persistent dedication to task completion. They understand leadership as a communication process, not an event or position. Transformational leaders are energetic, positive thinkers who act as visible role models in helping other nurses to develop leadership skills (Rolfe, 2011).

Structural Empowerment

Structural empowerment is a concept that describes the organizational commitments and configurations that give informational and supportive power to health care workers to accomplish their work effectively in significant ways. Complex health care issues require different types and levels of expertise, working together to achieve an outcome greater than the sum of individual efforts. Communication among health providers is open, and there is an appropriate mix of health care personnel to ensure quality care.

BOX 23.1 Nurses, Health, and Human Rights

CNA Position

- Nurses* are central to ensuring access to health care, which is a fundamental human right.
- As the Canadian Nurses Association (CNA) states in its *Code of Ethics for Registered Nurses*, "Nurses uphold principles of justice by safeguarding human rights, equity and fairness and by promoting the public good" (CNA, 2017, p. 15). Further, as the Code states, nurses must, as an ethical endeavour, do this by "maintaining awareness of broader global health concerns, such as violations of human rights, war, world hunger, gender inequities and environmental changes, and working and advocating (individually and with others) to bring about change locally and globally" (CNA, 2018, p. 18).

- A nurse's primary responsibility is to fulfil their professional duty to safeguard human rights, even if doing so conflicts with meeting an employer's obligations; nurses in such a conflict are solely responsible for their actions.
- Nursing organizations can use their influence to safeguard health as a human right. For example, they play a role by publicizing information (such as the Code of Ethics).
- It is the responsibility of governments to uphold human rights legislation and to comply with international declarations and treaties to which they are signatories.

*Unless otherwise stated, *nurse* or *nursing* refers to any member of a regulated nursing category (i.e., a registered nurse, nurse practitioner, licensed/registered practical nurse, or registered psychiatric nurse). This definition reflects the current situation in Canada, whereby nurses are deployed in a variety of collaborative arrangements to provide care.

From Canadian Nurses Association. (2017). *Code of ethics for registered nurses.* https://www.cna-aiic.ca/~/media/cna/page-content/pdf-en/code-of-ethics-2017-edition-secure-interactive; Canadian Nurses Association. (2018). *Nurses, Health and Human Rights. Position Statement.* https://www.cna-aiic.ca/-/media/cna/page-content/pdf-en/nurses-health-and-human-rights-position-statement_dec-2018.pdf?la=en&hash=F3E784558F08815146C4472003CBCA6434468226.

SIMULATION EXERCISE 23.3   **Characteristics of Exemplary Nurse Leaders**

Purpose

To help students distinguish leadership characteristics in exemplary leaders and managers encountered in everyday nursing practice. Identifying leadership characteristics helps students become aware of professional behaviours associated with achieving the mission of professional nursing.

Procedure

This exercise is most effective when the reflections take place prior to class time and findings are discussed in groups of four to six students.

1. Reflect on the professional characteristics and behaviours of a professional nurse you admire as a leader in your work or educational setting.
2. Write down what stood out for you about this person as a leader, in your mind. What specific characteristics

framed this person as a leader? How did this person relate to other health care providers, including students?

3. Share and discuss your findings with your small group. Have one student act as a scribe. Identify commonalities and differences in student perceptions.
4. Share small group findings with your larger class group.

Discussion

1. Describe specific behaviours associated with effective leadership.
2. Distinguish ways that nurses can demonstrate leadership in contemporary health care.
3. Evaluate ways nursing leadership is a dynamic, interactive process.
4. What are some of the ways nurses can demonstrate leadership in contemporary health care?

Communicating to Creating Safe, Supportive Work Environments

The acuity of people that nurses provide care for continues to rise over the decades. If there is a nursing shortage, this creates a great deal of stress for hospital administration and short-handed health care providers. Measures need to be implemented that attract nurses and improve clinical outcomes for the people they care for. Improving work environments in health care shapes outcomes for *both* nurses and the people they look after (Bianco et al., 2014).

Physical Space

Agency administrators have tried various strategies to promote healthy work environments that support easier communication among staff. Batch and Windsor's (2015) study found use of space integral to effective communication–for example, arranging inpatient beds and storing supplies in people's rooms to decrease the number of steps nurses walk. Communication devices such as smartphones or hands-free devices dated already allow nurses to locate other personnel more easily. Computers or tablets at bedsides promote easier record keeping. Refer to Chapters 26 and 27.

Climate

Beyond the physical arrangements, the work environment is patient-centred. There is a supportive atmosphere with a commitment to seek solutions, value nurses, and provide quality, patient-centred care. Likewise, nurses who are good communicators, competent, dependable, adaptable,

and responsible are key variables in creating a satisfying, quality work environment.

Open Communication

Collaborative relationships characterized by open communication are directly linked to optimal outcomes for people. Goals that focus on improvement rather than punitive measures are important to prevent future errors. Embracing use of technology also helps to reduce errors, such as barcoding for medicines or lab specimens.

Team Collaboration

Components of collaboration include working with other nurses who are clinically competent, with a supportive manager, and with team members who respect each other's roles and respond to errors in a facilitative, nonpunitive manner.

Manageable Workload

Safe work environments include safe staffing levels, provisions for adequate off-unit breaks, ongoing education, nurse autonomy and accountability, and adherence to standards of care with evidence-informed interventions (Amir, 2013).

Magnet Hospitals

The **Magnet Recognition Program** was created to develop and support quality work environments favourable to nurses and to recognize nursing role excellence. The designation is awarded through the American Nurses Association (ANA) credentialing centre. The application procedure is complex and demanding, and few hospitals achieve Magnet designation. The first Magnet hospital was designated in 1994, and non-American health care organizations were able to participate beginning in 2000. In the United States, approximately 6.61% of all registered hospitals have achieved Magnet Recognition status. In 2015, Mt. Sinai was the first and only Canadian hospital—and one of only eight institutions outside the United States—to achieve Magnet designation care (Mount Sinai Hospital, 2015).

Networking Roles

Networking is an essential component of professional role development and ultimately of advancing the status of professional nursing roles in health care delivery systems. *Professional networking* is defined as establishing and using contacts for information, support, and other assistance to achieve career goals (Canadian Nurses Association, 2021c). Nurses can use networking when they are in the market for a new job, need a referral, want to receive or share information about an area of interest, or need assistance with making a career choice. Networking is a two-way interactive process. As a form of communication, networking offers valuable professional opportunities for developing new ideas and receiving feedback that might not otherwise be available. Have your business cards with you. Follow up with contacts by sending a text, email, or other communication. Participating in activities of nursing organizations or continuing education events provides fertile ground for opportunities. Networking with health providers from other disciplines is also important.

Advocacy Roles

The goal of advocacy support of people you care for is to empower them and to help them attain the services they need for self-management of health issues. Nurses are advocates for people every time they protect, defend, and support a person's rights or intervene on behalf of people who cannot do so for themselves. The CNA (2021b) affirms advocacy as an essential role in its *Code of Ethics for Nurses*. People who benefit from advocacy fall into two categories: those who need advocacy because of vulnerability caused by their illness and those who have trouble successfully navigating the health care system. Nursing advocacy of people they care for includes facilitating access to essential health care services for people and acting as a liaison between people and the health care system to ensure quality care, improve health, and reduce health deviations. Nurses need to be aware of people's rights when advocating for them (Box 23.2). For more information on nurse involvement in community-based advocacy, see Chapter 25.

Advocacy should support autonomy. People need to be in control of their own destiny, even when the decision reached is not what you as the nurse would recommend. Referrals to community resources should be chosen based on compatibility with the person's expressed need, financial resources, accessibility (time as well as place), and ease of access.

Nurse–Person Role Relationships

Nurse Role

Professional performance behaviours in the nurse–person relationship include a sound knowledge base, technical competency, and interpersonal competency, as well as caring. On a daily basis, nurses must collect and process multiple, often indistinct, pieces of behavioural data. They problem solve with people and their families to come up with workable, realistic solutions. Through words and

---

BOX 23.2 Patient Rights

What Are Patient Rights?

Patient rights are those basic rules of conduct between patients and medical caregivers.

A patient is anyone who has requested to be evaluated by or who is being evaluated by any health care professional.

People don't always know that they have rights within the Canadian health care system, let alone what those rights are.

Here are some examples of your rights:

Patients in Canada have the right to the following:

1. To receive appropriate and timely care
2. To be treated with dignity and respect
3. To receive health services without discrimination
4. To have their personal and health information protected from disclosure
5. To have access to their health information unless, in the opinion of a relevant health professional, the disclosure could result in immediate and grave harm to the patient's health or safety
6. To refuse consent to any proposed treatment
7. To receive information relating to any proposed treatment and options
8. To the recognition of your representative or substitute decision maker
9. To the recognition of your advance directive
10. To a second opinion
11. To pain and symptom management

Each province and territory has its own unique documented patient rights.

Excerpted from Canadian Health Advocates. (2021). *Canadian Patient Rights.* https://canadianhealthadvocatesinc.ca/patient-rights/.

behaviours in relationship with other health care providers and agencies, nurses provide quality care and act as advocates for people and for the nursing profession.

Currently, nurses function in a high-tech, managed health care environment in which the human caring aspects of nursing are easier to overlook. Unique challenges to the nurse–person relationship in clinical practice include shorter in-person contacts, technology, and lower levels of trust in relation to these factors. The nurse–person relationship will become increasingly important in helping people feel cared for in a health care environment that sometimes neglects their psychosocial needs in favour of cost effectiveness.

The Role of People Receiving Care

In the current health care environment, people are expected to take an active role in self-management of their condition to whatever extent is possible. People receiving care also have rights (Box 23.2). Often, they are active members on hospital or hospital/university committees. The relational expectation is for an equal partnership, having shared power and authority as joint decision makers in their health care. Is the person-centred model of health care delivery actually true? Is every decision related to diagnosis and treatment based on combined input and joint responsibility for implementing the recommendations? Use of the person's self-knowledge and inner resources allows nurses to more effectively respond to their needs.

SUMMARY

How nurses perceive their professional role and how they function as a nurse in that role has a sizable effect on the success of their interpersonal communication. The professional nursing role should be evidenced in every aspect of nursing care but nowhere more fully than in the nurse–person relationship. A professional nurse's first role responsibility is to the person. Because hospitals no longer are the primary settings for nursing practice, nurse practice roles take place in nontraditional and traditional, community-based health care settings. Expanded nursing roles are described. Emphasis on health team roles and communicating with interdisciplinary team members will be further described in Chapter 24.

Socialization theory was described to explain the transition to the professional role. Among other theorists, focus was given to Benner's five developmental stages of increasing proficiency to describe the nurse's progression from novice to expert. Professional development as a nurse is a lifelong commitment. Mentorship and continuing education assist nurses in maintaining their competency and professional role development.

ETHICAL DILEMMA
What Would You Do?

As a new nurse on the unit, you witness people receiving diminished care quality due to poor communication and lack of provider continuity. If you raise the issue in a staff meeting with your supervisor and coworkers, you fear your opinion will not be taken seriously because the others have been working together for a much longer time than you. What should you do?

QUESTIONS FOR REVIEW AND DISCUSSION

1. Identify the critical indicators of professionalism in nursing.
2. Classify the skills you consider the most important in developing a collaborative team approach to clinical care.
3. Evaluate the statement, "Every nurse should be a leader," and explain how this idea might be realized in contemporary health care.
4. What do you conjecture as the distinct and collaborative contributions of different professional roles to providing care and health care delivery?

REFERENCES

American Association of Colleges of Nursing. (2004). *AACN position statement on the practice doctorate in nursing.* American Association of Colleges of Nursing. www.aacnnursing.org/DNP.

Amir, K. (2013). *Quality and safety for transformational nursing: Core competencies.* Pearson Education, Inc.

Amodo, A., Baker, D., Emery, D. et al. (2017, June 5). *TeamSTEPPS National Conference.*

Baldwin, A., Mills, J., Birks, M. et al. (2014). Role modeling in undergraduate nursing education: An integrative literature review. *Nurse Education Today, 34*(6), e18–e26.

Batch, M., & Windsor, C. (2015). Nursing casualization and communication: A critical ethnography. *Journal of Advanced Nursing, 71*(4), 870–880.

Bauer, T. N., & Erdogan, B. (2011). Organizational socialization: The effective onboarding of new employees. In S. Zedeck (Ed.), *APA handbook of industrial and organizational psychology* (Vol. 3, pp. 51–64). Author. http://doi.org/10.1037/12171-002.

Benner, P. (2001). *From novice to expert: Excellence and power in clinical nursing practice.* Prentice Hall. (Original work published 1984).

Bianco, C., Dudkiewicz, P. B., & Linette, D. (2014). Building nurse leader relationships. *Nursing Management, 45*(5), 42–48.

Bloomberg Faculty of Nursing. (2021). *Developing nursing leaders prepared to take their careers to the next level.* FAQ on Doctor of Nursing (DN) program. Lawrence S. Bloomberg Faculty of Nursing, University of Toronto. https://bloomberg.nursing.utoronto.ca/programs/doctor-of-nursing-dn/#content4.

Boamah, S. (2018). Linking nurses' clinical leadership to patient care quality: The role of transformational leadership and workplace empowerment. *The Canadian Journal of Nursing Research=Revue canadienne de recherche en sciences infirmieres, 50*(1), 9–19. https://doi.org/10.1177/0844562117732490.

Canadian Association of Schools of Nursing. (2012). *CASN nursing informatics: Entry-to-practice competencies for registered nurses.* https://www.casn.ca/2014/12/casn-entry-practice-nursing-informatics-competencies/.

Canadian Nurses Association. (2021a). *Advanced practice nursing.* https://www.cna-aiic.ca/en/nursing-practice/the-practice-of-nursing/advanced-nursing-practice.

Canadian Nurses Association. (2021b). *CNA learning centre.* https://www.cna-aiic.ca/en/professional-development/cna-learning-centre.

Canadian Nurses Association. (2021c). *Networking.* https://www.cna-aiic.ca/en/nursing-practice/career-development/career-planning/networking.

Canadian Patient Safety Institute. (2021a). *Use team strategies and tools to enhance performance and patient safety. TeamSTEPPS Canada.* https://www.patientsafetyinstitute.ca/en/education/TeamSTEPPS/Pages/default.aspx.

Canadian Patient Safety Institute. (2021b). *Policy brief.* https://www.patientsafetyinstitute.ca/en/toolsResources/HomeCareSafety/Documents/CrossSectorCollaborationbrief.pdf#search=interdisciplinary.

College of Nurses of Ontario. (2018). *RN and RPN Practice: The client, the nurse and the environment. Practice guideline.* https://www.cno.org/globalassets/docs/prac/41062.pdf.

deSwardt, H. C., van Rensburg, G. H., & Oosthuizen, M. J. (2017). Supporting students in professional socialization: Guidelines for professional nurses and educators. *International Journal of Africa Nursing Sciences, 6*, 1–7.

Dracup, K., & Bryan-Brown, C. W. (2004). From novice to expert to mentor: Shaping the future. *American Journal of Critical Care, 13*(6), 448–450.

Dreyfus, S. E., & Dreyfus, H. L. (1980). *A five-stage model of the mental activities involved in directed skill acquisition.* University of California at Berkeley.

Duchscher, J., & Kramer, M. (2012). *From surviving to thriving: Navigating the first year of professional nursing practice* (2nd ed.). Nursing the Future.

Farrell, K., Payne, C., & Heye, M. (2015). Integrating interprofessional collaboration skills into the advanced practice registered nurse socialization process. *Journal of Professional Nursing, 31*(1), 5–10.

Felstead, I. S., & Springett, K. (2016). An exploration of role model influence on adult nursing students' professional development: A phenomenological research study. *Nurse Education Today, 37*, 66–70.

Hesburgh, T. (1971). Presidential leadership. *Journal of Higher Education, 42*(9), 763–765.

Institute of Medicine. (2011). *The future of nursing: Leading change, advancing health.* Author.

Leininger, M. (1991). *Culture of care diversity and universality: A theory of nursing.* National League for Nursing.

Limoges, J., & Jagos, K. (2015). The influences of nursing education on the socialization and professional working relationships of Canadian practical and degree nursing students: A critical analysis. *Nurse Education Today, 35*, 1023–1027.

MacArthur, B. L., Dailey, S. L., & Vilagran, M. M. (2016). Understanding healthcare providers' professional identification: The role of interprofessional communication in the vocational socialization of physicians. *Journal of Interprofessional Education and Practice, 5*, 11–17.

McKenna, L., Brooks, I., & Vanderheide, R. (2017). Graduate entry nurses' initial perspectives on nursing: Content analysis of open-ended survey questions. *Nurse Education Today, 49*, 22–26.

Mount Sinai Hospital. (2015). *Mount Sinai first in Canada to achieve Magnet® Recognition for nursing excellence and patient care.* https://www.mountsinai.on.ca/about_us/news/2015-news/mount-sinai-first-in-canada-to-achieve-magnet-recognition-for-nursing-excellence-and-patient-care.

Oosterbroek, T., Yonge, O., & Myrick, F. (2017). Rural nursing preceptorship: An integrative review. *Online Journal of Rural Nursing and Health Care,* (17), 1.

Phillips, C., Esterman, A., & Kenny, A. (2015). The theory of organizational socialization and its potential for improving transition experiences for new graduate nurses. *Nurse Education Today, 35*, 118–124.

Rick, C. (2014). Competence in executive nursing leadership for the 21st century: The 5 eyes. *Nurse Leader, 12*(2), 64–66.

Rolfe, P. (2011). Transformational leadership theory: What every leader needs to know. *Nurse Leader, 9*(2), 54–57.

Sanner-Stiehr, E., & Ward-Smith, P. (2014). Lateral violence and the exit strategy. *Nursing Management, 45*(3), 11–15. https://doi.org/10.1097/01.NUMA.0000443947.29423.27.

Saskatchewan Registered Nurses Association. (2015). *Interpretation of the RN scope of practice.* https://www.srna.org/wp-content/uploads/2017/09/Interpretation_of_the_RN_Scope_2015_04_24.pdf.

Schoessler, M., & Waldo, M. (2006). The first 18 months in practice: A developmental transition model for the newly graduated nurse. *Journal for Nurses in Staff Development, 22*(2), 47e–554e.

Schot, E., Tummers, L., & Noordegraaf, M. (2020). Working on working together: A systematic review on how healthcare professionals contribute to interprofessional collaboration. *Journal of Interprofessional Care, 34*(3), 332–342. https://doi.org/10.1080/13561820.2019.1636007.

Shatto, B., Meyer, G., & Delicath, T. A. (2016). The transition to practice of direct entry clinical nurse leader. *Nurse Education in Practice, 19*, 97e–103e.

Strouse, S. M., & Nickerson, C. J. (2016). Professional culture brokers: Nurse faculty perceptions of nursing culture and their role in student formation. *Nurse Education in Practice, 18*, 10–15.

Sun, L., Gau, Y., Yang, J. et al. (2016). The impact of professional identity on role stress in nursing students: A cross-sectional study. *International Journal of Nursing Studies, 63*, 1–8.

Thomas, J., Jenks, A., & Jack, B. (2015). Finessing incivility: The professional socialization experiences of student nurses' first clinical placement: A grounded theory. *Nurse Education Today, 35*(12), e4–e9.

Yonge, O., Myrick, F., Ferguson, L. et al. (2012). Preceptorship and mentorship [Editorial]: *Nursing Research and Practice* (pp. 1–2). Hindawi Publishing Corporation. downloads. hindawi.com/journals/specialissues/389707.pdf.

World Health Organization. (2010). *Framework for action on interprofessional education and collaborative practice.* www. who.int/.

SUGGESTED READINGS

Benner, P. (2005). Using the Dreyfus model of skill acquisition to describe and interpret skill acquisition and clinical judgment in nursing practice and education. *Bulletin of Science, Technology & Society, 24*(3), 188–199.

Farag, A., & Tullai-McGuinness, S. (2017). Do leadership style, unit climate, and safety climate contribute to safe medication practices? *The Journal of Nursing Administration, 47*(1), 8–15.

WEBSITE/RESOURCES LIST

https://www.bccnp.ca/Standards/RN_NP/resourcescasestudies/ workplace/employedstudentnurses/Pages/preceptor.aspx.

https://bloomberg.nursing.utoronto.ca/programs/doctor-of-nursing-dn/#content4.

https://canadianhealthadvocatesinc.ca/patient-rights/.

https://www.casn.ca.

https://www.casn.ca/2014/12/casn-entry-practice-nursing-informatics-competencies/.

https://www.cihi.ca/en 2018.

https://www.cna-aiic.ca/en.

https://www.cna-aiic.ca/-/media/cna/page-content/pdf-en/ advanced-practice-nursing-framework-en.pdf?la=en&hash =76A98ADEE62E655E158026DEB45326C8C9528B1B.

https://www.cna-aiic.ca/en/nursing-practice/career-development/ career-planning/networking.

https://www.cna-aiic.ca/en/nursing-practice/the-practice-of-nursing/advanced-nursing-practice.

https://www.cno.org/globalassets/docs/prac/41062.pdf.

https://www.diabetes.ca.

https://www.ola.org/en/legislative-business/bills/parliament-36/ session-3/bill-9.

https://www.patientsafetyinstitute.ca/en/toolsResources/teamwork Communication/Documents/Canadian%20Framework%20 for%20Teamwork%20and%20Communications%20Lit%20 Review.pdf.

https://www.patientsafetyinstitute.ca/en/education/Team STEPPS/Pages/default.aspx.

https://www.srna.org/wp-content/uploads/2017/09/Interpretation_ of_the_RN_Scope_2015_04_24.pdf.

24

Interprofessional Communication

Olive Yonge

Originating US chapter by *Kathleen Underman Boggs*

OBJECTIVES

At the end of the chapter, the reader will be able to:

1. Discuss application of Team Strategies and Tools to Enhance Performance and Patient Safety (TeamSTEPPS) concepts of team communication and effects on safe care.
2. Identify communication barriers in interprofessional relationships, including disruptive behaviours.
3. Describe methods for handling conflict through interpersonal negotiation.
4. Discuss methods for communicating effectively with others in organizational settings (Canadian Interprofessional Health Collaborative [CIHC], 2010).
5. Discuss application of research to evidence-informed clinical communication, including TeamSTEPPS approach.

The World Health Organization (WHO) states that, to promote safety, people need to take ownership of their health care (2016). To be effective as a nursing professional, it is not enough to be deeply committed to person-centred care; proficient communication skills are necessary to function as a member of an interprofessional team to effectively provide quality care safely.

An essential communication skill is the ability to adapt your own communication style to meet the needs of team members and to mindfully and continually scan changing situations. This chapter focuses on principles of communication with other professionals. Strategies are suggested that you can use to function more effectively as an interprofessional team member and leader. Specific ways to communicate with other health care providers are described to help you remove communication barriers. Collaboration in health care teams are again discussed in Chapter 25.

BASIC CONCEPTS

Many experts cite effective communication as a bedrock principle of quality care. Effective communication is timely, accurate, complete, unambiguous, and understood by the recipient. Communication breakdowns can negatively affect people's care. For example, the literature shows that the greatest determinant of intensive care unit (ICU) death rates is how well nurses and physicians work together in planning and providing care. Effective communication prevents errors of all magnitudes. The Joint Commission (TJC) found that team communication breakdowns were the root cause of preventable sentinel events in 68% of cases (Canadian Patient Safety Institute [CPSI], 2021; TJC, 2015). Communication challenges are substantial when many different providers are involved. Deliberate and mindful use of strategies to improve communication is part of a nurse's job (Perry et al., 2016).

STANDARDS FOR A HEALTHY WORK ENVIRONMENT

Shared Mental Model

Increasing complexity of care characterizes all health care workplaces, usually requiring interprofessional teamwork to provide comprehensive care. Every team member needs to "buy in" to the collaborative team concept. Team functioning, especially in increasingly complex health situations, requires effective teamwork to ensure people's safety (Mace-Vadjunec et al., 2015; Polis et al., 2017). A good example of interprofessional collaboration is at the University of Toronto, where 11 health sciences programs all require the students to complete an Interprofessional Education (IPE) program as part of their curriculum (University of Toronto Centre for Interprofessional Education, 2016).

Open Communication

Open communication and trust are core elements for smooth and effective teamwork (Polis et al., 2017). A good example is the lack of compliance by health care workers to use good hand hygiene. Research results have shown it to be less than 40% (CPSI, 2020). The challenge is for health care workers to remind each other if they see lack of proper hand hygiene. Nurse Wang worked closely with a surgeon, Dr. Lui. Dr. Lui was always in a hurry to examine people postoperatively. Three factors drove him: genuine concern for people in his care, scarcity of time, and curiosity about the effectiveness of his surgery. One day, he touched and peeled back a corner of the bandage postoperatively of one of the people he had performed surgery on, and then he turned to examine another person in the same room. Nurse Wang quickly intervened and said, "You may need to sanitize your hands, and I just happen to have some hand sanitizer here. Just hold out your hand." Dr. Lui complied and later at the desk, thanked Nurse Wang for the intervention.

Collegiality

A culture of collegiality is essential for a work environment that is to provide high-quality care of people. The interprofessional team depends on an effective blending of the collective competencies of each provider to deliver quality health care. Collaboration begins with communicating an awareness of each other's roles, knowledge, and skills and continues with the development of shared values. If team members do not trust and respect each other and communicate in an open and respectful manner, they are more likely to make mistakes. Reflect on the following surgical unit case example.

Case Example: Conflict on a Surgical Unit

Two nursing teams work the day shift on a busy surgical unit. As nurse manager, Ms. Libby notices that both teams are arguing over computer use and have become unwilling to help cover people being looked after by the other team. It is now taking longer to complete assigned work. To achieve a more harmonious work environment, she arranges a staff meeting to get the teams to communicate. Rather than just

computer issues, multiple problems surface, suggesting inadequate time management and work overload. Ms. Libby listens actively, responds with empathy, and provides positive regard and feedback for solutions the group proposes. She asks the group to decide on two prioritized solutions. Recognizing that her staff feel unappreciated, and knowing that compromise is a strategy that produces behaviour change, she resolves to offer more frequent performance feedback, such as weekly evaluations via email, and to provide specific data on overtime. She herself assumes responsibility for requesting an immediate computer upgrade, using the unit budget's emergency funding allocation. A team member who serves on the employee relations committee assumes responsibility for requesting that the human services department schedule an in-service training on time management and stress reduction within the next month. The group agrees to meet in 6 weeks to evaluate.

Collegiality is discussed in Chapters 14 and 23, as are aspects of healthy work environments.

- Nurses must be as efficient in communication skills as they are in clinical skills.
- Nurses must be relentless in pursuing and fostering true collaboration.
- Nurses must be valued and committed partners in making policy, directing and evaluating clinical care, and leading organizational operations.
- Staffing must ensure the effective match between nurse competencies and the needs of people they provide care for.
- Nurses must be recognized and recognize others for the value each brings to the work of the organization.
- Nurse leaders must fully embrace the imperative of a healthy work environment, authentically live it, and engage others in its achievement.

Other professional nursing organizations have identified the following elements of a healthy workplace environment:

- Develop collaborative culture of trust
- Maintain respectful open communication and behaviour
- Provide a communication-rich culture that emphasizes trust and respect
- Define role expectations clearly, with accountability
- Maintain an adequate workforce
- Provide competent leadership
- Use shared decision making
- Participate in employee development
- Recognize workers' contributions

Code of Behaviour

The goal of collaboration is to communicate effectively with team members to provide safe, ethical, high-quality care. As part of creating a culture of teamwork where staff is valued, a standard across organizations should be zero tolerance for disruptive or bullying behaviours. To accomplish this, each organization needs one well-defined code of behaviour applied consistently to all staff. TJC mandates that each health care organization has a code of conduct defining acceptable and unacceptable behaviours, as well as an agency process for reporting and handling disruptive behaviours, discrimination, or disrespectful treatment (TJC, 2010). In Canada, the Canadian Nurses Association (CNA) has a Code that outlines for all nurses the importance of ethical relationships, behaviours, and decision making. The Code refers to the importance of being a colleague and working with others on the health team (Canadian Nurses Association, 2017).

Definitions for the word *collaboration* in the literature remain imprecise (Fewster-Thuente, 2015). Collaboration is a dynamic process in which work groups from different professional backgrounds cooperate and share expertise to deliver quality health care. This approach involves an integration of knowledge, skills, and attitudinal values. Complex health issues are best addressed by an interdisciplinary team approach (Farrell et al., 2015). This coordinated form of care delivery was advocated by the Institute of Medicine (IOM) 2011 Report. Ideally, each team member understands the roles of others and pools their own expertise with those of other team members.

The National Interprofessional Competency Framework "provides an integrative approach to describing the competencies required for effective interprofessional collaboration. Six competency domains highlight the knowledge, skills, attitudes and values that shape the judgements essential for interprofessional collaborative practice. The six competency domains are: 1) interprofessional communication 2) patient/client/family/community-centred care 3) role clarification 4) team functioning 5) collaborative leadership and 6) interprofessional conflict resolution" (CIHC, 2010).

The TeamSTEPPS program stresses the importance of developing a shared mental model (goal) for each person's care. In the program, health care providers learn how to adopt teamwork strategies within their own teams to build capacity and momentum (Canadian Patient Safety Institute, 2021).

Teamwork and Communication

Interprofessional team functioning is both a role-focused process and task-based skills–focused process. Team members have unique personalities, egos, and skill sets, yet all must work together. Playing to each team member's strengths enhances the ability to deliver safe, quality care. Collaborating in joint decision making and care coordination requires knowing when to hold and when to let go of ideas and opinions. Effective teamwork also requires individual members to have the requisite knowledge, skills, and attitudes (including collective efficacy, shared vision, team cohesion, mutual trust, and shared orientation) (Emanuel et al., 2011).

Teamwork and communication are recognized as key contributors to safe, high-quality care (Mchugh et al., 2020).

Barriers to Effective Team Communication

Barriers to effective team communication include not sharing information among team members; a hierarchical structure inhibiting some members from speaking up; variations in communication styles or vocabulary; and complacency, defensiveness, and conflict (TeamSTEPPS, 2017). Note that studies show that the vast majority of front-line staff report care not completed on the prior shift. Would open communication help resolve this?

Conflict Antecedents

Ineffective communication often leads to disagreements, injured feelings, and unsafe care. Poor communication is one of several factors frequently cited in the literature as an underlying cause of conflict (Almost et al., 2016; Trepanier et al., 2016). Refer to Box 24.1 for others. Misfeldt and colleagues (2017) applied a sociological model to analyze the functioning of primary health care teams in Canada. Their model lists effective team characteristics as effective formal and informal communication; mutual respect; team leadership and vision; and role clarity and accountability. Problems in any of these areas can be reflected as disruptive behaviour and can compromise safety.

Disruptive Behaviours

Conflict was defined in Chapter 14 as a hostile encounter. The nursing literature uses a variety of terms to refer to persistent, uncivil behaviours in the workplace: bullying; verbal abuse; horizontal violence; lateral violence; "eating your young"; in-fighting; and mobbing, harassment, or scapegoating. The term we use in this book is **disruptive behaviour**.

Disruptive behaviour is defined as a lack of civility or lack of respect that occurs within professional relationships as frequently as weekly and is repeated over time. Disruptive behaviours may include overt behaviours such as rudeness, verbal abuse, intimidation, or put-downs; angry outbursts, yelling, blaming, or criticizing team members in front of others; sexual harassment; or even threatening physical

BOX 24.1   Interpersonal Sources of Conflict in the Workplace: Barriers to Collaboration and Communication

1. Different expectations
   Role ambiguity
   Being asked to do something you know would be irresponsible or unsafe
   Having your feelings or opinions ridiculed or discounted
   Getting pressure to give more time or attention than you are able to give
   Being asked to give more information than you feel comfortable sharing
   Differences in language
2. Threats to self
   Maintaining a sense of self in the face of hostility or sexual harassment
   Being asked to do something concerning a person you are caring for that is in conflict with your personal or professional moral values
3. Differences in role hierarchy
   Differences in education or experience
   Differences in responsibility and rewards (payment)
   Lack of support from leadership or administration (or both)
4. Clinical situation constraints
   Emphasis on rapid decision making
   Complexity of care interventions
   Stressful workload

confrontations. Other disruptive behaviours are more covert; these include passive–aggressive communication, withholding need-to-know information, withholding help, assigning excessively heavy workloads, refusing to perform assigned tasks, impatience or reluctance to answer questions, refusal to return phone calls or pages, and speaking in a condescending tone. These behaviours threaten the well-being of nurses and the safety of the people they provide care for (Castronovo et al., 2016; Koh, 2016).

Disruptive behaviour is fairly common in large organizations, especially hospitals. Ranging from half to three-quarters of all nurses report being subjected to disruptive behaviour at some time, which they say compromised care and safety (Lyndon et al., 2015; Moore et al., 2017). TJC (2008) cites ineffective communication between team members as contributing to 60% of errors (Wilson & Rockstraw, 2012). This also affects student nurses, as seen in the Tee et al., 2016 study, in which half of student

nurses reported experiencing bullying or harassment. Most researchers have found that nurse-to-nurse disruptive behaviours occur more frequently than disruptive physician–nurse interactions and occur more often in high-stress areas such as surgical suites, psychiatric units, or emergency departments (Hutchinson & Jackson, 2013).

Outcomes for People Receiving Care

Disruptive behaviour is a barrier to effective health care and could even lead to serious medical errors (Kimes et al., 2015; Shahid & Thomas, 2018) and decreases person satisfaction (Mace-Vadjunec et al., 2015). For example, in Press and colleagues' 2015 study, disruptive behaviour was associated with increased levels of readmission to the hospital. Poor communication is associated with problems in safety. Good collaboration and communication have been shown to be associated with better outcomes, such as decreased infections (Boev & Xia, 2015).

Nurse Outcomes

As described earlier, failures in collaboration and communication among health team members are among the most common factors cited for nurse frustration, job stress, poor morale, job abandonment, lost productivity, loss of confidence, absenteeism, and task avoidance, and they adversely affect nurses' physical and mental health (Dzurec et al., 2017; Eriksen et al, 2016; Kimes et al., 2015).

Organization Outcomes

Costs to the agency focus on financial issues related to absenteeism, increased staff turnover, losses in productivity, as well as increases in care errors and even legal action. Other outcomes include decreases in care quality, increases in care errors, and adverse outcomes (Trepanier et al., 2016).

CREATING A COLLABORATIVE CULTURE OF REGARD TO ELIMINATE DISRUPTIVE BEHAVIOUR

To deliver safe, high-quality health care, the corporate climate now emphasizes a collaborative, **patient-centred care (PCC) model** in which the hierarchical power model is replaced by a model in which all team members are valued. Organizational support is essential for success. Collaboration is broadly defined as working with all members of the health care team to achieve maximum health outcomes for people the team is providing care for and includes the following:

1. Common goal: Developing a collaborative culture in which all team members keep the delivery of safe,

high-quality care foremost in mind requires that we trust and respect the decision making of all team members. Different professional groups were educated to hold differing beliefs and styles of communication. We need to develop an understanding of these various perspectives, not so we can change them, but so that we can utilize them.

2. Open, safe communication: Creating a communication-rich environment requires that all team members value open communication. We combine assertiveness (speaking up, giving and receiving feedback) with cooperation.

3. Mutual respect: Mutual respect involves appreciation for each member's value. An important part of working together is developing mutual trust; you trust coworkers to "have your back."

4. Shared decision making: The IOM (2011) says nurses should be full partners with other health team members. Leadership is required to avoid duplication of tasks and to ensure that all tasks are completed.

5. Role clarity: Members of a team that have been working well together generally have developed complementary roles. We know our role and that of other team members and recognize when we need to call on their expertise.

6. Message clarity: Message clarity is about focusing on salient facts and avoiding inconsequential comments.

Collaboration is a dynamic process benefiting from ongoing practice and evaluation. In the past, some organizations tolerated disruptive workplace behaviours. Pressures on nurses exist to increase productivity and cost-effectiveness. Accrediting organizations encourage agencies to practise zero tolerance of these behaviours. Individually, we need to become aware of how to discourage disruptive behaviours as we work to develop a healthy, collaborative workplace atmosphere to ensure high-quality care for people we look after. A few individuals can have a significant negative impact on the health care workplace, which threatens the safety of all (Health Quality Council of Alberta, 2013). A hallmark of a professional is acceptance of accountability for one's own behaviour. Preventing conflicts is accomplished by avoiding public criticism, cultivating an attitude of willingness to help, and doing one's fair share.

Respect

Feeling respected or not is an integral part of how nurses rate the quality of their work environment. Three key factors to feeling respected are a positive climate of professional practice, a supportive manager, and positive relationships with other staff. Nurses say they feel respected and appreciated if their opinions are listened to attentively and they receive feedback from authority figures as to the value of their work competence. When their opinions are discounted or ridiculed, they feel disrespected, angry, frustrated, and powerless. Such anger can be displaced toward others.

Factors that Affect Nurse Behaviour Toward Other Team Members

Team training has been instituted to educate all team members to work in a collaborative manner. But some factors may still negatively influence professional relationships.

Gender

Contemporary society is redefining traditional gender role behaviour, negating some of the traditional gender stereotypical behaviours.

Hierarchy

Because health care authority traditionally was vested in a hierarchical structure, control rested with the physician. Changes in the physician–nurse communication process are occurring as nurses become more empowered, more assertive, and better educated. Most nurses still occasionally encounter problems in the physician–nurse relationship, however. Differences in power, perspective, education, status, and pay may be barriers to workgroup communication and care.

Communication Silos

Traditionally, each health care profession was educated separately, evolving their own unique vocabulary. If you encounter a conflict situation at work, reflect on whether the problem is due to differences in communication style.

Generational Diversity

As mentioned, members of older and younger generations differ in their preferred communication styles. It is suggested that nurses adapt their communication style based on the communication method preferences of others.

Outcomes of Successful Team Training in Communication

Evidence from many studies on effects of team training shows improved efficiency and increased safety for the people the team cares for, with the team approach to health care. Refer to the TeamSTEPPS website for Team Strategies and Tools to Enhance Performance and Patient Safety (TeamSTEPPS)

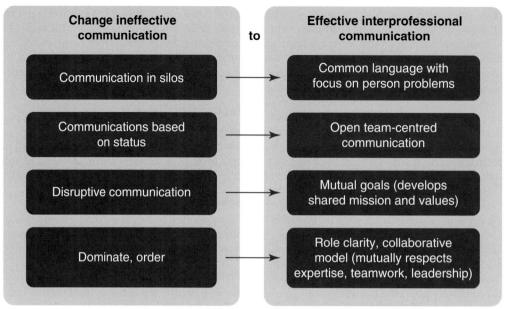

Fig. 24.1 Improve interprofessional communication

strategies https://www.ahrq.gov/teamstepps/instructor/essentials/pocketguide.html. Each nurse team member needs to participate and be accountable for facilitating team communication.

APPLICATIONS

As nurses, we can help to establish and sustain a healthy workplace. This requires continuous assessment of our own and others' current communication practices and implementation of "best practices" to prevent and deal with conflict. Communication and conflict-resolution strategies can be learned but require continued reinforcement through ongoing communication training. Improving communication has been shown to improve safety for people nurses provide care for. An essential component of communication on health care teams is for leadership to set goals, provide feedback (care outcome data), and facilitate conflict resolution.

CONFLICT RESOLUTION

As nurses, we have the responsibility to work effectively with others to provide care. Yet, whenever people work together, conflicts inevitably arise. Many of the same resolution concepts described in Chapter 14 can be applied to conflicts occurring among staff. Refer to Table 9.6 in Chapter 9 to clarify the differences between groups and teams. System conflicts arising from agency or system policies also need attention.

See Fig. 24.1 for strategies to change ineffective communication to effective interpersonal communication. These strategies can have a direct impact on reducing conflicts.

TeamSTEPPS: Team Strategies and Tools to Enhance Performance and Patient Safety

TeamSTEPPS is an evidenced-informed teamwork system program originally developed jointly by the Department of Defense (DoD) and the Agency for Healthcare Research and Quality (AHRQ), in the United States, to improve institutional collaboration and communication relating to the safety of people receiving care. The Canadian Patient Safety Institute (CPSI) was designated the national coordinating body for TeamSTEPPS Canada™. In collaboration with partners, including the Health Quality Council of Alberta, TeamSTEPPS Canada has been adopted and adapted by the Canadian Patient Safety Institute (CPSI) and made available to the Canadian health care field.

Tools and concepts learned in the TeamSTEPPS Canada program are applicable to all health care leaders, administrators, providers, and people and their families in any health care setting (Canadian Patient Safety Institute, 2021).

How many times do we say good communication is essential to effective team function? Effective communication skills convey accurate information and provide awareness of your role responsibilities. As a team member, you communicate to keep others informed, as noted in Fig. 24.2.

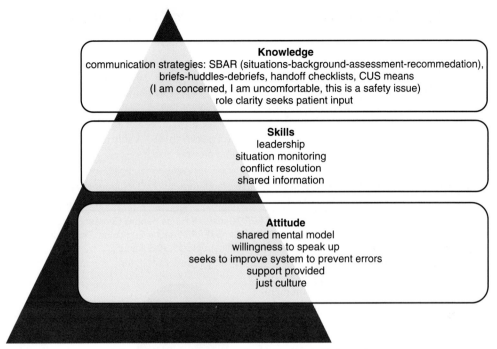

Fig. 24.2 Person-centred care team collaboration

Teamwork and collaboration is a major focus of TeamSTEPPS. Each team member shares a clear vision of expected outcomes for each person receiving care. TeamSTEPPS creates a transformed health care model. Tools and strategies are provided that can be used to develop better system-wide communication knowledge, skills, and attitudes. Communication clarity is an important goal, as is the conciseness found on checklists.

Case Example

Mr. Michaels is scheduled for discharge today. During morning team rounds, you notice redness at his intravenous (IV) site. Even though his temperature at 7 a.m. was recorded as 37.3°C, the resident wants to sign off on the discharge. You use the following assertive statements: state your concern, then why you are uncomfortable.

If the conflict is not resolved, state that there is a safety issue. Discuss in what way the concern is related to safety. If the safety issue is not acknowledged, a supervisor should be notified (Canadian Patient Safety Institute, n.d.). For this example, the nurse would say

"I am concerned about possible sepsis."

"I am uncomfortable discharging him today."

"This is a safety issue."

If the nurse is ignored, they could use the **two-challenge rule**, voicing the safety concern twice. The team leader would acknowledge the nurse's concern, but if the discharge is still scheduled, the nurse would use the chain of command and report this issue to the supervisor.

TeamSTEPPS teaches team members, including nurses, how to increase their competencies in leadership, situation monitoring, and use of mutual support strategies. Examples of leadership competency are clarifying team goals and roles. Competencies for situation monitoring include use of decision-making skills in emergent situations and providing corrective feedback. Mutual support skills include assisting others and using communication tools. Table 24.1 lists standards of effective communication for safer outcomes for people receiving care.

CONFLICT RESOLUTION STEPS

Many of the same strategies for conflict resolution discussed for conflicts between the person and nurse can be applied

Essentials of Communication	Sending Technique	Receiving Technique
TABLE 24.1 TeamSTEPPS: Using a Team Training Program Improves Team Communication		
Clear	Common language/terminology used	Validate: use feedback or "talk back" to confirm understanding
Brief	Communicate only information essential for this situation	Clarify any nonverbal information
Timely	Verify message is received; respond quickly to requests for additional information; provide updates	Verify receipt of information
Complete	Give all relevant information; use standardized communication tools	Document: essential information validated, understood, and recorded

Adapted from Canadian Patient Safety Institute. (n.d.) TeamSTEPPS Canada™ Fundamentals Course: Module 3 Communication. https://www.patientsafetyinstitute.ca/en/education/TeamSTEPPS/TeamSTEPPS-Canada-Curriculum/Documents/Module%203/TeamSTEPPS%20Canada%20Module%203%20Communication%20Instructors%20Guide.pdf.

to conflicts between the nurse and other health team members. Review the principles of conflict management in Fig. 14.1 in Chapter 14. As mentioned, conflict resolution can be a positive force for change. Instead of picturing a straight line of either "you win or I win," envision the outcome of conflict resolution as a triangle, with an outcome of mutual resolution as a peak, where you both have built something greater together (Fig. 24.3).

Step #1. Identify Sources of Conflict

Conflict often stems from miscommunication. Think through the possible causes of the conflict. Identify your own feelings about it and respond appropriately, even if the response is a deliberate choice not to respond verbally. Interpersonal conflicts that are not dealt with leave residual feelings that will re-emerge in future interactions.

Step #2. Set Goals

Goals should be immediate, specific, and measurable.

Step #3. Implement Solutions

Your primary goal in dealing with workplace conflict is to find a high-quality, mutually acceptable solution—a win–win strategy. Remembering that we all share the ultimate goal of delivering high-quality person-centred care may help us work together even if we personally do not like each other. In many instances, a better collaborative relationship can be developed through the use of the following conflict management communication techniques adapted from Johansen (2012):

- *Reframe* a clinical situation as a cooperative process in which the health goals and not the status of the providers becomes the focus.

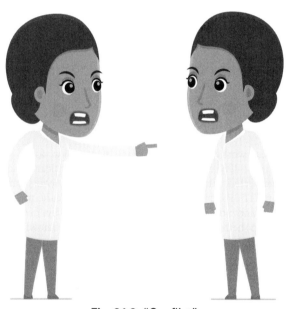

Fig. 24.3 "Conflict"

- *Assume responsibility* for your own behaviours and for maintaining a "blame-free" work environment.
- *Identify your goal.* A clear idea of the outcome you wish to achieve is a necessary first step in the process. Remember that the issue is the conflict, not your coworker.
- *Obtain factual data.* It is important to do your homework by obtaining all relevant information about the specific issues involved—and about the individual's behavioural responses to a health care issue—before engaging in negotiation.

- *Intervene early.* Be assertive. The best time to resolve problems is before they escalate to a conflict. Create a forum for two-way communication, preferably meeting periodically. Structured formats have been developed for you to use in conflict resolution, especially in team meetings.
- The DESC script can be used for both informational and interpersonal conflict but is most effective when conflict is of a personal nature.
  - D = describe the specific behaviour (the problem) using concrete data
  - E = express your concerns about the action, describing how this situation makes you feel
  - S = specify a course of action, suggesting alternatives, and state consequences to goals for people receiving care
  - C = obtain consensus; consequences should be stated (Canadian Patient Safety Institute, n.d.)
- *Avoid negative comments that can affect the self-esteem of the receiver.* Even when the critical statements are valid (e.g., "You do…" or "You make me feel…"), they should be replaced with "I" statements that define the sender's position. Otherwise, needless hostility is created and the meaning of the communication is lost.
- *Consider the other's viewpoint.* Having some idea of what issues might be relevant from the other person's perspective provides important information about the best interpersonal approach to use. In addition to dealing with your own feelings, you need an ability to deal with the feelings of the others. Be cooperative, acknowledging the team's interdependence and mutual goals.

Communicate to Promote Effective Collaboration: Avoid Barriers to Resolution

Refer to Box 24.2 for tips on how to turn conflict into collaboration.

Individual behaviours such as avoiding the use of negative or inflammatory, anger-provoking words, and avoiding phrases that imply coercion, have been described. Examples include: "We must insist that…" or "You claim that…" statements. Most individuals react to anger directed at them with a fight-or-flight-or-freeze response. Anyone can have a moment of rudeness, but monitor your own communications to avoid any pattern of abusive behaviours, including blaming or criticizing staff to others. When nurse supervisors become aware of how their behaviour affects their nurses, they can increase the nurses' performance, increase their job involvement, and increase organizational identification. Participating in mentoring newly hired nurses, even helping sustain internship programs for novice nurses, may help to avert conflict (Weaver, 2013).

BOX 24.2 Strategies to Turn Conflict Into Collaboration

1. Recognize and confront disruptive behaviours.
   Use conflict-resolution strategies.
   Take the initiative to discuss problems.
   Use active listening skills (refrain from simultaneous activities that interrupt communication).
   Present documented data relevant to the issue.
   Propose resolutions.
   Use a brief summary to provide feedback.
   Record all decisions in writing.
2. Create a climate in which participants view negotiation as a collaborative effort.
   Develop agency behaviour policies with stated zero tolerance for disruptive or bullying behaviours.
   Model communicating with staff in a respectful, courteous manner.
   Participate in organizational interdisciplinary groups.
   Solicit and give feedback on a regular, periodic basis.
   Clarify role expectations.

Physician–Nurse Conflict Resolution

Remarkable increases in safety in airline and space programs were achieved by creating a climate in which junior team members were free to question decisions of more senior, powerful team members. Health care is adopting a similar philosophy. The Code provides guidance for ethical relationships, behaviours and decision making. As well, nurses express and report their concern individually or collectively to the appropriate authority or committee to promote quality practice environments (Canadian Nurses Association, 2017, p. 11).

Nurses influence physician–person communication. Nurses assess what physicians tell people in their care, encouraging them to seek clarification, and support those people's right to ask questions. This is an important aspect of our belief that the person is a valued member of the health team.

Research showed that inadequate communication about people's medication across the levels of the health care system leads to numerous and potentially harmful medication errors (Frydenberg & Brekke, 2012). The link between miscommunication and poor outcomes has been well documented (The Joint Commission, 2015). Ineffective communication in health care results in delayed treatment, misdiagnosis, medication errors, and injury or death (Foronda et al., 2016).

Methods to improve safe communication are discussed in Chapter 2.

Make a Commitment to Open Dialogue

Foster a feeling of collegiality. Use strategies to defuse anger. During your negotiation, discussion should begin with a statement of either the commonalities of purpose or the points of agreement about the issue (e.g., "I thoroughly agree Mr. Smith will do much better at home. However, we need to contact social services and make a home care referral before we actually discharge him; otherwise, he will be right back in the hospital again."). Points of disagreement should always follow rather than precede points of agreement. Empathy and a genuine desire to understand the issues from the other's perspective enhance communications. Solutions that take into consideration the needs and human dignity of all parties are more likely to be considered as viable alternatives. Backing another health provider into a psychological corner by using intimidation, coercion, or blame is simply counterproductive. More often than not, solutions developed through such tactics never get implemented. The final solution derived through fair negotiation is often better than the one arrived at alone.

STRATEGIES TO REMOVE BARRIERS TO COMMUNICATION WITH OTHER PROFESSIONALS

Generally, conflict increases anxiety. When interaction with a certain peer or peer group stimulates anxious or angry feelings, the presence of conflict should be considered. Once it is determined that conflict is present, look for the basis of the conflict and label it as personal or professional. If it is personal in nature, it may not be appropriate to seek peer negotiation. It might be better to go back through the self-awareness exercises presented in previous chapters and locate the nature of the conflict through self-examination.

Sharing feelings about a conflict with others helps to reduce its intensity. It is confusing, for example, when nursing students first enter a nursing program or clinical rotation, but this confusion does not get discussed, and students commonly believe they should not feel confused or uncertain. As a nursing student, you face complex interpersonal situations. These situations may lead you to experience loneliness or self-doubt about your nursing skills compared with those of your peers. These feelings are universal at the beginning of any new experience. By sharing them with one or two peers, you usually find that others have had parallel experiences.

Individual Strategies to Deal With Workplace Conflicts

Consider using the behaviours listed in Table 24.2 when directly dealing with conflict in the workplace. Discussion of these behaviours may give you some ideas about how to implement them. Try Simulation Exercise 24.1.

Model Behaviours That Convey Respect

Prevent conflict by behaving with respect. Just as you treat people you provide care for with respect, you have an ethical responsibility to treat coworkers with respect. In a survey by Costello and colleagues (2011), 30% of surgical team respondents admitted to having treated coworkers with disrespect. Nurses need to be appreciated, recognized, and respected as professionals for the work they do. Unsupportive and uncivil coworkers and workplace conflicts negatively influence retention of nursing staff. Unprofessional communication can range from rudeness or gossip to overt hostile comments. Communication can become distorted rather than open when you are concerned about offending a more powerful individual. Strategies for dealing with disrespectful or disruptive behaviours include establishing common communication expectations and skills, teaching conflict resolution skills, and creating a culture of mutual respect within the health care system. Ideally, the system has ongoing education, leadership, and team collaboration support, as well as policies to evaluate behaviour violations.

Mentor New Nurses

Canadian data collected between 2005 and 2008 estimate the exit rate of RNs under the age of 30 varied between 11.58 and 14.51%, with an estimated mean of 13% exiting the nursing profession (Canadian Institute for Health Information, 2021). A number of these nurses transfer to other workplaces, but many actually abandon the nursing profession entirely. During the COVID pandemic, many nurses felt a high level of dissatisfaction with their employers due to lack of resources and support—including inadequate staffing—accelerating their departure from health care agencies. Chachula and colleagues (2015) used grounded theory to find out why nurses were leaving the profession. They found the participants had difficulties navigating the health care system, adjusting to shift work, experienced bullying and felt fearful and traumatized. To retain them in the workforce, they would have needed more effective mentoring, support, orientation, teamwork and to feel accepted as a colleague. They also very much wanted to engage with authentic nurse leaders.

Orientation of novice nurses is expensive for the institution. The IOM (2011) encourages agencies to establish internships or mentoring programs for the first 1 to 2 years of each novice nurse's employment. Furthermore, nursing associations need to provide leadership development, mentoring programs, and opportunities to lead for all their members (IOM).

TABLE 24.2 Examples of Reframing Unclear Communication

Situation	Cognitive Processes	Reframed to Improve Communication
Low self-disclosure	No one knows my real thoughts, feelings, and needs. *Consequently:* I think no one cares about me or recognizes my needs. Others see me as self-sufficient and are unaware that I have a problem. *Consequently:* Others are unable to respond to my needs.	Attitude: • Respect • Value working with others • Willingness to collaborateUse skills: • Open communication—I verbalize aloud my needs clearly so others can have an opportunity to respond, to speak up • Conflict-resolution strategies
Reluctance to delegate tasks	Other people think I do not believe that they can do the job as well as I can. *Consequently:* The others work at a minimum level. I do not expect or ask others to be involved. *Consequently:* Other people do not volunteer to help me. *Consequently:* I feel resentful, and others feel undervalued and dispensable.	Attitude: • Cooperate—I am part of a team • Trust—I need to assign team members to do the tasks they can complete competently Use skills: • Interdisciplinary communication
Making unnecessary demands	I expect more from others than they think is reasonable. *Consequently:* I feel the others are lazy and uncommitted and I must push harder. Others see me as manipulative and dehumanizing. *Consequently:* Others assume a low profile and do not contribute their ideas. *Consequently:* Work production is mediocre. Morale is low. Everyone, including me, feels disempowered.	Attitude: • Shared mental team model—accept team model and shared decision making • Willingness to listen • Acknowledge shared accountability—relinquish some autonomy Use skills: • Interdisciplinary communication strategies • Role clarity—I need to clearly define my expectations and capabilities; I need to set clear work goals and deadlines • Develop situational awareness—crosscheck and offer assistance when needed • Validation—I need to give feedback
Using communication styles unfamiliar to other disciplines	*Consequently:* Communication is unclear to others.	Attitude: • Willingness to reflect on personal communication style • Willingness to participate in conflict resolution Use skills: • Adapt own style to the needs of others on the health care team • Use standardized communication tools, especially during emergent situations

Clarify Communications

Poor communication is repeatedly cited as an influential factor leading to conflict (Almost et al., 2016). You can use the tools and skills taught throughout this textbook to improve both the clarity of message content and the emotional tone of interactions. Communication problems lead to a large percentage of disruptive behaviours, especially telephone communication. If miscommunication occurs, seek clarity by owning your part in misunderstandings. Message clarity is enhanced when standardized

SIMULATION EXERCISE 24.1   Interprofessional Communication Case

Purpose

To help students understand the basic concepts of advocacy for people they provide care for, communication barriers, and peer negotiation in simulated nursing situations.

Procedure

1. The following situation is an example of situations in which interprofessional communication barriers exist. Re-familiarize yourself with the concepts of professionalism, advocacy, communication barriers, and peer negotiation.
2. Formulate a response.
3. Compare your response with those of your classmates and discuss the implications of common and disparate answers. Sometimes, dissimilar answers provide another important dimension of a problem situation.

Situation

Dr. Tanlow interrupts Ms. Serf, RN, as she is preparing pain medication for 68-year-old Mrs. Gould. It is already 15 min late. Dr. Tanlow says he needs Ms. Serf immediately in Room 20C to assist with a drainage and dressing change. Knowing that Mrs. Gould, who has diabetes, will respond to prolonged pain with vomiting, Ms. Serf replies that she will be available to help Dr. Tanlow in 10 min (during which time she will have administered Mrs. Gould's pain medication). Dr. Tanlow, already on his way to Room 20C, whirls around, stating loudly, "When I say I need assistance, I mean now. I am a busy man, in case you hadn't noticed."

If you were Ms. Serf, what would be an appropriate response?

Reflective analysis: This situation could be discussed in class, assigned as a paper, or used as an essay exam.

1. Construct the best possible response.
2. Justify your response using the concepts of professionalism, advocacy, communication barriers, and peer negotiation.

---

formats such as SBAR, discussed in Chapter 2, are used: The nurse identifies self by name and position, the person by name, diagnosis, the problem (including current problem, vital signs, new symptoms, etc.), and clearly states their request. In interprofessional communication, message clarity is crucial (Fig. 23.1). Taking ownership of miscommunication allows recognition that no one is immune (Abourbih et al., 2015).

Clarify Roles

Since role ambiguity is a factor that frequently contributes to conflict (Almost et al., 2016), seek role clarity. Refer to Chapter 23 for an in-depth discussion of roles, so you can work toward role clarity.

Other Conflict-Resolution Strategies
Self-Reflection

Self-awareness is beneficial in assessing the meaning of a professional conflict. The strategies for communicating with angry people, as described in Chapter 14, can be applied when disrespect or anger is directed toward you from colleagues. First, take a moment to reflect on your own behaviours. Have you inadvertently triggered inappropriate behaviour in others? Take responsibility for how you communicate, both verbally and nonverbally. Do you

value the role of other team members? Do you treat each of them in a courteous manner?

Take Stress-Reduction Measures

Because we know that there is a higher risk for conflict if you are highly stressed, take whatever steps are needed to reduce personal stress.

Commit to a Collaborative Resolution Process

Just as the agency should have a code of conduct defining respectful behaviour, there should also be an established process for direct resolution of conflict issues, with support and even "coaches" who help staff resolve conflicts constructively (Box 24.3).

Process for Responding to Put-Downs

In addition, you need to develop a strategy to respond to unwarranted put-downs and destructive criticisms. Generally, the person delivering them has but one intention—to decrease your status and enhance their own. The put-down or criticism may be handed out because the speaker is feeling inadequate or threatened. Often, it has little to do with the actual behaviour of the nurse to whom it is delivered. Other times, the criticism may be valid, but the time and place of delivery are grossly inappropriate (e.g., in the middle of the nurses' station or in the presence of a person the nurse provides care for). In either case, the

BOX 24.3 Steps to Promote Conflict Resolution Among Health Care Team Members

1. Set the stage for collaborative communication.
   Self-reflection: Assume responsibility for own behaviour.
   Privacy: Meet in an appropriate venue, bringing together all involved groups.
   Acknowledge the conflict problem using clear communication.
   Allow sufficient time for discussion and resolution process.
2. Attitude: Maintain a respectful, nonpunitive atmosphere.
   Solicit the perspective of each team member.
   Define the problem issue and objectives clearly.
   Stay focused while respecting the values and dignity of all parties.
   Group members can be assertive but not manipulative.
   Remember to criticize ideas, not people.
3. Be proactive: Initiate early discussion.
   Use communication skills.
   Identify the conflict's key points.
   Have an objective or a goal clearly in mind.
   Seek mutual solutions.
   Have group members propose a solution: Identify the merits and drawbacks of each solution.
   Be open to alternative solutions in which all parties can meet essential needs.
   Depersonalize conflict situations.
4. Decide to implement the best solution.
   Specify persons responsible for implementation (role clarity).
   Establish timeline.
   Decide on the evaluation method.
   Emphasize a common goal—this is a shared value of quality care.
   Emphasize shared responsibility for team success.

automatic response of many nurses is to become defensive, embarrassed, or angry.

Recognizing a put-down or unwarranted criticism is the first step toward dealing effectively with it. If a comment from a coworker or authority figure generates defensiveness or embarrassment, it is likely that the comment represents more than just factual information about performance. If the comment made by the speaker contains legitimate information to help improve one's skill and is delivered in a private and constructive manner, it represents a learning response and cannot be considered a put-down. Learning to differentiate between the two types of communication helps the nurse to "separate the wheat from the chaff." Reflect on the Student Nurse case.

Student Nurse Case

You examine a crying child's inner ears and note that the tympanic membranes (eardrums) are red. You report to your supervisor that the child may have an ear infection.

A. *Response:* When a child is crying, the drums often swell and redden. How about checking again when the child is calm? *(Learning response)*

Or

B. *Response:* Of course, they're red when the child is crying. Didn't you learn that in nursing school? I haven't got time to answer such basic questions! *(Put-down response)*

Which response would you prefer to receive? Why? Whereas the first response allows the nurse to learn useful information to incorporate into practice, the second response serves to antagonize, and it is doubtful much learning takes place. What will happen is that the nurse will be more hesitant about approaching the supervisor again for clinical information. Again, it is the person receiving care who ultimately suffers.

Once a put-down is recognized as such, you need to respond verbally in an assertive manner, as soon as possible after the incident has taken place. Waiting an appreciable length of time is likely to cause resentment and loss of self-respect. It may be more difficult later for the other person to remember the details of the incident. At the same time, if your anger, not the problem behaviour, is likely to dominate the response, it is better to wait a few minutes for the anger to cool a little and then to present the message in a reasoned manner. Preparing your response is a form of "cognitive rehearsal." You can respond to put-downs in the following way:

- Address the objectionable or disrespectful behaviours first. Briefly state the behaviour and its impact on you. Emphasize the specifics of the put-down behaviour. Once the put-down has been dealt with, you can discuss any criticism of your behaviour on its own merits. Refer only to the behaviours identified.
- Prepare a few standard responses. Because put-downs often catch one by surprise, it is useful to have a standard set of opening replies ready. Examples might include the following:

"I found your comments very disturbing and insulting."

"I feel what you said as an attack. That wasn't called for by my actions."

Use Open Communication

Use Standardized Communication Tools and Standardized Lists

These tools have been especially found effective during handovers of people receiving care. They are effective in improving **interdisciplinary communication** (Foronda et al., 2016).

Criticize Constructively

Giving constructive criticism and receiving criticism is difficult for most people. Refer to Box 24.4. When a supervisor gives constructive criticism, some type of response from the person receiving it is indicated. Initially, it is crucial that the conflict problem be clearly defined and acknowledged. To help handle constructive criticism, nurses can do the following:

- Schedule a time when you are calm.
- Request that supervisory meetings be in a place that allows privacy.
- Defuse personal anxiety.
- Listen carefully to the criticism and then paraphrase it.
- Acknowledge that you take suggestions for improvement seriously.
- Discuss the facts of the situation, but avoid becoming defensive.
- Develop a plan for dealing with similar situations; become proactive rather than reactive.
- Maintain open dialogue.

Document and Report Disruptive Behaviours

A crucial aspect of sustaining quality care is the ability to confront a team member whose behaviours violate accepted norms. Studies show that reporting a colleague to an authority figure without talking over the objectionable behaviour with them is not effective in restoring harmony. Yet surveys show that the vast majority of physicians and nurses are reluctant to either confront or report. If your attempts to directly discuss behaviour with the involved person fail to achieve behaviour change, then you need to follow the agency's process and report the problem. In handling disruptive behaviour occurrences, documentation is a key step. Hopefully the agency has a no-blame process, but remember that when pushed, many people will retaliate. Be aware!

> **BOX 24.4   Constructive Criticism Example**
>
> **Steps in Giving:**
> 1. Express caring. *Sample statement:* "I understand that things are difficult at home."
> 2. Describe the behaviour. *Sample statement:* "But I see that you have been late coming to work three times during this pay period."
> 3. State expectations. *Sample statement:* "It is necessary for you to be here on time from now on."
> 4. List consequences. *Sample statement:* "If you get here on time, we'll all start off the shift better. If you're late again, I'll have to report you to the personnel department."
>
> **Steps in Receiving:**
> 1. Listen and paraphrase. If unclear, ask for specific examples. *Sample reply:* "You're saying being late is not acceptable."
> 2. Acknowledge you are taking suggestions seriously. *Sample comment:* "I hear what you're saying."
> 3. Give your side by stating supportive facts, without being defensive. *Sample comment:* "My car would not start."
> 4. Develop a plan for the future. *Sample plan:* "With my next pay, I'll get my car repaired. Until then, I'll ask Mary for a ride."

Some agencies may hold "communication training sessions" after the offenses have been documented. Simulations such as Simulation Exercise 24.2 have you practise strategies to promote a healthy workplace.

DEVELOP A SUPPORT SYSTEM

Collegial relationships are an important determinant of success for professionals. Since lack of support is associated with workplace conflicts (Almost et al., 2016), you need to make positive efforts to create a support system network. Don't just passively wait and hope it happens. Integrity, respect for others, dependability, a good sense of humour, and an openness to sharing with others are communication qualities people look for in developing a support system.

Positive Reinforcement

Everyone likes to be recognized for their efforts. Simple steps such as saying "thank you" or texting a "job well done" message to colleagues is appreciated. In organizations that

SIMULATION EXERCISE 24.2 Communication to Promote a Healthy Work Environment

Purpose

To brainstorm ideas about communicating with team members and administration to facilitate a healthier workplace

Directions

Gather in small groups to role-play ways to communicate that might help promote a pleasant, healthy work environment.

Reflect, then compare ideas.

Suggestions include negotiating with nurse administrators to avoid being assigned to multiple shifts or allowing small breaks every few hours to recharge; texting or posting affirmation (positive) messages for all the staff to read; saying or texting a message of "good job" or "thank you" to a team member; using humour; putting a smile on your face.

---

have integrated team training and safety initiatives, participation in team activities is integrated into job evaluations. In some agencies, positive evaluations are tied to bonuses. Other organizations hold formal and informal affairs to recognize and celebrate efforts to improve communication and safety.

ORGANIZATIONAL STRATEGIES FOR CONFLICT PREVENTION AND RESOLUTION

Organizational Climate

The CNA and the Canadian Federation of Nurses Unions (CFNU) believe that all nurses have the right to work in a respectful environment that is free from any form of violence and bullying and to work where these are not tolerated as part of a nurse's job (Canadian Nurses Association, 2014).

Specific strategies mentioned by Dzurec et al. (2017), OSHA (2015), and many others include the following:

- Zero tolerance policy for disrespect (organizations' Code of Conduct)
- Continuing education programs to raise awareness and teach conflict intervention skills
- Accountability follow-up
- Creation of a corporate climate conveying respect for all workers

Nursing students are likely to be emotionally bullied by other students, their teachers, and nurses on the wards. The effects of emotional bullying is greater than being physically assaulted (Magnavita & Heponiemi, 2011). Seibel and Fehr (2018), using a workshop format with students to enact bullying scenarios, discovered that the way educators gave feedback to students undermined and hurt them.

The following strategies would assist educators in diminishing bullying in their institutions:

1. Empowerment of nursing students should be the core concept guiding curriculum.

2. Introduce bullying education early and proactively.
3. Educators must practise self-awareness and be encouraged to consider how they communicate nursing culture to students.
4. Provide students with opportunities to practise skills for managing bullying.
5. Communicate clearly and transparently about policies and procedures, available supports, communication techniques and skills, and the nature of bullying.
6. Utilize student-centred learning approaches.
7. Consider students' unique characteristics in education strategy development. (Sidhu & Park, 2018)

Promote Opportunities for Interdisciplinary Communication

Creating opportunities for interdisciplinary groups to get together is a highly effective strategy for enhancing collaboration and communication. Ideas for opportunities to get together include collaborative rounds, huddles, team briefings and debriefings, and committee meetings to discuss problems. Some studies associate daily team rounds and joint decision making with shorter hospital stays and lower hospital charges.

Promote Understanding of the Organizational System

Whenever you work in an organization, you automatically become a part of a system that has norms for acceptable behaviour. Each organizational system defines its own chain of command and its rules about social processes in professional communication. Even though your idea may be excellent, failure to understand the chain of command, or an unwillingness to form the positive alliances needed to accomplish your objective, dilutes the impact.

Although sidestepping the identified chain of command and going to a higher or more tangential resource in the hierarchy may appear less threatening initially, such action may not resolve the difficulty. Furthermore, the trust needed for serious discussion becomes limited. Some of

DEVELOPING AN EVIDENCE-INFORMED PRACTICE

Team Communication and Collaboration

There is a correlation between supportive relationships and care quality in the health care system. Conversely, the rise in workplace aggression and bullying has also been extensively documented. The aim of this study was to investigate the subtle forms of workplace mistreatment (bullying and incivility) on Canadian nurses' perceptions of safety risk to people they provide care for and, ultimately, nurse-assessed quality and prevalence of adverse events. To achieve this goal, a survey was sent to 336 nurses in Ontario with questions pertaining to their perceived levels of incivility and safety to people they care for.

Results

The results proved that bullying and incivility from nurses, physicians, and supervisors have significant direct and indirect effects on nurse-assessed adverse events and perceptions of care quality, primarily through perceptions of increased safety risk to people they look after.

Application to Your Workplace

The results of this study confirm that bullying and incivility among health care workers are a detriment to the efficiency of a workplace by impeding communication, collaboration and workplace satisfaction. To achieve a high quality of care, workplaces need to focus on improving the relationship conditions. Leadership, workplace civility interventions and zero-tolerance workplace bullying policies are some tactics that may be adopted to combat incivility.

Adapted from Laschinger, H. K. (2014). Impact of workplace mistreatment on patient safety risk and nurse-assessed patient outcomes. *JONA: The Journal of Nursing Administration, 44*(5), 284–290. doi:10.1097/nna.0000000000000068.

the reasons for avoiding positive interactions stem from an internal circular process of faulty thinking. Because communication is viewed as part of a process, the sender and receiver act on the information received, which may or may not represent the reality of the situation.

Promote Clear Policies

As mentioned earlier, regulatory bodies are requiring that health care organizations have written codes of behaviour and internal processes to handle disruptive behaviours.

Canadian Centre for Occupational Health and Safety (CCOHS) has a vision: the elimination of work-related illnesses and injuries (Canadian Centre for Occupational Health and Safety, 2021). Prevention strategies might include participation in assertiveness training, in-services, or participation in the TeamSTEPPS Canada program. Educational interventions that increase staff awareness are extremely effective, as are simulations similar to the exercises in this book. It is not enough to offer an educational intervention once; team ongoing training is necessary. Literature recommends periodic reassessment of need and offering reviews of communication skills and conflict management strategies.

SUMMARY

In this chapter, the same principles of communication used with conflicts in the nurse–person relationship are broadened to examine the nature of communication among health providers on the health care team. Most nurses experience conflicts with coworkers at some point during their careers. The same elements of thoughtful purpose, authenticity, empathy, active listening, and respect for the dignity of others that underscore successful nurse–person relationships are needed in relations with other health providers. Building effective communication with colleagues involves concepts of collaboration, coordination, and networking. Modification of barriers to professional communication includes negotiation and conflict resolution. Learning is a lifelong process, not only for nursing care skills but for communication skills. These will develop as you continue to gain experience working as part of an interdisciplinary health care team.

ETHICAL DILEMMA

What Would You Do?

You are working a 12-hr shift on a labour and delivery unit. Today, Mrs. Kalim is one of the assigned people you will look after. She is fully dilated and effaced, but contractions are still 2 minutes apart after 10 hours of labour. Mrs. Kalim, her obstetrician, Dr. Mar, and you have agreed on her plan to have a fully natural delivery without medication. However, her obstetrician's partner is handling a day shift today. This new obstetrician orders you to administer several medications to Mrs. Kalim to strengthen contractions and speed up delivery because he has another person across town to help deliver. Your unit adheres to an empowering model of practice that believes in person advocacy. How will you handle this potential physician conflict? Is this a true moral dilemma?

QUESTIONS FOR REVIEW AND DISCUSSION

1. Reflect on a time someone tried to intimidate or bully you. How did you feel? Assemble and support some productive strategies for responding in such situations.
2. Develop a list of strategies that seem to work best when communicating with team members from outside nursing to facilitate a collaborative environment.

REFERENCES

Abourbih, D., Armstrong, S., Nixon, K. et al. (2015). Communication between nurses and physicians: Strategies to surviving in the emergency department trenches. *Emergency Medicine Australasia, 27*, 80–82.

Almost, J., Wolff, A. C., Stewart-Pyne, A. et al. (2016). Managing and mitigating conflict in healthcare teams: An integrative review. *Journal of Advanced Nursing, 72*(7), 1490–1505.

Boev, C., & Xia, Y. (2015). Nurse-physician collaboration and hospital acquired infections in critical care. *Critical Care Nurse, 35*(2), 66–72.

Canadian Centre for Occupational Health and Safety. (2021). https://www.ccohs.ca/.

Canadian Institute for Health Information. (2021). https://www.cihi.ca/en.

Canadian Interprofessional Health Collaborative (CIHC). (2010). A national interprofessional competency framework. Her Majesty the Queen in Right of Canada. https://drive.google.com/file/d/1Des_mznc7Rr8stsEhHxl8XMjgiYWzRIn/view.

Canadian Nurses Association. (2014). Workplace violence and bullying. Joint position statement. https://cna-aiic.ca/~/media/cna/page-content/pdf-en/Workplace-Violence-and-Bullying_joint-position-statement.pdf.

Canadian Nurses Association. (2017). *Code of Ethics. 2017 Edition.* https://www.cna-aiic.ca/-/media/cna/page-content/pdf-en/code-of-ethics-2017-edition-secure-interactive.pdf?la=en&hash=09C348308C44912AF216656BFA31E33519756387.

Canadian Patient Safety Institute. (n.d.). TeamSTEPPS Canada fundamentals course: Module 6 Mutual Support. https://www.patientsafetyinstitute.ca/en/education/TeamSTEPPS/TeamSTEPPS-Canada-Curriculum/Documents/Module%206/TeamSTEPPS%20Canada%20Module%206%20Mutual%20Support%20Instructors%20Guide.pdf.

Canadian Patient Safety Institute. (2020). *The need for better hand hygiene in healthcare.* https://www.patientsafetyinstitute.ca/en/toolsResources/Hand-Hygiene-Fact-Sheets/Pages/The-Need-for-Better-Hand-Hygiene-in-Healthcare.aspx.

Canadian Patient Safety Institute. (2021). Use team strategies and tools to enhance performance and patient safety. TeamSTEPPS Canada. https://www.patientsafetyinstitute.ca/en/education/TeamSTEPPS/Pages/default.aspx.

Castronovo, M. A., Pullizzi, A., & Evans, S. (2016). Nurse bullying: A review and a proposed solution. *Nursing Outlook, 64*(3), 208–214.

Chachula, K. M., Myrick, F., & Yonge, O. (2015). Letting go: How newly graduated registered nurses in Western Canada decide to exit the nursing profession. *Nurse Education today, 35*(7), 912–918. https://doi.org/10.1016/j.nedt.2015.02.024.

Costello, J., Clarke, C., Gravely, G. et al. (2011). Working together to build a respectful workplace: Transforming OR culture. *AORN Journal, 93*(1), 115–126.

Dzurec, L. C., Kennison, M., & Gillen, P. (2017). The incongruity of workplace bullying victimization and inclusive excellence. *Nursing Outlook, 65*(5), 588–598. https://dx.doi.org/10.1016/j.outlook.2017.01.012.

Emanuel, L. L., Taylor, L., Hain, A. et al. (2011). The patient safety education program—Canada (PSEP—Canada) curriculum. PSEP—Canada.

Eriksen, T. L., Hogh, A., & Hansen, A. M. (2016). Long-term consequences of workplace bullying on sickness absence. *Labour Economics, 43*, 129–150.

Farrell, K., Payne, C., & Heye, M. (2015). Integrating interprofessional collaboration skills into the advanced practice registered nurse socialization process. *Journal of Professional Nursing, 31*(1), 5–10.

Fewster-Thuente, L. (2015). Working together toward a common goal: A grounded theory of nurse-physician collaboration. *MedSurg Nursing, 24*(5), 356–362.

Foronda, C., MacWilliams, B., & McArthur, E. (2016). Interprofessional communication in healthcare: An integrative review. *Nurse Education in Practice, 19*, 36–40.

Frydenberg, K., & Brekke, M. (2012). Poor communication on patients' medication across health care levels leads to potentially harmful medication errors. *Scandinavian Journal of Primary Health Care, 30*(4), 234–240. https://doi.org/10.3109/02813432.2012.712021.

Health Quality Council of Alberta. (2013). *Managing disruptive behaviour in the healthcare workplace. Provincial Framework.* https://hqca.ca/wp-content/uploads/2020/01/HQCA_Disruptive_Behaviour_Framework_041113.pdf.

Hutchinson, M., & Jackson, D. (2013). Hostile clinician behaviours in the nursing work environment and implications for patient care: A mixed-methods systematic review. *BMC Nursing, 12*(1), 25. https://doi.org/10.1186/1472-6955-12-25.

Institute of Medicine. (2011). *The future of nursing: Leading change, advancing health.* The National Academies Press. https://doi.org/10.17226/12956.

Johansen, M. L. (2012). Keeping the peace: Conflict management strategies for nurse managers. *Nursing Management, 43*(2), 50–54.

Kimes, A., Davis, L., Medlock, A. et al. (2015). 'I'm not calling him!': Disruptive physician behaviour in the acute care setting. *MedSurg Nursing, 24*(4), 223–227.

Koh, W. M. S. (2016). Management of workplace bullying in hospital: A review of the use of cognitive rehearsal as an alternative management strategy. *International Journal of Nursing Sciences, 3*(2), 213–222.

Lyndon, A., Johnson, M. C., Bingham, D. et al. (2015). Transforming communication and safety culture in intrapartum care: A multi-organization blueprint. *JOGNN, 44*(3), 341–349.

Mace-Vadjunec, D., Hileman, B. M., Melnykovich, M. B. et al. (2015). The lack of common goals and communication within a Level I trauma system: Assessing the silo effect among trauma center employees. *Journal of Trauma Nursing, 22*(5), 274–281.

Magnavita, N., & Heponiemi, T. (2011). Workplace violence against nursing students and nurses: An Italian experience. *Journal of Nursing Scholarship, 43*(2), 203–210. https://doi.org/10.1111/j.1547-5069.20.11.01392.x.

Mchugh, S. K., Lawton, R., O'Hara, J. K. et al. (2020). Does team reflexivity impact teamwork and communication in interprofessional hospital-based healthcare teams? A systematic review and narrative synthesis. *BMJ Quality & Safety, 0*, 1–12. https://doi.org/10.1136/bmjqs-2019-009921.

Misfeldt, R., Suter, E., Oelke, N. et al. (2017). Creating high performing primary health care teams in Alberta, Canada: Mapping out the key issues using a socioecological model. *Journal of Interprofessional Education & Practice, 6*, 27–32.

Moore, L. W., Sublett, C., & Leahy, C. (2017). Nurse managers speak out about disruptive nurse-to-nurse relationships. *JONA, 47*(1), 24–29.

Occupational Safety and Health Administration. (2015). *Guidelines for preventing workplace violence for healthcare & social workers.* OSHA Publication No. 3148. Author.

Perry, V., Christiansen, M., & Simmons, A. (2016). A daily goals tool to facilitate indirect nurse-physician communication during morning rounds on a medical-surgical unit. *MedSurg Nursing, 25*(2), 83–87.

Polis, S., Higgs, M., Manning, V. et al. (2017). Factors contributing to nursing team work in an acute care tertiary hospital. *Collegian, 24*(1), 19–25.

Press, M. J., Gerber, L. M., Peng, T. R. et al. (2015). Post-discharge communication between home health nurses and physicians: Measurement, quality, and outcomes. *JAGS, 63*, 1299–1305.

Seibel, L., & Fehr, F. (2018). "They can crush you": Nursing students' experiences of bullying and the role of faculty. *Journal of Nursing Education and Practice, 8*(6). https://doi.org/10.5430/jnep.v8n6p66.

Shahid, S., & Thomas, S. (2018). Situation, background, assessment, recommendation (SBAR) communication tool for handoff in health care—A narrative review. *Safety in Health, 4*(1). https://doi.org/10.1186/s40886-018-0073-1.

Sidhu, S., & Park, T. (2018). Nursing curriculum and bullying: An integrative literature review. *Nurse Education Today, 65*, 169–176. https://doi.org/10.1016/j.nedt.2018.03.005.

TeamSTEPPS. (2017). National TeamSTEPPS conference, June 13, 2017. Cleveland, OH.

Tee, S., Üzar Özçetin, Y. S., & Russell-Westhead, M. (2016). Workplace violence experienced by nursing students: A UK survey. *Nurse Education Today, 41*, 30–35. https://doi.org/10.1016/j.nedt.2016.03.014.

The Joint Commission. (2008). *Behaviors that undermine a culture of safety (40).* Sentinel Event Alert. http://www.jointcommission.org/assets/1/18/SEA_40.pdf.

The Joint Commission. (2010). *Preventing violence in the health care setting. (45).* Sentinel Event Alert. http://www.jointcommission.org/assets/1/18/sea_45.pdf.

The Joint Commission. (2015). *Advancing effective communication, cultural competence, and patient- and family-centered care.* http://www.jointcommission.org/Advancing_Effective_Communication/.

Trepanier, S., Fernet, C., Austin, S. et al. (2016). Work environment antecedents of bullying: A review and integrative model applied to registered nurses. *International Journal of Nursing Studies, 55*, 85–97.

University of Toronto Centre for Interprofessional Education. (2016). *Interprofessional education at the University of Toronto.* https://ipe.utoronto.ca/.

Weaver, K. B. (2013). The effects of horizontal violence and bullying on new nurse retention. *Journal for Nurses in Professional Development, 29*(3), 138–142.

Wilson, L., & Rockstraw, L. (2012). *Human simulation for nursing and health professions.* Springer.

World Health Organization. (2016). *Setting priorities for global patient safety.* Italy: Conference Florence. www.who.int/patientsafety/.

WEBSITE/RESOURCES LIST

https://www.ccohs.ca/.

https://www.cihi.ca/en.

https://www.cna-aiic.ca/-/media/cna/page-content/pdf-en/code-of-ethics-2017-edition-secure-interactive.pdf?la=en&hash=09C348308C44912AF216656BFA31E33519756387.

https://cna-aiic.ca/~/media/cna/page-content/pdf-en/Workplace-Violence-and-Bullying_joint-position-statement.pdf.

https://drive.google.com/file/d/1Des_mznc7Rr8stsEhHxl8XMjgiYWzRIn/view.

https://www.healthcareexcellence.ca/en/what-we-do/what-we-do-together/hand-hygiene-fact-sheets/?utm_source=patientsafetyinstitute.ca&utm_medium=CTA&utm_campaign=Migration&utm_content=handhygiene-en.

https://hqca.ca/wp-content/uploads/2020/01/HQCA_Disruptive_Behaviour_Framework_041113.pdf.

https://ipe.utoronto.ca/.

https://www.patientsafetyinstitute.ca/en/education/TeamSTEPPS/Pages/default.aspx.

https://www.patientsafetyinstitute.ca/en/education/TeamSTEPPS/TeamSTEPPS-Canada-Curriculum/Documents/Module%203/TeamSTEPPS%20Canada%20Module%203%20Communication%20Instructors%20Guide.pdf.

https://www.patientsafetyinstitute.ca/en/education/TeamSTEPPS/TeamSTEPPS-Canada-Curriculum/Documents/Module%206/TeamSTEPPS%20Canada%20Module%206%20Mutual%20Support%20Instructors%20Guide.pdf.

https://www.patientsafetyinstitute.ca/en/education/TeamSTEPPS/TeamSTEPPS-Canada-Curriculum/Pages/Module-3-Communication.aspx.

25

Communicating for Continuity of Care

Olive Yonge

Originating US chapter by *Elizabeth C. Arnold*

OBJECTIVES

At the end of the chapter, the reader will be able to:

1. Explain the concept of continuity of care (COC) in contemporary health care systems.
2. Describe current challenges in the health care system, related to COC.
3. Discuss applications of relational continuity in person-centred care and interdisciplinary team collaboration.
4. Apply informational continuity concepts in transitional and discharge planning processes.
5. Discuss applications of management continuity related to case management, care coordination, and navigation of the health care system.

The Canadian Oxford Dictionary's (n.d.) definition of a *paradigm shift* is "a fundamental change (in approach, philosophy, etc.)." There has been the strong realization that health care systems organized around acute, episodic care no longer suffice as a primary service model. The complexity of contemporary health care requires a different care process to match new health realities (Mitchell et al., 2012). There are several reasons for the dramatic shift to community-based health models as a primary source of health care delivery. Examples include longer lifespans, demographics of the population with greater ethnic and racial diversity, skilled provider shortages, and cost.

Technology advances in diagnosis and treatment and discovery of novel medications and treatments have reduced the incidence of premature death from acute health conditions. Instead, chronic disorders account for people now self-managing previously untreatable cancers and other conditions as chronic health conditions, with a good quality of life for longer periods of time, as the rule rather than the exception. Thus, attention has turned to chronic disease management, early detection, and interventions to enhance lifestyle health behaviours within a shared care process.

People are discharged earlier and sicker, often with complex medication and treatment regimens, which need to be followed in the community in primary care settings.

This chapter explores the concept of continuity of care (COC) as the foundation in collaborative health team functionality, central to its structure, and operations across contemporary health care systems. COC has a conceptual framework for the study and application of COC strategies (Health Quality Council of Alberta, 2016). Addressing the role of communication in achieving the purposes of COC is essential to ensuring quality, safety, and satisfaction across contemporary health care systems.

BASIC CONCEPTS

Worldwide, chronic diseases account for up to 60% of deaths (Paquette-Warren et al., 2014). However, as people live longer, there is a higher incidence of chronic conditions requiring an array of supportive health care services. The focus on care provision has shifted from the hospital to the community and a public health focus, using an integrated service framework (World Health Assembly, 2016). Providing a continuum of aggregated services offers the most comprehensive option for care of people with chronic physical and mental health conditions (Stans et al., 2013; Porter-O'Grady, 2014).

CONCEPTS

COC describes a multidimensional, longitudinal process construct in health care that emphasizes seamless provision and coordination of person-centred quality care across clinical settings (Haggerty et al., 2013). COC operates across three dimensions: relational, informational, and management continuity. These constructs are unique; they are related to each other but do not completely overlap. They are essential components of care. (Health Quality Council of Alberta, 2016).

Relational continuity can be defined as " the ongoing, trusting therapeutic relationship between a person and a primary care physician and their team, where the person sees this primary care physician the majority of the time. This approach results in improved health outcomes, decreased mortality, better quality of care, reduced health care costs, increased person and provider satisfaction, fewer emergency department visits and hospital admissions" (Top Alberta Doctors, 2019). Frequent team communication about all aspects of care helps to ensure relational continuity among treatment teams.

Informational continuity refers to the use of data to tailor current treatment and care to each person's evidenced needs. The concept includes accurate record sharing and technology to allow real-time communication exchanges between providers and with people in remote sites. It is a primary communication vehicle during care transitions and is used to help people and their families make quality care decisions.

Management continuity refers to a consistent, coherent, person-specific care management approach, which can be flexibly adjusted as a person's needs change. Care coordination and case management have emerged as significant methodologies associated with management continuity.

The COC process is concerned with the safety and quality of care. COC links acute care with primary care approaches for people, through coordinated, acute care, and community-based health services. The overarching goal of COC is to ensure reliable, coordinated transition of people from one health care setting to another, such that care in each setting continues to provide a secure, trustworthy health safety net for individuals and their families that they can rely on for support and information.

A scoping review of 55 articles on COC yielded some important results. The authors stated that those using the concept of COC in research or policy papers must provide an explicit definition. They suggested the definition be the provision of coordinated care and services over time and across levels and disciplines, which is coherent with a person's health needs and personal circumstances. The definition provides a framework whereby there are three key components:

- Longitudinal care (repeated visits over time)
- The nature of the person–provider relationship (based on trust, familiarity, and knowledge co-production)
- Coordinated care (consistent across levels and disciplines for a unified treatment plan with proper information management) (Meiqari et al., 2019).

COC decreases the potential for service duplication, conflicting assessments, and gaps in service. It reduces the use of preventable acute care services and lessens medication and treatment errors. Continuity provides timely follow-up and can ease transitions between care settings. For people with chronic conditions and older people, COC means that they are more likely to have health care providers who are familiar with their overall history, who can notice subtle changes in health status. These people want a trusting relationship between themselves and their physicians that in turn would result in greater honesty, transparency, and preventive care (Crooks et al., 2012).

COC: Treatment Pathway of Choice for Chronic Conditions

COC is the treatment model of choice for **chronic health conditions** in primary care. The National Center for Chronic Disease Prevention and Health Promotion defines chronic disease as conditions that last one year or more and require ongoing medical attention or limit activities or both (CDC, n.d.). Examples of chronic illness include asthma, fibromyalgia, arthritis, osteoporosis, cancer, multiple sclerosis, diabetes, serious persistent mental health disorders, chronic obstructive pulmonary disease (COPD), and congestive heart failure.

Chronic illness is a major cause of death and disability, nationally and globally. Roberts, and colleagues (2015, p. 1) found that 2.9% of Canadians report two or more chronic diseases, and 3.9% report three or more chronic diseases. Those reporting three or more were more likely to be female, older, living in the lowest income quintile, and to have not completed high school. "Having two or more chronic diseases concurrently, referred to as *multimorbidity*, adds another layer of complexity to their prevention and management, in part because people with multiple diseases are at a greater risk of adverse health outcomes, more frequent hospitalizations and greater health care needs" (Boyd & Fortin, 2010, p. 451). People with chronic illnesses typically have periods of exacerbations and remissions and have their lives disrupted in multiple ways. They experience multiple losses, may have fears about financial security, and experience shifts in relationships (Potter et al., 2019). They share a requirement for ongoing health support and self-care management (Franek, 2013). Kleinman (1988) explains the impact in this way: "The undercurrent of chronic illness is like the volcano: it does not go away, it menaces. It erupts. It is out of control … confronting crises is only one part of the total picture. The rest is coming to grips with the mundaneness of worries … Chronic illness also means the loss of confidence in one's health and normal bodily processes" (pp. 44–45).

The COC construct is based on an expanded version of the chronic care model originally developed by Wagner and associates (2001). This model, as presented later, is designed to foster productive interactions between informed people and families and prepared, proactive practice teams to produce improved clinical outcomes. Application of the chronic care model within the primary health care system functions as a safety net and support. This is achieved by empowering individuals and families to assume primary responsibility for self-management of chronic illness, in partnership with ongoing professional support from skilled providers across selected health care settings. This shared responsibility helps to bridge the gap between diminishing financial support for chronic care and its multifaceted care demands, which can last for years. Relevant primary care strategies focus on ensuring that patients—who are always the priority—are consulted about the design and delivery of team-based care, and teams are in turn supported to give this team-based care (Schottenfeld et al., 2016).

Medical Home in Primary Care

Primary care, described as the hub of community-based care, provides a wide range of integrated health care services delivered in a single community-based setting. The medical home in primary care serves as the first point of entry for people receiving primary care. The staff in the medical home offer diagnosis and treatment of common non-acute illnesses. Services also include health promotion education, preventive screenings, and health maintenance care. Community resource support, integrated decision making, and information technology work together to strengthen person-centred relationships and improve health outcomes (Green et al., 2012).

Key features of the medical home in primary care include the following:

- Person-centredness, with sustained continuity of relationships between provider and person
- Functions as a first contact point, with easy access services for common health care problems
- Comprehensive care, which can meet many of the person's needs without referral
- A highly personalized form of care related to a stronger knowledge about individual health care needs and responses over time (IOM, 2012; Smith, 2013).

≫ DEVELOPING AN EVIDENCE-INFORMED PRACTICE

Objective

The objective was to determine "if continuity of care (COC) is associated with decreased health resource utilization, improved outcomes, and person satisfaction" (p. 4).

Method

The research question was as follows: Is higher COC effective at reducing health resource utilization and improving outcomes? MEDLINE, EMBASE, CINAHL, the Cochrane Library, and the Centre for Reviews and Dissemination databases were searched for studies on COC and chronic disease, published from January 2002 until December 2011. Review methods, systematic reviews, randomized controlled trials, and observational studies were eligible if they assessed COC in adults and reported health resource utilization, outcomes, or person satisfaction (p.4).

Findings

Eight systematic reviews and 13 observational studies met the criteria for examining the effectiveness of COC. Essentially, there is a weak association between COC and outcomes. The researchers using observational research methods identified that COC was associated with people who had fewer hospitalizations and emergency department visits. For three systematic reviews, the researchers found greater person satisfaction.

Implications for Clinical Practice

No data was found to examine the relational aspects such as the trust or confidence people had with their provider. There was one finding that supports the development of programs, and that was the association between high COC and person satisfaction. More research is needed in this area.

From Health Quality Ontario. (2013). Continuity of care to optimize chronic disease management in the community setting: An evidence-based analysis. *Ontario Health Technology Assessment Services, 13*(6), 1–41. http://www.hqontario.ca/en/documents/eds/2013/full-report-OCDMcontinuity-of-care.pdf.

APPLICATIONS

Coping with chronic conditions is embedded within the context of the larger life patterns and availability of health-related resources. "A common trap in primary care is to consider problems in isolation, failing to respect its multidimensional and longitudinal nature" (Ferrer & Gill, 2013, p. 301). COC recognizes the need to provide structured, collaborative efforts in creating workable solutions for people over time and space.

COC offers a care pathway to safeguard care stability and to provide a secure health safety net for individuals and families that they can rely on for support and information. Each dimension of COC—relational, informational, and management continuity—ideally works together to set directions and implement coordinated interventions throughout the health care system. COC needs to be considered from both the person and provider perspectives. This makes sense given the level of partnership needed to ensure continuity and a seamless experience for the person (Health Quality Council of Alberta, 2016).

RELATIONAL CONTINUITY

Relational continuity refers to the interpersonal elements of the COC model across time and care settings. The term applies to nurse–person and family relationships, team relationships, and relationships between health system providers and community-based supports. The stronger the relationships, the greater is the potential for quality-coordinated care. Respect for person and family values, beliefs, knowledge, cultural background, and preferences are fundamental aspects of person-centred relational continuity. Trusting relationships with a primary provider or "medical home" health care team gives people confidence that their care needs will be consistently met.

The goal of relational COC is to develop sustained person–provider relationships in which informed, motivated people interact with prepared, proactive professional health care teams to achieve identified health goals for chronic health conditions. The Joint Commission person-centred communication standards include data on communication with physicians and nurses, responsiveness of staff, communication about medications, pain management, and discharge planning as measurable outcomes (The Joint Commission, 2013). Increasing the level of collaboration among health care providers is identified as a primary strategy for improving the level of continuity needed for successful health care outcomes (WHO, 2018).

NEW ROLES IN CONTINUITY OF CARE

Continuity of care is described as "the connectedness between different stages in the health care system among the patient, health care professionals, and the organization" (Renholm et al., 2016, p. 2). Health care reform has led to the development of new professional relational roles and service delivery approaches to better address the nation's health needs. Innovative roles include the hospitalist, the medical home, and collaborative, interdisciplinary, team-based care delivery. When thinking about COC, nurses and other health professionals should consider the health experience as a whole and be guided by **team-based principles**.

Hospitalist

A professional role designed to improve COC in acute care settings is that of the hospitalist. A **hospitalist** may be a physician or nurse practitioner employed by the hospital to clinically manage a person's medical care. The hospitalist specializes in medical care of hospitalized people and assumes *full* responsibility for coordinating care, ordering and integrating diagnostic test results, making decisions, presenting options to the person and family, and communicating with other professionals who may be or will become involved in the person's care after discharge. The specific dimensions of the hospitalist role are determined by the care site rather than clinical specialty (Fox, 2014). Specialty physicians function as consultants.

Nurses play an important communication role with hospitalists. They function as key informants, skilled practitioners, advocates, and supporters of coordinated care in hospital settings. People receiving care do not have a relationship with the hospitalist prior to or post-hospitalization. As the person's nurse, you are responsible for carrying out the hospitalist's orders. Nurses should be proactive by talking informally with hospitalists about people in their care and presenting information formally in collaborative team meetings.

As a person's condition changes, the hospitalist meets with the family to discuss changes, treatment options, and family concerns. Even in the best of circumstances, these meetings with the person and family, hospitalist, and health care team, to discuss sensitive health issues such as discontinuing life support or transfer of people, can be intimidating. Nurses can help people and their families by continuing conversations after the hospitalist or health care team leaves, answering questions and providing support.

Medical Home

The **medical home** is considered a "concept" as well as a "place" in primary care. As a concept, it has particular relevance for increasing access to primary care in the public sector (Crabtree et al., 2010). A medical home accepts responsibility for providing regular, accessible, comprehensive primary care services for designated people and their families within a single familiar setting. It serves as a central first point of contact in primary care through which the majority of the person's health needs are met (College of Family Physicians of Canada, 2019); Keeling & Lewenson, 2013).

People depend on their medical home as a first-line treatment resource. Physicians, nurse practitioners, physician's assistants, nurses, social workers, dentists, and other health care providers can provide better-quality care because they have ongoing knowledge of the person's medical and lifestyle issues. Subtle changes in the person's situation or health status are recognized in subsequent care visits.

External coordination of health care services with specialists and community agencies expand the capabilities of the medical home. Because they are part of a larger health system in many cases, referrals are accomplished efficiently. Information passes swiftly and accurately between providers. There is less chance of duplicative or unnecessary medical appointments because care is coordinated through the person's medical home. A critical element is that professional recipients of people's data must maintain confidentiality and privacy. Quality and safety are essential characteristics of primary care medical homes (see Chapter 2 for general principles associated with safety).

Relational Continuity on Collaborative Health Teams

Relational continuity on collaborative health teams describes an active, ongoing alliance between health care providers from different disciplines who work together in complementary roles to provide integrated health care services. Each team member brings skills to address different aspects of a person's illness experience, but the team is expected to act as a coordinated unit. Some functions overlap; others are complementary. All functions must be coordinated so that the team functions as an integrated unit. Team meetings allow skilled professionals to develop mutual understandings developed about common problems as a foundation for generating stronger innovative solutions. Professional health care team collaboration is an important contributor to total quality management and is identified as a nursing "quality and safety education for nurses" competency (see Chapter 2).

Special function teams engage in coordinated activities to ensure that COC meets targeted person-centred needs. Examples of special function teams include disaster response teams, acute care hospital teams, medical home–based and home care teams, mental health emergency teams, and palliative care teams (Mitchell et al., 2012). Collaborative health care teams are broadly classified as multidisciplinary, interdisciplinary, and transdisciplinary, with the expectation that care will be provided through the combined collaborative efforts of two or more skilled clinical practitioners.

Interdisciplinary team relationships take into account the diverse standards and behaviours associated with each clinical discipline, while emphasizing a common mission of working together to resolve complex clinical problems (Cohen, 2014). Team members are expected to value and respect diversity in the personal, cultural, and experiential backgrounds of each professional.

In formal meetings, relational continuity is encouraged by setting a direction, prioritizing agenda items and activities, and establishing realistic boundaries about care contributions. Members monitor potential relationship safety issues, such as status differences and receptiveness to taking interpersonal risks when others disagree. When interprofessional team members deal with relational group process issues successfully, members experience higher levels of learning and satisfaction with team care outcomes.

ESSENTIAL ELEMENTS OF RELATIONAL CONTINUITY

Development of therapeutic relationships with known providers offers a consistent, fundamental communication channel that people can use to secure better health care services, which are tailored to their specific health needs. The interpersonal process relations required for relational COC involve the three C's—person-centredness, collaboration, and coordination—in a shared enterprise of therapeutic care delivery across multiple systems (Stans et al., 2013).

Fig. 25.1 presents components of person-centred care. People should be key informants, active negotiators, final decision makers, and engaged participants in evaluating treatment outcomes (Gallivan et al., 2012; WHO, 2016). They need to be actively involved in defining and updating realistic treatment goals. Person-centredness is evidenced in a partnership characterized by mutual valuing and safeguarding of the legitimate interests of the provider and the person in creating and managing health care decisions.

Shared decision making is a key element of relational continuity with people receiving care and with the entire team. The decision-making process starts with providing each person with sufficient information tailored to their

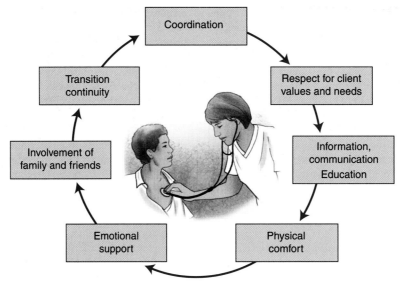

Fig. 25.1 Dimensions of person-centred care in continuity of care (COC)

unique circumstances to make an *informed* decision. The information must be in a format and language that is easily understandable to the person. Information should be relevant to each person's diagnosis, treatments, and treatment options. The first question you should consider is: What *essential* information does this person need to have in order to make an informed decision? Some people value knowing as much as possible; others want just the basic facts. Another may need to have essential information developed in steps and spread over several encounters. This accommodation allows for better processing and formulation of related questions. Cultural norms also can dictate levels of information and to whom the information should be given (see Chapter 7).

A second query is: What level of information does the person desire *at this point in time?* For example, someone with newly diagnosed terminal ovarian cancer focuses on a long trip she wants to take in the future. She suggests several times that she is going to make it and not die from her cancer. Empathetic acceptance of the person as she is processing a diagnosis is more helpful than presenting her with "facts" that she is not willing to accept at the current moment. Other professionals should be alerted to differences in people's informational needs or consulted so that all caregivers are on the same page.

To ensure that care decisions respect the person's values, needs, and preferences, care providers need to observe and listen carefully to the person's description of their health experience. These data become the basis for providing people and their families with the tailored education and

support they need to make reasoned health care decisions. Relevant information includes the following:

- Detailed information on diagnosis
- Options for treatment and what to expect
- Risks and benefits of each treatment approach
- Anticipated clinical outcomes
- Treatment and care processes required to achieve desired clinical outcomes

Consistency of personnel over time allows people and the professional team to share a stronger investment in achieving personalized quality health outcomes. Providers and people receiving care learn to know, value, and respect each other. Box 25.1 identifies essential competencies for the Interprofessional Competency Framework, released by the Canadian Interprofessional Health Collaborative (CIHC).

COLLABORATION

The second C in relational continuity is collaboration. "The Canadian Nurses Association (CNA) believes that interprofessional collaborative models for health service delivery are critical for improving access to client-centred health care in Canada. The responsiveness of the health system can be strengthened through effective collaboration among health professionals, regulators, educators, and professional associations" (Canadian Nurses Association, 2011). People need an integrated, consistent flow of informed communication among providers and community agencies about their treatment and care.

BOX 25.1 Interprofessional Competency Framework

The six competencies outlined in the Interprofessional Competency Framework released by the Canadian Interprofessional Health Collaborative (CIHC) have been adopted by Alberta Health Service and are described as follows:

1. Role Clarification: Learners and providers understand their own role and the roles of those in other professions and use this knowledge appropriately to establish and achieve person/client/family and community goals.
2. Individual/Client/Family and Community-Centred Care: Learners and providers seek out, integrate, and value, as a partner, the input and engagement of the person/client/family/community in designing and implementing care and services.
3. Team Functioning: Learners and providers understand the principles of teamwork dynamics and group/team processes to enable effective interprofessional collaboration.
4. Collaborative Leadership: Learners and providers understand and can apply leadership principles that support a collaborative practice model.
5. Interprofessional Communication: Learners and providers from different professions communicate with each other in a collaborative and responsible manner.
6. Interprofessional Conflict Resolution: Learners and providers actively engage self and others, including the client and family, in positively and constructively addressing disagreements as they arise.

Excerpted from Canadian Interprofessional Health Collaborative (CIHC). (2010, February). A National Interprofessional Competency Framework. University of British Columbia, Vancouver, Canada. https://drive.google.com/file/d/1Des_mznc7Rr8stsEhHxl8XMjgiYWzRln/view

Interdisciplinary collaboration enables practitioners to learn new skills and approaches and encourages synergistic creativity among professionals. As different disciplines work closely together, they build new understandings about each other's expertise and trust in each other to develop consensus about the best approaches to each person's unique health care situation. Each discipline member is cognizant of unique and shared spheres of responsibility with team members from other disciplines. Structured team collaboration decreases fragmentation and duplication of effort and promotes safe quality care (see Chapter 2). Fig. 25.2 presents desired characteristics of relational interprofessional collaboration.

The level of collaborative team communication between people and providers and between providers affects treatment outcomes and satisfaction. Receiving care within an ongoing therapeutic relationship with the same group of providers over time, with care that follows the person across primary and secondary care settings, enhances the person's confidence. Mitchell et al. (2012) identify five principles of collaborative team effectiveness: "shared goals, clear roles, mutual trust, effective communication, and measurable processes and outcomes" (p. 6). Setting forth measurable process and outcome benchmarks from the outset of care planning helps all involved participants to keep an eye on the goal, with formative evaluations along the way to correct for error.

COORDINATION

The third C of relational COC is coordination. Effective coordination depends on the development of dynamic relationships among involved professionals. Relationships are as important to success as content. Shared goals and basic knowledge regarding each provider's work such that each provider knows how that work fits together as a whole is key to understanding coordination and its role in facilitating positive clinical outcomes. Havens and colleagues (2010) suggest that relational understanding is particularly important as "participants from different disciplines often reside in different

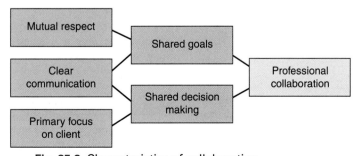

Fig. 25.2 Characteristics of collaboration.

'thought worlds' because of differences in training, socialization and expertise" (p. 928). The other knowledge requirement for active coordination relates to factors concerning the people receiving care—preferences, financial resources, access to care, support systems, and so on—because any of these can result in an unintended misalliance. Developing shared goals allows for effective coordination for treatment of chronic conditions.

Shared Goals

Shared goals are an essential product of effective person-centred collaboration and coordination. The person and family should be critical team members in determining, refining, and updating goals. Their inclusion as a collaborative team member allows for a more realistic assessment of a person's needs, preferences, resources, and personal goals. They can provide important input into how things are going and can sensitize providers to realistic needs and priorities.

People and their families are unique members of the care team. Usually, they lack formal training in health care and may not always understand the medical language used in team meetings. Although the same team members interact with each other on a regular basis informally in the care of people, this is not true of the people themselves. Nurses are an essential resource in helping to orient and introduce nonprofessional team members to the roles and expectations of collaborative teamwork and to adapt medical language so that it is easily understood (Mitchell et al., 2012).

Discussion at team meetings should focus on shared goals developed by the person and professional team members. Carefully defining the person's health problems and identifying possible contributing factors is an essential first step before moving on to brainstorming potential solutions. Unrelated data can compromise the concentration of the team on key person and family needs and solutions.

Problem-solving communication should be respectful, accurate, timely, and frequent. Aim for developing shared meanings rather than simple information exchanges. Mutual trust and respect for differences offer powerful reinforcement for open dialogue. Once agreement is reached, the entire team, including the person receiving care, needs to take full responsibility for implementing clearly described action plans.

Role Clarity

Role clarity is an essential prerequisite for relational continuity on interdisciplinary health care and community-based family care teams. Effective collaborative participation requires a clear understanding of one's own discipline's values and expected level of skill and **scope of practice**, *plus* a knowledge of and mutual respect for other team member disciplines' roles, professional responsibilities, and expertise (Hudson et al., 2017; Busari et al., 2017).

Team members function both as an individual professional representing a distinct discipline *and* as a collaborative **health care team** member. Mosser and Begun (2014) note that "the roles, education and values of different health professions give each profession a distinctive character on teams" (p. 55). Each discipline has its own set of behavioural norms and professional ethics. Although they may be similar, they are not identical in either scope or implementation of care. Studies of provider perspectives on effective team functioning identify role understanding and interpersonal communication as being the most important variables affecting role functioning on interdisciplinary teams (Cramm & Nieboer, 2011).

Even when core personal and professional values, attitudes, and practices are not at odds with each other, professional training and interpretations of standards can shape how professional values are prioritized (Shahriari et al., 2013). Team role confusion, fueled by professional rivalries, territoriality, and lack of clarification about job responsibilities, is identified as a potential barrier to effective team communication (Conference Board of Canada, 2012). Simulation Exercise 25.1, Learning About Other Health Professions, offers an opportunity to understand roles of different health professions.

Mutual Trust

In time, health providers from different disciplines learn to trust and rely on each other's competence and it becomes easier to support each other's efforts (Bosch & Mansell, 2015). This is unlikely to happen without regularly scheduled interdisciplinary team meetings. Unless there is a formal time and place for collaborative dialogue, the necessary professional connectivity for interdisciplinary collaboration will not take place in a meaningful way. Team meetings allow different disciplinary professionals to get to know each other. They also provide a forum for discussion of potential conflicts. People receiving care can sense when their care team is having conflicts. This tends to make the team's comments less credible, leading to potential confusion and adverse outcomes. Consistent consultations offer a scheduled opportunity to develop team-working processes, discuss potential conflicts, and reinforce commitment to delivering quality collaborative health care.

Effective Communication

Team communication skills include ones that are similar to those you would use in any professional health care situation. Added to these are specialized team communication

SIMULATION EXERCISE 25.1   Learning About Other Health Professions

Purpose

To familiarize students with differences and similarities in education and skill sets of key interdisciplinary health team members

Procedure

1. Break the class into groups of four to six students. Assign each student group a professional role to explore by describing the educational preparation and expected skill set of one of the following professional disciplines: physician, pharmacist, occupational therapist, speech pathologist, lab technologist, social worker, nurse practitioner.
2. (Initial research can be done as an out of class assignment.) Write a concise description about your assigned discipline that can be easily explained to your group members.

3. Identify and agree upon 10 to 12 key descriptors related to your findings and the dominant features of the profession within your group.
4. Each discipline group should present its findings to the larger class group.

Discussion

1. Compare and contrast similarities and differences in education and expected skill sets identified by each group.
2. In what ways might the skill set of the different disciplines complement each other in person-centred clinical care and decision making?
3. How could you use what you learned in this exercise to create better communication with other health care professionals?

---

skill sets, which include flexibility and openness, critical discernment skills, reading and writing proficiency, speaking, and nonverbal communication skills.

Interdisciplinary team meeting communication differs from other forms of work group communication, although similar group development processes occur (see Chapter 9). The focus of team group meetings is always on the immediate care issues of the person receiving the care. Each team member, including the person, is accountable for sharing relevant information about the person, listening to the comments of others, and actively participating in focused problem solving and decision discussions. In team group meetings, it is important to respect the diversity, professional values, and ideas of each team member, even when you do not agree with them. It is important to respect and consider the input of other team members who may approach the same situation from a very different perspective.

Here are some simple tips you can use in team meetings to enhance communication in team and task groups:

- *Listen before you speak.* Attentive listening is one of the strongest collaborative communication skills. When you take a measured listening stance, you show respect for the speaker. As you hear the other person's words, visually attend to the attitudes and nonverbal behaviours of the speaker and other team members. These are important information-transmitting factors that can influence understanding, allowing you to respond appropriately.
- *Know what you are talking about.* When you share clinical observations and professional opinions in team meetings, be as informed, authentic, specific, and descriptive as possible. Honest feedback and genuine

sharing builds trust and strengthens professional relationships, even when ideas are being challenged. Evidence-informed data provide an underpinning for interdisciplinary discussions. Nurses can communicate a critical appraisal of a person's presenting issues, health needs, preferences, values, and personal responses. This is your forte. Nurses spend the most time with people in their care and have the most "talking and observing" sustained contact with them.

- *Use your voice wisely.* Nurses' active participation in formal team meetings is essential. You do not have to comment on everything, but your input is unique and critical to the discussion. Information about the person receiving care, and human responses to illness and treatment represent data nurses are best positioned to share.
- *Be open to different ideas.* A strong advantage of team communication is that it allows more than one viewpoint to bear on a health situation. Exploration of different ideas and perspectives enriches the problem-solving approaches needed to develop a coordinated, consistent, and workable approach to difficult issues related to the person receiving care. Be knowledgeable about the differences in role responsibilities and common values of other disciplines so you can better frame messages and can understand their perspective. Recognize your limitations, as well as your strengths, and how you might be able to incorporate the expertise of other disciplines in total care for the person.
- *Ask for feedback.* Encourage other team members with whom you interact to provide relevant feedback—for example, "I'd like to hear what you think about this."

Analyze the information you receive, and ask relevant, open-ended questions. Brainstorming and problem-solving processes are indispensable to developing the most workable solutions. Interdisciplinary team decisions should be negotiated, not dictated, with all members being mindful of working through their individual differences in a respectful manner. Consensus solutions work best and are more easily implemented.

- *Work within the system.* Although the people receiving care are the core focus of care, health care centres are part of much larger health care management systems, which influence team functions and outcomes (Ginter et al., 2013). System factors beyond the control of the person receiving care and the direct care team will influence what is and is not possible in a given health care situation. Valuable time is saved when team members are knowledgeable about the constraints and opportunities available within their delivery system.

CONTENT VERSUS COMMUNICATION PROCESSES IN TEAM MEETINGS

Content and process are interwoven in effective team meetings. Content should be focused, with each team member as fully prepared as possible. This means that you need to understand what you do know and what you do not know about the person's situation. Scheduled team meetings should have clear agendas, with the time to be spent on each item identified. Structure keeps people on track. The agenda can be brief. Additional critical items can be added at the beginning of the meeting, if needed. Minutes taken at each meeting highlight decisions made, identify action items to be completed, and specify individual team member responsibilities for tasks, when indicated. Rotation of leadership and scribe roles help

team members share the workload and build a sense of collaborative team responsibility. Clarifying roles and expectations and identifying the scope of functional activities helps to direct attention to what is important and meaningful; it also helps to save time.

Sharing ideas with professional tact is an art. Skills can be learned. If someone makes a point that is particularly relevant, acknowledge its merit. If members have reservations about an idea, they should be encouraged to speak up. Presenting a concern or an alternative with a rationale is different from judging the rightness or wrongness of another team member's ideas, and it is easier to hear. Explain your rationale in neutral terms about the issue, not about the person. Learning to deal with conflict is as essential to team building as it is to individual professional collaborative conversations (see Chapter 24).

Smoothly run collaborative care meetings are those in which each team member understands and agrees to support the team mission of quality coordination of care. Time is a precious commodity for busy health care providers; team meetings should begin and end on time. An agenda keeps all team members focused on the business at hand. Simulation Exercise 25.2 provides an opportunity for students to understand collaboration skills in team decision making.

INFORMATIONAL CONTINUITY

Informational continuity refers to data exchanges among providers and provider systems, and between providers and people receiving care, for the purpose of providing continuously coordinated quality care. Instant electronic transmission of data ensures that the same information is available to all providers, it is seamless, and tests or other results are available to all in a timely manner (Canadian Nurses Association, 2013). Ideally, there is an

---

SIMULATION EXERCISE 25.2 Collaborative Decision Making

Purpose
To help students discover how they can work together to achieve consensus about an uncertain situation

Procedure
Break up the class into groups of three to four students. Identify one student for each group to act as scribe.
1. Each group member presents a real-time clinical scenario related to a person with complex medical needs, in one or two paragraphs.
2. Each student presents their scenario for group consideration. Other group members can ask questions.

3. The group should choose one of the scenarios and provide a rationale for its choice.

Discussion
1. How did each group reach its decision?
2. What was it like to know you had to make a team decision about an issue for which there is no perfect answer?
3. What factors made collaborative discussion and decision making easier or harder?
4. What did you learn from doing this exercise about how people function as a team in making a difficult decision within a short time frame?

uninterrupted flow of data and clinical impressions among health care providers and agencies, with people and their families, over time and space. Specific information follows the person from primary to secondary care settings. An electronic health record (EHR) provides secure, always up-to-date, and accurate information about the person. It prevents duplication of assessments among caregivers (Canadian Nurses Association, 2013). Data about possible medication interactions, start and stop dates, and personal responses to specific medications are easily accessible.

Informational continuity is critical to providing safe, quality care. Gaps can occur as a result of misplaced clinical records, inadequate discharge planning or referral data, deficient or delayed authorization for treatment, and a lack of understanding by the person about their illness, treatment, or self-management. Lack of information at the time of transfer can result in treatment delays, which increases the person's and family's anxiety unnecessarily.

Information continuity provides a safety net for people who often become overwhelmed with the number of procedures, appointments, and providers involved with their care. The capacity to communicate directly with various providers and treatment centres—and feeling comfortable that everyone involved in their care has the same information—is one less thing people and providers have to worry about.

Immediate forms of informational continuity within hospital units include interdisciplinary team meetings, huddles, comfort rounds, and progress notes. Handovers, discharge plans, referral contacts, and summaries are used for transfers of people from one care setting to another.

In the community, informational continuity can empower people through appointment reminders and call-back checks, careful instruction about diagnosis and care options, and accurate EHRs, shared with people and providers. The goal for informational continuity is to help ensure that everyone involved in the care of a person is on the same page. Sharing health and treatment information with people and their families should be consistent, complete, accurate, value neutral, and delivered in an easily understandable and supportive manner. Knowing what to expect, with contingency plans in place, increases the person's security (Haggerty et al., 2013). Notifying the family of changes in the person's condition or treatment recommendations is an essential part of ensuring informational continuity, particularly if the family is not in close contact with the person. Informational COC facilitates effective and efficient transition of care from one clinical setting to another. Receiving consistent information from different providers bolsters the person's confidence and is more likely to be believed.

Transition and Discharge Planning in Continuity of Care

Rhudy and colleagues (2010) identify improving the quality of transitions of people across health care settings as a national priority. People with complex chronic conditions typically experience multiple care transitions in their health experience. Unfortunately, changeovers between care settings are associated with a larger number of "avoidable adverse events" and "near misses" (Health Quality Council [Saskatchewan], 2018; Mitchell et al., 2012). Accurate recording of information and sharing it between the giving and receiving institutions are part of information continuity, but there is a relational aspect, too (Box 25.2).

A transfer from one care setting to another often is precipitated by a change in health, functional status, or the complexity of the person's needs rather than by the person's choice. Care transition, whether from the hospital to home or to a rehabilitation centre, assisted living setting, or whether from a community setting to a hospital, is an emotional as well as a physical event for people and their families. It is a vulnerable time. People and families caring for them are anxious because they do not know what to expect (Health Quality Council [Saskatchewan], 2018).

NURSING ROLE IN TRANSITIONAL CARE

Transitional care is defined as a "broad range of time-limited services designed to ensure health care continuity, avoid preventable poor outcomes among at-risk populations, and promote the safe and timely transfer of patients from one level of care to another or from one type of setting to another. Transitional care is complementary to but not the same as primary care, care coordination, discharge planning, disease management or case management. The hallmarks of transitional care are the focus on highly vulnerable, chronically ill patients throughout critical transitions in health and health care, the time-limited nature of services, and the emphasis on educating patients and family caregivers to address root causes of poor outcomes and avoid preventable rehospitalizations" Naylor et al., 2011, p. 747). Transitional care begins in the hospital and represents an expansion of the nurse's traditional role in hospital care. Successful transitions consider the combined needs of the person and family, which are paired with the resources of an agency or health care provider to realistically identify and meet identified care needs. Table 25.1 identifies key elements in effective transitional care.

Acute care hospitals are intended for short-term stays. When people require skilled medical and nursing care beyond a designated time period, they may be transferred

BOX 25.2   Core Functions for Transitional Sending and Receiving Teams

Transition of the Person

If you are working with an individual to transition them to a new provider, team, or program, you should do the following:

- Establish goals for the transition with the individual and family.
- Assess the individual for readiness for transition.
- Co-create a care transition plan with the individual, family, and receiving service or provider.
- Provide all referral information to the receiving provider and individual.
- Ensure that the individual is informed about what the transition might look like.
- Connect with the new provider, team. or program and ensure that they have all of the correct and up-to-date information about the individual's plan for care and recovery, and answer any questions they might have.
- Help to coordinate the transition from one service, unit, or facility to another.
- Notify the primary care physician, as appropriate, of the care transition plan.

As the receiver of transition information, you should:

- Ensure you receive all relevant transition and recovery plan information for the individual coming to your area.
- Acknowledge receipt of the referral.
- Correspond with the transitioning team or individual involved about any questions or clarification required, to do with the transition plan.
- Confirm a date, time, and location for the individual's first meeting or appointment with you.
- Communicate with the sending provider or primary care physician (or both), if the individual does not attend their initial appointment.
- Meet with the individual to welcome them and introduce them to the new facility, unit, service, and team.
- Follow-up with the individual to see if they have any questions about the new service.

Hospital Transfer

1. In discussion with the person and family, complete Hospital Transfer–Patient Snapshot form, which includes a complete identification of all variables connected to transfer for people identified as T-3 in their transportation process. Ensure communication has occurred with the person and family.
2. Ensure communication occurs with people and their family members:

    Reason for anticipated transfer

    Plan for care at receiving site—provide information and answer questions from the person or family about the care they will receive at the receiving site.

    Transportation options and costs—Offer a choice: How will the person be transferred? Will the family participate or be present during the transfer?

    Other supports required—What supports do the person and family feel they need?

    Obtain consent to proceed
3. Include the name of the primary nurse so the receiving region knows who to contact for care information.
4. Collate snapshots by region and send to the central point of transfer for those regions with identified T-3 people.
5. Central point of contact participates in the regional huddle validating existing snapshots on T-2/T-1 people. Identify any changes in the person's information.

Essential Tasks: Receiving Region

1. Receive snapshot of T-3 people. Identify any potential barriers to providing care for the person to be transferred and alert sending site of any concerns through daily huddles.
2. Update local physicians of impending transfers. Identify the potential Most Responsible Physician (MRP). Notify the person's family provider of pending transfer and to which site.
3. Participate in the region-to-region huddle, updating T-2/T-1 snapshots. Discuss any care changes.

From Alberta Health Services. (2021). *Transitions in Care.* https://www.albertahealthservices.ca/assets/info/amh/if-amh-ecc-transitions-in-care.pdf; https://hqc.sk.ca/Portals/0/documents/Patient%20Flow%20Toolkit%20April%202016.pdf?ver=2016-05-05-093704-600.

to a long-term care or rehabilitation hospital. People and their families need to know what parameters will be used for discharge as soon as this is known. They need face-to-face and real time conversations (Health Quality Ontario, n.d.). Usually, the hospital has a care coordinator, but nurses are often involved in arranging for the care coordinator to see the person and in working with follow-up concerns. All recommendations for transfer should be thoroughly

discussed with the person and family and included in the person's treatment plan.

Nurses play a crucial role in planning transitions between care settings. Early planning for transition to a different care setting is essential. This planning time gives people and significant caregivers a better chance to develop a realistic plan consistent with the person's care needs, strengths, preferences, and financial means—a plan that all

TABLE 25.1 Key Elements of a Coordinated Plan

Key Element	Primary Activities	Areas for Implementation and Measurement
1. Care coordination needs assessment	Family-driven Goal setting Assign roles and responsibilities to team	Use a structured tool to identify needs. Involve families as active participants in setting shared goals. Communication: ask families if their needs have been met.
2. Care planning and communication	Care team and family develop care plans together	Engage family in care plan development. Monitor, refine, and update care plan to track progress continually. Make care plan accessible to all team members.
3. Facilitating care transitions	Engage family to align plan with family goals and needs Timely information transfers	Track referrals with outside health entities. Ensure timely communication of information across transitions. Ensure required information is available at transition points.
4. Connecting with community resources and schools	Facilitate connections with support organizations	Ask the family if they have all the connections they need. Coordinate services needed and link to family partners and agencies. Ensure bidirectional communications work.
5. Transitioning to adult care	Foster self-care skills, communication skills, and self-advocacy	Co-develop written plans with people transitioning to adult care. Have health summary available at transition.

Adapted from Massachusetts Health Quality Partners. (2014). "Key Elements" Framework V3 (4.21.14). Key Elements Framework from the Care Coordination Task Force, Massachusetts Child Health Quality Coalition. http://www.masschildhealthquality.org.

those involved can feel is right and the best solution at the time. Follow-up plans are better negotiated if people have sufficient time to consider all aspects of potential choices and to think them through carefully before making significant decisions. Transition planning from the person's perspective also allows nurses to uncover hidden issues such as the person's fear of being abandoned or of receiving substandard care in an unknown setting.

Nonroutine discharges in which the person needs a postdischarge, rehabilitative or subacute placement, additional health support services, or equipment at home require a more complex discharge planning process for optimum results. If the discharge is to home, involved family members should be part of the discussion and decision because they will intimately be involved in care provision.

A complex discharge planning process begins with a careful review of initial admission data and continues as a thread with each subsequent review. Starting early in the hospitalization allows time for people and their families to become physically and emotionally prepared for transition and to have needed support available postdischarge.

Informal discussions can be introduced during routine care. Other times, education can be offered to the person in a more concentrated way, with a **teach-back method** and return demonstrations. Frequent check-ins with people and their families encourages them to ask questions and express concerns in a supportive environment. Box 25.3 presents nursing actions associated with complex discharges.

Simulation Exercise 25.3 provides practice with discharge planning processes.

The goal of discharge planning is to provide people and their families with the level and kind of information they need to secure their recovery and maintain health status during the immediate post-hospital period. Research shows that having discharge plans tailored to the individual needs of the person seems to have an effect on reduced hospital stay and readmission rates and increases people's satisfaction (Shepperd et al., 2013).

If the person is to be discharged to home, medication reconciliation and teach-back strategies discussed in Chapter 16 should be part of the discharge planning. Specific instructions for postdischarge care and contact arrangements with external care providers should be shared with people and families. Offering choices about available

and appropriate post-acute providers represents a unique form of advocacy for people and their families.

Medication reconciliation is an important dimension of admission and discharge planning. The Joint Commission specifically identifies it as National Patient Safety Goal No. 8. People may come into a care setting on a wide variety of medications. Some medications may be changed or discontinued; others may be added. When the person is being discharged, a medication reconciliation, including the name of the medication, generic and prescribed name, dosage, frequency, and the time each medication was last taken should be entered into the EHR, with a computer-generated or written list given to the person. Go over the list with the person and designated caregiver, if applicable. Medication reconciliation also should be done periodically with the person in primary care settings, especially if the person is seeing more than one provider (Mitchell et al., 2013; Accreditation Canada, the Canadian Institute for Health Information, the Canadian Patient Safety Institute, and the Institute for Safe Medication Practices Canada, 2012).

Crucial questions are who in the person's close support system is available to help the person in the immediate postdischarge period and what arrangements are in place if additional care support is required? It is important to ask open-ended questions about the home environment and the support the person has. This information needs to be precise. Just because a person has family in the area does not mean that they would be available to the person for direct support. You will need to identify the name of a primary support person or specific post-hospital arrangements in the person's EHR. Very important is asking people about their concerns and expectations after discharge. People discharged to home and their caregivers

---

BOX 25.3   Nursing Actions in Comprehensive Discharges

- Assess the person's understanding of the discharge plan by asking them to explain it in their own words.
- Advise the person and family of any tests completed at the hospital with pending results at time of discharge. Also notify appropriate clinicians of this contingency.
- Schedule follow-up appointments or tests after discharge, if needed. Provide relevant contact numbers.
- Provide information about home or health care services, if needed and if not initiated prior to discharge.
- Confirm the medication plan, ensuring that the person and family understand any changes (e.g., medication in the hospital not available or accessible in the community).
- Review written summary care instructions with the person and family and go over in detail what to do if a problem develops.
- Identify the responsible caregiver in the home as well as transportation arrangements.
- Expedite transmission of the discharge summary to health care providers and case managers accepting responsibility for the person.

SIMULATION EXERCISE 25.3   Using a Discharge Planning Process

Purpose

To provide an opportunity for students to develop an experiential understanding of a discharge planning process

Procedure

Using the guideline data, develop a simple discharge planning report for a newly admitted person on your unit, or use the following case study.

Jeff O'Connor is a 66-year-old man originally admitted to the emergency department with severe chest pain, shortness of breath, dizziness, and intermittent palpitations. He was diagnosed with a myocardial infarction and admitted to the coronary care unit. He was placed on oxygen and remained on the unit for several days because his serum markers continued to rise. He received morphine

for pain and sedatives to keep him comfortable. He is currently stabilized with digoxin, demonstrates a normal sinus rhythm, and is being transferred to the step-down unit this afternoon. His wife and daughter have visited him several times each day. His wife states she is exhausted but glad he is being transferred. Jeff has long-standing coronary artery disease and a family history of cardiac events. This is his first heart attack.

Discussion

If this is the only information you have on Jeff, what other data might you need to develop a full transitional report using the SBAR (situation, background, assessment, recommendation) format described in Chapter 4?

need specific instruction to successfully self-manage recovery and chronic health problems at home, not just once but several times. Written instructions should be verbally explained and given to each person. Arrangements and referrals for essential support or training needs to be in place before discharge.

Discharge Summary

The Joint Commission (2013) mandates that discharge summaries be completed within 30 days of hospital discharge. A discharge summary has diagnostic findings, hospital management, and plans for follow-up at the end of a person's hospitalization. Well written summaries assist in preventing readmissions and adverse effects like medication mismanagement, and overall, increase person and caregiver satisfaction and security (Newnham et al., 2017). Content mandated for each person's written discharge summary includes the following:

- Reason for hospitalization
- Significant findings
- Procedures and treatment provided
- The person's condition at discharge
- Instructions for the person and family (as appropriate)
- The attending physician's signature

Nurses are accountable for verbally reviewing discharge summaries with the person or caregiver (or both), providing written instructions, and completing discharge documentation in the chart. People and their significant caregiver(s) are given a copy of the discharge summary and encouraged to keep it in a safe place. People should bring their discharge summary to initial follow-up appointments. Although the physician is responsible for initiating and signing discharge summaries and orders, nurses play a critical role in their discharge.

Discharge instructions are not the same as discharge orders or discharge summaries. Specific, *written* discharge instructions should include a basic follow-up plan identifying diet, activity level, weight monitoring, what to do if symptoms develop or worsen, and the contact numbers of relevant hospital and primary care providers. Written instructions needs to be be simple and concrete—for example, "Call the doctor if you gain more than 2 pounds in 1 week." A written list of all medications prescribed at discharge, including prescription and over-the-counter medications, vitamins, and herbals to be given to the person and caregiver. Use teach-back methods (see Chapter 16) to ensure that discharge home management instructions are understood. Relational continuity helps ensure that the coaching and health teaching (presented in Chapter 16) get shared across all involved agencies.

Subheadings help to organize and highlight pertinent information for follow-up care. Discharge documentation in the person's chart includes the person's condition or functional status at time of discharge, followed by a summary of the treatment and nursing care provided and discharge instructions given to the person and family, along with the person's responses. Clearly identify the intermediate placement (nursing home, rehabilitation centre) or home. The health care staff need to document that the person or caregiver (or both) was physically given a copy of the discharge instructions.

MANAGEMENT CONTINUITY

The Canadian Nurses Association established a National Expert Commission in 2011. They produced a report called A Nursing Call for Action. Based on the Institute for Healthcare Improvement's triple aim initiative, they recommended, "Better health, better care, better value, best nursing" (Canadian Nurses Association, 2012). The aim of transformational approaches required to overhaul the health care system is to improve care experiences (including quality and satisfaction), cultivate overall population health, and reduce the per capita cost of health (Brandt et al., 2014).

Strong system-based management continuity facilitates self-care management. *Management continuity* involves ongoing communication across health care teams, institutions, and professions, and the focus of the communication is always on the person (Health Quality Council of Alberta, 2016). As a longitudinal approach to the clinical management of chronic illness in the community, management continuity involves aligning the person's needs with community support through care coordination and case management. *Care coordination* is the term used to describe "management of interdependencies among tasks" (Yang & Meiners, 2014, p. 96).

CARE COORDINATION AND SYSTEM NAVIGATION*

The basic goals of care coordination and system navigation are to proactively guide people through the barriers in complex health systems, decrease fragmentation, coordinate services, and improve health outcomes. Care coordinators are responsible for ensuring that the plan of care developed by the provider is carried out in partnership with the person. This process begins with developing a nonjudgemental, collaborative relationship with the person to identify health goals and any barriers that could impede success. Care coordinators are responsible for identifying

---

* Joseph, 2014.

an individual's health goals and coordinating services and providers to meet those goals. They must learn to be adept at navigating complex systems and communicating with people, their families, and professionals involved with the person's care. Coordination activities include the following:

- Establishing relationships based on trust
- Communicating with people, families, providers, and community resources that lead to shared expectations for communication and care
- Providing health education
- Assessing strengths, challenges, needs, and goals
- Implementing a proactive plan of care
- Monitoring progress and assisting with follow-up
- Supporting self-management goals
- Facilitating informed choice, consent, and decision making
- Facilitating transitions in care
- Linking people to community resources
- Aligning resources to meet the person's needs
- Developing connectivity that provides pathways that encourage timely and effective information flow between all entities involved, including the person

Effectively establishing and maintaining professional boundaries are essential when working with people and families to coordinate care. Boundaries provide the limits that enable care coordinators to maintain professionalism and secure an environment where both the person and care coordinator are mutually respected. Listed next are some important tips on maintaining boundaries.

- Always work within the treatment recommendations of the person's provider. The care coordinator should never give any recommendations contrary to the recommendations of the provider.
- The care coordinator is in a position of influence, and the person is in a vulnerable position. Overinvolvement with a person can be draining on the care coordinator and can interfere with the important tasks of the job.
- Assess your cultural ideas and prejudices. Know your community.

The success of care coordination depends to a large extent on the strength of the interpersonal relationships between individual clinicians and community support organizations. Without familiarity and shared objectives, the administrative transfer of information will not occur or be sustained. Ongoing use of the broad stakeholder group (the medical neighbourhood) and joint review of performance data at care coordination meetings can help to foster a community of continuous **quality improvement** among multiple providers. Routine performance measurement and reporting about the effectiveness and quality of care coordination are critical to understand if people's needs are being met.

CASE MANAGEMENT

Case management is an organizational and structured approach of responding to the complex needs of very vulnerable clients. It promotes self-management support and better integration of health care services (Hudon et al., 2015). It has a strong record of success as a strategy to reduce fragmentation in health care delivery and has been proven effective in reducing emergency department use and lower health costs (Woodward & Rice, 2015). Whether nurses work in the hospital or in a primary care setting, they should all have knowledge of how case management works and how it fits into COC.

Case management, also known as *care coordination*, is a professional support intervention, which assists people in self-managing their health. It makes a unique contribution to the health, social care, and participation of vulnerable people with complex health conditions. The goal of case management strategies is to help people function at their highest possible level in the least restrictive environment. Case management strategies are designed with the following purposes:

- To enhance the person's quality of life
- To use collaboration and effective communication in all aspects of care
- To promote the person's safety
- To decrease fragmentation and duplication of health delivery processes
- To contain unnecessary health care costs

Case management allows people with multiple or serious chronic physical and mental health conditions to stay in their homes and function in the community (Tortajada et al., 2017). People need a case manager when they are unable to safely establish or maintain self-management of a chronic health condition in a consistent manner without external support. Included in the population group served by case managers are older people, people with mental health disorders or dementia, and people with chronic physical disabilities affecting activities of daily living (ADLs).

Team-based case management is an effective care strategy that improves adherence and health outcomes and can decrease overall medical care costs. Knowledge of community resources to facilitate health care delivery in **primary care** settings allows case managers to consistently deliver the right care at the right time to the right person and family. Standards of practice for case management related to quality of care, collaboration, and resource utilization are consistent with National Patient Safety goals developed by The Joint Commission (2013).

Case Example

Ray Bolton is a 48-year-old man with severe chronic Crohn's disease. He has a permanent ileostomy, is on multiple medications, and suffers from periodic exacerbations of his condition, resulting in hospitalization. Ray's only source of income is from a Canadian disability program. He has neurological symptoms affecting his balance and gait that cause him significant pain. He has difficulty sleeping and is socially isolated. He lives by himself, with his cat. Apart from his 80-year-old mother, who lives in another province, Ray has no support system except for his nurses and physicians. He was referred for case management, following his latest hospitalization. Simulation Exercise 25.4 provides an opportunity to assess and plan for care using a case management approach.

CASE MANAGEMENT PRINCIPLES AND STRATEGIES

Case management strategies are designed to coordinate and manage care across a wide continuum of health care services and community supports. Case management models follow the nursing process as a structural framework. Strategies incorporate COC concepts related to communication, team building, and data sharing with all members of the multidisciplinary care team, including the person and family caregivers.

Case finding is a proactive case management strategy to identify individuals at high risk for potential health problems (Health Council of Canada, 2013). The manner in which a care provider approaches the person will determine the completeness of information they receive.

An intake assessment should include the names, addresses, and phone numbers of the person's health care providers, social service representatives, school or work contacts (if applicable), and health insurance information. Availability of social supports and religious affiliations, previous hospitalizations and history of treatment, current medications and allergies, advance directives and do not resuscitate (DNR) status, cognitive and mental status, mobility status, and functional assessment of Activities of Daily Living (ADLs) are other pieces of case management assessment data. Identifying potential barriers to treatment adherence, including the impact that the person's diagnosis has on family members and coworkers, is important. Case managers interact directly with all members of the collaborative health team, people, and families on a regular basis. The case manager works with an assigned person to identify the individual needs and health goals. Operationalizing self-management of chronic conditions requires special attention to empowering people related to role and emotional self-management, as well as the person's medical or behavioural management needs (McAllister et al., 2012). Case management treatment strategies are customized for each person, based on personal needs, values, and preferences, using a rehabilitative strength-based focus. Because case management represents a longitudinal treatment management process, care plans will likely need adjustment from time to time to reflect changes in the person's situation. People who are competent, capable of making valid judgements, should have final responsibility for decision making.

Case managers help people to coordinate services and overcome barriers. They provide people with the essential support to assume as much responsibility as possible in the self-management of their health issues. They meet with people at scheduled intervals to monitor the person's progress and provide suggestions, as needed. When single-agency resources are insufficient to meet complex health needs, case managers help people and their families to identify

---

SIMULATION EXERCISE 25.4 Planning Care for Ray Bolton

Case Management Approaches

Purpose
To provide practice with assessing and planning care for a person (Ray Bolton), using a case management approach

Procedure
(Initial consideration of Ray's issues can be completed as an out-of-class assignment.) In groups of four to five students, consider the case example of Ray Bolton in this chapter (see p. 16).
Each group should identify:
• Relevant assessment data
• The best ways to address Ray's complex health needs and why

• What kinds of resources Ray will need to effectively self-manage his multiple chronic health problems

After 15 to 20 minutes' discussion, have each student group share with the rest of the students what their plan would be, the resources they will need to accomplish the task, and why.

Discussion
1. What was your experience of doing this exercise?
2. What were the commonalities and differences developed by different student teams?
3. Were you surprised by anything in doing this exercise?
4. What are the implications for your future practice?

and coordinate services with other agencies. Networking and communication with other health providers involved with the person help to prevent, or minimize, emergence of full-blown health problems. Strategies include guidance or referrals to social supports such as legal aid, social security benefits and disability, safe affordable housing, social services, and mental health and addictions services. To be effective, case managers need a strong understanding of community resources' strengths and weaknesses, including accessibility, availability, affordability, how systems work, and how people and families can best make use of them.

Case managers have an advocacy role, too. They educate community workers who work with people with disabilities or chronic conditions about the social aspects of disability, to facilitate understanding and acceptance of the person's problems. Goodman (2014) suggests that the opportunities for nursing advocacy are boundless, depending on a nurse's personal interests and skills. For example, nurses often speak before legislative and other funding sources to advocate for essential services. Their testimony is believable because of their close relationship in caring for people in these vulnerable populations. Case managers sometimes negotiate on a person's behalf with insurance companies and equipment suppliers, as a supportive adjunct, when a person is unable to do so.

Case managers evaluate outcomes in terms of the person's satisfaction, clinical outcomes, and cost. Recommendations for treatment planning variations should correspond with observed changes in the person's situation or health condition, or in health care resources. Documentation from external providers and agencies needs to be included in the person's case management record, as do variances from the treatment plan, reasons for the variance, and plans for modification in care plans.

MANAGEMENT CONTINUITY RESOURCE FOR FAMILY CAREGIVERS

Case managers provide ongoing support and encouragement for family caregivers. The focus is on ensuring that care is coordinated and based on quality, safety, and access (Katz et al., 2017). Living with chronic illness increasingly is a home care responsibility, with family members as informal caregivers providing most of the care. Family caregiving is neither a career choice nor a role for which one can prepare. It is more intensive, complex, and long-lasting than in the past (Katz et al.; Schulz & Eden, 2016). Simulation Exercise 25.5 offers insights into the role of family caregivers from the caregiver perspective.

Caring for people with significant disability at home has positive and negative aspects. Being cared for at home offers stronger COC management because home is associated with personal identity, security, and relationships with people who genuinely care about the person. Variation exists in a family member's capacity to be supportive, especially if the caregiver's health is not optimal, the care is labour intensive and time consuming, they lack the skills to meet the demands, they are strained financially, or the relationship with the person is conflictual. Case managers can fill in essential information gaps for family caregivers, through careful questioning, observation, validation about feelings and observations, and consultation about emerging

---

SIMULATION EXERCISE 25.5   Understanding the Role of a Family Caregiver

Purpose

To help students understand the caregiver role from the perspective of family caregivers

Procedure

1. Interview the family caregiver of a person with a long-standing chronic condition or mental health disorder, and write a summary of the caregiver's responses.
2. Use the following questions to obtain your data.
   a. Why and how did you assume responsibility for caregiving?
   b. In what ways has your life changed since you became a caregiver for your parent, spouse, child or adult family member with a disability, or family member with a mental health disorder?
   c. What do you find most challenging about the caregiving role?
   d. What do you find rewarding about the caregiving role?

   e. How do you balance caring for your family member with caring for yourself?
   f. What advice would you give someone who is about to assume the caregiving role for a family member with a disability or chronic condition?
3. Three students should be asked to report to the class their findings from the interviews.

Discussion

- What was it like to get a picture of the caregiver role?
- Were you surprised by any of the caregiver's responses?
- What were the similarities and differences in caregiver responses?
- What are some of the reasons for any of the variation among student reports?
- How could you incorporate what you learned doing this exercise in your clinical practice?

health issues. Working with families should include providing educational information on medications, signs and symptoms of impending problems and potential adverse reactions, and when to call a health care provider. Names, locations, and phone numbers of primary care and follow-up providers should be discussed and the information provided in written form to the caregiver.

CASE MANAGEMENT FOR PEOPLE WITH HISTORY OF A MENTAL HEALTH DISORDER

COC is essential for effectively caring for people with history of a mental health disorder in the community, particularly if trusting relationships can be formed between the person and their informal caregivers. This relationship allows for COC and comprehensiveness, which can counter the complexities of chronic comorbidities (College of Family Physicians of Canada, 2016). These people find that fulfilling even basic needs for shelter, food, clothing, and transportation to be quality-of-life issues. People with chronically mentally health disorders and people with substance dependencies often function at a marginal level because of their symptoms. Many experience homelessness and are in poor physical health. These people often do not seek out help proactively. Yet, as A. C. Benson (n.d.) notes, "People seldom refuse help, if one offers it in the right way."

Case management for people with chronic mental health disorders is key to providing quality health care, particularly for youths and older people in the public sector (Woodward & Rice, 2015). Case managers provide people with mental health disorders with mentoring, coaching, and referrals for job training services. They help people avert crisis relapses that precipitate rehospitalization. Case managers use recovery principles of care, such as linking people with counselling and alternative treatment services, social services, and community networks.

COC for people with mental health disorders and people with dual diagnoses includes formal wraparound support services for children and families and case management for adults and children. Wraparound services for children use a strengths-based format, which involves the family, community, school, and service providers in the child's environment. Professionals work with the family and other social providers to promote adaptive functioning. Strengthening family ties to supportive people within the family's social environment is deliberately included in wraparound services to help strengthen social support (Thomas et al., 2017).

▌ SUMMARY

COC is a dynamic, multidimensional concept, consisting of relational, informational, and management continuity

and focused on assisting individuals and families with the resources they need to manage chronic illness within and across clinical settings. The goal of COC is to ensure a seamless continuum of quality care for people, provided through coordinated, community-based health services. COC integrated delivery systems focus on what really matters to a person and family and have the capacity to provide services to meet the person's needs.

Relational continuity embraces collaborative relationships and shared decision making among health care providers and people. Successful outcomes also depend on interdisciplinary collaboration and interprofessional team communication caring for the person, family, or community in need of care.

Informational COC allows for an uninterrupted flow of data and clinical impressions between health care providers and agencies, with people and their families, in a care experience that is connected and coherent over time. Informational COC is a critical component in effective transition and discharge planning.

Case management is a major vehicle in ensuring management continuity for individuals who otherwise might not be able to function independently in the community because of a physical or mental health disorder. Care coordination and service navigation in public sector health care helps people and families to get the support they need when multiple service providers are involved.

👤 ETHICAL DILEMMA
What Would You Do?

Paul is ready to be discharged from the hospital, but it is clear that he can no longer live independently. He has had several heart attacks in the past, with significant heart damage, and currently suffers from serious chronic obstructive pulmonary disease (COPD). His recent hospitalization was for uncontrolled diabetes. Paul has difficulty complying with diet restrictions and his need to take daily insulin. He is not an easy person to live with, but Paul is sure that his daughter will welcome him into her home because he is "family."

Although his daughter agrees to assume care for her father, she does so reluctantly. She has her own life and does not have a positive relationship with her father. She resents that he just assumes that she will take care of him. Without her support, Paul cannot live independently in the community. What would you do as the nurse in this situation to help them resolve this dilemma? What are the implications of this situation as an ethical dilemma?

QUESTIONS FOR REVIEW AND DISCUSSION

1. What do you see as facilitators and barriers for COC in your current care setting?
2. In what ways do different interdisciplinary roles influence and complement each other in complex clinical care situations?
3. In what ways does COC support the triple aim of effective health care? What do you understand better about COC as a result of reading this chapter?

REFERENCES

Accreditation Canada, the Canadian Institute for Health Information, the Canadian Patient Safety Institute, and the Institute for Safe Medication Practices Canada. (2012). *Medication Reconciliation in Canada: Raising The Bar—Progress to date and the course ahead.* https://www.ismp-canada.org/download/MedRec/20121101MedRecCanadaENG.pdf.

Benson, A.C. (n.d.). *A. C. Benson quotes.* BrainyQuote.com. http://www.brainyquote.com/quotes/quotes/a/acbenson101010.html.

Bosch, B., & Mansell, H. (2015). Interprofessional collaboration in health care: Lessons to be learned from competitive sports. *Canadian Pharmacists Journal/Revue des Pharmaciens du Canada, 148*(4), 176–179. https://doi.org/10.1177/1715163515588106.

Boyd, C., & Fortin, M. (2010). Future of multimorbidity research: How should understanding of multimorbidity inform health system design? *Public Health Review, 32*(2), 451–474.

Brandt, B., Lutfiyya, M., King, J. et al. (2014). A scoping review of interprofessional collaborative practice and education using the lens of the triple aim. *Journal of Interprofessional Care, 28*(5), 393–399.

Busari, J. O., Moll, F. M., & Duits, A. J. (2017). Understanding the impact of interprofessional collaboration on the quality of care: A case report from a small-scale resource limited health care environment. *Journal of Multidisciplinary Healthcare, 10,* 227–234. https://doi.org/10.2147/JMDH.S140042.

Canadian Oxford Dictionary. (n.d.). Paradigm shift.

Canadian Nurses Association. (2011). *Interprofessional Collaboration.* Position Statement. https://www.cna-aiic.ca/-/media/cna/page-content/pdf-en/interproffessional-collaboration_position-statement.pdf?la=en&hash=5695B7264EB8EE6FA1A4B1A73A44A052F0FEA40F.

Canadian Nurses Association. (2012). *A nursing call to action: The health of our nation, the future of our health system.* Prepared by the National Expert Commission. Canadian Nurses Association. https://www.cna-aiic.ca/~/media/cna/files/en/nec_report_e.pdf.

Canadian Nurses Association. (2013). *Integration: A new direction for Canadian health care. A report on the health provider summit process.* Canadian Nurses Association—Canadian Medical Association—Health Action Lobby. https://www.colleaga.org/sites/default/files/attachments/cna_cma_heal_provider_summit_transformation_to_integrated_care_e%20%281%29%202.pdf.

Centers for Disease Control and Prevention: The National Center for Chronic Disease Prevention and Health Promotion. (n.d.) *About chronic diseases.* https://www.cdc.gov/chronicdisease/about/index.htm.

Cohen, M. (2014). *How can we create a cost-effective system of primary and community care built around interdisciplinary teams?* https://www.policyalternatives.ca/publications/reports/ccpa-bc-submission-select-standingcommittee-health.

College of Family Physicians of Canada. (2016). *Best advice: Chronic care management in a patient's medical home.* College of Family Physicians of Canada. https://patientsmedicalhome.ca/files/uploads/BAG_ChronicCare_ENG_Jun22.pdf.

College of Family Physicians of Canada. (2019). *A new vision for Canada: Family practice—The patient's medical home.* College of Family Physicians of Canada. https://patientsmedicalhome.ca/files/uploads/PMH_VISION2019_ENG.pdf.

Conference Board of Canada. (2012). *Improving primary health care through collaboration briefing 2—Barriers to successful interprofessional teams.* https://professionals.wrha.mb.ca/old/professionals/collaborativecare/files/IPHCTC-Briefing2.pdf.

Crabtree, B., Nutting, P., Miller, W. et al. (2010). Summary of the national demonstration project and recommendations for the patient-centered medical home. *Annals of Family Medicine, 8*(Suppl. 1), 580–590.

Cramm, J., & Nieboer, A. (2011). Professional views on interprofessional stroke team functioning. *International Journal of Integrated Care, 11*(25), 1–8.

Crooks, V. A., Agarwal, G., & Harrison, A. (2012). Chronically ill Canadians' experiences of being unattached to a family doctor: A qualitative study of marginalized patients in British Columbia. *BMC Family Practice, 13*(1). https://doi.org/10.1186/1471-2296-13-69.

Ferrer, R., & Gill, J. (2013). Editorial: Shared decision making, contextualized. *Annals of Family Medicine, 11*(4), 303–305.

Fox., K. (2014). The role of the acute care nurse practitioner in the implementation of the Commission on Cancer's Standards on palliative care. *Clinical Journal of Oncology Nursing, 18*(S1), 39–44. https://doi.org/10.1188/14.cjon.s1.39-44.

Franek., J. (2013). Self-management support interventions for persons with chronic disease: An evidence-based analysis. *Ont Health Technol Assess Ser, 13*(9), 1–60. http://www.hqontario.ca/en/documents/eds/2013/full-report-OCDM-self-management.pdf.

Gallivan, J., Kovacs Burns, K., Bellows, M. et al. (2012). The many faces of patient engagement. *Journal of Participatory Medicine, 4,* e32.

Ginter, P., Duncan, W. J., & Swayne, L. (2013). *Strategic management of health care organizations* (7th ed.). Jossey-Bass.

Goodman, T. (2014). Guest editorial: The future of nursing: An opportunity for advocacy. *Association of Operating Room Nurses Journal, 99*(6), 668–670.

Green, M. E., Hogg, W., Savage, C., et al. (2012). Assessing methods for measurement of clinical outcomes and quality of care in primary care practices. *BMC Health Serv Res, 12,* 214. https://doi.org/10.1186/1472-6963-12-214.

Haggerty, J. L., Roberge, D., Freeman, G. K., et al. (2013). Experienced continuity of care when patients see multiple clinicians: A qualitative metasummary. *Annals of Family Medicine, 11*(3), 262–271.

Havens, D., Vasey, J., Gittell, J. et al. (2010). Relational coordination among nurses and other providers: Impact on the equality of patient care. *Nursing Management, 18*(8), 926–937.

Health Council of Canada. (2013). *A scoping review of screening in Canada.* https://healthcouncilcanada.ca/files/A_Scoping_Review_of_Screening_in_Canada_EN.PDF.

Health Quality Council of Alberta. (2016). *Understanding patient and provider experiences with relationship, information, and management continuity.* https://www.hqca.ca/wp-content/uploads/2018/05/Relationship_Information_Management_Continuity_Aug2016-1.pdf.

Health Quality Ontario. (n.d.) *Adopting a common approach to transitional care planning: Helping health links improve transitions and coordination of care.* http://ontariostrokenetwork.ca/wp-content/uploads/2014/05/bp-traditional-care-planning-1404-en.pdf.

Hudon, C., Chouinard, M. C., Diadiou, F. et al. (2015). Case management in primary care for frequent users of health care services with chronic diseases: A qualitative study of patient and family experience. *Annals of Family Medicine, 13*(6), 523–528. https://doi.org/10.1370/afm.1867.

Hudson, C., Gauvin, S., Tabanfar, R. et al. (2017). Promotion of role clarification in the health care team challenge. *Journal of Interprofessional Care, 31*(3), 401–403. https://doi.org/10.1080/13561820.2016.1258393.

Institute of Medicine. (2012). *Primary care and public health: Exploring integration to improve population health.* National Academy Press.

Joseph, M.J. (2014). Center for Health Improvement, Primary Care Coalition of Montgomery County. (Unpublished manuscript)

Katz, A., Herpai, N., Smith, G. et al. (2017). Alignment of Canadian primary care with the patient medical home model: A QUALICO-PC study. *Annals of Family Medicine, 15*(3), 230–236. https://doi.org/10.1370/afm.2059.

Keeling, A., & Lewenson, S. (2013). A nursing historical perspective on the medical home: Impact on health care policy. *Nursing Outlook, 61,* 360–366.

Kleinman, A. (1988). *The illness narratives: Suffering, healing, and the human condition.* Basic Books.

McAllister, M., Dunn, G., Payne, K. et al. (2012). Patient empowerment: The need to consider it as a measurable patient-reported outcome for chronic conditions. *BMC Health Services Research, 12,* 157.

Meiqari, L., Al-Oudat, T., Essink, D. et al. (2019). How have researchers defined and used the concept of 'continuity of care' for chronic conditions in the context of resource-constrained settings? A scoping review of existing literature and a proposed conceptual framework. *Health Research Policy and Systems, 17*(1). https://doi.org/10.1186/s12961-019-0426-1.

Mitchell, J. I., Owen, M. M., Colquhoun, M. H. et al. (2013). Medication reconciliation: A prescription for safer care. *Healthcare Quarterly (Toronto, Ont.), 16*(4), 10–13. https://doi.org/10.12927/hcq.2014.23659.

Mitchell, P., Wynia, M., Golden, R. et al. (2012). *Core principles & values of effective team-based health care.* Discussion Paper. Institute of Medicine. www.iom.edu/tbc.

Mosser, G., & Begun, J. (2014). *Teamwork in health care.* McGraw Hill.

Naylor, M. D., Aiken, L. H., Kurtzman, E. T. et al. (2011). The importance of transitional care in achieving health reform. *Health Affairs, 30*(4), 746–754. https://doi.org/10.1377/hlthaff.2011.0041.

Newnham, H., Barker, A., Ritchie, E. et al. (2017). Discharge communication practices and healthcare provider and patient preferences, satisfaction and comprehension: A systematic review. *International Journal for Quality in Health Care, 29*(6), 752–768. https://doi.org/10.1093/intqhc/mzx121.

Paquette-Warren, J., Roberts, E., Fournie, M. et al. (2014). Improving chronic care through continuing education of interprofessional primary care teams: A process evaluation. *Journal of Interprofessional Care, 28*(3), 232–238.

Porter-O'Grady, T. (2014). From tradition to transformation: A revolutionary moment for nursing in age of reform. *Nurse Lead, 12*(1), 65–69.

Potter, P. A., Perry, A. G., Stockert, P. A. et al. (2019). *Canadian fundamentals of nursing* (6th ed). Canada: Elsevier.

Renholm, M., Suominen, T., Puukka, P. et al. (2016). Nurses' perceptions of patient care continuity in day surgery. *Journal of Perianesthesia Nursing, 1*(10).

Rhudy, L., Holland, D., & Bowles, K. (2010). Illuminating hospital discharge planning: Staff nurse decision making. *Applied Nursing Research, 23*(4), 198–206.

Roberts, K., Rao, P., Bennett, T., et al. (2015). Prevalence and patterns of chronic disease multimorbidity and associated determinants in Canada. *Health Promot Chronic Dis Prev Can. 35*(6), 87–94. https://www.ncbi.nlm.nih.gov/pmc/articles/PMC4910465/.

Schottenfeld, L., Petersen, D., Peikes, D. et al. (2016). *Creating patient-centered team-based primary care.* AHRQ Pub. No. 16-0002-EF. Agency for Healthcare Research and Quality.

Schulz, R., & Eden, J. (2016). Family caregiving roles and impacts. In *Families caring for an aging America.* The National Academies Press.

Shahriari, M., Mohammadi, E., Abbaszadeh, A. et al. (2013). Nursing ethical values and definitions: A literature review. *Iranian Journal of Nursing and Midwifery Research, 18*(1), 1–8.

Shepperd, S., Lannin, N., Clemson, L., et al. (2013). Discharge planning from hospital to home. *Cochrane Database of Systematic Review, 1,* CD000313.

Smith, M. D. (2013). *Best care at lower cost: The path to continuously learning health care in America.* National Academies Press. doi. https://doi.org/10.17226/13444.

Stans, S. E., Stevens, J. A., & Beurskens, A. J. (2013). Interprofessional practice in primary care: Development of a tailored process model. *Journal of Multidisciplinary Healthcare, 6,* 139–147.

The Joint Commission. (2013). *Comprehensive accreditation manual for hospitals: The official handbook (CAMH).* Joint Commission on Accreditation of Health Care Organizations. https://ijc.org/en.

Thomas, P. A., Liu, H., & Umberson, D. (2017). Family relationships and well-being. *Innovation in Aging, 1*(3), igx025. https://doi.org/10.1093/geroni/igx025.

Top Alberta Doctors. (2019). Toward optimized practice (TOP) relational continuity working group. Relational continuity clinical practice guideline, p. 5. https://actt.albertadoctors.org/file/Relational-Continuity-CPG.pdf.

Tortajada, S., Giménez-Campos, M. S. Villar-López, J., et al. (2017). Case management for patients with complex multimorbidity: Development and validation of a coordinated intervention between primary and hospital care. *International Journal of Integrated Care, 17*(2), 4. https://doi.org/10.5334/ijic.2493.

Wagner, E., Austin, B., Davis, C. et al. (2001). Improving chronic illness care: Translating evidence into action. *Health Aff, 20*(6), 64–78.

Woodward, J., & Rice, E. (2015). Case management. *Nursing Clinics of North America, 50,* 109–121.

World Health Assembly. (2016). Framework on integrated, people-centred health services: Report by the Secretariat. World Health Organization. https://apps.who.int/iris/handle/10665/252698.

World Health Organization. (2016). Patient engagement. In *Technical series on safer primary care.* World Health Organization.

World Health Organization. (2018). *Continuity and coordination of care: A practice brief to support implementation of the WHO framework on integrated people-centred health services.* World Health Organization. https://apps.who.int/iris/bitstream/handle/10665/274628/9789241514033-eng.pdf?ua=1.

Yang, Y. T., & Meiners, M. (2014). Care coordination and the expansion of nursing scopes of practice. *Journal of Law, Medicine & Ethics, 42*(1), 93–103.

WEBSITE/RESOURCES LIST

https://actt.albertadoctors.org/file/Relational-Continuity-CPG.pdf.

https://www.albertahealthservices.ca/assets/careers/ahs-careers-stu-supporting-interprofessional-placements.pdf.

https://apps.who.int/iris/bitstream/handle/10665/274628/9789241514033-eng.pdf?ua=1.

https://www.cdc.gov/chronicdisease/about/index.htm 2019.

https://www.cmsa.org/who-we-are/what-is-a-case-manager/.

https://www.cna-aiic.ca/-/media/cna/page-content/pdf-en/interproffessional-collaboration_position-statement.pdf?la=en&hash=5695B7264EB8EE6FA1A4B1A73A44A052F0FEA40F.

https://www.cna-aiic.ca/~/media/cna/files/en/nec_report_e.pdf.

https://www.colleaga.org/sites/default/files/attachments/cna_cma_heal_provider_summit_transformation_to_integrated_care_e%20%281%29%202.pdf.

https://content.oma.org//wp-content/uploads/coordinatedcareplan_june2014-1.pdf.

https://www.cpha.ca/caregiver-burden-takes-toll-mental-health.

https://www.hqca.ca/wp-content/uploads/2018/05/Relationship_Information_Management_Continuity_Aug2016-1.pdf.

https://www.hqontario.ca/Portals/0/documents/qi/health-links/bp-improve-package-cdm-en.pdf.

https://www.ismp-canada.org/download/MedRec/20121101MedRecCanadaENG.pdf.

https://www.longwoods.com/content/17216/healthcarepapers/towards-a-canadian-model-of-integrated-healthcare.

http://ontariostrokenetwork.ca/wp-content/uploads/2014/05/bp-traditional-care-planning-1404-en.pdf.

https://patientsmedicalhome.ca/files/uploads/BAG_ChronicCare_ENG_Jun22.pdf.

https://patientsmedicalhome.ca/files/uploads/PMH_VISION2019_ENG.pdf.

https://professionals.wrha.mb.ca/old/professionals/collaborativecare/files/IPHCTC-Briefing2.pdf.

e-Documentation in Health Information Technology Systems

Claire Mallette

Originating US Chapter by *Kathleen Underman Boggs*

OBJECTIVES

At the end of the chapter, the reader will be able to:
1. Identify purposes for documentation.
2. Discuss electronic health/medical records (EHRs and EMRs) and computerized provider order entry (CPOE) systems as part of larger electronic health information technology (HIT) systems, evaluating whether "meaningful use" requirements have improved care quality.
3. Draw conclusions as to how clinical pathways, decision support, CPOE, and other aspects of HIT systems improve person and safety outcomes.
4. Identify health outcomes and legal aspects of documenting in electronic records.

Two key elements of collaborative work are communication and documentation (Chao, 2016).

The process of obtaining, organizing, and conveying people's health information to others in print or electronic format is referred to as **documentation**. Fig. 26.1 illustrates the purposes of electronic documentation, especially in terms of improved communication and evidence gathered from aggregated electronic health records (EHRs) to establish "best practice" interventions for quality improvement.

The process of interdisciplinary communication has been increasingly integrated into EHRs as the method nurses use to document outcomes of care given. However, EHRs are only a component of the larger **health information technology (HIT)** system (Rodrigues et al., 2016). Use of **computerized provider order entry (CPOES) systems** are also described in this chapter. Your use of HIT technology to communicate and manage the person's health information is a competency skill specifically cited in the Canadian Association of Schools of Nursing (2012). The overarching competency identifies the use of information and communication technologies to support information synthesis, in accordance with professional and regulatory standards in the delivery of care. Regulatory and ethical implications of documentation

will also be described in this chapter, concluding with a brief discussion of coding and nursing taxonomies. New technology and devices for health communication at the point of care, clinical decision support systems (CDSSs), remote monitoring, secure messaging, and telehealth are discussed in Chapter 27.

BASIC CONCEPTS

Computerized Health Information Technology (HIT) Systems

Computers make information more accessible to all who are involved, including the person being cared for. *Health information technologies (HIT)* are the hardware, software, and infrastructure required to collect, store, access, and exchange electronic health information in clinical practice (Chang & Gupta, 2015). The use of HIT can improve people's safety and health outcomes and assist providers in being more efficient and effective (Tepper, 2018).

HIT is also making care safer by engaging people as partners in their health care, promoting better communication, and increasing use of preventive practices and evidence-informed "best practices" (Dolin et al., 2014). Use

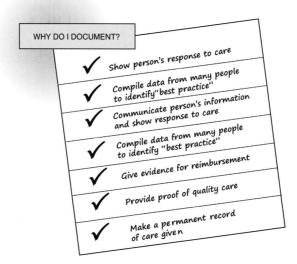

Fig. 26.1 Why do I document?

of HIT skills is an expectation of nurses, even as students and novice nurses. Nurses need to know how to incorporate technology into their practice to support their work (Strudwick & Booth, 2020). Studies show that knowledge and skills related to the use of electronic health/medical records (EHR/EMR) can be successfully integrated into simulations labs teaching these skills (Georges et al., 2016).

Meaningful Use

Adoption of HIT creates an interactive, computerized information and communication system. Far more complex than just putting existing paper documentation on a computer, HIT systems are designed to support the multiple information needs required by today's complex health care, provide you and others on the health team with *clinical decision support*, and achieve safer care for the person receiving that care.

Within HIT, there are different electronic health records, with similar but different information. They are known as **electronic health records (EHRs)**, **electronic medical records** (EMRs), **electronic patient records** (EPRs), and **personal health records** (PHRs). (See Box 26.1 for definitions of each). The term *EHR* is increasingly used to refer to the lifetime record of all health care occurrences. Ideally, EHRs have portability and can follow the person to other health care providers, specialists, hospitals, or nursing homes. Presently, the six core EHR components are: person and provider demographics, diagnostic imaging in hospitals, profiles of dispensed drugs, laboratory test results,

clinical reports, and immunizations (Canada Health Infoway, 2018). The term *EMR* describes the digital record that is used in primary health practitioner offices or in clinics (Naigle, 2007). The *EPR* is used by health care providers in facilities such as hospitals and long-term care. For the purposes of this chapter, the term EMR will be used to describe both health information from physicians' offices and clinics (EMRs), and from hospitals and long-term care facilities (EPRs). The PHR is controlled by the person and can integrate information from a variety of sources, such as medical records, multiple health care providers, and the person (Canada Health Infoway, 2018).

In Canada, as a result of decentralized health care administration from the federal government, to provinces and territories, to local regions, there are multiple EHRs and EMRs that are not compatible across systems (Chang & Gupta, 2015). In 2001, Canada Health Infoway was created to work toward the ability to exchange health information safely across systems. Canada Health Infoway's (n.d.-a) purpose is to "realize the vision of healthier Canadians through innovative digital health solutions through working with partners to accelerate the development, adoption and effective use of digital health solutions across Canada." The type of information captured in EHR/EMR systems can vary with types of information included, such as the person's demographics, health history, progress and procedure notes, health issues, medications, and allergy lists, including immunization status, laboratory test results, key clinical reports, diagnostic images, and advanced directives (Strudwick & Booth, 2020).

BOX 26.1   Understanding EHR, EMR, EPR, and PHR

Electronic Health Record (EHR): An electronic health record (EHR) refers to the systems that make up the secure and private lifetime record of a person's health and health care history. These systems store and share such information as lab results, medication profiles, key clinical reports (e.g., hospital discharge summaries), diagnostic images (e.g., X-rays), and immunization history. The information is available electronically to authorized health care providers.

Electronic Medical Record* (EMR): An electronic medical record (EMR) is an office-based system that enables a health care provider such as a family physician or a physician in a clinic to record the information gathered during a patient's visit This information might include a person's weight, blood pressure, and clinical information, and would previously have been handwritten and stored in a file folder in a physician's office. Eventually, the EMR will also allow the physician to access information about a patient's complete health record, including information from other health care providers that is stored in the EHR.

Electronic Patient Record* (EPR): An electronic or digital record that is used by health providers involved in the person's care in a health care organization such as a hospital or long-term care organization.

Personal Health Record (PHR): A complete or partial health record under the custodianship of a person(s) (e.g., a patient or family member) that holds all or a portion of the relevant health information about that person over their lifetime. This is also a person-centric health record, but unlike the EHR, the person has control or "custodianship" over the record, rather than the health care provider.

*For the purposes of this chapter, the term *EMR* is used to capture both health information from the EMRs from physician's offices and EPRs from hospitals and long-term care facilities.

Adapted from: Canada Health Infoway. (n.d.-b). Understanding EHRs, EMRs, and PHRs. infoway-inforoute.ca/en/solutions/digital-health-foundation/understanding-ehrs-emrs-and-phrs#:~:text=At%20Canada%20Health%20Infoway%2C%20the%20terms%20are%20defined%20as%20follows%3A&text=Electronic%20Medical%20Record%3A%20An%20electronic,gathered%20during%20a%20patient's%20visit; and Barry, M. A. (2019). Documenting and Reporting. In P. A. Potter, A. G. Perry, P. Stockert et al. *Canadian fundamentals of nursing* (6th ed.). Elsevier.

Three Keys to Electronic Records

The three keys to electronic records are **interoperability**, portability, and ease of access.

Interoperability (Interagency Accessibility)

Exchanging health information among agencies is critical to smoothly delivering comprehensive person-centred care. *Interoperability* means different systems can "talk to each other" to share person information. This is essential if we are to reduce costs by eliminating redundancy. For example, when the person's laboratory results or imaging files are available to multiple providers, unnecessary repetition of tests or procedures can be eliminated and costs reduced. Canada Health Infoway tracks the availability of provincial and territorial data. In 2017, there were an estimated 301000 health care providers accessing one or more sources for people's information in the EHR. Regions have also focused in recent years on increasing access to connected health information, from acute care settings to community and long-term care settings. Approximately 42% of nurses and primary care physicians reported having access to provincial/territorial information systems (Canada Health Infoway, 2018).

Case Example: Mrs. Levine's Case

Mrs. Levine's laboratory results can be directly entered into her primary provider's electronic health record by an outside laboratory and then you, the nurse, can access them from your clinic. With interoperability, health information flows to providers as needed, allowing seamless transitions. With interoperability we can have "anytime, anywhere access" of health care records using remote devices. In some cases, Mrs. Levine can access her health care provider's portal using her home computer to read case notes, look at her lab test results, and schedule another appointment if needed. For example, if Mrs. Levine was accessing health care at University Health Network in Toronto, Ontario, she would have access to four centres (two acute care hospitals, one cancer centre, and one rehabilitation institute). With that access, Mrs. Levine could see her appointments, as well as her lab, pathology, and imaging results from the four centres and clinics as soon as they are ready, through the patient portal (University Health Network, 2020).

Portability

Electronic records are more durable than paper charting and are portable—they are easily transferable. As there is presently no single national EHR in Canada, access to health information by others is limited. For example, if you had an accident, the health care providers who are treating you would most likely not be able to access your health information. Even if your family physician is using an EMR system, there is no access by other health care providers to the information. The health care facility treating your injuries would have to contact your family physician for a copy of your health records. This is often still done by information sent through fax machines, as there is a belief that this is more secure than email or secure websites (Goldman, 2019).

Alberta is making inroads in creating better access of health information across the province. Alberta Netcare Portal was launched in 2006, in which all health care facilities keep their own records of health services provided to people. They then send key health information to Alberta Netcare. Key health information includes medication information; laboratory test results; diagnostic images and reports; hospital visits; surgeries; drug alerts, allergies, and intolerances; personal demographic information; and immunizations. This procedure allows health care providers across the province the ability to access this information whenever needed (Alberta.ca, n.d.).

Ease of Access

Ideally, ease of access means access at the point of care or remotely using various digital devices. While maintaining health record security, people can give permission for access by multiple caregivers for anytime, anywhere communication. As just described, the ease of access varies depending on province or territory, health care organizations, electronic health and medical records, and availability of patient portals.

HIT system barriers preventing better access currently include cost, incompatible hardware and software, federal and provincial government funding, privacy regulations, and most importantly, the great difficulty in keeping stored data secure.

DOCUMENTING INFORMATION IN ELECTRONIC RECORDS

HIT systems compile records of people's health care. Yet the effects on nurse–person communication during the process of entering data into electronic records are less well known. Canada Health Infoway, in collaboration with the Canadian Nurses Association (CNA) and the Canadian Nursing Informatics Association (CNIA), did a survey in 2020, examining the adoption and use of electronic and clinical information by nurses across Canada. The survey explored nurses' views (n = 1642 with 1132 providing direct patient care) on the adequacy of the electronic/clinical information systems for nursing practice and confidence in the systems. The findings indicated that the majority (59%) of nurses are providing direct care in Canada using a combination of paper and electronic tools for their documentation. Nurses' positive perception of the impact of electronic records on the quality of nursing and their practice productivity, and satisfaction with their current electronic/clinical information system, has increased since 2014 (Canada Health Infoway, 2020).

Advantages to Electronic Health Records

Improved Information Flow

A comprehensive computer information system changes the way information flows through the health care delivery system. Communication is streamlined rapidly. HIT can simultaneously communicate to nurses, physicians, people receiving care, and families, across agencies. See the Case Example on Ms. Thibault, describing the information flow in a comprehensive computer information system.

Case Example: Ms. Thibault

Ms. Thibault develops trouble breathing. She is admitted via the emergency department (ED) to a medical unit at a general community hospital, at 11 a.m., with a diagnosis of congestive heart failure. Her ED physician accessed her prior electronic health record (EHR), updated the information, and documented the physician's notes and Ms. Thibault's electrocardiogram (ECG) results. The ED nurse documented medications and treatments given. The health information technology (HIT) system alerts the family physician, who comes in to examine Ms. Thibault and enters diagnostic and treatment orders using a CPOE system. The family physician does not need to repeat the ECG, because the system already contains these data. These orders are simultaneously and instantly transmitted to the pharmacy, the laboratory, and radiology, as well as to you, the nurse assigned to care for Ms. Thibault on your unit.

IMPROVED COMPLETENESS OF NURSING DOCUMENTATION

We need to ensure accurate communication of the care people receive, verbally and through our documentation. Timely and accurate documentation of care given is critical to providing team members with the information they need to make informed decisions. The primary purpose of documentation is to maintain an exchange of information about the person among all care providers, including nurses at the point of care. Documentation in EMRs supports the continuity, quality, and safety of your care. Quality documentation not only improves communication about the admitting health issues and diagnosis but also may increase recognition of comorbid conditions that can then also be treated (Towers, 2013).

Is it possible to fully document all nursing care given? Lack of visibility seems to be a recurring theme. Nurses report that the individualized care they provide is not visible in the format demanded by the EMR standardized documentation systems, especially when a checklist format is used for care. Nurses also report that drop-down checklists often do not adequately capture the person's health issues. In these cases, nurses usually have the ability to include a narrative note (Strudwick & Booth, 2020). Nurses additionally rely on "informal" communication passed along during change of shift, as well as the information on the person's EMR. Records that are inaccurate, incomplete, or not reinforced verbally can compromise clinical decisions and quality of care reporting. Nurses need to communicate the person's current condition information and response to treatment, both in the record and verbally. It is also very important to remember that nursing documentation is a formal legal document that captures the person's health care experience. All provincial and territorial nursing regulatory bodies have documentation standards that must be followed.

PARTNERING IN DOCUMENTING WITH PEOPLE RECEIVING CARE

Studies repeatedly show that when people are actively involved in decision making about their health, they self-manage their health issues better, following the mutually agreed-upon self-management strategies. Access to patient **portals**, where available, allow the person to view their health information. Some PHRs even allow the person to enter information into their medical record. The PHR is controlled by the person and can integrate information from a variety of sources such as medical records, multiple health care providers, and the person (Canada Health Infoway, n.d.-b). MYChart™ is an example of a PHR that is being adopted in health care organizations across Ontario and at Fraser Health in British Columbia. This PHR allows people to review information such as their test results, discharge reports and relevant health information. MYChart™ also allows the person to enter their own information—for example, record their

symptoms or keep track of other health-related factors that could influence their health and treatments. People can also share their health information with whoever they choose (Registered Nurses' Association of Ontario, 2018).

Essentials of Nursing Documentation

Our documentation is guided by nursing regulatory standards and is a formal legal document. Every health care agency has its own version of what constitutes complete clinical documentation. Nursing documentation contains a daily record of the person's progress and evaluation of outcomes. Daily records may include flow sheets, nursing notes, intake and output forms, and medication records. Some data, such as vital signs, may be automatically recorded into the EMR.

Clarity

Information should flow in an efficient and effective manner so all health team members have access to current data to do ongoing evaluations of treatment outcomes. Such improvements in communication lead to improved outcomes for people. Try thinking of it this way: every task sequence you perform requires you to access data before and after completion to maintain continuity. As you document continually, entering information into the system, communication among the health team is improved. In one example, home care nurses in a study by Nemeth et al. (2007) accessed current laboratory test results at the point of care, allowing them to discuss changes in care during home visits. A specific example might be instant access to laboratory results on blood clotting time, allowing you to contact the physician for a change in anticoagulation medication levels while you are still at the person's home.

Clear documentation means using standardized terms that are understood by every member of the health team. Documentation of care must be accurate, based on your assessments. For example, you are expected to document the presence on admission of catheters and intravenous lines, as well as facts about the status of any decubitus ulcers (bedsores).

Efficiency

Some literature suggests that nurses feel caught between the demands for meeting people's care needs and the agency requirements for complete documentation. However, the majority of evidence shows that EMRs actually save time, allowing staff nurses more time at the point of care, especially when devices for charting are at the bedside (Yee et al., 2012). The Canada Infoway (2020) survey findings indicated that nurses primarily have access to stationary laptop computers, with only limited access to mobile devices. A majority of respondents believe that it is essential to have access to mobile devices to provide and document direct care, communicate with team members, and facilitate day-to-day communication.

The potential impact of EMRs on nursing efficiency is measured by a reduction in the amount of time spent doing activities other than direct nursing care. Concerns about documentation time may be alleviated in the future, as access to computers become more available and as they are able to use voice entry through the use of speech recognition software that then converts spoken words to computer readable input (Strudwick & Booth, 2020). Computerization improves the efficiency and quality of charting, by prompting for information needed while eliminating duplication. For example, instead of re-questioning the person about health history, this information is already available on their EMR. Efficiency is increased because health care providers all across the agency have immediate access to information. The literature lists HIT benefits that improve nursing efficiency in other "downstream" ways (i.e., that happen later in the process), beyond what is apparent in documentation activities, such as medication record resolution, automatic medication calculations, automatic downloading of bedside monitoring records, and automated nursing discharge summaries.

Safety

As discussed in Chapter 2, HIT systems have made care safer. HIT systems force standardization of nursing terminology, eliminate use of inappropriate abbreviations, and avoid problems of illegibility. Errors are prevented because assistance is given with drug calculations as well as with decision support, such as checking drug incompatibility and allergies. Studies of the medication process show errors or potential errors cut by half with the use of HIT (Radley et al., 2013). Improved communication and continuity of care between health care providers through the use of HIT systems have also been reported.

ENHANCED QUALITY OF CARE

There are many secondary uses of data contained in people's health records. Standardized clinical data can provide data that informs effective care practices and areas for improvement (Canadian Nursing Informatics Association, 2019). When masses of data are analyzed, information is generated to add to our knowledge of what care measures lead to improved and effective nursing "best practice" care (American Nurses Association [ANA], 2017).

Documentation to demonstrate quality assurance. Access time to EHR and EMR data should be enhanced using HIT systems. For example, using paper files, it took a long time to do audits for quality assurance (QA) activities.

Health care has shifted to emphasize measurement of quality outcome indicators. Reviews are done to determine the extent to which evidence-informed care standards are being met and can be improved upon in health care organizations, and at provincial or territorial and national levels. Assessments as to quality of care are based on what was documented and coded. Clear documentation also provides evidence of effective care and outcomes during accreditation reviews. Evidence is accumulating that shows that data retrieved from HIT systems can make health care more person centred, promote better coordination of care, and make communication more effective.

Health outcomes. HIT systems offer ease of access to **aggregated data** from many people for reports and disease surveillance, to determine health outcomes and issues, and to research "best practice" nursing care and interventions that need to be changed. For example, you can obtain information about the number of postoperative infections that have occurred on your unit. Or you may want to find out how many people with diabetes in your primary care practice failed to return for follow-up teaching and then generate a list to follow up with them. HIT systems can be used to obtain reports about predictors of health outcomes in home health care. By combining data, nurses identify better treatment methods and evaluate the outcomes of their interventions on groups of people.

Epidemiological data. Combining data from many care recipients quickly can speed identification of adverse outcomes. Public health agencies analyze information to identify disease trends to generate epidemiological information. The Public Health Agency of Canada (PHAC), in partnership with others, focuses activities on preventing disease and injuries, promoting good physical and mental health, and providing information to support informed decision making (Government of Canada, 2020). The data obtained during the COVID-19 pandemic in 2020 by the PHAC and equivalent agencies in each province and territory were pivotal in decision making related to how to manage COVID-19 outbreaks. Another organization is the Canadian Institute for Health Information (CIHI) that provides comparable data and information that can be used to accelerate improvements in health care, health system performance, and population health across Canada, and inform policy decisions (CIHI, n.d.).

Use of Computerized Provider Entry Systems

Computerized provider order entry (CPOE) refers to the HIT that providers such as nurse practitioners, physicians, physician assistants, or sometimes nurses at the point of care, use to directly enter their orders for diagnosis or treatment. The information is then transmitted directly to the recipient responsible for carrying out that order, such as the pharmacy, the laboratory, or radiology. At a minimum, this aspect of the system ensures that orders are complete, use standard terms, and are available in a legible format. This system not only processes an order, it cross-compares it with data in the person's electronic health/medical record, such as whether the person is allergic to a newly ordered medication, has a potential for a drug–drug adverse interaction, or whether the dose or route ordered exceeds standard guidelines for safety. CPOE may also check for errors of omission. For example, it would give a "prompt" about a need to also order a laboratory test to verify an acceptable blood level of the new medication. CPOE systems are usually paired with computer-assisted **clinical decision support systems (CDSSs)**, which are discussed in Chapter 27.

Outcomes for use of computerized provider entry. Evidence is beginning to suggest that use of CPOE systems improves the appropriateness of orders, positively affects communication, and improves outcomes, particularly by reducing medical errors and adverse drug events and even increasing compliance (Agency for Healthcare Quality Research [AHRQ], n.d.; Charles et al., 2014). However, there is still potential for error, such as entering data on the wrong person. This potential to make mistakes requires nurses to continually use critical thinking skills to evaluate for safe practice, especially in the area of medication administration.

Other Formats for Documenting Nursing Care

Use of structured documentation has been found to be associated with more complete nursing records, better continuity of care, more meaningful nursing data, and better outcomes. In charting electronically, the nurse can call up a template to record the day's or the health experience's data.

Flow sheets or checklists. Electronic charting can use **flow sheets** with predefined progress parameters, based on written standards with preprinted categories of information. Flow sheets contain documentation of repetitive care, such as activities of daily living and daily assessments of normal findings. For example, in assessing lung sounds, the nurse needs to merely indicate "clear" if that information is normal. Deviations from normal must be completely documented. By marking a flow sheet or checklist, you are identifying that all care was performed according to existing agency protocols.

Plan of Care

Nursing care plans are still valued by nursing instructors as a tool for student learning. However, in the age of electronic records in hospitals, clinics, and long-term care facilities, the traditional nursing care plans for each person are being replaced by electronic clinical pathways. Clinical pathways stating daily goals for people have mostly either been incorporated into the EMR or been replaced by electronic prompts.

CLINICAL PATHWAY PLANS OF CARE

Clinical pathways (also known as *care maps*) are standardized care processes for specific patient populations and are a patient-informed knowledge translation tool, either paper or electronic based, to ensure that people receive the best evidence-informed care (Lawal et al., 2016). Clinical pathways have the ability to foster standardized, evidence-informed strategies and patient safety and health efficiencies, and to support health care teams to provide key treatment priorities in a timely fashion (Jabbour et al., 2018). As nurses, it is important to recognize that, while critical pathways provide evidence-informed best practices, each person is unique and the clinical pathway may need to be modified to address the person's health care needs.

Standards: Ethical, Regulatory, and Professional

Standards of documentation must meet the requirements of government, health care agency, and professional standards of practice. The use of EMRs, and the storage of personal health information in computer databases, have refocused attention on the issues of ethics, security, privacy, and confidentiality that are described earlier in this book. For example, a nurse in one unit of a hospital who accesses the EMR of a person in another unit and for whom the nurse has no responsibilities for care is violating confidentiality. Ethical professional practice requires that you do not allow others to use your access logon. Other ethical issues with electronically generated care plans and standard orders centre on how to determine who is responsible for the computer-generated care decisions.

Confidentiality and Privacy

As discussed in Chapter 3, confidentiality is the act of limiting disclosure of private matters appropriately, maintaining the trust that an individual has placed in an agent entrusted with private matters. All provinces and territories have legislation regulating access to personal health information guiding the disclosure of health information. Electronic storage and transmission of health records have sparked intense scrutiny over privacy protection. Many breaches have been reported in popular media. In the United States, more than 70% of consumers have expressed concerns that their PHRs, stored in EHRs or EMRs with Internet connections, will not remain private, and as a result, 89% say they withhold health information (Gordon, 2017). In Canada, there was a large digital health data breach in 2019, when there was a cyber attack that involved unauthorized access to LifeLabs data, including people's names, addresses, emails, logins, passwords, dates of birth, health card numbers, and test results (Webster, 2020). Experts say a breach of your health records is in all likelihood not a matter of whether it will occur, but a matter of when.

Ethical and legal parameters limit when you can share personal information. When computers are located at the bedside, the screen displays information to anyone who stops by the bedside. You need to be alert to this potential privacy violation. Violations of confidentiality because of unauthorized access or distribution of sensitive health information can have severe consequences for people. It may lead to discrimination at the workplace, loss of job opportunities, or loss of some insurance benefits. Personal information in health records such as social insurance numbers, home address, and so on can be used in identity theft. Issues of privacy will dominate how nurses and other health care providers address clinical documentation in the years ahead. Hardware safeguards such as workstation security, keyed lock hard drives, and automatic log-offs are used in addition to user identification and passwords to prevent unauthorized access. Some advocate that individuals be able to choose how much of their information is shared and be notified when their information is accessed. In Canada, laws requires people to be notified in the event of a breach of their personal health information. Refer to Chapter 3 for provincial and territorial health information privacy regulations.

Legal Aspects of Charting

Nursing literature emphasizes the need for quicker documentation that still reflects the nursing process. At the same time, documentation must be legally sound. The legal assumption is that the care was not given unless it is documented in the record, which is a legal document, even though it is digital (Merriweather, 2017). Nurses have been deemed negligent based on having failed to document safe, effective care.

"If it was not charted, it was not done." This statement stems from a legal case *(Kolesar v. Jeffries)* heard before Canada's Supreme Court, in which a nurse failed to document the care of a person on a Stryker frame before they died. Because the purpose of the health record is to list care given and outcomes, any information that is clinically significant must be included. There is always the potential that every nurse could have their documentation records subpoenaed at some time during their nursing career (refer to Box 26.2 for recommendations for EHR use).

BOX 26.2 Tips for Electronic Health Record Use That Promote a Culture of Person Safety	
Do	**Do Not Do**
Change your electronic health record (EHR) password frequently	Do not share your EHR password. Do not rush: ask for administrative time for data entry
	Do not rush when typing data
	Avoid shortcuts such as "copy and paste"
Enter notes in "real time" as much as possible (chart promptly)	Avoid saving all charting until end of shift; do not make "untimely" entries (after another shift has charted)
Maintain confidentiality (e.g., enter data in way that visitors cannot see)	Do not just rely on the "sleep" screen
Verbalize a summary of what you enter at the bedside, so the person can validate the information	Avoid cutting and pasting, a common data entry workaround
Explain to the person the e-documentation process, letting them know they can ask questions as you enter data	
Review or read back crucial data you have entered	
Make eye contact with the person, periodically	Try not to depersonalize by ignoring the person as you type or by having your back to the person as you face the screen
Document progress; all changes in the person's condition	Do not fail to record any ordered care that was not done or who was notified of the omission
Verbally reinforce important information with staff, even if you entered it into the person's record	Do not let confusing or contradictory information be unexplained in the documentation
Participate in all offered e-training updates	
Correct errors per agency protocol, usually by adding an addendum to your notes, listing correct information with an explanation	Avoid using "soft" or "hard" delete to remove documentation errors

Any method of documentation that provides comprehensive, factual information is legally acceptable. This includes graphs and checklists. By signing a protocol, check sheet, pathway, and medication record, you are documenting that every step was performed. If a protocol exists in a health care agency, you are legally responsible for carrying it out.

 DEVELOPING AN EVIDENCE-INFORMED PRACTICE

Health communication literature frequently alludes to the effects the use of computers has on nurse–person–family interactions. One common theme: Does documenting people's information on computers interfere with our interpersonal relationship with the person? Mayor and Bietti (2017) examined 40 journal articles describing nurse–person conversations.

Results:

Despite our commitment to person-centred care, their analysis reveals interaction asymmetry, with nurses dominating the flow of communication. Nurses were found to exert control over most of the progress of an interaction, including setting the topic of conversation. People's participation in health care centres showed nurse-directed communications focusing on collection of clinical information. However, the opposite was found when the interaction occurred in the person's own home. With increased use of technology-mediated interactions, there is the risk that the use of technology limits the possibilities for meaningful interactions with people.

Implications for Your Clinical Practice:

If the person's EHR/EMR prompts you with a set checklist of needed information, how could you ensure the person's participation? Mayor and Bietti recommend that nurses compiling person-generated information into a computerized health record first encourage the person to tell their entire story, before using the computer tool to record data. Others have suggested allowing the person to see what you are typing, using this as a conversation booster. What suggestions might realistically work, considering the workload demands made on many nurses?

From Mayor, E., & Bietti, L. (2017). Ethnomethodological studies of nurse-person and nurse-relative interactions: A scoping review. *International Journal of Nursing Studies, 70*, 46–57.

Accountability

We in health care will increasingly focus on measures that matter. HIT allows us to develop data for multiple levels of accountability, including for individual health care providers, health and government agencies, and policymakers. The data obtained from HITs can inform and improve evidence-informed practices, population based health outcomes, and policymaking.

APPLICATIONS

Computer Literacy

One of the Canadian Association of Schools of Nursing competencies expected of the new graduate nurse is the ability to use informatics. *Nursing informatics* is defined as follows: "Nursing informatics science and practice integrates nursing, its information and knowledge, and their management with information and communication technologies to promote the health of people, families, and communities worldwide" (CNA, 2017, p.1). To practise nursing in the coming years, you will need to continually upgrade your technology skills to practise in the complex contemporary health care environments of today and the future.

Communicating Medical Orders
Written Orders

Nurses are required to question orders that they do not understand or those that seem to be unsafe. Failure to do so puts the nurse at *legal risk*. "Just following orders" is not an acceptable excuse. Conversely, nurses can be held accountable if they arbitrarily decide not to follow a legitimate order, such as choosing to withhold ordered pain medication. Reasons for such a decision would have to be explicitly documented. With computerization, it is possible to have standing orders, such as for administering vaccines. The computer is programmed to recognize the absence of a vaccination and then to automatically write an order for a nurse to administer. What might the legal implications be? What would the nurse have to assess and confirm with the electronic order, prior to implementing the order and with the person who is supposed to receive the vaccine?

While many health agencies are moving to computerized provider entry systems for medications and orders, there are still agencies that continue to be paper based. You will have to consider the policies and standards on transcribing and implementing paper-based orders in the health care organization if that is the system they use.

The physician or nurse practitioner may need to send faxed orders or health information when there is not a way to access the information electronically. Because faxes are a form of written order, they have been shown to decrease the number of errors that occur when transcribing verbal or telephone orders. However, there is the risk for violating confidentiality when faxing health-related information. One of the primary sources of error is when the person sending the fax enters the wrong fax number. In the United Kingdom, the use of fax machines was banned by 2020, with health organizations required to use modern communication methods such as secure emails to improve upon patient information safety and cyber security (Department of Health & Social Care, 2018).

Verbal Orders

Often, a change in a person's condition requires the nurse to text or telephone the nurse practitioner, primary physician or hospital staff resident to obtain new orders. Most primary providers work in group practices, so it is necessary to determine who is "on call" or who is covering for the person when the primary provider is unavailable. It may be necessary to call for new orders if there is a significant change in the person's physical or mental health condition as noted by vital signs, laboratory value reports, treatment or medication reactions, or response failure. Before calling for verbal orders, access the person's EMR and familiarize yourself with current vital signs, medications, infusions, and other relevant data. Read Chapter 2 on using the SBAR (situation, background, assessment, recommendation) format to communicate with physicians and other health providers.

With the increased use of CPOE systems, where the health provider enters the order from wherever they have computer access, verbal orders are becoming less acceptable to use. It will be important for you to know the health care organization's policies and procedures regarding when and how to accept verbal orders.

It is not acceptable to chart for others. Reflect on what you would do in the following case if you were called by Juanita Diaz, RN.

Case Example: Juanita Diaz

Juanita Diaz worked the day shift. At 6 p.m., she calls you and says she forgot to chart Mr. Reft's preoperative enema. She asks you to chart the procedure and his response to it. Can you just add it to your notes? In court, this would be portrayed as an inaccuracy. The correct solution is to add an addendum to your EHR notes, as follows: "1800: Nurse Juanita Diaz called and reported …"

WORKLOAD AND WORKAROUNDS

Workaround behaviours are those that bypass or temporarily fix an actual or perceived workflow block. Workarounds are done to solve problems, sidestep problematic rules, bypass workflow blocks created for safety, address poor workflow designs, save time, compensate for inadequate technology, and as a result of addressing organizational and system issues (Debono et al., 2013). To avoid work burden and allow for task completion, some nurses create shortcuts to bypass aspects of the computerized system, known as "workarounds." These shortcuts raise safety concerns and may alter a system that is designed to improve safety, making it less safe (Finkel & Galvin, 2017). It is important to report system problems and errors so that a safer system can be created rather than implementing workarounds.

Documenting on a Person's Health Record

Documenting electronically requires learning the specific system used at your agency. There is a learning curve; that is, initially it may take longer, but as you become familiar with each agency system, EMRs should increase your nursing efficiency. Electronic charting for nurses usually combines dropdown boxes with forced choice pick lists with free text boxes for narrative information. Keep in mind the need to use standardized terminology and, where possible, to use checklists. These allow for combining information into large data sets to examine outcomes for the purpose of establishing "best practices."

Although it is recognized that for some, entry of e-data takes longer, the need to do so is a question of safety (Finkel & Galvin, 2017). Refer to Box 26.2 for some EHR tips regarding safety. To describe changes in the person's health issues, you would document completely the changes in the narrative section. Remember that free text boxes may have word count limits. In addition, narrative comments may provide needed detail, but they may also perpetuate the electronic invisibility of nursing unless information can be captured into categories to be extracted for aggregate data on nursing practices and outcomes by using standardized terminology. Tips for efficient documentation include not repeating checklist information, use of proofreading narrative comments, checking all numbers to detect data entry errors, and avoiding unacceptable abbreviations.

Maintaining Therapeutic Communication While Doing Computerized Charting

Nurses have also reported concerns about unintended effects on their communication when they use technology while caring for the person. How would you manage therapeutic communication during an interview, when the HIT system keeps prompting you to obtain data and you are entering the information into the system? Try to focus primarily on the person and the secondarily on the technology. One suggestion is to face the computer terminal toward the person, so you do not turn your back while typing information and they can see what is being entered. Some nurses comment aloud about the general information they are inputting, stopping every minute or so to make eye contact with the person. Asking for information and then typing can help the person feel like they are actively contributing to their EMR information. In addition, explaining about how these entries are keeping the team aware of updated information about the person's condition may help them to value the process.

Coding

Coding allows nursing information to be easily communicated and extracted from HIT systems for the purpose of compiling information to make cross-comparisons—evaluations, audits, and research—and to develop standards of care. A prerequisite for the use of coding was to change nursing terminology to a standard taxonomy. It is crucial to nursing that nursing terminologies become embedded into HITs, both to improve communication between nurses, such as at change of shift, and to allow data to be extracted to describe and provide evidence related to nursing care and health outcomes (Fig. 26.2).

Coding Nursing Practice Provides Information:

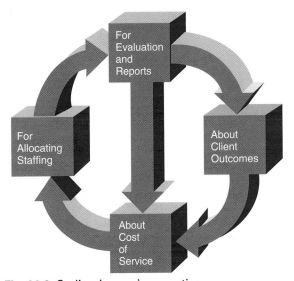

For
Evaluation
and
Reports

About
Client
Outcomes

For
Allocating
Staffing

About
Cost
of
Service

Fig. 26.2 Coding in nursing practice

Classification of Care: Use of Standardized Terminologies and Taxonomies

In the past, nursing has been invisible in data sets such as the Canadian Institute for Health Information (CIHI) Management Information Systems (MIS) and Discharge Abstract Database (DAD), leading to an inability based on evidence to describe nursing's effect on health outcomes or its contributions to quality in providing nursing care (Strudwick & Booth, 2020). In home care health records, nurses most often document nursing issues related to the medical diagnosis and physiological health needs, with nursing practices such as health teaching and support of the person and family managing health issues at home not being captured or measured. Capturing and measuring these practices in HITs requires a set of nursing data standards to guide what data elements and standardized terminology should be used (Strudwick & Booth).

Taxonomies: Standardized Language Terminology in Nursing

Nursing classification systems provide a standard and common language for nursing care so that nursing contributions to people's care become visible, promote "best practices," and define professional practice. The nursing profession has been developing standardized terminology and taxonomies, to be captured in health information technologies. **Taxonomy** is defined as a hierarchical method of classifying a vocabulary of items according to certain rules. A nursing taxonomy allows nursing data to be extracted from health records to improve communication, make nursing practice visible within (computerized) health information systems and assist in establishing evidence-informed nursing practice. The International Council of Nurses (ICN) developed a unified nursing language system, the International Classification for Nursing Practice (ICNP). The ICNP provides agreed-upon terminology to document assessments and interventions across the world that can be used for data extraction (International Council of Nurses, n.d.). The **North American Nursing Diagnosis Association International (NANDA-I)** is an internationally implemented nursing classification system, particularly in the United States. In Canada, the Canadian Nurses Association (CNA) was very concerned about nursing's invisibility in Canadian data sets and convened the first Nursing Minimum Data Set (NMDS) conference in the early 1990s, to promote the entry of nursing practices with standardized terminology and data accessibility (Strudwick & Booth, 2020).

Since the initial NMDS conference, the work to build capacity within Canadian HITs to capture nursing practice continues. The CNA and CNIA (2017) joint position statement states that nursing informatics competencies are essential for nurses in today's and the future advancing, complex, technological health care environments. The joint position statement advocates for both the Systematized Nomenclature of Medicine-Clinical Terms (SNOMED CT)—a computer-accessible international collection of medical terms used in clinical documentation and reporting—and the ICNP to be adopted to represent nursing documentation in EHRs in Canada. This would enable visibility of nurses' communication and practice, and aggregating and analyzing nurse's roles in people's care across the health continuum.

The joint position statement also recommends the adoption of standardized assessment methodologies and documentation tools such as the Canadian Health Outcomes for Better Information and Care (C-HOBIC) and the Logical Observation Identifiers Names and Codes (LOINC) Nursing Physiological Assessment Panel and InterRAI instruments that nurses could use to guide quality care across the health continuum. The C-HOBIC has adopted the SNOMED CT and ICNP to document a standardized nursing assessment (CNA & CNIA, 2017). C-HOBIC's concepts by category specific to nursing practice are outlined in Table 26.1.

Advantages and Disadvantages of Nursing Classification Systems

Nursing terminology standards are an essential requirement for a computer-based health record, yet they continue to not be incorporated into HIT systems. Adopting ICNP and SNOMED CT as well as standardized approaches to nursing documentation in all clinical practice settings across Canada using C-HOBIC and the LOINC Nursing Physiological Assessment Panel will provide nursing data and evidence to improve clinical outcomes and support decision making. This will also provide the ability to share data across health care settings (CNA & CNIA, 2017).

TABLE 26.1   C-HOBIC Concepts by Category

Functional status & continence (ADLs* & IADLs*) *ADLs: Activities of daily living that are basic self-care tasks *IADLs: Instrumental activities of daily living that are more complex (e.g., planning and preparing meals, managing your budget, doing own shopping)	• Bathing • Personal hygiene • Walking • Toilet transfer • Toilet use • Bed Mobility • Dressing • Eating • Bladder Continence
Symptoms	• Pain: frequency • Pain: intensity • Fatigue • Dyspnea • Nausea
Safety	• Falls • Pressure ulcer
Therapeutic self-care	• Knowledge of current medications • Knowledge about why you are taking current medications • Ability to take medications as prescribed • Recognition of changes in body (symptoms) related to health • Ability to carry out treatments to manage symptoms • Ability to do everyday things, like bathing, shopping • Access to someone you can call if help is needed • Knowledge of whom to contact in case of medical emergency

Adapted from: Canadian Nurses Association. (2015). *Canadian health outcomes for better information and care: C-HOBIC phase 2 final report.* https://www.cna-aiic.ca/-/media/cna/page-content/pdf-en/2015jan_chobic-phase2-final-report.pdf?la=en&hash=F857E FEFDB59BDE71130CAE5BA713DEAE45DC724.

SIMULATION EXERCISE 26.1 Understanding and Application of Knowledge in Using Health Information Technology (HIT) Documentation Systems

Purpose

To increase your awareness and understanding of the importance of HIT documentation systems and the current differences in clinical practice

Procedure

Reflect on the type of health records you have seen and used during your clinical experiences in answering the following questions:

1. What were the documentation systems? Were they paper records, electronic records, or a hybrid (paper and electronic)?
2. What did you like about the documentation system? Identify any barriers in using the system.
3. What training did you receive in order to have access to the documentation systems? What surprised you about the training experience? Why?

4. How did the documentation format influence your ability to follow your nursing regulatory, legal, and organizational standards for documentation?

Discussion

1. Discuss in groups of 3–4 your experiences, based on your reflections.
2. Explore how documentation systems could be improved upon.
3. Identify why it is important for interoperability, portability, and ease of access of electronic health records to be available across Canada.
4. Discuss why is it important for nursing data to be accessed from health records. How could this data be used to inform health outcomes and nursing practice?

Simulation Exercise 26.1 assists in applying your knowledge when documenting in clinical practice using different HIT systems.

SUMMARY

This chapter focuses on electronic documentation of care in the nurse–person relationship. Documentation refers to the process of obtaining, organizing, and conveying information to others through access to people's health records. The broad aspects of health information systems, as well as the nurse's role in using health information technologies, were discussed. Emphasis on the EHR and EMR roles in reducing redundancy, improving efficiency, reducing cost, decreasing errors, and improving compliance with standards of practice was emphasized. The many secondary uses of the data gathered from electronic records for generation of knowledge were described, especially those that identify with nursing care practices that produce best health and practice outcomes. Standardized terminology and the need for standardized approaches to nursing documentation in all clinical practice settings across Canada, using C-HOBIC and the LOINC Nursing Physiological Assessment Panel with the incorporation of SNOMED CT and ICNP, were also explored. Chapter 27 discusses technology that can facilitate communication among health care workers, increase health education and increased engagement, and assist providers of health care with decision making.

ETHICAL DILEMMA
What Would You Do?

A coworker mentions that a staff nurse you both know, Alice Jarvis, RN, has been admitted to the medical floor for some strange symptoms and that her laboratory results have just been posted in her electronic medical record (EMR), showing she is positive for hepatitis C, among other things.

1. Identify at least two alternative ways to deal with this ethical dilemma. (What response would you make to your coworker who retrieved information from the computerized system? What else might you do?)
2. What ethical principle and regulatory standards can you cite to support each answer?

From Sonya R. Hardin, RN, PhD, CCRN.

QUESTIONS FOR REVIEW AND DISCUSSION

1. Explain why "use of technologies to assist in effective communication in a variety of health care settings" is listed as an expected nurse competency by CASN, CNA, and province and territorial nursing regulatory associations.
2. Documentation is an important aspect of your nursing. Of the reasons to document, determine the one of greatest concern to the novice nurse. How does the use of technology influence your concern? Defend your selection.

REFERENCES

Agency for Healthcare Quality and Research. (n.d.). *PSNet Patient Safety Network: Computerized provider order entry*. https://psnet.ahrq.gov/primer/computerized-provider-order-entry.

Alberta.ca (n.d.). *Alberta Netcare EHR*. https://www.albertanetcare.ca/WhatIsAnEHR.htm.

American Nurses Association. (2017). *Electronic health record: ANA position statement*. Author. http://nursingworld.org/MainMenuCategories/Policy-Advocacy/Positions-and-Resolutions/ANAPositionStatements/.

Canada Health Infoway. (n.d.-a). *About Canada health infoway*. https://www.infoway-inforoute.ca/en/about-us.

Canada Health Infoway. (n.d.-b). *Understanding EHRs, EMRs, and PHRs*. infoway-inforoute.ca/en/solutions/digital-health-foundation/understanding-ehrs-emrs-and-phrs#:~:text=At%20Canada%20Health%20Infoway%2C%20the%20terms%20are%20defined%20as%20follows%3A&text=Electronic%20Medical%20Record%3A%20An%20electronic,gathered%20during%20a%20patient's%20visit.

Canada Health Infoway. (2018). *Connected health information in Canada: A benefits evaluation study*. https://www.infoway-inforoute.ca/en/component/edocman/resources/reports/benefits-evaluation/3510-connected-health-information-in-canada-a-benefits-evaluation-study-document.

Canada Health Infoway. (2020). *2020 National survey of Canadian nurses: Use of digital health technology in practice*. https://www.infoway-inforoute.ca/en/component/edocman/3812-2020-national-survey-of-canadian-nurses-use-of-digital-health-technology-in-practice/view-document?Itemid=0.

Canadian Association of Schools of Nursing. (2012). *Nursing informatics entry-to-practice competencies for registered nurses*. https://www.casn.ca/wp-content/uploads/2014/12/Infoway-ETP-comp-FINAL-APPROVED-fixed-SB-copyright-year-added.pdf.

Canadian Institute for Health Information. (n.d.). *About CIHI*. https://www.cihi.ca/en/about-cihi.

Canadian Nurses Association and Canadian Nursing Informatics Association. (2017). *Joint position statement: Nursing informatics*. https://www.cna-aiic.ca/-/media/cna/page-content/pdf-fr/nursing-informatics-joint-position-statement.pdf.

Canadian Nurses Association and Canadian Nursing Informatics Association. (2017). *Joint position statement: Nursing informatics*. https://www.cna-aiic.ca/-/media/cna/page-content/pdf-fr/nursing-informatics-joint-position-statement.pdf..

Canadian Nursing Informatics Association. (2019). *Advancing an essential clinical data set in Canada*. https://cnia.ca/resources/Documents/Advancing%20an%20Essential%20Clinical%20Data%20Set%20in%20Canada%20-%20Infographic%20ENG.pdf.

Chang, F., & Gupta, N. (2015). Progress in electronic medical record adoption in Canada. *Canadian Family Physician*, *61*(12), 1076–1084.

Chao, C. (2016). The impact of electronic health records on collaborative work routines: A narrative network analysis. *International Journal of Medical Informatics*, *82*, 418–426.

Charles, K., Cannon, M., Hall, R. S., et al. (2014). Can utilizing a computerized provider order entry (CPOE) system prevent hospital medical errors and adverse drug events? *Perspectives in Health Information Management*, *11*(Fall) (1b). e-collection 2014. https://www.ncbi.nlm.nih.gov/pmc/articles/PMC4272436/.

Debono, D. S., Greenfield, D., Travaglia, J. F., et al. (2013). Nurses' workarounds in acute healthcare settings: A scoping review. *BMC Health Services Research*, *13*(175). https://bmchealth servres.biomedcentral.com/articles/10.1186/1472-6963-13-175.

Department of Health & Social Care. (2018). *Health and Social Care Secretary bans fax machines in NHS*. https://www.gov.uk/government/news/health-and-social-care-secretary-bans-fax-machines-in-nhs.

Dolin, R. H., Goodrich, K., & Kallem, C. (2014). Getting the standard: EHR quality reporting rises in prominence due to meaningful use. *Journal of AHIMA*, *85*(1), 42–48.

Finkel, N., & Galvin, H. (2017). EHRs: Medication decision support for inpatient medicine. *Hospital Medicine Clinics*, *6*(2), 204–215.

Georges, N. M., Drahnak, D. M., Schroeder, D. L., et al. (2016). Enhancing prelicensure nursing students' use of an EHR. *Clinical Simulation in Nursing*, *12*, 152–158.

Goldman, B. (2019, January 14). *A national electronic health record for all Canadians*. CBC White Coat, Black Art. https://www.cbc.ca/radio/whitecoat/a-national-electronic-health-record-for-all-canadians-1.4976932#:~:text=In%20Canada%2C%20health%20care%20may,but%20health%20records%20are%20not.&text=It's%20a%20pan%2DCanadian%20institution,to%20the%20provinces%20and%20territories.

Gordon, L. T. (2017). Connecting consumers to their health information. *Journal of AHIMA*, *88*(3), 13.

Government of Canada. (2020). *Public Health Agency of Canada*. https://www.canada.ca/en/public-health.html.

International Council of Nurses. (n.d.). *About ICNP*. https://www.icn.ch/what-we-doprojectsehealth-icnptm/about-icnp.

Jabbour, M., Newton, A. S., Johnson, D., et al. (2018). Defining barriers and enablers for clinical pathway implementation in complex clinical settings. *Implementation Science*, *13*(139). https://doi.org/10.1186/s13012-018-0832-8.

Lawal, A. K., Rotter, T., Kinsman, L., et al. (2016). What is a clinical pathway? Refinement of an operational definition to identify clinical pathway studies for a Cochrane systematic review. *BMC Medicine*, *14*, 35.

Mayor, E., & Bietti, L. (2017). Ethnomethodological studies of nurse-patient and nurse-relative interactions: A scoping review. *International Journal of Nursing Studies*, *70*, 40–57.

Merriweather, K. (2017). CDI in the outpatient setting: Finding the hidden gems of opportunity for improvement. *Journal of AHIMA*, *88*(7), 48–51.

Naigle, L. (2007). Informatics: Emerging concepts and issues. *Nursing Leadership*, *20*(1), 30–32.

Nemeth, L. S., Wessell, A. M., Jenkins, R. G., et al. (2007). Strategies to accelerate translation of research into primary care with practices using electronic medical records. *Journal of Nursing Care Quality, 22*(4), 343–349.

Radley, D. C., Wasserman, M. R., Olso, L., et al. (2013). Reduction in medication errors in hospitals due to adoption of computerized provider order entry systems. *Journal of the American Medical Informatics Association, 20*, 470–476.

Registered Nurses' Association of Ontario. (2018). *Patient-centred health records.* Queen's Park on the Road 2018. https://rnao.ca/sites/rnao-ca/files/Patient-centred_health_records_QPOR_2018_public.pdf.

Rodrigues, J. P. C., Compte, S. S., & de la Torra Diez, I. (2016). *E-Health systems: Theory and technical applications.* Elsevier.

Strudwick, G., & Booth, R. (2020). Caring and communication in nursing with technology. In J. Wadell & N. A. Walton (Eds.), *Yoder-Wise's leading and managing in Canadian nursing* (2nd ed., pp. 249–272). Elsevier.

Tepper, J. (2018). Putting a quality lens on health technology. Health Quality Ontario: Blog. https://www.hqontario.ca/Blog/quality-improvement/putting-a-quality-lens-on-health-technology.

Towers, A. (2013). Clinical documentation improvement—A physician perspective. *Journal of AHIMA, 84*(7), 34–43.

University Health Network. (2020). *About myUHN Patient Portal.* https://www.uhn.ca/PatientsFamilies/myUHN.

Webster, P. (2020). Canadian digital health data breaches: Time for reform. *The Lancet.* https://www.thelancet.com/pdfs/journals/landig/PIIS2589-7500(20)30030-3.pdf.

Yee, T., Needleman, J., Pearson, M., et al. (2012). The influences of integrated EMRs and computerized nurses' notes on nurses' time spent in documentation. *Computers, Informatics, Nursing, 30*(6), 287–292.

27

Digital Health and Communication Technology

Claire Mallette

Originating US Chapter by *Kathleen Underman Boggs*

OBJECTIVES

At the end of the chapter, the reader will be able to:

1. Evaluate use of digital health technology applications and their effects on nurse–person communication.
2. Discuss the advantages and disadvantages of various technologies for continual communication at point of care, as well as anytime, anywhere access.
3. Describe nurse advantages in using clinical guidelines and clinical decision support systems in regard to increasing efficiency in delivery of safe, quality health care.
4. Analyze strengths and weaknesses of various health technologies in improving communications and facilitating people's self-management.

Advances in technology continue to revolutionize health care through digital communication. This chapter will focus on the use of digital health and the **Internet of Things (IoT)**, a term used to describe smart devices used for a variety of purposes. **Smart devices** are defined as a "device in the real world that is able to communicate" (Paré et al., 2017, p. 5).

We have entered a new era, in which smart device applications with biomedical sensors are becoming widely used by people to communicate with health providers (Topol, 2015). In his book, *The Patient Will See You Now*, Topol (2015) describes the emergence of smart devices into health care as an unparalleled opportunity to change the way health care is delivered. Nurses are playing an active role in changing the focus from illness care to health care. We employ the latest in technology to communicate with other health providers and with people receiving care. Smart devices such as portable laptops and tablets are more frequently being used at the **point of care**, be it at the acute care bedside, in the person's home or in the community. Mobile devices such as tablets and smart devices are becoming indispensable for engaging people in their own health care. We communicate with people for health care, for health promotion, to support their self-management activities, and to connect them to e-support groups. Mobile

devices and voice-activated systems allow continual, real-time interactive communication of information, customized clinical decision making, and **decentralized remote access** to information at the point of care. Technology enhances our work flow through expanded use of devices that input data automatically, provide "alerts," and enable us to give remote care via telehealth. Since our focus is nurse communication, this chapter describes digital technologies. We also discuss technology support for safe practice, through access to computerized clinical decision support systems (CDSSs), secure messaging, remote monitoring, and use of Internet-based clinical practice guidelines.

BASIC CONCEPTS

Competency Expectations

As discussed in Chapter 26, nursing organizations such as the Canadian Association of Schools of Nursing (CASN) advocate informatics proficiency for student nurses, to promote safe, high-quality care. Novice nurses are expected to be proficient in the use of digital technologies for communication and for information management (CASN, 2012). In addition to the electronic health records and electronic medical records (EHRs/EMRs), technology management includes monitoring systems, medication systems, and continual updating on new technologies associated with our nursing care. Electronic collection of people's outcome data should lead us to critically analyze "best practice" evidence to make better decisions. Using digital health technology can also meet the expectation of person-centred care by integrating the person and caregiver as active partners in their health management. Other expected outcomes of improved communication are decreases in health care costs over the long term and primary access to health care in homes and communities, rather than only in acute care organizations. These rapidly evolving technologies offer new ways to deliver health care.

Digital Health

The term **digital health** care means the use of any wireless device and its downloaded health-related applications (apps). These use the Internet and are independent of location. The Internet of Things (IoT) describes networks of both physical and digital devices that are interlinked and communicate to one another. Examples of IoT that are increasingly being used are types of wearable devices such as Fitbits and smart watches (Strudwick & Booth, 2020). Smart clothing is also being developed that communicates with smart devices to process physiological data such as heart rate, temperature, respirations, and stress (Fernández-Caramés & Fraga-Lamas, 2018).

Internet Use. Globally, 6 in 10 people around the world use the Internet, with 60% of the world's population being online (Kemp, 2021). In 2020, it is anticipated that there will be 31 billion IoT devices in use with an estimated 127 new IoT devices connected to the web every second (Security Today, 2020). Statistics Canada reported in 2019 that 91% of Canadians aged 15 and older used the Internet, with 94% reporting home Internet access. Reasons for not having the Internet were the cost (28%), access to equipment (19%) and the unavailability of Internet service (8%) (Statistics Canada, 2019).

Communication Facilitation

Technologies such as digital health foster "anywhere, anytime" communication, with access to health providers and health information. Evidence shows that technologies facilitate our communication and teamwork to provide more effective, safe care. Ideally, we work to establish fully integrated computerized systems that share information across the entire health care system. Globally, health care focus is shifting toward being person-centred, with people actively participating in their own care (Anwar et al., 2015). Technology helps us shift from providing just "sick" care to a focus on health promotion.

Hand-held, wireless Internet devices are small enough to be easily carried. Decentralized access to information and ability to document your care at the person's location are referred to as point-of-care capability. You can use your smartphone or tablet to access nursing information databases to obtain evidence-informed clinical care interventions. You can also document at the "point of care," either at people's bedsides or in their homes.

As the use of health technology and IoT rapidly advances, the exchange of information, the way it is conveyed, and how care is delivered will continue to change. While the case example on Sam Sulif doesn't yet fully exist in Canada, some technology does and it could and should exist in the future.

Case Example: Sam Sulif

A nurse is employed by Medical Centre on a medical unit. This Centre is made up of three hospitals, all of which use a fully integrated computer system. The nurse is notified at 08:00 that there will be a new admission, Samantha (Sam) Sulif, who is down in admissions getting a barcoded name bracelet. Sam uses the pronoun *he*. In admissions, Sam is entering his own history information into a tablet that has also scanned and uploaded his health history and information from his own smart health card into the electronic medical record (EMR). Dietary is flagged because Sam Sulif has nut allergies. Preadmission laboratory results are already in the EMR, having been uploaded by a lab tech, who notes that the system has flagged a low hematocrit result and sent an alert to the admitting nurse and physician. The nurse is also advised of the need for accessible equipment for Sam. On the unit by 08:45, a robot has delivered equipment to the room while the nurse has summoned a personal support worker by text to help lift Sam into bed; he is wearing hospital pajamas that were stored right in the room. The nurse reviews the reason for admission, discusses the history with Sam, and enters additional information at the bedside using a tablet, correcting some minor misinformation. Dr. Chi, the intensivist physician, arrives to examine Sam. Dr. Chi enters the medical orders into the computerized provider order entry (CPOE) system, which simultaneously notifies the lab and pharmacy. The nurse then prints out barcoded labels with Sam Sulif's identity number, gets a urine sample from Sam and sends it off for analysis. The nurse also checks for robot delivery of the STAT medications, which are administered after scanning the name band and double verifying Sam Sulif's name orally. The nurse uses the tablet to find the latest clinical guidelines associated with Sam Sulif's diagnosis.

1. How much of the technology and methods of communication exchange described in this case example already exist in your health care system?
2. What are reasons for why either the technology presently exists in your health care system or is still not available?
3. How safe and efficient is the care described in the case example?
4. What additional steps could make care safer or more efficient?
5. When it is time for Sam's discharge and follow-up by a home health nurse? What other communication should occur?

Technology continues to drive major shifts in our nursing practice and communication methods. Digital health technologies useful in health education, self-monitoring, and support are expanding rapidly. Digital health devices promote greater control of a person's own care, potentially improving health outcomes. As people are using more technology apps (application programs) on their mobile devices to communicate and to actively participate in their own care, what nursing interventions can we adopt to increase their engagement in health-related activities?

Decentralized Access: Technology for Communicating at the Point of Care

Nurses believe that technology should be designed to reduce the burden associated with work flows in documentation, medication administration, communication, orders, and obtaining equipment and supplies. Nurses also say it is essential to have smart, portable, point-of-care devices to document and transmit information. But this technology must be user friendly, easily accessible, and function well, and it must not add to existing workload. For technology to be effective and congruent with nursing expectations, nurses need to seek input into software design (Zadvinskis et al., 2014). If use is cumbersome, nurses will devise workarounds so they can complete their assigned care in a timely manner. Some workarounds are potentially unsafe, as described in Chapter 2.

"Smart" devices allow nurses decentralized access to people's records, incorporating point-of-care information and documentation. Mobile wireless devices allow continual use of updated information and reference material at any location where nursing care is being delivered. Communication in a timely manner is a standard of effective communication. Communication in real time is the hallmark of bedside nursing in the age of technology. Refer to Fig. 27.1. With fiscal cutbacks, increased nurse–person

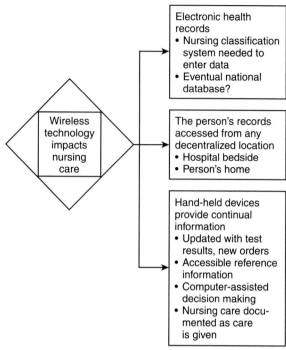

Fig. 27.1 Health information technology: Wireless technology impacts nursing care.

assignments, and increased acuity of conditions, use of technology can enhance critical thinking, clinical decision making, and delivery of safe, efficient care (HealthIT.gov, 2017).

Information can be stored and sent to your agency computer or directly to a printer for information collection. You can update the person's records, including history, your assessment, the health issue list, or other data and nursing notes. Your wireless device can also be used to track information such as a person's medications and dosages or laboratory test results, in a flow sheet format. For example, a nurse practitioner using a hand-held device can call up previous prescriptions, renew them at a touch, record this new information in the agency server, correctly calculate the dosage of a new medication, write the order, and send this prescription to the person's pharmacy, instantly—all without writing anything on paper.

Digital Health Devices
Cell Phones

Ordinary cell phones can be used to locate clinicians or verify and clarify information. While some agencies ban them, perhaps fearing non–job-related distraction or bacterial transmission from the cell phone to care providers' hands, resulting in health care–associated infections, others are issuing mobile phones to staff nurses so they can directly contact physicians or hospital departments from the bedside, give condition updates, or obtain orders.

Smart devices

Smart devices represent the convergence of cell phones, other smart devices such as tablets, and complex computer systems. In addition to making calls, these devices have other functions useful to nurses. They enable you to download and access information resources, use health care apps, have Internet access to the person's health information (new laboratory results or physician orders), and do instant messaging (IM) such as to update the physician of a person's changing condition. Some downloaded apps provide alerts by beeping when there are new orders or newly available test results. In addition to housing downloaded reference programs, smart devices may even have computer-assisted clinical decision support systems (CDSSs). For example, an app that has a drug information program not only provides drug information but when you type in the person's information such as age, weight, and diagnosis, the app provides you with guidelines for correct dosage, contraindications, and side effects. New information alerts are sent to your device in a timely manner. Guidelines for best practice can also be downloaded.

Tablets and Laptop Computers

Laptop computers are more powerful than tablets, yet both are still small and portable enough to be taken into the person's hospital room or home. Using tablets to chart and transmit and receive data are described throughout this book. Try Simulation Exercise 27.1.

Smart Health Cards

In the future, all of a person's health history could be carried on a smart health card. When the person accesses health care, their health data could be entered into the health care facility's integrated computer information system by scanning the person's smart health card. When the person travels outside their health care system, their personal health information could also be accessed through their smart health card.

Smart health cards containing the person's health information do not presently exist in Canada. In order to have access to publicly funded health care under the provinces' or territories' health insurance program, you must have a provincial or territorial health card to demonstrate your eligibility. This health card is not a smart card containing personal health information.

Mobile Biomedical Sensors

Topol writes that biomedical sensors interfacing with smart devices are changing communication (2015). Sensors can be part of smart devices, including phones or interfaced as an attachment. Some sensors are worn on your body (such as a Fitbit or Apple Watch) or are types of nanotechnology that are being researched for delivery of drugs across the blood–brain barrier to treat brain tumours or central nervous system diseases (Canadian Medical Association [CMA], 2018). People in the community, using sensors in conjunction with smart devices, monitor their own health data and communicate this data to health providers (or to their computers). Examples include measurement of heart rate or blood pressure, blood glucose or oxygenation, lung function, or eye pressure. Other sensors can obtain and transmit ultrasounds, image organs, or obtain electrocardiograms. Sensors can be applied to the skin or embedded into medication. Some sensors can automatically alert a preferred contact if the person is in trouble or signal emergency services to come to the location recorded on the device. Sensors can also provide continuous data collection for analysis by health care providers to better understand the person's health issues (McCradden, 2020). Algorithms designed to manage big data receive and analyze this data. The term **health data ecosystem** is increasingly being used to describe the complex web of health data sources, stakeholders, and applications associated with health (CMA, 2018). What roles do you see evolving for nurse–person communication as all this data accumulates? (Fig. 27.2).

SIMULATION EXERCISE 27.1 Using SBAR on Mobile Communications

You are making your home visit to Mr. Jackson. He is 78 years of age and has terminal lung cancer. He has stopped taking oral fluids and has had no urine output in the last hour. His wife is requesting placement of a feeding tube.

Have another student role-play Dr. Holle while you try using SBAR format to make a call, email, and text to let Dr. Holle know Mr. Jackson's status.

Reflective analysis: Which contact method worked best in SBAR format? If you are emailing or texting, what do you have to consider before communicating in this way?

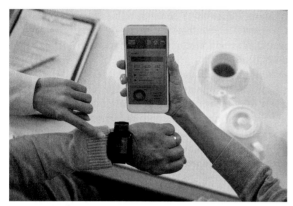

Fig. 27.2 Phone screen and smart watch with health data. Copyright © DragonImages/iStock.com

Enhanced Work Flow

Remote Site Monitoring, Diagnosis, Treatment, and Communication

Technological innovations can help make our care more efficient. Formerly, staff nurses in hospitals spent less than 40% of their day actually caring for people and at least 25% of their time doing such activities as walking to answer phones, obtain charts, gather supplies, and locate other staff. Nurses now can use new technology systems to improve their work flow and allow them more time at the bedside. Remote-site self-monitoring of health conditions and treatment progress can allow people more timely, early interventions, the ability to remain at home longer, and less time in hospital. Technology innovations are coming so fast, this chapter cannot be all inclusive. The following sections describe some examples of health care technology related to nurse–person communication.

Hands-Free Communication

Voice-activated communication systems use wearable, hands-free devices that use existing wireless networks to support instant voice communication and messaging among staff within an agency. The nurse wears a small, lightweight badge that permits one-button voice access to other users of the system. It also connects to the phone and EHR system. One example of this type of system is Vocera, which is being used mostly in the United States. It is said to reduce the time for key communications, such as looking for the medication keys, looking for others (a 45% reduction), paging doctors, or walking to the nursing station phone (a 25% reduction). Nurses report that voice-activated communication results in fewer interruptions, promotes better continuity of care, and improves their work flow. Sioux Lookout Meno Ya Win Health Centre (SLMHC),

in northern Ontario, announced in 2019 that they were implementing the new Vocera Smartbadge for care team communication. The Smartbadge was implemented hospitalwide, to standardize care team communication, provide clinicians more agility, and improve people's care and satisfaction (Canadian Healthcare Technology, 2019).

Robotics

Robotic technology in health care is also being developed at a rapid pace. By 2025, it is estimated that US $50 billion will be spent on building personal care robots (Tanioka et al., 2017). One of the key reasons for this plan is that the global aging population will require an increased demand in health care, and it is projected there will be a shortage of people to care for them (Tanioka et al., 2017). Robots are being developed to perform roles such as personal service robots, social robots, and to carry out activities in health care settings. An example of a social robot is Pepper, a humanoid robot that speaks a variety of languages and can socialize with people (Strudwick & Booth, 2020). Archibald and Barnard (2018) describe "nurse robots" that are presently being developed to assist with activities of daily living (ADLs), medication administration, feeding people, assisting with ambulation, and engaging in supportive communication.

With the increasing development and introduction of robots in the health care environment, it is anticipated that the nursing role will change, and nurses will be freed up from doing ADL tasks, allowing them to focus more on knowledge and skills in the areas of complex interactions that care robots and technology cannot perform. These interactions include communication, assessments, critical thinking, collaborating, navigating, negotiating, documentation, and the qualities of compassionate care by implementing empathy and promoting values, dignity, and trust (Mallette et al., 2020).

In-Hospital Biomedical Monitoring

When the point of care is at the hospital bedside, several of the technologies already mentioned, such as noninvasive automatic recording of vital signs, wireless telemetry, or the use of "smart" beds with sensors, automatically transmit and upload data into the person's electronic health/medical record (EHR/EMR). In another example, telemetry sensors might monitor information such as whether nurses wash their hands. Or you might receive a signal if a person falls and does not get up.

Care in the Community

Wireless technology extends into the person's home. **E-visits** offer opportunities for diagnosis, treatment, and monitoring of the person's status via Internet portals. This makes care more affordable and convenient. A person may use intelligent vital monitoring products to obtain updates such as blood pressure, blood glucose levels, or current electrocardiogram strips. The person then transmits this information to you, allowing you to assess it without having to make a home visit. E-visits are usually done by home care nurses. Studies show positive outcomes including major reductions in hospital admissions and in the number of actual home visits required.

Information can also be communicated to providers via data transmitted by **radio frequency identity (RFID) chips** or sensors. RFID can be used for tracking and locating equipment and supplies more efficiently. Staff nurses spend a large amount of time and walk hundreds of kilometres a year trying to locate and gather equipment and supplies they need to carry out their bedside care. RFID technology could instantly locate equipment, such as a needed infusion pump stored in the supply room or the location of specimens and laboratory results. RFID has also been considered for tracking people. For example, people with Alzheimer's disease who tend to wander off could wear a RFID badge that would assist in finding their location. However, there are privacy and ethical concerns related to tracking a person without their known consent that need to be considered.

Computer-Mediated Communication in the Community

Telehealth

Telehealth, also called *telemedicine, telenursing,* or *eHealth,* is changing the way health care is delivered. Canada was an early adopter in the use of telehealth, via the use of telephone technology in the 1970s. Dr. Maxwell House of Memorial University in Newfoundland provided virtual consultations over the phone to remote sites across the province (Canadian Medical Association, 2019). Since then, telehealth is available in every province and territory and provides greater access to specialized care, via the phone and increasingly through the use of the Internet. *Telehealth* is a general term for any real-time interactive use of the Internet for delivery of health care or diagnosing and treating health issues across a distance, resulting in decreased travel costs and time saved not sitting in a physician's office (Canada Health Infoway, n.d.). The ability to use telehealth requires Internet access and high-definition visual and audio two-way communication, allowing the telehealth nurse to see, monitor, and remotely interact with people using their own devices. Advanced practice nurses can monitor diagnostic and lab tests and assess for physiological changes remotely, even for people requiring intensive care. For the nurse using telehealth, clinical skill expertise and communication skills are indispensable (Kleinpell et al., 2016; Van Houwelingen et al., 2016).

Information is exchanged across geographic distances and is often used for specialist consultations. The consultant can manipulate ophthalmoscope or stethoscope attachments to assess retinas or lung sounds or do diagnostic tests. Use of this communication technology is becoming commonplace. Studies tend to show telehealth decision making and diagnosing improves health outcomes, with no difference between face-to-face encounters and remote intervention (Raskas et al., 2017a, 2017b). Telehealth has also been found to maximize access to care, making health care delivery more efficient and equitable. Telehealth originated at health facilities, but now, it often originates from the person's home, using cameras in smart devices. Refer to the case of Mr. Dakota.

Case Example: Mr. Dakota

Jim Dakota, age 69 years, runs a bed and breakfast business in rural Saskatchewan. He recently was discharged after bowel surgery, from a hospital 3 hours away. Instead of closing his business and travelling 3 hours to the health centre, he is able to self-manage his wound healing by taking "selfie" photos of his wound to send to his nurse, allowing her to provide guidance and monitor for complications remotely.

What other telehealth applications can you identify that can enable access to health care while saving travel costs and time off work?

Home-Based Telehealth Monitoring Unit

Although results are mixed, more studies show use of telehealth technology reduces hospitalizations, increases quality of care and person satisfaction, decreases emergency department visits, and decreases health care costs. Not to mention eliminating the extensive travel costs to people. With the COVID-19 pandemic in 2020, virtual health consultations, meetings, education, and social gatherings become the norm and were conducted via video conferencing applications such as Zoom or health networks in each province, such as the Ontario Telemedicine Network (OTN). Maintaining people's privacy and protecting people health information using videoconferencing applications, must be ensured.

Computerized Clinical Decision Support Systems

Decision Support System Information to Assist Critical Thinking and Decision Making

An important asset of health information technology adoption is the provision of computerized clinical decision support systems (CDSSs). CDSSs are cloud-based information programs designed to assist in decision-making (Lugtenberg et al., 2015). The person's information is inputted and the database provides you with person-specific care guidelines. By doing so, CDSS enhances the quality of your care as well as its safety. CDSS is often integrated with order entry systems in the hospital, but versions can be available to nurses working in the community. Key CDSS issues are speed and ease of access. CDSSs are useful but do not take the place of your own clinical critical thinking. The following case about Ms. Kravchenko is an example of how this technology is designed to assist you in delivering better and safer nursing care, more efficiently.

Case Example: Ms. Kravchenko Case

Michael Wagner, RN, is assigned to Ms. Kravchenko as one of the six people he is caring for on an obstetrical unit. Ms. Kravchenko is in preterm labour. Michael's clinical decision support system (CDSS) automatically lists desired health outcomes for the people he is caring for, lists best practice interventions based on his work assignment, and then gives real-time feedback about outcomes. A tablet receives electronic prompts to assist in clinical decision making. For example, the hospital's CDSS program calculates expected delivery date for Ms. Kravchenko and supplies the correct dose of the prescribed medication based on the weight entered into the EMR. The CDSS alerts Michael if the prescribed dose he intends to administer exceeds maximum standard safety margins and also cross-checks this new drug for potential drug interactions with the ones Ms. Kravchenko is already taking. The CDSS also pops up a screening tool for Michael to use to assess Ms. Kravchenko's current status and then alerts Michael if today's results are not documented.

The more sophisticated CDSSs give interactive advice after comparing entries of your data with a computerized knowledge base. The information offered to you is personalized to the person's condition (filtered) and is offered at appropriate times in your workday.

Since the National Academies of Science, Engineering and Medicine (formerly the Institute of Medicine IOM) and the Canadian Institutes of Health Research began advocating CDSS programs or supporting research into the effect of CDSSs on care, the suggested types of data in the CDSS have come to include the following:

- Diagnosis and care information displays with care management priorities listed
- A method for communication—that is, for order entry and for entering data (system offers prompts so you enter complete data; offers smart or model forms)

- Automatic checks for drug–drug, drug–allergy, and drug–formulary interactions
- Ability to send reminders to people according to their stated preference
- Medication reconciliations and summary of care at transitions of care
- Ability to send electronic alerts or prompts if problems occur or you have not acknowledged receipt of information, such as the person's laboratory test results

The hardware can be a computer terminal on your hospital unit or wireless hand-held device. A software database can be information residing in the agency server or a central repository such as a disease registry or government database.

For the nurse, some CDSS software can generate specific information for the person you are caring for, including assessment guidelines and forms, analyses of their laboratory test results, and use of best practice protocols to make specific recommendations for safe care. Ideally, this information is integrated into the electronic health/medical record system your agency is using. Ease of use is crucial. Studies continue to show that the majority of time, staff nurses still prefer to rely on colleagues to validate their decisions.

Based on input about the person's current condition, the CDSS is programmed to provide you with appropriate reminders or prompts. For example, after you complete care for your first assigned person, specific information is presented to you if you have not yet documented a needed intervention. This prompt assists you in preventing treatment errors or omissions and helps improve your documentation. More timely interventions should lead to fewer health complications. The central focus remains person-centred care, so it is important to include the person's preferences in our clinical decisions.

Outcomes of Computerized Clinical Decision Support Systems (CDSS)

CDSS technology is slowly being adopted. Early systems were stand-alone, but technology is rapidly advancing, leading to more user-friendly systems integrated into health information technology to provide timely, relevant content. Because the system stores the information about your activity, you can, for example, obtain reports about your overall compliance with standards of care or provide data for research.

Constant improvements to our electronic health care technologies are geared to improving the flow of communication, increasing safety, and improving the quality of our care. As an example, Fogel (2013) reported that people who were critically ill had significantly better blood glucose control when providers used a CDSS. In fact, reviewers who analyzed more than 15 000 articles found strong evidence that using CDSSs effectively improves health outcomes on a range of measures for people in diverse settings (Agency for Healthcare Research and Quality [AHRQ], 2012).

The literature shows mixed results when reminders or alerts are sent. Nurses have been found to be more likely to chart when an electronic reminder is received. Also, people respond positively to reminders of their self-management strategies, such as texts and to CDSS coaching about their self-care.

Clinical Practice Guidelines: Access to Online Information

By standardizing interventions based on outcome evidence, practice guidelines promote quality and safety. Nurses have the opportunity to search databases when they need information, using computers or smart devices. **Clinical practice guidelines** need to be easily accessible and usable in your daily practice, with content from trusted, credible sources. Clinical guideline databases should allow input from you about the person you are caring for and then provide customized clinical decision guidance. Clinical databases have been systematically developed to provide appropriate care recommendations for the person's specific diagnoses, based on available research evidence.

Apps for Health Care Providers

Apps useful to nurses are accessible in iOS and Android operating systems. Health apps have been developed for health care providers to access, related to pharmaceutical and diagnostic aids, clinical guidelines, and evidence-informed information. Nurses also have access to apps that can assist in calculating drug doses, assist in clinical decision making and document clinical observations (Canadian Nurses Protective Society [CNPS], n.d.-a). When using apps, it is important to critically assess whether the app's information is accurate and safe to use. Those apps developed by reputable organizations, that link to up-to-date current guidelines and databases based on clinical practice and are approved by Health Canada, carry minimal risk to using them. It is important to know that there is no requirement for apps to go through Health Canada approval; they may be developed by designers without any health care knowledge or education, and not evaluated for currency, accuracy, and safety. When downloading apps to assist in your clinical practice it is recommended that you examine the source of the application, and be aware that commercial apps vary in quality. Apps should never be used as a substitute for critical clinical judgement. The risk of privacy breaches by entering a person's health information can also exist when using apps (CNPS, n.d.-a). See Box 27.1 for precautions to consider when using digital health applications.

BOX 27.1 Current Best Practices for Digital Health Apps

- Consider the source and any other information available about the app's reliability before downloading it.
- Use mobile health care apps that have been reviewed and approved by your employer.
- Consider whether you have sufficient training and knowledge to use the app accurately and appropriately in your clinical area.
- Frequently update any apps used, to ensure all data is current.
- Avoid relying on the app to complete a task you could not otherwise complete on your own.
- Evaluate apps recommended to people to ensure they are reliable and appropriate.
- Take appropriate steps to maintain the privacy of personal health information collected through the use of the app.
- Review and set appropriate privacy settings on the app and your mobile device.
- Know what permissions you are giving the app, and don't install it if you don't feel comfortable giving the app the access it is requesting.
- Review the app's privacy policy to determine whether third parties have access to information obtained and, if so, whether users have the ability to opt out.

Adapted from Canadian Nurses Protective Society. (n.d.-a.) *Current best practices for mobile health-care apps.* https://cnps.ca/article/mobile-healthcare-apps/.

Person Engagement

In Canada and around the world, there has been a shift in health care practices to improve the quality and delivery of health care by supporting and enacting person-centred care and engagement (Registered Nurses' Association of Ontario [RNAO], 2015). Use of newer technologies can foster this goal of greater person engagement. In addition to the use of email, texting, and Internet e-referrals, people can use "portals" or personal health records, allowing them to use provincial and territory privacy-secure platforms to communicate with nurses and physicians in order to gain information, make appointments, or view their records (including lab test results).

Digital technology has not only changed the way we document, it now provides communication resources we can use for health education with the people we provide care for. This information can be specifically tailored for each individual person.

To review technologies involved in nurse–person communication, it is important to remember that when using these forms of communication, the person's consent, privacy, and confidentiality must be maintained. You should also avoid using personal digital health devices and identifiers such as your email address and social media sites, and instead, use professional ones.

Email can be a convenient, rapid, inexpensive method of communicating between providers and people. Yet, while most people express a desire to communicate with their health care providers via email, not all providers choose to do so, citing concerns about confidentiality, liability, and time factors. Read the case about Ms. Trooper.

Case Example: Trooper Case

Ms. Trooper, RN, a community nurse, uses email for posting test results, providing prescription refills or health reminders, and doing follow-ups. For example, she tracks the response of people who are on new medications, instead of waiting until their next office appointment.

What privacy and confidentiality concerns need to be considered when communicating with someone using email? Examine whether your province or territory has nursing standards related to digital health communication.

Texting, or instant messaging (IM), is commonly used in daily life. Secure IMs can be used to improve communications between members of the health team or between people and providers. For example, you could IM the person's health provider that the prescribed pain medication is not relieving the person's pain. While you can't receive a texted pain medication order, you can let the health care provider know you need one. IM can be used by people to communicate self-monitored information to their care provider. In the previous case, Ms. Trooper could text reminders to monitor blood glucose to a person who was recently diagnosed with diabetes.

Technology for People's Health Self-Management

Digital health apps are perfect for anytime, anywhere learning. Because tablets and smart devices have mobility, available health apps for these devices have become common (Cho, 2016). They provide effective communication at minimal cost. Try downloading an app for monitoring your diet, or share information about how your wearable device monitors your exercise.

Online learning has been found to be as effective as traditional learning for people to gain information as part of their health management. Most people have searched the Internet for health information, using one of the many consumer health information sites. There is strong potential for improved health learning associated with interactive computer teaching programs.

Active participation is said to increase the likelihood of producing positive health outcomes. Surveys show that consumers hold positive attitudes toward use of technology, including digital apps. They can use apps to record data such as glucose levels, dietary intake, sleep deprivation, and so on. The Agency for Healthcare Research and Quality's analysis of 146 studies of the impact of computer health modules on outcomes found that these programs succeeded in engaging people's attention, but more significantly, they improved people's health (AHRQ, 2009). Just as studies have documented positive health outcomes after phone support from nurses, contact with providers using interactive computer programs for health education or to provide answers to health-related questions lead to positive health outcomes.

Just as many of us use wearable devices like a Fitbit or an Apple Watch to encourage exercise, devices and websites increase the person's knowledge about health promotion. Information about health conditions has been shown to positively impact outcomes. Nurses should recommend reliable Internet sites to people, helping them avoid inaccurate information.

Other Technology for Assisting People in Self-Management

Portal Technology to Assist People to Communicate and to Self-Manage

Portals are provincially or territorially privacy-secure, software gateways that interface with a person's electronic health/medical record's information, giving health providers and people they care for a shared view of that person's health. Portals can be "view only," or they can be "interactive." People have continuous access to their health information, such as immunizations or lab results. As described in Chapter 26, some health care organizations in Canada, such as University Health Network in Toronto, Ontario, have portals on which people can see their appointments, and lab, pathology, and imaging results.

More sophisticated interactive portals allow the person to record and share results of their home monitoring, and to schedule appointments. They also provide a mechanism for secure texting between the person and health providers and for downloading personalized health information or requesting prescription refills. Studies report the highest use by consumers is in viewing lab tests, making appointments, and viewing visit summaries. Providers use portals to send reminders about appointments. The portals are important for care coordination and allow us to give self-management support to people (AHRQ, 2017). Insurance and pharmaceutical companies have portals that provide consumer and health care provider access to drug information. People sign on and click on various menu bars to access areas of their electronic health/medical records or to access customized educational information (Nambisan, 2017). Some services provide access to physicians or nurses to answer questions or even make diagnoses after the person answers a series of questions about their condition. Potentially, their care provider could make a diagnosis, order treatment, write a progress note in the electronic health/medical record, and reply to the person. This not only decreases use of staff time such as to answer phone calls, but it also records that this person accessed and received certain information (HealthIT.gov, 2017).

Canadian private health care websites are becoming available, where people can connect with a physician or nurse practitioner via video or text. The health care provider can diagnose health conditions, write prescriptions, and order diagnostic lab tests virtually. People using these websites need to be aware that these types of health services are not part of our publicly funded health care system and they will have to pay for the health services received. There are provincially funded virtual websites such as Telehealth, in Ontario, and telemedicine systems in some areas in British Columbia that are covered under the provincial health care plans.

Personal Health Records (PHRs)

The literature speaks of portals and personal health records (PHRs) as being similar. PHRs are records of one's health history that the person maintains, entering data to provide a lifelong medical history record that can be accessed by all providers; these are described in Chapter 26. This system allows people to control their own data and is said to assist them in self-management (Laugesen & Hassanein, 2017). PHRs are seen as a tool to overcome the fragmentation of information that occurs when a person is seen by multiple providers and agencies. They are intended to be a centralized source for self-management, to provide communication tools similar to portals for making appointments, receiving reminders for prescription refill, and decision-support tools. To be effective and to appeal to users, they need to be a seamless component of the person's health record, perhaps in the form of a compatible app.

Nursing Outcomes of Digital Technology Use

For nurses, technology is said to improve work flow, provide safer care, provide automatic monitoring and documentation of some of the person's data, allow more nurse autonomy, and improve communications among team members. Many acute care providers have adopted wireless devices at the bedside for communication. Evidence is mixed about the effects of technology. There is an expectation that it will decrease long-term costs. Generally, it seems to improve the flow of communications. But some negative outcomes include perceptions that electronic communication damages the team interpersonal relationships and can be a barrier in nurse–person communication if the focus is on the technology rather than on the person (Wu et al., 2011). Does new technology assist or impede work flow? Evidence is mixed, particularly when there is no access to wireless devices at the point of care. Nurses are also assuming increased responsibilities for interpretation of transmitted data and for instituting interventions.

Nurse–Person Communication Outcomes

Few studies are available that show effects of technology on nurse–person communication. Generally, care may be less labour intensive and easier if delivered remotely via smart devices. Technology is said to facilitate self-monitoring, improve self-management, improve cognitive functioning, reduce time spent in physician offices, provide needed information, provide support, decrease rehospitalization, increase quality of life, and improve timely communication with health providers. Smartphone apps are effective methods for teaching preventive care. For some people, nursing care delivered remotely via smart devices may be the preferred modality. When deciding on how best to provide nursing care, it is important to remember that each person's needs are unique, and some may not have the access or ability to use smart devices in managing their health care.

APPLICATIONS

Technology Use

Technology cannot replace your accumulated knowledge and expertise in making a decision, but it can provide supplementary tools to help make these decisions. Competency in health information technology use has broadly been cited by national, provincial, and territorial nursing organizations, accrediting agencies, and policy organizations as an essential of basic nursing practice. Use of informatics is a CASN expected competency for new nurse graduates. The overarching competency is to have the ability to use information and communication technologies to support information synthesis in accordance with professional and regulatory standards in the delivery of care of people, families, and communities. There is also an expectation that the use of technology is in accordance with professional and regulatory standards and workplace policies (CASN, 2012). As self-regulated professionals, we are responsible for maintaining this competency in our nursing practice.

DEVELOPING AN EVIDENCE-INFORMED PRACTICE

Telehealth Outcomes

This article contains evidence-mapped systematic reviews of 58 studies from over 1000 articles, describing key characteristics of telehealth use to inform practice, policy, and research decisions.

Results:

Overall, use of telehealth technology produced positive health improvements when used for person monitoring for several chronic conditions, such as cardiovascular or respiratory disease, as well as for delivering psychotherapy. The most consistent benefit across studies was when telehealth was used for communication and counselling for people with chronic conditions. Authors suggest the next step is to broaden research to decrease barriers to this method of delivering health care.

Application to Your Practice:

Consider opportunities for using technology to reach people virtually. How can technology help your practice? The Canadian Nurses Association (CNA, 2010) defines evidence-informed practice as "the ongoing process that incorporates evidence from research, clinical expertise, client preferences and other available resources to make nursing decisions about clients" (p. 3).

Try using one or more apps to find evidence-informed guidelines to guide your next interventions. What apps did you use? How did you assess the reliability of the information on the site?

From Totten, A. M., Womack, D. M., Eden, K. B. et al. (2016). Telehealth: Mapping the evidence for patient outcomes from systematic reviews. *Agency for Healthcare Research and Quality*, Publ No.16-EHC034-EF.

Standards of care are applicable to electronic nursing just as they are to bedside care. General standards are discussed in Chapter 2. More specific standards may be available from nursing organizations such as the CNA, along with your provincial or territorial nursing standards.

In electronic care, as in all our care, we need to be aware of the person's preferences; we also need to consider their ability to use digital health technology.

Point of Care

Wireless entry of data at the point of care can increase your access to and use of evidence-informed resources in your practice. If smart devices are used for personal activities, as well as in work situations, secure separate email or messaging accounts (or both) will be needed. Hand-held devices at point of care provide timely access to the person's information, are convenient, and are cost effective in the long run. Their prompts should help you provide safer, more comprehensive care.

Device Use Guidelines

Infection Control

Prevention of device contamination is a concern. Some studies identify that approximately 9 to 15% of mobile communication devices carry pathogenic bacteria (Corrin et al., 2016). When we are giving hands-on care or setting our device down in a person's space, we need to avoid contamination by disinfecting before and after use. Some areas have cleansing disinfectant wipes that are safe to use on technology. Some suggest using an inexpensive plastic

bag to encase the device. Hand hygiene is crucial alongside restricting the use of devices in high-risk areas and cleaning them with 70% isopropyl alcohol (Corrin et al.).

Electronic Mail Guidelines

While emailing and texting are becoming more acceptable in health care provider practice, it is important to remember that any personal health information sent is governed by your province or territory's health information privacy legislation. Internet-based email systems generally do not provide the security required for transmitting personal health information. Errors can occur, such as sending the email to the wrong email address. Even if you have the person's consent to correspond by email, you are responsible for protecting personal health information and preventing any unauthorized access (Canadian Nurses Protective Society, n.d.-b). If you are using emails to communicate directly with people, it is recommended that you inform them when you will be available to respond to their emails. Nurses are also encouraged to put copies of their email communication in either the person's electronic or paper chart as these communications are considered legal documentation and can be used in legal proceedings (Canadian Nurses Protective Society, n.d.-c).

Nursing students are responsible for protecting the health information of the people they care for. One area where a breach could occur is in students' course assignments, where they have to reflect on their practice or demonstrate application of knowledge in caring for the person. A student could inadvertently create a privacy breach if they do not keep the person's name confidential and report personal health information as part of their assignment.

Smartphone Use Guidelines

While every nursing student has seen or used a wireless device, not everyone has used them as an aid to their nursing practice. There are still hospitals that prohibit nurses from using cell phones, even though studies show these devices can save time, decrease errors, and simplify information retrieval at the point of care. Ethically, you should not use electronic devices in your workplace for personal, nonprofessional use. All information and use needs to follow your province or territory's privacy and confidentiality health regulations and the health care facility's policies.

Texting and e-Messaging Personal Use Guidelines

In the work environment, electronic provider–person IM can be used to communicate simple data. Both phone and IM have been shown to be as effective as in-person education for people with chronic conditions. Texts are used to remind people of appointments and services, to take a medication, or to perform self-monitoring care. This approach may promote better quality care and improved utilization. When texting, you need to consider all the privacy issues surrounding this practice. Also, by texting, you don't know if, when, and to whom a message has been sent. There also may be no way to include the message in the person's electronic or paper health record. If you are texting in relation to your practice, you need to consider whether you have your employer's consent, following the organization's policies, and whether the communication is on a secure network (Canadian Nurses Protective Society, 2014).

Multiple articles in the literature describe the efficacy of using personalized IM for helping people manage their conditions, as illustrated in the following case example.

Case Example

Mr. Simpson, 47 years, is newly diagnosed with hypertension. Mr. Simpson is taking a new medication and texts his self-monitored blood pressure readings daily to the nurse. Using text messaging, the nurse could text message a reminder to take his evening dose. Next, the nurse texts a reminder to Ms. Patel, who has diabetes, that she has forgotten to submit her blood glucose level this morning. What are the concerns related to doing these practices? Other concerns involve threats to safety and confidentiality. Also, when an incoming message distracts a nurse during a crucial procedure, this distraction could potentially contribute to making an error (Shaw & Abbott, 2017).

Use of Social Media

Social media sites are powerful communication platforms, using Internet-based venues to communicate, strengthen interpersonal relationships, and even disseminate information for education. Social media and portable devices with downloadable apps are revolutionizing our communication with people. Social media sites provide opportunities for health education, obtaining information to make more educated health choices and obtain input from supportive "friends." Unfortunately, there is also a lot of incorrect information available. Use of social media may improve our nursing practice by increasing access to information and support.

Guidelines for using social media were discussed in Chapter 3. Ensure that you review and enact your school's social media policies, organization policies, and your provincial or territorial professional association's social media standards and guidelines. For example, the College and Association of Registered Nurses of Alberta (2020) document, *Social Media: e-Professionalism for Nurses*, outlines the importance of nurses developing social media competence and understanding their professional and ethical obligations to protect the public and maintain online their professional trustworthiness and integrity. Nurses must also understand the differences between the general open-to-all social sites, such as Instagram and Twitter, from secure sites with restricted access such as those created by health care organizations as internal professional staff social networks.

Clinical Decision Support System (CDSS) Use

While use of CDSSs never eliminates the need for us to think critically, such systems are another tool to help us manage our nursing care. Use of CDSSs allows you to align your clinical decisions for the specific person with best practice guidelines, as in the case of Ms. Esteves.

Case Example: Ms. Esteves's case

As 'the staff nurse in the cardiac care unit, you sign on to Ms. Esteves's electronic record. The CDSS offers you a reminder (alert) about a medication order. You are given information about possible harmful interactions with other medications she is already taking. This CDSS reminder then gives you a suggestion to obtain a lab INR result prior to considering giving this medication. Thus, the CDSS is integrated with your work flow, giving you suggestions about interventions based on evidence-informed best practice. Perhaps the CDSS next reminds you that later medications should be held since Ms. Esteves has an NPO (nothing by mouth) order beginning at midnight.

It might offer you a suggested alternative if you fail to document this intervention.

In another example, it used to be that nurses working with children needed to use calculators to determine correct fractional dosage based on the child's weight. Now, instead, they can use an automated CDSS because it automatically predetermines the correct doses, which reduces medication calculation errors.

More studies are needed to examine effects of CDSS on communication, but data suggest a positive effect. In Canada, nurses use mobile devices to access the Registered Nurses' Association of Ontario best-practice guidelines, to look up timely information specific to the people they are caring for. Try Simulation Exercise 27.2 to explore usability.

Clinical Decision Support System Concerns

A common problem is that the CDSS might send you so many alerts that you learn to ignore them. Alarm fatigue is a commonly reported problem. This is particularly true for drug–drug interactions. Studies suggest that as many as 90% of alarm alerts are overridden. Customizing alerts to the person's medication needs or setting parameters into low-priority (warning but no alarm) and high-priority (audible alarm) might overcome this.

Cost and ease of use are the main concerns in adopting CDSS types of technology.

Access at the point of care to databases containing evidence-informed guidelines for care means you have resources specifically tailored to suggest interventions for a specific person.

Criteria to consider for downloadable clinical practice guidelines include the following:

- They are evidence-informed, with current (within the last 5 years, depending on the issue), quality-referenced information demonstrating clinical effectiveness.
- They are easily accessible on your wireless device.

- They allow you to enter personal data to customize the interventions (data from the electronic health/medical record), yet maintain privacy and confidentiality of the person and follow organization policies and professional nursing standards.
- They contain hotlinks to allow you to obtain and print more information.

Digital Health: Technology for Person Engagement

Use of Health and Lifestyle Monitoring Apps

Wearable devices, such as smart watches, make wellness and diagnostic apps even easier to use (Box 27.2). This chapter describes possible app uses, but of course, use of apps is not quite as easy as it sounds, requiring devices, science-based programs, and user skills. Would you recommend to consumers owning smart devices to download apps that assist them in tracking their self-assessment? For example, should a person with diabetes try using FreeStyle Libre that automatically measures and continuously stores glucose readings, day and night? Or maybe uChek, a digital log of urinalysis testing results, with data entered using the smartphone camera to record urine dipstick results? What factors would you consider before making this recommendation? The Canadian Medical Association (2015) advises that if you are recommending health apps for use, they should be created or endorsed by a recognized professional association or society or have gone through a peer review process.

Outcomes of Digital Health

Virtual Health Education for Health Promotion

There is considerable evidence about the efficacy of providing health care education and information online. See Chapter 15 for discussion of health promotion concepts.

SIMULATION EXERCISE 27.2   Critique of an Internet Nursing Resource Database

Purpose:
To encourage students to gain familiarity and critically assess Internet resources

Procedure:
As an in-class or out-of-class assignment, access a nursing resource database for information related to nursing practice (for example, professional standard or professional practice, a chronic health condition,

leadership, work issues etc.), preferably using a smartphone or tablet.

Reflective Analysis and Discussion:
1. How did you go about searching for the information?
2. What surprised you about doing the search?
3. Discuss results, listing sites you think are useful.
4. Evaluate each website's credibility for professional use.

BOX 27.2 Use of Digital Devices (Wireless, Wi-Fi-Enabled, Hand-Held Devices)

Advantages

- Improve the flow of communication as well as work flow
- Easily portable; can be used at the point of care (person's bedside, in the home, etc.)
- Quick documentation when nurse enters information by tapping menu selections
- Can contain reference resources about treatment, for medication dosage, and so forth, if uploaded
- Assists with customized decision making, reminders about standards of care; sends alerts
- Instant communication (e.g., nurse is signalled by beep regarding receipt of new information)
- Provide quick access to person records
- Provide people with self-management tools
- Build support networks
- Provide a method of connecting with people who are hard-to-reach

Disadvantages

- Possible threats to person's legal privacy rights
- Access issues related to equity, marginalization, and location
- Nurse does not have a printed copy of information (until downloaded to agency printer)
- Small screen does not allow view of entire page of information
- Technical problem may result in dysfunction or downtime

New technology increases our options for providing needed information. One example is unit-owned tablets containing health management information in skill-based learning modules that are lent to people while in hospital. Similar modules could be provided after discharge. Use of national website-based modules would eliminate the need for each agency to develop their own programs.

Health information about controlling chronic health conditions can be provided to people effectively, quickly, and inexpensively, via the Internet. Nurse-provided information sent to a person's mobile device allows them to make better self-management decisions. For example, reminding a person with diabetes that their glycated hemoglobin (A1C), which measures the average blood glucose control for the last 2–3 months, needs to be done. Actively engaging and assisting in decision support is another way to provide person-centred care, by shifting the focus

to self-care in the person's own home. One problem in accessing Internet health information is that not all online information is accurate or easy to verify in measurable outcomes. See Chapter 16 for health teaching concepts.

Documentation of each person's education session should contain the following:

- The topic discussed
- The time spent and when it occurred
- Your mutual behavioural goal(s) for the session
- Your assessment of the person's knowledge of their health issue and their readiness to learn
- Your assessment about the person's level of understanding of their health issue and the education session

Virtual Care in Canada

Virtual care in Canada is not as advanced as in other countries such as the United States. The Virtual Care Task Force, guided by Canadian physician groups, examined the issue of virtual care in Canada and identified that part of the reason it is not as advanced as elsewhere is that there are no national standards for access to health information or for the safety and quality of virtual care (Vogel, 2020). This is also a result of decentralized health care administration and funding, from the federal government, to provinces and territories, to local regions. Electronic health systems are also designed locally or regionally and often are not compatible with one another (Chang & Gupta, 2015).

Group E-support

Smart devices are used to mediate support groups for families and people with various health issues. These formal Internet groups provide information, but, importantly, they have also been shown to provide improved social support for those with health issues. Studies show group participants report decreased stress, less depression, increased quality of life, and improved ability to manage their health condition. Participants can also learn how others have coped with similar issues, and access to the groups is not limited by geographical boundaries. There are limitations to online support groups, such as inaccurate and outdated information being used, or the development of excessive reliance on online support resources (Chung, 2013). Online chat rooms are usually synchronous, in real time, providing immediate feedback. Usually, discussion forums are asynchronous, with time delays between postings and responses, allowing for more reflection before posting. More studies are needed before we can specify the needed frequency, duration, and quality of content for optimal support.

Caregivers of people with chronic health conditions can use Internet support groups, chat rooms, email, or direct communication with care providers to gain support.

Nurses can gain insight and better understand the "lived experiences" of people by participating in these Internet opportunities. Internet or phone support has been shown to be a cost-effective method for improving functioning and quality of life for people with chronic health conditions, and similar beneficial effects in nurse–caregiver relationship support are occurring (Solli et al., 2015). Do you believe support group chat rooms can improve nurse–person communication?

Outcomes

Early evidence shows that use of devices, portals, and apps can result in improved health outcomes (AHRQ, 2017). Nurses can recommend quality, approved sites, preferably interactive ones, on the Internet, that people can use to have a positive impact on their health. Laptops, notebooks, and smart devices can be used for anywhere, anytime learning. Online learning has been repeatedly shown to be as effective as or superior to traditional forms of learning. For example, have you used podcasts or webinars to assist in your learning and understanding of health issues?

Issues

The main concerns with technology are interoperability and security. There are also other considerations:

Cautions or barriers to application of new technologies include access, inability to use technology, and literacy issues. The transition to use of digital health technology in nursing implies a learning curve. Some providers and users cite issues such as the time involved in learning how to use the technology, cost, equipment design limitations, access issues, interference with work flow, and fears about losing hand-held devices. In all cases, communication needs to be tailored to the needs and abilities of the person being cared for.

For nurses, rapid advances in technology mean we need to continuously transform the way we communicate. For people receiving care, new technology offers tools to become more engaged in self-management of their own health. Information needs to be in a context they understand. Emerging are verbal avatars, graphics, and video-based formats that can also provide this context (Morrow et al., 2017).

Guidelines for professional relationships apply to use of electronic media. Caution is advised in communicating with people outside the professional relationship. Online contact with former people you have cared for blurs the relationship boundary and can violate professional nursing standards.

Major costs are involved in developing and obtaining software and hardware and creating interoperability among different systems. A consideration for providers is also cost

recovery. How will physicians, nurses, dietitians, therapists, and so on be acknowledged and paid for the time devoted to interacting with people using Internet modalities?

Use of the Internet presents many questions about how to maximize its communication potential while maintaining professional standards, privacy, and confidentiality and providing appropriate documentation.

Separate organizations providing care to the same person need to share information securely. Any information you learn during the course of treatment must be safeguarded. With any computer use, we are concerned about maintaining security. Many surveys of consumer concerns cite breach of privacy as their biggest concern. As health information technology systems become more sophisticated and accessibility is a top priority, mechanisms and regulations to ensure privacy become more complex. As digital devices, wearable devices, and implanted devices interconnect on the Internet, there is potential for harm from unintended or malicious acts. Major breaches of health care databases have occurred, and attempts are likely to increase with the recognition of the value of access to personal identity and health information (Williams, 2017).

Security experts recommend data encryption and always using a required login password, one that is changed frequently. Refer to Chapter 3 for discussion of national, provincial, and territorial privacy regulations. These concerns are why you have sign-on pass codes for portable computer terminals or automatic screen saver modes to darken screens, preventing visitors from reading records.

Professionally, you are bound by laws for privacy protection. Except for sharing information with other health team members, a nurse can reveal person information only in very limited, specific situations: when failure to disclose would result in significant harm or when legally required to do so. One example would be if you recognize signs of physical abuse in a child or a person tells you they are going to die by suicide.

SUMMARY

Digital health is transforming the ways nurses communicate with other professionals, people they provide care for, and data. Technology provides nurses with new tools to deliver nursing at the person's point of care. Hand-held and wearable devices, and use of portals, provide people with easy access to be able to communicate with health care providers. It is anticipated that use of health information technology will improve the quality of care, giving us new ways to partner with the people we care for, to educate them and so they can actively manage their own care.

👤 ETHICAL DILEMMA

What Would You Do?

One of the staff nurses you work with "friends" you on Facebook. When looking at the posts on her page, you read a post by a student nurse assigned to the nursing unit. The student made a post saying that the person she was caring for that day told her that they were going to die by suicide. You do not personally know either the student nurse or the person she referred to.

1. Since this information is now openly available on the Internet, what ethical responsibility do you have to intervene?
2. What professional nursing standards did the nursing student violate?
3. If you were the student who made the post, what steps should you have taken as soon as you received this information?
4. If it was your Facebook page where the post was made, what should you do?

QUESTIONS FOR REVIEW AND DISCUSSION

1. Social media sites have become a prominent component of our society. Identify any future professional uses for social media that you can envision.
2. Construct a set of criteria for determining whether websites are providing reliable information for your clinical practice.
3. Identify the advantages and disadvantages of virtual and telehealth care. What is the role for nurses in today's and in future health care systems, using virtual and telehealth care?
4. The nurse–person relationship is changing to the nurse–person–technology relationship. How do you envision this will change how you provide nursing care and your relationships with health care providers and the people and families you care for, in the future?

REFERENCES

Agency for Healthcare Research and Quality. (2009). *Impact of consumer health informatics applications. Evidence Report, Publication No.10–E019.* www.ahrq.gov/professionals/clinicians-providers/guidelines-recommendations.index.html.

Agency for Healthcare Research and Quality. (2012). *Healthcare decision-making. Publication No.12-E0001-EF.* www.ahrq.gov/research/findings/evidence-based-reports/er203-abstract.html.

Agency for Healthcare Research and Quality. (2017). *A national web conference on effective design and use of patient portals and their impact on patient-centered care.* www.ahrq.gov/.

Anwar, M., Joshi, J., & Tan, J. (2015). Anytime, anywhere access to secure, privacy-aware health care services: Issues, approaches and challenges. *Health Policy and Technology, 4,* 299–311.

Archibald, M. M., & Barnard, A. (2018). Futurism in nursing: Technology, robotics and the fundamentals of care. *Journal of Clinical Nursing, 27*(11–12), 2473–2480.

Canada Health Infoway. (n.d.). *Telehealth.* https://www.infoway-inforoute.ca/en/solutions/digital-health-foundation/telehealth.

Canadian Association of Schools of Nursing. (2012). *Nursing informatics entry-to-practice competencies for registered nurses.* https://www.casn.ca/wp-content/uploads/2014/12/Infoway-ETP-comp-FINAL-APPROVED-fixed-SB-copyright-year-added.pdf.

Canadian Healthcare Technology. (2019). *Meno Ya Win Health Centre implements Vocera.* https://www.canhealth.com/2019/09/11/meno-ya-win-health-centre-implements-vocera/.

Canadian Medical Association. (2015). *Guiding principles for physicians recommending mobile health applications to patients.* https://policybase.cma.ca/documents/PolicyPDF/PD15-13.pdf.

Canadian Medical Association. (2018). *The future of technology in health and health care: A primer.* cma.ca/sites/default/files/pdf/health-advocacy/activity/2018-08-15-future-technology-health-care-e.pdf.

Canadian Medical Association. (2019). *CMA health summit virtual care in Canada: Discussion paper.* https://www.cma.ca/sites/default/files/pdf/News/Virtual_Care_discussionpaper_v2EN.pdf.

Canadian Nurses Association. (2010). *Evidence-informed decision-making and nursing practice.* https://www.cna-aiic.ca/-/media/nurseone/page-content/pdf-en/evidence-informed-decision-making-and-nursing-practice.pdfCanadian.

Canadian Nurses Protective Society. (n.d.-a) *Current best practices for mobile health-care apps.* https://cnps.ca/article/mobile-healthcare-apps/.

Canadian Nurses Protective Society. (n.d.-b). *Legal risks of email—Part 1: Privacy concerns.* https://cnps.ca/article/legal-risks-of-email-part-1-privacy-concerns/.

Canadian Nurses Protective Society. (n.d.-c). *Legal risks of email—Part 2: Practical considerations.* https://cnps.ca/article/legal-risks-of-email-part-2-practical-considerations/.

Canadian Nurses Protective Society. (2014). *Ask a lawyer: Texting updates to other health professionals.* https://cnps.ca/article/ask-a-lawyer-texting-updates-to-other-health-professionals/.

Chang, F., & Gupta, N. (2015). Progress in electronic medical record adoption in Canada. *Canadian Family Physician, 61*(12), 1076–1084.

Cho. J. (2016). The impact of post-adoption beliefs on the continued use of health apps. *International Journal of Medical Informatics, 87,* 75–83.

Chung. E. J. (2013). Social interaction in online support groups: Preference for online social interaction over offline social interaction. *Computers in Human Behavior, 29,* 1408–1414. https://www.sciencedirect.com/science/article/pii/S0747563213000228?casa_token=oKZbZG6juQ4AAAAA:I

1a8HbVwZAwBxob-Mke5qtLYckCRex1IxHESK4xEuCzNa-Zs6kLQ_lg7omIA5vz1pGMOxcw3nMir.

College and Association of Registered Nurses of Alberta. (2020). *Social media: e-professionalism for nurses.* https://nurses.ab.ca/docs/default-source/default-document-library/social-media-e-professionalism-for-nurses-(march-2020).pdf?sfvrsn=6a120897_8.

Corrin, T., Lin, J., MacNaughton, C. et al. (2016). The role of mobile communication devices in the spread of infections within a clinical setting. *Environmental Health Review, 59*(2), 63–70. https://pubs.ciphi.ca/doi/pdf/10.5864/d2016-014.

Fernández-Caramés, T. M., & Fraga-Lamas, P. (2018). Towards the Internet-of-smart-clothing: A review on IoT wearables and garments for creating intelligent connected e-textiles. *Electronics, 7*(405). https://pdfs.semanticscholar.org/fa6e/2bf1fa214d0756ca5a05371aac972dfc8675.pdf.

Fogel, S. L. (2013). Effects of computerized decision support systems on blood glucose regulation in critically ill surgical patients. *Journal of the American College of Surgeons, 216*(4), 1–2.

HealthIT.gov. (2017). *Benefits of EHRs.* https://www.healthit.gov/topic/health-it-and-health-information-exchange-basics/benefits-ehrs.

Kemp, S. (2021). *Digital 2021 April Global Statshot Report.* https://datareportal.com/reports/digital-2021-april-global-statshot.

Kleinpell, R., Barden, C., Rincon, T. et al. (2016). Assessing the impact of telemedicine on nursing care in intensive care units. *American Journal of Critical Care, 25*(1), e14–e20.

Laugesen, J., & Hassanein, K. (2017). Adoption of personal health records by chronic disease patients: A research model and an empirical study. *Computers in Human Behavior, 66*, 256–272.

Lugtenberg, M., Weenink, J., van der Weijden, T. et al. (2015). Implementation of multiple-domain covering computerized decision support systems in primary care: A focus group study on perceived barriers. *BMC Medical Informatics and Decision Making, 15*, 1–11.

Mallette, C., Rose, D., & Spadoni, M. (2020). Compassion and health professional education. In B. Hodges, G. Paech, & J. Bennett (Eds.), *Without compassion there is no healthcare* (Chapter 5). McGill-Queen's University Press.

McCradden. M. (2020). *Empowering patients and caregivers to engage with digital health: A briefing document.* AMS Healthcare. http://www.ams-inc.on.ca/wp-content/uploads/2020/04/200327-empowering-PAPER-en-1.pdf.

Morrow, D., Hasegawa-Johnson, M., Huang, T. et al. (2017). A multidisciplinary approach to designing and evaluating electronic medical record portal messages that support patient self-care. *Journal of Biomedical Informatics*, e1–e16. https://doi.org/10.1016/j.2017.03.015.

Nambisan, P. (2017). Factors that impact patient web portal readiness (PWPR) among the underserved. *International Journal of Medical Informatics, 102*, 62–70. https://doi.org/10.1016/j.ijmedinf.2017.03.004.

Paré, G., Bourget, C., Aguirre, M. et al. (2017). *Diffusion of smart devices for health in Canada. CEFRIO: The digital experience.* Canada Health Infoway. https://www.infoway-inforoute.ca/en/component/edocman/resources/reports/benefits-evaluation/3366-the-diffusion-of-smart-devices-for-health-in-canada-study-final-report.

Raskas, M. D., Gali, K., Schinasi, D. A. et al. (2017a). Reporting live from your stomach. *Journal of AHIMA, 88*(8), 56.

Raskas, M. D., Gali, K., Schinasi, D. A. et al. (2017b). Telemedicine and pediatric urgent care: A vision into the future. *Clinical Pediatric Emergency Medicine, 18*(1), 24–31.

Registered Nurses' Association of Ontario. (2015). *Clinical best practice guidelines: Person-and family-centered care.* https://rnao.ca/sites/rnao-ca/files/FINAL_Web_Version_0.pdf.

Security Today. (2020). *The IoT rundown for 2020: Stats, risks and solutions.* https://securitytoday.com/Articles/2020/01/13/The-IoT-Rundown-for-2020.aspx?Page=2&p=1.

Shaw, P. A., & Abbott, M. (2017). Distracted nursing: Strategies to teach nursing students about mobile devices. *Nurse Educator, 42*(4), 203.

Solli, H., Hvaloik, S., Bjork, I. T. et al. (2015). Characteristics of the relationship that develops from nurses-caregiver communication during telehealth. *Journal of Clinical Nursing, 24*, 1995–2001.

Statistics Canada. (2019). *Canadian Internet use survey.* https://www150.statcan.gc.ca/n1/daily-quotidien/191029/dq191029a-eng.htm.

Strudwick, G., & Booth, R. (2020). Caring and communication in nursing with technology. In J. Wadell & N. A. Walton (Eds.), *Yoder-Wise's leading and managing in Canadian nursing* (2nd ed., pp. 249–272). Elsevier.

Tanioka, T., Yasuhara, Y., Osaka, K. et al. (2017). *Nursing robots: Robotic technology and human caring for the elderly.* Fukuro Shuppan.

Topol, E. (2015). *The patient will see you now.* Basic Books.

Van Houwelingen, C. T. M., Moerman, A. H., Ettema, R. G. A. et al. (2016). Competence required for nursing telehealth activities: A Delphi study. *Nurse Education Today, 39*, 50–62.

Vogel, L. (2020). Canada has long way to go on virtual care. *Canadian Medical Association Journal, 192*(2), E227–E228. https://www.cmaj.ca/content/192/9/E227.

Williams, P. A. H. (2017). Standards for safety, security and interoperatability of medical devices in an integrated health environment. *Journal of AHIMA, 88*(4), 32–35.

Wu, R., Rossos, P., Quan, S. et al. (2011). An evaluation of the use of smart devices to communicate between clinicians: A mixed-methods study. *Journal of Medical Internet Research, 13*(3), e59.

Zadvinskis, I. M., Chipps, E., & Yen, P. (2014). Exploring nurses' confirmed expectations regarding health IT: A phenomenological study. *International Journal of Medical Informatics, 83*(2), 89–98.

A

Accommodation   A desire to smooth over a conflict through cooperative but nonassertive responses.

Acculturation   How a person from a culture other than the dominant one initially learns the behaviour norms and values of that culture and begins to adopt its behaviours and language patterns.

Active listening   A communication skill that embodies listening with full attention on the other person for the purpose of developing and understanding collaboratively constructed meanings.

Acute grief   Somatic distress that occurs in waves, with feelings of tightness in the throat, shortness of breath, an empty feeling in the abdomen, a sense of heaviness and lack of muscular power, and intense mental pain.

Acute stress   Intense anxiety that disables the individual.

Adaptation   A physiological, whole-body response to stress, primarily through the endocrine and autonomic nervous systems.

Advance directive   A legal document executed by a competent individual or legal proxy, specifically identifying individual preferences for level of treatment at the end of life, should the person become unable to make valid decisions at that time.

Advanced practice nurse   A registered nurse with a baccalaureate degree in nursing and an advanced degree in a selected clinical specialty, with relevant clinical experience.

Advocacy   Interceding or acting on behalf of another person or other people to provide the highest quality of care obtainable.

Affective domain   The learning domain concerned with emotional attitudes related to acceptance, compliance, and taking personal responsibility for health care.

Ageism   Discrimination against older people based on their age.

Aggregated data   Compilation of multiple bits of factual information into large groupings, allowing analysis.

Aggressive behaviour   A response in which individuals act to defend themselves, deflecting the emotional impact of personal attack with an extreme reaction.

Ally/enacting allyship   Recognizing the privilege that settler cultures have and take for granted; implies challenging and working toward breaking down those barriers that continue to colonize and negatively impact Indigenous communities. Being an ally and practising allyship require social action, strength, courage, humility, and a support network.

Andragogy   The art and science of helping adults learn.

Anticipatory grief   An emotional response that occurs before the actual death of a family member with a degenerative or terminal condition.

Anticipatory guidance   A proactive provider strategy of sharing information to help people cope effectively with stressful situations, thereby reducing unnecessary stress.

Anxiety   A vague, persistent feeling of impending doom.

Aphasia   A language disorder that results from damage to one or more of the language areas of the brain, most often following a stroke; most people with aphasia have at least some difficulty with communicating verbally, understanding when others speak, writing, and understanding what they read.

Apraxia   An impairment of the ability to perform preplanned, volitional, purposeful movements even when the symptoms can't be explained by paralysis, weakness, sensory loss, or comprehension deficits.

Art of nursing   A seamless, interactive process in which nurses blend their knowledge, skills, and scientific understandings with their individualized knowledge of each person they care for, as a unique human being.

Assertive behaviour   Behaviours that convey confidence, including setting goals; acting on those goals in a clear, consistent manner; and taking responsibility for the consequences of those actions.

Authenticity   The capacity to be true and congruent to one's values and beliefs, personality, spirit, and character within the nurse–person relationship.

Authoritarian leadership   A leadership style in which leaders take full responsibility for group direction and control group interaction.

Autonomy   An individual's right to self-determination.

B

Behavioural emergency   Crisis escalation to the point that the situation requires immediate intervention to avoid injury or death.

Beneficence   An ethical principle guiding decisions, based on doing the greatest good for the greatest number and avoiding malfeasance.

Best practice   Nursing interventions derived from research evidence, demonstrating successful outcomes for people receiving care.

Biofeedback   Immediate and continuous information about a person's physiological responses; auditory and visual signals that increase one's response to external events.

Body image   People's perceptions, thoughts, and behaviours associated with their appearance.

Body language (also kinesics)   The conscious or unconscious perceptions, thoughts, and behaviours associated with one's appearance or body.

Boundary crossings   A deviation from the therapeutic relationship that is harmless and has the potential to be innovative and supportive of the therapeutic alliance.

Boundary violations   Violations of distance within a professional relationship interaction that can represent a conflict of interest and may be harmful to the goals of the therapeutic relationship.

Briefing   An oral statement of roles and responsibilities prior to activity.

Burnout   A state of fatigue or frustration brought about by devotion to a cause, way of life, or relationship that fails to produce an expected reward; often used in relation to work-related stress.

C

Callouts A call to the team to review the situation aloud.

Caring An intentional human action characterized by commitment and a sufficient level of knowledge and skill to allow nurses to support the basic integrity of the person.

Case finding A proactive strategy to identify individuals at high risk.

Case management A collaborative process of assessment, planning, facilitation, and advocacy for options and services to meet an individual's health needs that is used to promote quality, cost-effective outcomes.

Catastrophic reactions Emotional overreactions to situations that appear like temper tantrums; can occur with dementia.

Chronic health conditions Health conditions that last one year or more and require ongoing medical attention or limited activities, or both.

Chronic sorrow A normal grief response associated with an ongoing living loss that is permanent, progressive, recurring, and cyclic in nature.

Circular questions A question format that focuses on family interrelationships and the effects of a serious health alteration on individual family members and the equilibrium of the family system; fosters conversations among the group.

Civil laws A body of rules and legal principles that oversee relations, rights, and obligations among individuals, corporations, or other institutions.

Clan Social groups whose members trace the descent from their ancestors; used in some Indigenous groups.

Clarification A therapeutic, active listening strategy designed to aid in understanding communication by asking for more information or for elaboration on a point.

Clinical Decision Support Systems (CDSSs) Software programs that input specific information about a person, analyze it, and make recommendations for care based on best practice outcomes, as established by research.

Clinical practice guidelines Protocols listing standardized recommended care.

Clinical preceptor An experienced nurse, chosen for clinical competence, who supports, guides, and evaluates clinical competence within a formal relationship with a student nurse.

Closed-ended questions A question format that requires a yes or no or other one-word response; used in emergency situations to quickly gather information.

Coaching A teaching strategy that provides information and support, teaching self-management and problem-solving skills to people and their families experiencing unfamiliar tasks and procedures.

Cognition The thinking processes people use; includes processes such as perception, attention, memory, language, imagination, reasoning, and problem solving.

Cognitive dissonance The sense of discomfort felt when holding two or more conflicting values at the same time.

Cognitive distortions Faulty or negative thinking that causes a person to interpret neutral situations in an unrealistic, exaggerated, or negative way.

Cognitive restructuring A stress-reducing technique that replaces stressful thoughts and beliefs with more balanced, positive ones.

Cohesiveness An essential curative factor in therapeutic groups that encompasses the value a group holds for its members and underscores the level of member commitment to the group.

Commendations The practice of noticing, drawing forth, and highlighting previously unobserved, forgotten, or unspoken family strengths, competencies, or resources.

Communication A combination of verbal and nonverbal behaviours integrated for the purpose of sharing information that is timely, accurate, complete, unambiguous, and understood by the receiver.

Communication aids Augmentative or alternative communication methods to support or replace spoken language, for people with communication disorder; encompasses a broad range of low-tech (e.g., letter boards, symbol charts) and high-tech (e.g., electronic devices that use switches, eye gaze, joysticks) methods.

Communication disorder An impairment in the ability to receive, send, process, and comprehend concepts or verbal, nonverbal, and graphic symbol systems.

Community Any group of citizens that have either a geographic, population-based, or self-defined relationship and whose health may be improved by a health promotion approach.

Compassion fatigue A syndrome associated with serious spiritual, physical, and emotional depletion related to caring for people who are seriously ill. It can also be apathy or indifference toward the suffering of others as the result of overexposure to tragic news stories and images and subsequent appeals for assistance.

Compassionate witnessing Noticing and feeling empathy for others, which helps to support and broaden one's perspective.

Competency A set of knowledge, skills, and attitudes.

Complicated grieving A form of grief distinguished by being unusually intense, lasting significantly longer than other types of grief, and being emotionally incapacitating.

Computerized provider order entry systems (CPOE) Part of the health information system that allows providers to order tests and treatments.

Confidentiality The obligation to respect another person's privacy that involves holding and not divulging information given in confidence, except in case of suspected abuse, commission of a crime, or threat of harm to self or others.

Conflict resolution The informal or formal process that two or more parties use to find a peaceful solution to their dispute.

Connotation A more personalized meaning of a word or phrase.

Continuity of care A multidimensional, longitudinal construct in health care that emphasizes seamless provision and coordination of person-centred, quality care across clinical settings.

Coping Any response to external life strains that serves to prevent, avoid, or control emotional distress.

Countertransference Feelings representing unconscious attitudes or exaggerated feelings that nurses may develop toward a person in their care.

Crisis A stressful life event that overwhelms an individual's ability to cope effectively in the face of a perceived challenge or threat.

Crisis de-escalation The process for strategically defusing and resolving a crisis to reduce the intensity of the conflict or of a potentially violent situation.

Crisis intervention The systematic application of problem-solving techniques, based on crisis theory, designed to help an individual move through the crisis process as swiftly and painlessly as possible, with a return to their pre-crisis functional level.

Crisis state An acute, normal human response to severely abnormal circumstances; not a mental health disorder.

Critical incident stress debriefing A strategy used to help a group of people who have witnessed or experienced a mass trauma crisis event to externalize and process its meaning.

Critical thinking An analytical process that purposefully uses specific thinking skills to make complex clinical decisions.

Cultural competence A complex process of critical reflection and action, taking into account the cultural, social, and political dimensions of care, to respond, respectfully and effectively, when providing culturally safe and congruent care, in partnership with the health experiences of individuals, families, and communities (Blanchet Garneau & Pepin, 2015[1]; Danso, 2016[2]).

Cultural diversity The existence of a variety of cultural groups within a society.

Cultural humility An ongoing, lifelong commitment to having the humility to learn from others and critical self-reflection to identify and acknowledge biases, prejudices, attitudes, and behaviours in addressing power imbalances within relationships (Foronda et al., 2016[3]; Nguyen et al., 2020[4]).

---

[1]Blanchet Garneau, A., & Pepin, J. (2015). Cultural competence: A constructivist definition. *Journal of Transcultural Nursing, 26*(1), 9–15. 10.1177/1043659614541294.

[2]Danso, R. (2016). Cultural competence and cultural humility: A critical reflection on key cultural diversity concepts. *Journal of Social Work, (0)*, 1–21. 10.1177/1468017316654341.

[3]Foronda, C., Baptiste, D. L., Reinholdt, M. M. et al. (2016). Cultural humility: A concept analysis. *Journal of Transcultural Nursing, 27*(3), 210–217. 10.1177/1043659615592677.

[4]Nguyen, P. V., Naleppa, M., & Lopez, Y. (2020). Cultural competence and cultural humility: A complete practice. *Journal of Ethnic & Cultural Diversity in Social Work, 30*(3), 273–281. 10.1080/15313204.2020.1753617.

Cultural safety An approach that considers historical and social contexts as well as structural and interpersonal power imbalances, social relationships, and social justice, all of which shape health and health care services.

Cultural sensitivity Awareness of a person's culture and being tolerant and sensitive to the person's differences from those of people in the dominant culture.

Culture A complex social concept that encompasses the values and beliefs, practices, characteristics, and knowledge of a group of people, encompassing historical context, language, customs, and socioeconomic and political systems.

CUS A communication tool used by team members to promote safe care; stands for "I am Concerned; I am Uncomfortable; this is a Safety issue."

D

Debriefing A short meeting after an event to review the incident.

Decentralized remote access The use of Internet devices to view or document health information.

Decolonization The undoing of colonial processes through which a nation re-establishes cultural practices, languages, traditions, ceremonies, land, water, and traditional governance and maintains governance of their territories.

Delegation The transfer of responsibility for the performance of an activity from one individual to another, while retaining accountability for the outcome.

Democratic leadership A leadership style in which the leader involves members in active, open discussion and shared decision making. Democratic leaders are goal directed and flexible and preserve individual member autonomy.

Denial An unconscious refusal to allow painful facts, feelings, and perceptions into conscious awareness.

Denotation The generalized meaning assigned to a word.

Deontological model (duty-based model) A model for making ethical decisions based on the decisions being morally required or being required to fulfil a duty.

Digital health The use of electronic communication tools, including wireless devices and their downloaded

health-related applications (apps) in the delivery of health care services.

Discharge planning A process of concentration, coordination, and technology integration, through the cooperation of health care providers as well as people receiving care and their families, to ensure that people receive the appropriate continuing care after they leave the hospital.

Discrimination The unfair or prejudicial treatment of people and groups based on characteristics such as race, gender, age, or sexual orientation.

Disease prevention A concept concerned with identifying modifiable risk and protective factors associated with diseases and disorders.

Disenfranchised grieving Feelings of loss experienced by a nurse following the death of someone they were caring for.

Disruptive behaviour Conduct that interferes with safe care by negatively affecting the team's ability to work together—for example, bullying, harassment, blaming.

Distress A negative stress that causes a high level of anxiety and is perceived as exceeding the person's coping abilities.

Documentation The process of obtaining, organizing, and conveying health information to others, in print or electronic format.

Dysfunctional conflict Conflict in which information is withheld, feelings are expressed too strongly, the problem is obscured by a double message, or feelings are denied or projected onto others.

E

Ecomap A graphical representation that illustrates the shared relationships between family members and the external environment.

Ego defence mechanisms Conscious and unconscious coping methods people use to protect themselves, by changing the meaning of a situation in their minds.

Ego integrity The capacity to look back on your life with satisfaction and few regrets.

Elder Respected older community member known for their knowledge of language, culture, ceremonies, and traditions specific to their nation. The naming of an Elder is done through the traditional systems and is not based merely on advanced age.

Electronic health record (EHR) Systems that make up the secure and private lifetime record of a person's health and health care history.

Electronic Medical Record (EMR) A digital record that is used in primary health practitioner offices or clinics (Naigle, 2007[5]).

Electronic Patient Record (EPR) Records used by health care providers in facilities such as hospitals and long-term care.

Emotion-focused coping:Empathy The sensitivity and ability to communicate understanding of another person's feelings.

Empowerment The interpersonal process of providing the appropriate tools, resources, and environment to another person to build, develop, and increase the ability to set and reach goals; helping another person become a self-advocate.

Environment The internal and external context of an individual, as affected by their health care situation.

Ethics The study of questions that are morally good or bad or are morally right or wrong.

Ethical dilemma (also moral dilemma) The conflict of two or more moral issues; a situation in which there are two or more conflicting ways of looking at a situation.

Ethnicity Shared cultural heritage with others based on common racial, geographical, ancestral, religious, or historical bonds.

Eustress A short-term, mild level of stress.

Evidence-based practice A "problem-solving approach to the delivery of health care that integrates the best evidence from well-designed studies and patient care data and combines it with clinical expertise and patient preferences and values" (Melnyk et al., 2010, p. 51[6]).

Evidence-informed practice A holistic approach that moves beyond evidence-based practice to incorporate both

research and practice knowledge as well as evidence from local ways of knowing, Indigenous knowledge, cultural and religious norms, and clinical judgement (LoBiondo-Wood et al., 2018[7]; Mackey & Bassendowski, 2017[8]).

E-visits Home-based health care that uses wireless technology and that offers opportunities for diagnosis, treatment, and monitoring of the person's status via the Internet.

F

Family A self-identified group of two or more individuals whose association is characterized by special terms, who may or may not be related by bloodlines or law but who function in such a way that they consider themselves to be a family.

Family projection process An unconscious casting of unresolved family emotional issues or attributes of people from the past onto a child.

Feedback Information sought, shared, or offered about a person's performance of a task or their engagement in a process. The intention is to assist in changing or improving behaviours.

Feminist Ethics An approach to ethics that recognizes that moral dilemmas involve human relationships, with a greater emphasis on values, feelings, and desires and on creating a path to end social and political oppression of women.

Flow sheets Charting that organizes people's status information in preprinted categories of information.

Focused questions Questions that require more than a yes or no answer, but they place limitations on the topic to be addressed.

Functional status A broad range of purposeful abilities related to physical health maintenance, role performance, cognitive or intellectual abilities, social activities, and level of emotional functioning.

G

Genogram A standardized set of connections used to graphically record basic information about family members and their relationships over three generations.

Good death A death that is free from avoidable distress and suffering for people, their families, and their caregivers, in general accord with their wishes and those of their families and in a way that is reasonably consistent with clinical, cultural, and ethical standards.

Grief A holistic, adaptive process that a person goes through following a significant loss.

Group dynamics Communication processes and behaviours that occur during the life of a group.

Group norms The unwritten behavioural rules of conduct expected of group members. Norms can be universal (present in all groups) or group specific (those constructed by group members).

Group process The structural development of small group relationships (i.e., forming, storming, norming, performing, and adjourning).

Groupthink The support of decisions that group members fundamentally disagree with, just for the sake of harmony, due to the extreme cohesiveness that occurs when the approval of other group members becomes too important.

H

Hand-held, wireless Internet devices Wireless Internet devices small enough to be easily carried—for example, tablets, smartphones.

Hand-offs (also handovers) The transfer process that takes place when people being cared for are reassigned to another team of health care providers.

Health A multidimensional concept with physical, psychological, sociocultural, developmental, and spiritual characteristics that is used to describe an individual's state of well-being and level of functioning.

Health care team A coordinated group of professionals with complementary skills who collaborate to give care and are mutually committed to specific performance goals, with shared accountability for goal achievement.

[5]Naigle, L. (2007). Informatics: Emerging concepts and issues. *Nursing Leadership, 20*(1), 30–32.

[6]Melnyk, B. M., Fineout-Overholt, E., Stillwell, S. B. et al. (2010). Evidence-based practice: Step by step: The seven steps of evidence-based practice. *American Journal of Nursing, 110*(1), 51–53.

[7]LoBiondo-Wood, G., Haber, J., Cameron, C. et al. (2018). *Nursing research in Canada: Methods, critical appraisal and utilization* (4th ed.). Elsevier.

[8]Mackey, A., & Bassendowski, S. (2017). The history of evidence-based practice in nursing education and practice. *Journal of Professional Nursing, 33*(1), 51–54. https://doi.org/10.1016/j.profnurs.2016.05.009.

Health data ecosystem The complex web of health data sources, stakeholders, and applications associated with health (CMA, 2018[9]).

Health information technology (HIT) The hardware, software, and infrastructure required to collect, store, access, and exchange electronic information in clinical practise.

Health literacy The cognitive and social skills that determine people's motivation and ability to access, understand, and use information in ways that promote and maintain good health and allow them to make appropriate health decisions.

Health promotion The process of enabling people to take control over and improve their health.

Health teaching A specialized form of teaching; the focused, creative, interpersonal interventions that provide people with information, emotional support, and health-related skill training.

Hierarchy Complex layers of smaller systems that exist within a system.

Homeostasis (also dynamic equilibrium) A person's sense of personal security and balance.

Hospitalist A physician or nurse practitioner employed by a hospital to clinically manage people's medical care. This provider assumes *full* responsibility for coordinating care for those people.

Huddle A brief, informal health team gathering to review a course of action.

Human rights–based model A model based on the belief that each person has basic rights.

I

Identity An internal construct about one's abilities, self-image, and characteristics.

Informational continuity Data exchanges between providers, provider systems, and people receiving care, for the purpose of providing coordinated care.

Informed consent A focused communication process in which a health provider discloses all relevant information related to a procedure or treatment, with full opportunity for dialogue, questions, and expressions of concern, prior to asking for a person's signed permission.

Interagency accessibility Transmission and availability of people's health information across different health agency systems.

Interdisciplinary communication A dynamic process involving two or more health providers with complementary backgrounds and skills, sharing common health goals and exercising concerted physical and mental effort in assessing, planning, or evaluating care.

Internet of Things (IOT) Networks of both physical and digital devices that are interlinked and communicate to one another.

Interoperability The ability for different systems to "talk to" one another, to share a person's health information.

Interpersonal competence The ability to interpret the content of a message from the point of view of each participant in an interaction and the ability to use language and nonverbal behaviours to achieve the goals of the interaction. Interpersonal competence develops as you come to understand the complex cognitive, behavioural, and sociocultural factors that influence communication.

Interprofessional education The learning experiences that occur when two or more health providers interact to improve collaboration and the quality of care.

Interprofessional health team collaboration A coordinated group of health providers with complementary skills, all of whom are valued, sharing goals and accountability for goal achievement.

J

Just culture A work environment in which staff are empowered to speak about their concerns, especially regarding safety.

Justice An ethical principle that guides decision making through fairness and impartiality; also a legal term.

K

Knowledge Keeper A respected community member known for their developing knowledge of language, culture, ceremonies, and traditions specific to their nation. They are typically groomed and mentored by Elders in the community to demonstrate and apply protocols in respectful engagement with other Indigenous and non-Indigenous people.

L

Laissez-faire leadership A "hands off" leadership style that allows group members to decide how to complete a task within the defined time frame.

Leadership Interpersonal influence that is exercised in situations and directed through the communication process toward attainment of a specified goal or goals.

Learning readiness A person's mindset and openness to engage in a learning or counselling process for the purpose of adopting new behaviours.

Licensed practical nurses (LPNs) Health care providers who who work in health promotion and illness prevention. They assess, plan, implement, and evaluate care for people in collaboration with the health care team. Currently, LPNs are regulated in all 13 provinces and territories. Note: In Ontario, these nurses are called *registered practical nurses*.

Lifestyle Patterns of choices about the way people live, made from the alternatives available to them.

Linear communication model A communication model that consists of a sender, message, receiver, channel, and context.

M

Magnet recognition program A unique national program that recognizes quality care and nursing excellence in health care institutions and agencies, by identifying them as work environments that act as a "magnet" for professional nurses desiring to work there because of their excellence.

Management continuity A management strategy of developing pathways and aligning resources to encourage a timely, effective information flow between all entities involved in facilitating person-centred care.

Marginalization Treatment of a person, group, or concept as insignificant or peripheral.

[9]Canadian Medical Association. (2018). *The future of technology in health and health care: A primer.* cma.ca/sites/default/files/pdf/health-advocacy/activity/2018-08-15-future-technology-health-care-e.pdf.

Meaning-focused coping   The act of appraising the meaning of a significant stressor in a person's life, based on the person's values and life purpose and what matters to them.

Medical home   A place that serves as a central, first contact point in primary care and that provides regular, accessible, comprehensive primary care services for designated people and families within a single familiar setting.

Mentoring   A special type of informal, professional relationship in which an experienced nurse or clinician (mentor) assumes a role responsibility for guiding the professional growth and advancement of a less-experienced person (protégé).

Message   The transmitted verbal or nonverbal expression of thoughts and feelings.

Message competency   The ability to use language and nonverbal behaviours strategically in the intervention phase of the nursing process to achieve the goals of the interaction.

Metacommunication   Broadly, all of the verbal and nonverbal factors used to enhance or negate the meanings of words.

Metaparadigm   The global concepts that identify the phenomena of central interest to a discipline, the global propositions that describe the concepts, and the global propositions that state the relationships between the concepts. The four core nursing constructs—person, environment, health, and nursing—make up the metaparadigm for professional nursing.

Microaggressions   Communication of subtle and often unintentional discrimination pertaining to self-concepts of race, ethnicity, gender, sexual orientation, or any other cultural contexts; includes microassaults, microinsults, and microinvalidations.

Microassault   Explicit negative verbal or nonverbal communication that marginalizes an individual through criticism, racial stereotyping, or purposeful prejudicial actions.

Microinsults   Verbal, nonverbal, and environmental communications that convey rudeness and insensitivity and put down a person's culture or identity.

Microinvalidations   Communications that discount or invalidate a person's values, culture, or lifestyle.

Mindfulness meditation   A combination of mindfulness and meditation, whereby a person is truly present and has moment-to-moment awareness of the here and now. It is highly effective for stress management.

Minimal cues   The simple, encouraging phrases, body actions, or words that communicate interest and encourage people to continue with their story.

Moral distress   A feeling that occurs when nurses, guided by their own moral judgement, are not able to do what they believe is right, leading them to experience physical and emotional suffering, resulting in feelings of anger, frustration, and guilt.

Moral uncertainty   A difficulty in deciding which moral rules (e.g., values or beliefs) apply to a given situation.

Motivation   The forces that activate behaviour and direct it toward one goal instead of another.

Multigenerational transmission   The emotional transmission of behavioural patterns, roles, and communication response styles, from generation to generation.

Mutuality   An agreement on problems and the means to resolve them; a commitment by two parties to enhance well-being.

N

Near-miss incidents   A "patient safety incident that did not reach the patient and therefore no harm resulted" (CPSI, 2020[10]).

Noise   Any distraction that interferes with one's ability to pay full attention to a discussion.

Nonmaleficence   The obligation to act in a way that avoids bringing harm to another person.

Nonverbal communication   Physical expressions and behaviours that are the part of the message but not expressed in words and that help people understand the emotional meanings of messages.

North American Nursing Diagnosis Association International (NANDA-I)   An internationally implemented nursing classification, used primarily in the United States.

Nuclear family emotional system   The way family members relate to one another within their immediate family, when stressed.

Nurse practitioners (NPs)   Nurse practitioners (NPs) provide direct care to people to diagnose and manage disease and illness, prescribe medications, order and interpret laboratory and diagnostic tests, and refer people to specialists. In Canada, NPs are licensed by jurisdictional nursing regulators and work in a variety of health care settings, such as community care (community clinics, health care centres, physicians' offices, and people's homes), long-term care (nursing homes), hospitals (outpatient clinics, emergency departments, and other areas where people receive care) and NP-led clinics.

Nursing informatics   Nursing informatics science and practice that integrates nursing information and knowledge management with communication technologies to promote the health of people, families, and communities worldwide (CNA, 2017).[10a]

Nursing process   A process that embodies five phases of health care delivery: assessment, problem identification and diagnosis, planning, implementation, and outcome evaluation.

O

Open-ended questions   A question format designed to help individuals express health problems and needs in their own words. Open-ended questions are open to interpretation and cannot be answered with a yes or no or other one-word response.

P

Palliative approach   An approach that uses palliative care principles (i.e., dignity, hope, comfort, quality of life, relief of suffering) with people facing chronic, life-limiting conditions at all stages, not just at the end of life.

Palliative care   Person-centred care with an emphasis on care of people with diagnosed, progressive, life-limiting health conditions. The focus is on the comfort, pain control, management of physical symptoms, and easing of psychosocial and spiritual distress experienced by people and their families as they come to terms with coping with a life-limiting illness.

[10]Canadian Patient Safety Institute. (2020). *Glossary*. https://www.patientsafetyinstitute.ca/en/toolsResources/PatientSafetyIncidentManagementToolkit/Pages/Glossary.aspx.

[10a]Canadian Nurses Association and Canadian Nursing Informatics Association. (2017). Joint position statement: *Nursing informatics*. https://www.cna-aiic.ca/-/media/cna/page-content/pdf-fr/nursing-informatics-joint-position-statement.pdf.

Paralanguage   The verbal delivery of a message expressed through means other than words, (e.g., tone of voice and inflection, sighing, crying).

Paraphrasing   Transforming a person's words into the nurse's words while keeping the meaning intact.

Patient-centred care (PCC) model   A model that includes clinical collaborative team partnership with people receiving care, according to their preferences, needs, and values.

Patient education   A set of planned educational activities that result in changes in knowledge and health-related behaviours and attitudes.

Patterns of knowing   Multiple integrated knowledge data patterns—empirical, personal, aesthetic, ethical, and emancipatory—that nurses use to provide effective, efficient, and compassionate care, based on the needs of the person receiving care, individuality, complexity, and situational contexts.

Pedagogy   The theory, practices, and processes involved in teaching.

Perception   A cognitive process by which a person transforms external sensory data into personalized images of reality.

Person-centred care (PCC)   A model of care that focuses not only on health issues but also on the person's social care, influenced by cultural contexts, values, family, diversity, social circumstances, and lifestyles (Hafskjold et al., 2015[11]; Kuluski et al., 2016[12]).

Personal health record   A record of a person's health history that the person maintains and that can include information from a variety of sources, such as medical records, multiple health care providers, and the person themselves (Canada Health Infoway, 2018[13]).

[11]Hafskjold, L., Sundler, A. J., Homstrom, I. K. et al. (2015). A cross-sectional study on person-centred communication in the care of older people: The COMHOME study protocol. *BMJ Open 5*(4).

[12]Kuluski, K., Peckham, A., Williams, A. P. et al. (2016). What gets in the way of person-centred care for people with multimorbidity? Lessons from Ontario, Canada. *Healthcare Quarterly, 19*(2), 17–23. https://www.longwoods.com/content/24694.

[13]Canada Health Infoway. (2018). *Connected health information in Canada: A benefits evaluation study.* https://www.infoway-inforoute.ca/en/component/edocman/resources/reports/benefits-evaluation/3510-connected-health-information-in-canada-a-benefits-evaluation-study-document.

Personal Information Protection and Electronic Documents Act (PIPEDA)   A federal act that requires private sector organizations to protect personal information collected for the purpose of commercial activities.

Personal space   The invisible and changing boundary around an individual that provides a sense of comfort and protection to the person and is defined by past experiences and culture.

Point of care   The location in which the nurse provides care, whether at the bedside in a hospital room, in an outpatient clinic, or even in someone's home.

Point-of-care information   Health information updated via wireless Internet devices, at any location.

Portals   An agency website that provides opportunities for consumers to use hyperlinks to access a variety of information, receive cyber support, make appointments, pay bills, and more.

Possible selves   A concept used to explain the future-oriented component of self-concept.

Potlach   A ceremony used in the governing structure, culture, and spiritual First Nations traditions.

Power of attorney   A document that gives another party the legal authority to act on a person's behalf, to manage their legal and financial affairs.

Prejudices   Stereotypes based on strong emotions, preconceived ideas, and opinions about people.

Presbycusis   Age-related hearing loss.

Presbyopia   An age-related condition in which the eyes lose the ability to focus.

Primary care   A wide range of integrated ambulatory health care services delivered in community-based settings.

Primary prevention   Actions taken to preclude illness or prevent the natural course of illness from occurring; strategies target modifiable risk factors with health education, to promote a healthy lifestyle.

Privacy   The right to have control over personal information; contrasts with *confidentiality*, which refers to the obligation not to divulge anything shared in a nurse–person relationship.

Problem-focused coping   Strategies to cope with stress that involve the person directly confronting stressors.

Professional boundaries   The invisible structures imposed by legal, ethical, and professional standards of nursing that respect the rights of the nurse and the person receiving care and protect the functional integrity of their alliance.

Professional communication   A specialized form of communication that is a complex, interactive process used in clinical settings to help individuals achieve health-related goals.

Professional standards   Professional expectations for a competent level of professional knowledge, skills, and attitudes needed to provide quality, safe care. All provincial and territorial regulatory bodies have their own professional standards that registered nurses and student nurses must follow.

Protective factors   Behavioural activities or conditions that delay the emergence of chronic disease or lessen its impact.

Proxemics   The study of an individual's use of space between themselves and others.

Psychomotor domain   The domain of learning focused on learning a skill through hands-on practice.

Punishment   Actions taken after a behaviour has occurred, to keep the behaviour from occurring again. Positive punishment involves presenting an aversive stimulus (e.g., receiving a speeding ticket); negative punishment involves taking away a desirable stimulus (e.g., a student missing recess).

Q

Quality improvement (QI)   A framework used to improve the delivery of health care through the combined efforts of health care providers, people and their families, researchers, policymakers, and educators to make changes that result in better clinical outcomes and system performance.

Quality of life   A personal experience of subjective well-being and general satisfaction with life that includes, but is not limited to, physical health.

R

Race   Grouping of humans based on biological and physical characteristics such as skin colour and eye shape, as well as some social qualities.

Racialize   Categorize or divide according to race.

Racism   Prejudice or discrimination directed against a person or people on the basis of their membership in a racial or ethnic group.

Radio frequency identity (RFID) chips   Small, embedded computerized chips that can be tracked remotely.

Reflection   A listening response focused on the emotional implications of a message; used to help people clarify important feelings related to message content.

Reflexivity   Related to reflective practice, the ability to understand and question your own contexts, attitudes, values, beliefs, assumptions, and experiences of advantage and disadvantage that have shaped the way you understand the world and in relation to others (Landy et al., 2016[14]; Verdonk, 2015[15]).

Registered nurses (RNs)   Nurses who deliver direct health care services to people at all stages of life and in all situations of health, illness, injury, and disability; registered nurses also coordinate care and support people in managing their own health. RNs contribute to the health care system through their leadership across a wide range of settings, in practice, education, administration, research, and policy. They are currently regulated in all 13 provinces and territories.

Registered psychiatric nurses (RPNs)   Nurses who focus on mental and developmental health, mental health disorders, and addictions, while integrating physical health and utilizing biopsychosocial and spiritual models for a holistic approach to care. Registered psychiatric nurses are currently regulated in the four Western provinces—Manitoba, Saskatchewan, Alberta, and British Columbia—as well as in Yukon. Note: RPNs are educated and trained independently of the registered nursing class.

Reinforcement   Establishing consequences for performing targeted behaviours; reinforcement increases the probability of a response—positive reinforcement does so through reward, and negative reinforcement does so by removing an aversive consequence.

Relational communication   Communication processes in professional relationships to achieve optimal health outcomes.

Relational continuity   A shared enterprise of therapeutic care delivery relationships across multiple systems, characterized by person-centredness, collaboration, and coordination.

Relational practice   Practice that is "guided by conscious participation with clients using a number of relational skills including listening, questioning, empathy, mutuality, reciprocity, self-observation, reflection and sensitivity to emotional contexts" (College of Nurses of Ontario, 2018, p.11[16]).

Relationality   A philosophy that describes the interconnections between all of creation and kinship and consists of family, community, and all extended human and more-than-human relations" (Campbell et al., 2020, p. 8)[17].

Resilience   Strength and stability during change and stressful life events, with rapid recovery from adversity.

Role   A multidimensional psychosocial concept that describes a traditional pattern of behaviour and self-expression performed by or expected of an individual within a given society.

Role modelling   A teaching strategy that involves demonstrating a behaviour for others to learn through observation and questioning.

S

Safe Place/Space   An area where cultural practices such as smudging can be performed; an area with adequate ventilation that will not set off fire alarms and is designated as culturally safe. Also, a space that allows for the practice of cultural practices. In communication, a nurse creates an openness and a trusting environment where individuals are more apt to share their cultural practices or desire to practise them (or both), while undergoing care in a health care organization, community health setting, or palliative care centre.

Safety   A focus on reduction and mitigation of unsafe acts within the health care system, as well as the use of best practices shown to lead to optimal outcomes (Canadian Patient Safety Institute, 2020)[18].

SBAR (situation, background, assessment, recommendation)   A standardized verbal communication tool with a structured format to create a common language among nurses, physicians, and other members of the health team to convey critical information; especially useful when brief, clear communication is needed in acute situations.

Scope of practice   The legal and ethical boundaries of practice for professional nurses, defined in written statutes.

Secondary prevention   Interventions designed to promote early diagnosis of symptoms, through health screening or timely treatment, after the onset of disease, thereby minimizing their effects on a person's life.

Self-awareness   An intrapersonal process in which a nurse reflects on how their own feelings and beliefs influence professional behaviours.

Self-concept   People's complex understanding of their cultural heritage, environment, upbringing and education, basic personality traits, and cumulative life experiences.

Self-determination   A concept that describes how individuals and groups of a culture define their existence through their traditional practices, knowledge, ceremonies, language, laws, and ways of being.

[14] Landy, R., Cameron, C., Au, A. et al. (2016). Educational strategies to enhance reflexivity among clinicians and health professional students: A scoping study. *Forum: Qualitative Social Research, 17*(3), Article 14.

[15] Verdonk, P. (2015). When I say…..reflexivity. *Medical Education, 49*, 147–148.

[16] College of Nurses of Ontario. (2018). *Entry-to-practice competencies for registered nurses.* https://www.cno.org/globalassets/docs/reg/41037-entry-to-practice-competencies-2020.pdf.

[17] Campbell, E., Austin, A., Bax-Campbell, M. et al. (2020). Indigenous relationality and kinship and the professionalization of a health workforce. *Turtle Island Journal of Indigenous Health, 1*(1), 8–13. https://doi.org/10.33137/tijih.v1i1.34016.

[18] Canadian Patient Safety Institute. (2020). *Glossary.* https://www.patientsafetyinstitute.ca/en/toolsResources/PatientSafetyIncidentManagementToolkit/Pages/Glossary.aspx.

Self-differentiation A person's capacity to define themselves within the family system as an individual having legitimate needs and wants.

Self-efficacy A person's perceptual belief about their capability to perform tasks and execute courses of action successfully.

Self-esteem A person's personal sense of worth and well-being; related to multiple factors connected to childhood development and life experiences.

Self-management The tasks and strategies that an individual carries out to live well with chronic health conditions, including increasing confidence to cope with medical treatments and the change in roles, and managing emotions associated with having a chronic health condition.

Self-reflection A process of linking past, present, and future experiences, allowing you to integrate the values, beliefs, attitudes, and emotions you felt during an experience to understand and examine that experience through multiple perspectives. This process helps you recognize how the experience could be understood in different ways, identify the lessons learned, and identify how your behaviours could be changed in the future as the result of the reflective practice.

Self-talk A cognitive process people use to lessen cognitive distortions.

Sentinel event A life-changing health care occurrence; to refer to serious errors in health care that harm people.

Shaping The use of reinforcement to gradually increase target behaviours.

Sharing Circles Circle meetings that provide an opportunity for all voices in the circle to be heard, have equal time and space, and be respected and valued. They are an essential part of the oral tradition of Indigenous communities.

Situating Self A protocol of introduction to Indigenous peoples to relay one's cultural lineage and geographical location, as a foundation on which to build relations.

Smart Devices Electronic devices that are connected to other devices or networks, such as laptops, tablets, smartphones, and complex computer systems that allow nurses decentralized access to a person's records, incorporating point-of-care information and documentation.

Smudging The practice of burning select medicines and herbs (e.g., sage, cedar, tobacco). The smoke from the burning of the medicines is either cupped in the hands or fanned with a sacred feather to wash it over areas of the body. Smudging is said to assist with cleansing the mind, spirit, heart, and body by washing away negative energy, and it readies people for holistic health and healing.

Social cognitive competency The ability to interpret message content within interactions from the point of view of each participant.

Social determinants of health A wide range of contextual factors that influence the health and well-being of individuals and communities, such as where a person is born, grows up, lives, and works, as well as their economic status, education, sexual orientation, and social inclusion.

Social support The social connections available to people to assist them.

Societal emotional process Parallels that Bowen found between the family system and the emotional system operating at the institutional level in society.

Spirituality A unified concept, closely linked to a person's world view, providing a foundation for a personal belief system about the nature of God or a higher power, moral–ethical conduct, and reality.

Standardized communication tools Uniformly used formats for communication of information about people receiving care, among all care providers—for example, the SBAR tool.

Statutory laws Legislated laws; formal written sets of rules passed by a legislative body to regulate a particular area—for example, the acts that regulate the nursing profession in each province and territory. (Also called *legislation*.)

Stereotyping The process of attributing characteristics to a group of people as though all persons in the identified group possessed them.

Stress A natural physiological, psychological, and spiritual response to the presence of a stressor.

Stressor A demand, situation, internal stimulus, or circumstance that threatens a person's personal security or self-integrity.

Summarization An active listening skill used to pull several ideas and feelings together, either from one interaction or a series of interactions, into a few succinct sentences.

Sundowning Episodic agitated behaviour occurring later in the day, in people with dementia.

T

Taxonomy A hierarchical method of classifying vocabulary.

TCAB An acronym for the program, Transforming Care At the Bedside, which empowers nurses to make changes to provide care that is safe, team-based, person-centred, and value-added.

Teach-back method A teaching strategy used in patient education to evaluate and verify the person's understanding of the health teaching; the learner's ability to repeat a demonstration of requisite knowledge and skills.

Team-based principles Group collaboration by all professionals giving care, which includes shared goals, clear roles, mutual trust, and effective communication.

TeamSTEPPS™ A program that emphasizes improving outcomes by improving communication; stands for Team Strategies and Tools to Enhance Performance and Patient Safety.

Telehealth Any real-time interactive use of the Internet for delivery of health care or diagnosing and treating health issues across a distance (Also known as *telemedicine, telenursing, ehealth*).

Tertiary prevention Rehabilitation strategies that focus on minimizing the damaging effects of a disease or injury once it has occurred.

Therapeutic communication A goal-directed form of communication used in health care to achieve objectives that promote the person's health and well-being.

Therapeutic relationship A professional alliance in which the nurse and person join for a defined period to achieve health-related treatment goals.

Time-out A communication tool used by teams to stop and review a situation.

Transactional communication models Communication models that employ systems concepts to describe communication context, feedback loops, and validation; each person influences the other and is both a sender and receiver, simultaneously within the interaction.

Transference   Projecting emotions and feelings, often unconsciously, from one person to another—for example, in therapy sessions, a person may apply certain feelings or emotions toward the therapist.

Transitional care   A set of actions designed to ensure the coordination and continuity of health care as people transfer between locations or different levels of care within the same location.

Triage   A method used by health care providers to sort out the severity of a person's (or of people's) multiple needs to determine the priority of treatments in a crisis situation.

Triangles   A defensive way of reducing, neutralizing, or defusing heightened anxiety between two family members by drawing a third person or object into the relationship.

Trust   A dynamic relational process involving perceptions of reliance, reflecting the deepest needs and vulnerabilities of individuals.

Two-challenge rule   A safety communication tool in which a team member states their concern twice.

U

Unregulated care providers (UCPs)   Health care providers who are not registered with a regulatory body; UCPs assist with, or perform, certain aspects of care traditionally provided by regulated health care providers. Nurses are often expected to teach, supervise, or assign health care duties to UCPs.

Utilitarian or goal-based model   A framework for making ethical decisions in which the rights of the person and the duties of the nurse are determined by what will achieve maximum welfare or overall good.

V

Validation   A focused form of feedback involving confirming, verbally and nonverbally, that both participants in an interaction have the same basic understanding of a message. Feedback loops allow people to validate the information or make corrections to it.

Values   A concept or standard that has significant importance to an individual, a group, or society. Values—both personal and professional—shape who you are. In Canada, we value diversity, health and well-being, and equal access to health care.

Values acquisition   The conscious assumption of a new value—for example, a new value acquisition would be values related to privacy and confidentiality of the people being cared for.

Values clarification   A process that encourages one to clarify one's own values by sorting them through, analyzing them, and setting priorities.

Vicarious trauma   Trauma that is experienced or realized through imaginative or sympathetic participation in the experience of another.

Violence   "The intentional use of physical force or <u>power</u>, threatened or actual, against oneself, another person, or against a group or community, which either results in or has a high likelihood of resulting in injury, death, psychological harm, maldevelopment, or deprivation" (WHO, 2002[19]).

Visible minority   In the sense used by the *Employment Equity Act* and Statistics Canada, "persons, other than Aboriginal peoples, who are non-Caucasian in race or non-White in colour"; implies that people are being compared to the perceived dominant group in Canada.

W

Well-being   A person's subjective experience of satisfaction about their life, related to six personal dimensions: intellectual, physical, emotional, social, occupational, and spiritual.

Wisdom   Aristotle stated wisdom is the ability to deliberate well about which courses of action would be good and expedient. Per *Oxford Dictionary*, it is the quality of having experience, knowledge, and good judgement; the quality of being wise.

Workarounds   Use of unapproved shortcuts in giving health care.

World view   The way people tend to look out upon their world or their universe to form a picture or value stance about life or the world around them.

[19]World Health Organization. (2002). World report on violence and health: Summary. World Health Organization. https://www.who.int/violence_injury_prevention/violence/world_report/en/summary_en.pdf.

INDEX

Note: Page numbers followed by *b* indicate boxes *f* indicate figures, and *t* indicate tables.

NOTES

NOTES

NOTES

NOTES

NOTES

NOTES